Creating the Health Care Team of the Future

Chapter 1

Gases and the Kinetic-Molecular Theory

Temperature and Pressure

1.1 TEMPERATURE SCALES

The fixed points on the *Celsius* or *centigrade scale* are exactly 0 °C and 100 °C for the freezing and boiling points, respectively, of pure water at 1 atm. The *absolute Kelvin scale* is defined by

$$T(\text{K}) = T(°\text{C}) + 273.15° \tag{1.1}$$

The fixed points on the *Fahrenheit scale* are exactly 0 °F for the freezing point of a saturated NaCl-water solution and 212 °F for the normal boiling point of pure water.

EXAMPLE 1.1. If the freezing point of a saturated NaCl-water solution is −17.8 °C, derive an equation relating the Celsius and Fahrenheit temperature scales.

The above data indicate that 0 °F = −17.8 °C and 212 °F = 100 °C. The relative size of the respective degrees is found by comparing the number of degrees for the same span, giving

$$\frac{212.0\ °\text{F} - 0.0\ °\text{F}}{100.0\ °\text{C} - (-17.8\ °\text{C})} = 1.800\ °\text{F}\ °\text{C}^{-1}$$

The general form of the desired relation between the scales is

$$T(°\text{F}) = (1.800\ °\text{F}\ °\text{C}^{-1})\,T(°\text{C}) + k$$

where k corrects for the difference between the zero points of the scales. This constant can be evaluated by substituting the boiling-point temperature, giving

$$212.0\ °\text{F} = (1.800\ °\text{F}\ °\text{C}^{-1})(100.0\ °\text{C}) + k$$

$$k = 212.0\ °\text{F} - 180.0\ °\text{F} = 32.0\ °\text{F}$$

The desired equation is

$$T(°\text{F}) = (1.800\ °\text{F}\ °\text{C}^{-1})\,T(°\text{C}) + 32.0\ °\text{F} \tag{1.2}$$

1.2 PRESSURE

Pressure is defined as a force distributed over an area. Commonly used units for expressing pressure include the SI unit of a *pascal*, which is equal to a newton meter^{-2}; an *atmosphere*, which is 1.01325×10^5 N m^{-2}; a *torr*, which is equal to the pressure exerted by a 1-mm column of mercury (133.3224 N m^{-2}); a *pound-per-square-inch*, which is equal to 6894.7572 N m^{-2}; and a *bar*, which is 1×10^5 N m^{-2}. The *absolute pressure* of a system is defined as the gauge pressure plus the ambient atmospheric pressure.

EXAMPLE 1.2. If there are 760.0 torr in an atmosphere, calculate the height of a column of water equivalent to one atmosphere.

The heights of various liquids that are equivalent to the same pressure are inversely proportional to the densities of the liquids, so

$$h_{H_2O} = h_{Hg}\frac{d_{Hg}}{d_{H_2O}} = (760.0\ \text{mm})\frac{13.6 \times 10^3\ \text{kg m}^{-3}}{1.00 \times 10^3\ \text{kg m}^{-3}} = 10.3\ \text{m} = 33.9\ \text{ft}$$

Laws for Ideal Gases

1.3 BOYLE'S LAW

For a fixed mass of gas under isothermal (constant-temperature) conditions,

$$PV = \text{constant} \tag{1.3}$$

where P is the absolute pressure and V is the volume occupied by the gas.

EXAMPLE 1.3. Calculate the pressure necessary to compress isothermally a 105-dm³ sample of air at one atmosphere to 35 dm³. (Note: 1 dm³ = 1 liter.)

For the fixed amount of gas, (*1.3*) gives $P_1V_1 = P_2V_2$, or

$$P_2 = P_1\frac{V_1}{V_2} = (1.00\text{ atm})\frac{105\text{ dm}^3}{35\text{ dm}^3} = 3.0\text{ atm}$$

EXAMPLE 1.4. Assuming the constant in (*1.3*) to be 22.4 dm³ atm for 1 mole of gas at 273 K and 224 dm³ atm at 2730 K, prepare isothermal plots of V against P for values of P between 0 and 100 atm.

Substituting $P = 0.01, 0.05, 0.1, 1, 5, 10, 50$ and 100 atm into $V = (22.4\text{ dm}^3\text{ atm})/P$ gives $V = 2240, 448, 224, 22.4, 4.5, 2.2, 0.4$ and 0.2 dm³, respectively, at 273 K. These results and the results of calculations for 2730 K are graphed in Fig. 1-1.

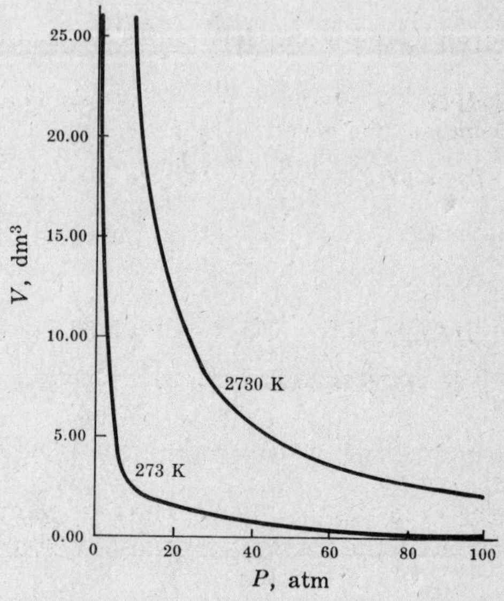

Fig. 1-1

1.4 CHARLES'S OR GAY-LUSSAC'S LAW

For a fixed mass of gas under isobaric (constant-pressure) conditions,

$$\frac{V}{T} = \text{constant} \tag{1.4}$$

where V is the volume and T is the absolute temperature.

EXAMPLE 1.5. Calculate the resulting temperature change if a 52-dm³ sample of gas at 25 °C is isobarically expanded to 104 dm³.

For a fixed amount gas, (*1.4*) gives $V_1/T_1 = V_2/T_2$, or

$$T_2 = T_1\frac{V_2}{V_1} = (25° + 273°)\frac{104\text{ dm}^3}{52\text{ dm}^3} = 596\text{ K}$$

The temperature change is

$$\Delta T = T_2 - T_1 = 596\text{ K} - 298\text{ K} = 298\text{ K}$$

EXAMPLE 1.6. Equation (*1.4*) can be stated as $V = V_0(1 + \alpha T')$, where V_0 is the volume of the gas at 0 °C, α is a constant, and T' is the temperature in °C. Find the value of α.

Equations (*1.4*) and (*1.1*) give

$$V = V_0\frac{T}{T_0} = V_0\frac{T' + 273°}{0° + 273°} = V_0\left(1 + \frac{T'}{273°}\right)$$

Upon comparison of terms within the parentheses, $\alpha = 1/273° = 3.66 \times 10^{-3}\ °\text{C}^{-1}$.

1.5 COMBINED GAS LAW

Combining (*1.3*) with (*1.4*) gives

$$\frac{PV}{T} = \text{constant} \tag{1.5}$$

for a fixed amount of gas. Under Avogadro's hypothesis that equal volumes of all ideal gases under identical pressure and temperature conditions contain equal numbers of molecules, it can be shown that (*1.5*) becomes

$$\frac{PV}{nT} = R \tag{1.6}$$

where n is the number of moles of gas and R is the gas constant.

EXAMPLE 1.7. Consider a 42.5-dm^3 sample of gas at 25 °C and 748 torr. If the volume is expanded to 52.5 dm^3 and the pressure changed to 760.0 torr, what is the final temperature of the gas?

For a fixed amount of gas, (*1.5*) gives $P_1V_1/T_1 = P_2V_2/T_2$, or

$$T_2 = T_1\frac{P_2}{P_1}\frac{V_2}{V_1} = (298\text{ K})\frac{760.0\text{ torr}}{748\text{ torr}}\frac{52.5\text{ dm}^3}{42.5\text{ dm}^3} = 374\text{ K}$$

1.6 DALTON'S LAW OF PARTIAL PRESSURES

The total pressure, P_t, of a mixture of r gases is given by

$$P_t = \sum_{i=1}^{r} P_i \tag{1.7}$$

where P_i is the partial pressure of component i in the mixture. If P_t and the molar composition of the mixture are known, P_i can be calculated from

$$P_i = x_i P_t \tag{1.8}$$

where x_i, the mole fraction for component i, is defined as

$$x_i = \frac{n_i}{\sum_{i=1}^{r} n_i} = \frac{n_i}{n_{\text{total}}} \tag{1.9}$$

EXAMPLE 1.8. The vapor pressure, P_v, of a material can be measured by passing an inert gas over a sample of the material and analyzing the composition of the gaseous mixture. For these conditions, (*1.8*) and (*1.9*) become

$$\frac{P_v}{P_t} = \frac{n}{n + n_{\text{inert}}}$$

Calculate P_v for Hg at 23 °C if a 50.4-g sample of nitrogen-Hg at 745 torr contains 0.702 mg of Hg.

The numbers of moles of gases in the mixture are

$$n_{\text{Hg}} = \frac{7.02 \times 10^{-4}\text{ g}}{200.59\text{ g mol}^{-1}} = 3.50 \times 10^{-6}\text{ mol}$$

$$n_{N_2} = \frac{50.4 - 7.02 \times 10^{-4}}{28.0134\text{ g mol}^{-1}} = 1.799\text{ mol}$$

giving

$$P_v = (745\text{ torr})\frac{3.50 \times 10^{-6}}{3.50 \times 10^{-6} + 1.799} = 1.45 \times 10^{-3}\text{ torr} = 0.193\text{ N m}^{-2}$$

1.7 GRAHAM'S LAW OF EFFUSION

In a gaseous mixture, the rate at which molecules leak out, or *effuse*, one by one through an orifice of molecular size is given by

$$\frac{\text{rate}_1}{\text{rate}_2} = \frac{P_1/M_1^{1/2}}{P_2/M_2^{1/2}} \tag{1.10a}$$

where P_i is the partial pressure of the ith gas and M_i is its molecular weight. Under identical pressure conditions for each gas, (*1.10a*) becomes

$$\frac{\text{rate}_1}{\text{rate}_2} = \left(\frac{M_2}{M_1}\right)^{1/2} = \frac{u_1}{u_2} = \frac{t_1}{t_2} = \left(\frac{d_2}{d_1}\right)^{1/2} \qquad (1.10b)$$

where u_i is the speed, t_i is the time required for the gas to effuse from the container, and d_i is the density. Equations (*1.10*) are also valid for comparing the effusion rates of pure gases from the same container under identical temperature conditions.

EXAMPLE 1.9. Assuming an equal mixture of N_2 and He, how many times faster will the He initially leak through a pinhole in the container? Repeat the calculation for a mixture such that $x_{\text{He}} = 0.75$.

Substituting molecular weights into (*1.10b*) gives for the equal mixture

$$\frac{\text{rate}_{\text{He}}}{\text{rate}_{\text{N}_2}} = \left(\frac{28.0134}{4.0026}\right)^{1/2} = 2.6455$$

Recognizing that $x_{\text{He}} = 0.75$ implies that $P_{\text{He}} = 3P_{\text{N}_2}$, we have from (*1.10a*):

$$\frac{\text{rate}_{\text{He}}}{\text{rate}_{\text{N}_2}} = \frac{3P_{\text{N}_2}/\sqrt{4.0026}}{P_{\text{N}_2}/\sqrt{28.0134}} = 7.9366$$

Real Gases

1.8 VAN DER WAALS EQUATION

The van der Waals equation of state

$$\left(P + \frac{an^2}{V^2}\right)(V - nb) = nRT \qquad (1.11)$$

corrects the combined gas law, (*1.6*), for the excluded volume of the molecules, b, and the force of interaction between the molecules, a.

EXAMPLE 1.10. Using (*1.6*) and (*1.11*), calculate the volume that 1.50 moles of $(C_2H_5)_2S$ would occupy at 105 °C and 0.750 atm. Assume that $a = 18.75\ \text{dm}^6\ \text{atm mol}^{-2}$ and $b = 0.1214\ \text{dm}^3\ \text{mol}^{-1}$.

Assuming the gas to be ideal, (*1.6*) gives

$$V = (1.50\ \text{mol})(0.0821\ \text{dm}^3\ \text{atm mol}^{-1}\ \text{K}^{-1})\frac{378\ \text{K}}{0.750\ \text{atm}} = 62.1\ \text{dm}^3$$

On the other hand, (*1.11*) gives

$$\left(0.750 + \frac{42.2}{V^2}\right)(V - 0.1821) = 46.6$$

or

$$0.750\,V^3 - 46.7\,V^2 + 42.2\,V - 7.68 = 0$$

Of the several ways to solve a polynomial equation for the various roots, one of the most useful is known as the *Newton-Raphson iterative process*. For the equation $f(x) = 0$, the $(n+1)$th estimate of the root is given by

$$x_{n+1} = x_n - \frac{f(x_n)}{f'(x_n)} \qquad \text{where} \qquad f'(x_n) = \left.\frac{df}{dx}\right|_{x=x_n} \qquad (1.12)$$

Denoting the left-hand side of the above equation for volume as $f(V)$, we have

$$f'(V) = 2.250\,V^2 - 93.4\,V + 42.2$$

and (*1.12*) becomes

$$V_{n+1} = V_n - \frac{0.750\,V_n^3 - 46.7\,V_n^2 + 42.2\,V_n - 7.68}{2.250\,V_n^2 - 93.4\,V_n + 42.2}$$

Assuming for V_1 the value predicted by (*1.6*), the second estimate is

$$V_2 = 62.1 - \frac{(0.750)(62.1)^3 - (46.7)(62.1)^2 + (42.2)(62.1) - 7.68}{(2.250)(62.1)^2 - (93.4)(62.1) + 42.2}$$

$$= 62.1 - \frac{2131}{2919} = 61.4 \text{ dm}^3$$

The third estimate, and the answer to three significant figures, is

$$V_3 = 61.4 - \frac{f(61.4)}{f'(61.4)} = 61.4 - \frac{133}{2789} = 61.4 \text{ dm}^3$$

1.9 VIRIAL EQUATIONS

There are two virial equations, one describing PV as a function of $1/V$ and the second using the variable P. For one mole of gas, these are

$$P\bar{V} = A_v + B_v(1/\bar{V}) + C_v(1/\bar{V})^2 + \cdots \qquad (1.13)$$

$$P\bar{V} = A_p + B_pP + C_pP^2 + \cdots \qquad (1.14)$$

Here $\bar{V}$ is the molar volume, and A_v, B_v, etc., are constants for a particular gas. The values of these virial coefficients can be determined from the van der Waals constants, statistical mechanics, or from experimental data.

EXAMPLE 1.11. Evaluate A_v and A_p in (*1.13*) and (*1.14*), assuming that a real gas will approach ideality as $(1/V) \to 0$ and as $P \to 0$.

As the limits of zero are approached, the polynomial terms in (*1.13*) and (*1.14*) become insignificant and both equations approach (*1.6*), giving $A_v = A_p = RT$.

1.10 COMPRESSIBILITY FACTOR

The *compressibility factor, z,* is an empirical correction for the nonideal behavior of real gases which allows the simple form of the combined gas law to be retained. Thus, we write for a real gas

$$PV = znRT \qquad (1.15)$$

The factor z is determined by first calculating the *reduced temperature,* T_r, and the *reduced pressure,* P_r, defined as

$$P_r = \frac{P}{P_c} \qquad (1.16)$$

$$T_r = \frac{T}{T_c} \qquad (1.17)$$

where the *critical pressure,* P_c, and the *critical temperature,* T_c, are constants for the gas. Then the value of z is read from a graph of z plotted against P_r for various reduced temperatures (Fig. 1-2).

EXAMPLE 1.12. Using (*1.15*), repeat the real-gas calculations in Example 1.10 if $P_c = 39.1$ atm and $T_c = 283.8$ °C for $(C_2H_5)_2S$.

Using (*1.16*) and (*1.17*) gives

$$P_r = \frac{0.750 \text{ atm}}{39.1 \text{ atm}} = 1.92 \times 10^{-2} \qquad T_r = \frac{105° + 273°}{283.8° + 273.2°} = 0.679$$

From Fig. 1-2, $z = 0.99$, so (*1.15*) gives

$$V = (0.99)(1.50 \text{ mol})(0.0821 \text{ dm}^3 \text{ atm mol}^{-1} \text{ K}^{-1})\frac{378 \text{ K}}{0.750 \text{ atm}} = 61.4 \text{ dm}^3$$

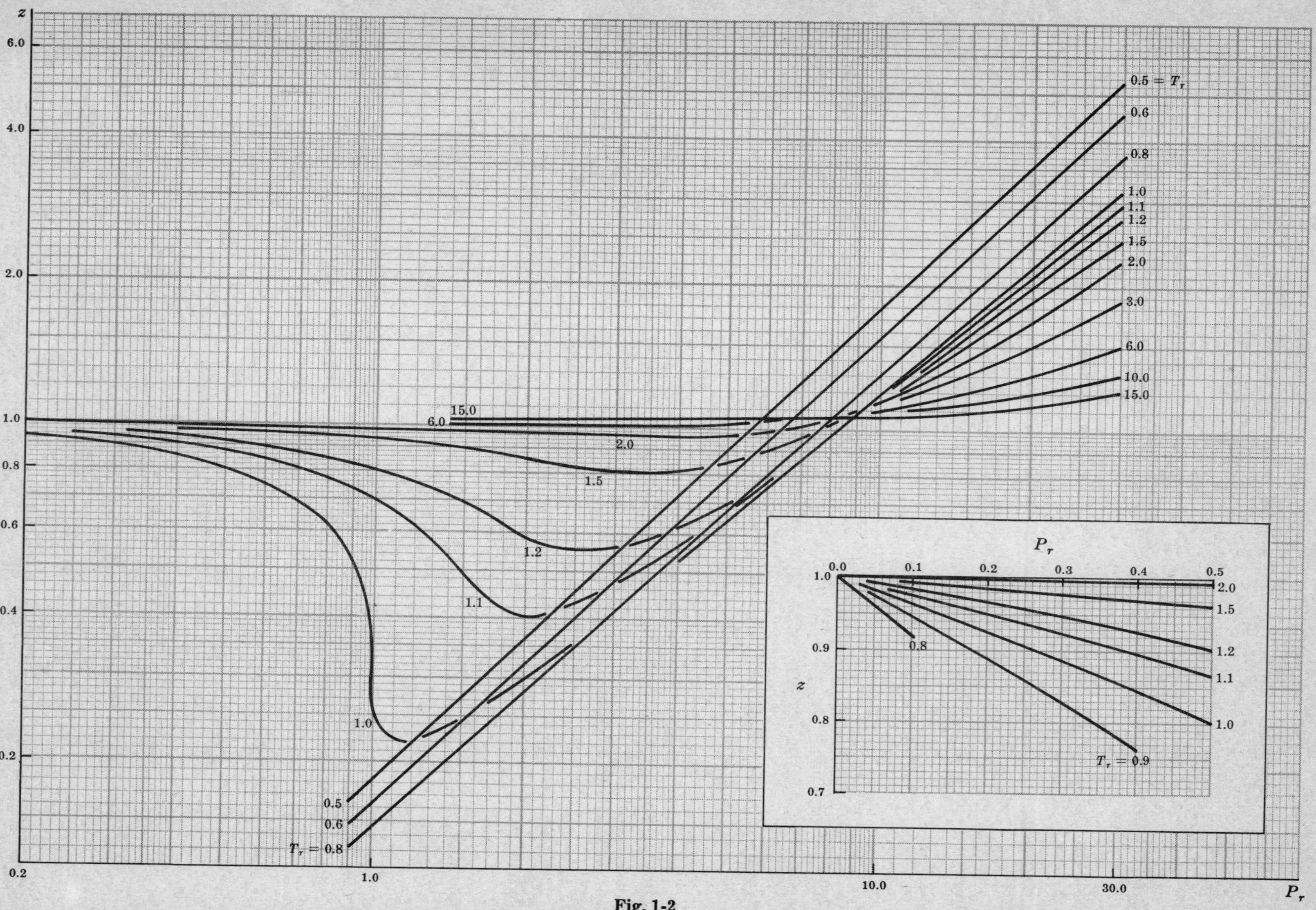
z
6.0
4.0
2.0
1.0
0.8
0.6
0.4
0.2
0.2
1.0
10.0
30.0
P_r
$0.5 = T_r$
0.6
0.8
1.0
1.1
1.2
1.5
2.0
3.0
6.0
10.0
15.0
15.0
6.0
2.0
1.5
1.2
1.1
1.0
0.5
0.6
$T_r = 0.8$
P_r
0.0
0.1
0.2
0.3
0.4
0.5
1.0
0.9
0.8
0.7
z
2.0
1.5
1.2
1.1
1.0
0.8
$T_r = 0.9$

Fig. 1-2

1.11 CRITICAL POINT

As real gases are cooled, the nicely-shaped isotherms shown in Fig. 1-1 become distorted. The isotherm which exhibits a point of inflection, i.e. $\partial P/\partial V = \partial^2 P/\partial V^2 = 0$, corresponds to the critical temperature. The values of P and V at the point of inflection are P_c and V_c, respectively.

EXAMPLE 1.13. Critical-point data can be used to determine approximate values of the van der Waals constants. Derive these values.

Solving (*1.11*) for P and taking the necessary derivatives gives, for 1 mole,

$$P = \frac{RT}{\bar{V} - b} - \frac{a}{\bar{V}^2}$$

$$\left(\frac{\partial P}{\partial V}\right)_T = \frac{-RT}{(\bar{V}-b)^2} + \frac{2a}{\bar{V}^3} = 0$$

$$\left(\frac{\partial^2 P}{\partial V^2}\right)_T = \frac{2RT}{(\bar{V}-b)^3} - \frac{6a}{\bar{V}^4} = 0$$

Assigning the values of P, $\bar{V}$ and T as P_c, $\bar{V}_c$ and T_c and solving the three simultaneous equations gives

$$b = \frac{\bar{V}_c}{3} \qquad a = 3P_c\bar{V}_c^2 \qquad R = \frac{8P_c\bar{V}_c}{3T_c}$$

Because R is usually determined from other sources, the value of $\bar{V}_c$ can be eliminated, giving

$$a = \frac{27R^2T_c^2}{64P_c} \qquad b = \frac{RT_c}{8P_c}$$

EXAMPLE 1.14. Any equation of state containing R and two coefficients may be written in reduced form if the expressions for R and the coefficients in terms of the critical constants are substituted into the equation and reduced variables are introduced. Determine the reduced form of the van der Waals equation of state.

Substituting a, b and R from Example 1.13 into (*1.11*), we find

$$\left(P + \frac{3P_c\bar{V}_c^2}{\bar{V}^2}\right)\left(\bar{V} - \frac{\bar{V}_c}{3}\right) = \left(\frac{8P_c\bar{V}_c}{3T_c}\right)T$$

which upon multiplication of both sides by $3/P_c\bar{V}_c$ gives

$$\left(\frac{P}{P_c} + \frac{3\bar{V}_c^2}{\bar{V}^2}\right)\left(\frac{3\bar{V}}{\bar{V}_c} - 1\right) = \frac{8T}{T_c}$$

Introducing reduced variables gives

$$\left(P_r + \frac{3}{V_r^2}\right)(3V_r - 1) = 8T_r$$

Molecular Weights

1.12 MOLECULAR WEIGHT OF AN IDEAL GAS

Substituting $n = m/M$ into (*1.6*) gives

$$M = \frac{mRT}{PV} \tag{1.18}$$

or, in terms of density,

$$M = \frac{dRT}{P} \tag{1.19}$$

EXAMPLE 1.15. If the density of dry air at 740 torr and 27 °C is 1.146 g dm^{-3}, calculate the composition of air assuming only N_2 and O_2 to be present.

The "molecular weight" of air can be calculated from *(1.19)* as

$$M = \frac{(1.146\text{ g dm}^{-3})(0.0821\text{ dm}^3\text{ atm K}^{-1}\text{ mol}^{-1})(300\text{ K})}{(740\text{ torr})(1\text{ atm}/760\text{ torr})} = 28.99\text{ g mol}^{-1}$$

Assuming the mass fraction of N_2 to be w,

$$w(28.0134) + (1-w)(31.9988) = 28.99 \quad \text{or} \quad w = 0.755$$

Thus, air is 75.5% N_2 and 24.5% O_2 by weight.

1.13. MOLECULAR WEIGHT OF A REAL GAS

For n moles of a real gas at rather low pressures, *(1.14)* becomes

$$PV = n(RT + B_pP)$$

Upon substituting $n = m/M$ and $d = m/V$, the above equation becomes

$$\frac{d}{P} = \frac{M/RT}{1 + (B_pP/RT)}$$

At low pressures, $[1 + (B_pP/RT)]^{-1} \approx 1 - (B_pP/RT)$ and

$$\frac{d}{P} = \frac{M}{RT} + \left(\frac{M}{RT}\right)\left(\frac{-B_p}{RT}\right)P \qquad (1.20)$$

Thus an isothermal plot of d/P against P will have a slope of $(M/RT)(-B_p/RT)$ and an intercept of M/RT.

EXAMPLE 1.16. E. Moles reports the following density-pressure data for SO_2 at 0 °C:

P, atm	1.000	0.500	0.100	0.010	0.001	0.0001
d/P, g dm^{-3} atm^{-1}	2.926682	2.892407	2.864974	2.858800	2.858183	2.858121

Determine the molecular weight for SO_2 from these data.

A plot of d/P against P gives the intercept as 2.858114 g dm^{-3} atm^{-1}; thus

$$\begin{aligned} M &= (\text{intercept})(RT) \\ &= (2.858114\text{ g dm}^{-3}\text{ atm}^{-1})(0.0820568\text{ dm}^3\text{ atm mol}^{-1}\text{ K}^{-1})(273.15\text{ K}) = 64.0612\text{ g mol}^{-1} \end{aligned}$$

Kinetic-Molecular Theory

1.14 POSTULATES OF KMT FOR GASES

The model for an ideal gas is based on the assumptions that (1) the gas consists of sufficiently many particles to allow statistical averaging to be performed; (2) the intrinsic volume of the particles is small compared to the distances between the particles and negligible relative to the volume of the container, which implies that the particles may move freely throughout the entire volume; (3) the particles are in random motion and have no mutual attractions; (4) the collisions between the particles and between the particles and the walls of the container are elastic, which implies conservation of energy and momentum; and (5) the average translational kinetic energy of the particles is proportional to the absolute temperature.

EXAMPLE 1.17. The average kinetic energy for a molecule, $\overline{\text{ke}}$, is given by

$$\overline{\text{ke}} = \frac{1}{2}m\overline{u^2}$$

where m is the molecular mass and $\overline{u^2}$ is the average of the square of the velocity. If $\overline{u^2} = 3kT/m$, where k is *Boltzmann's constant*, calculate the ratio of the kinetic energies at 200 °C and 100 °C.

$$\frac{\overline{\text{ke}}_{200}}{\overline{\text{ke}}_{100}} = \frac{\frac{1}{2}m(3kT/m)_{200}}{\frac{1}{2}m(3kT/m)_{100}} = \frac{473\text{ K}}{373\text{ K}} = 1.27$$

1.15 P-V-KE RELATIONSHIPS

The KMT implies the following series of relationships for one mole of an ideal gas:

$$P\bar{V} = \frac{1}{3}M\overline{u^2} = \frac{2}{3}\overline{\text{KE}} = RT \tag{1.21}$$

where $\overline{\text{KE}}$ is the average kinetic energy for one mole of gas and the other terms have been defined previously.

EXAMPLE 1.18. For oxygen molecules at 25 °C, find the root mean square speed, rms, which is defined by

$$\text{rms} = (\overline{u^2})^{1/2} \tag{1.22}$$

Substituting (*1.21*) into (*1.22*) gives

$$\text{rms} = \left(\frac{3RT}{M}\right)^{1/2} = \left[\frac{3(8.314\text{ J mol}^{-1}\text{ K}^{-1})(298\text{ K})}{32.0\times10^{-3}\text{ kg mol}^{-1}}\right]^{1/2} = 4.82\times10^{2}\text{ m s}^{-1}$$

1.16 VELOCITY DISTRIBUTION

The Maxwell relation gives the fraction of molecules in a mole, dN/L, having a velocity in the x-direction between u_x and $u_x + du_x$ as

$$\frac{dN/L}{du_x} = Ae^{-\frac{1}{2}mu_x^2/kT} \tag{1.23}$$

where A is a constant and L is Avogadro's number. In three dimensions, the Maxwell-Boltzmann relation for the fraction of molecules in a mole, dN/L, having a speed between u and $u + du$ is

$$\frac{dN/L}{du} = 4\pi u^2\left(\frac{m}{2\pi kT}\right)^{3/2} e^{-\frac{1}{2}mu^2/kT} \tag{1.24}$$

EXAMPLE 1.19. Evaluate the constant A in (*1.23*) based on the property that $\int dN = L$.

Dividing $\int dN = L$ by L gives

$$1 = \int \frac{dN}{L} = A\int_{-\infty}^{\infty} e^{-\frac{1}{2}mu_x^2/kT}\,du_x$$

Transforming variables by letting $z = (m/2kT)^{1/2}u_x$ gives

$$1 = A\left(\frac{2kT}{m}\right)^{1/2}\int_{-\infty}^{\infty} e^{-z^2}\,dz$$

The integral is equal to $\pi^{1/2}$, giving

$$A = \left(\frac{m}{2\pi kT}\right)^{1/2}$$

EXAMPLE 1.20. Derive an expression for rms in terms R, T and M using (*1.24*).

With respect to the speed distribution (*1.24*), the average value of any function $h(u)$ is defined as

$$\bar{h} = \int_0^\infty h(u)\, dN/L$$

In particular, for $h(u) = u^2$ we have

$$\overline{u^2} = \int_0^\infty u^2\, dN/L = 4\pi\left(\frac{m}{2\pi kT}\right)^{3/2} \int_0^\infty u^4 e^{-\frac{1}{2}mu^2/kT}\, du$$

The integral can be transformed by letting $z^2 = \frac{1}{2}mu^2/kT$, which gives

$$\overline{u^2} = 4\pi\left(\frac{m}{2\pi kT}\right)^{3/2}\left(\frac{2kT}{m}\right)^{5/2} \int_0^\infty z^4 e^{-z^2}\, dz$$

The integral is equal to $3\pi^{1/2}/8$, giving

$$\overline{u^2} = 4\pi\left(\frac{m}{2\pi kT}\right)^{3/2}\left(\frac{2kT}{m}\right)^{5/2}\frac{3\pi^{1/2}}{8} = \frac{3kT}{m}$$

So for rms, (*1.22*) gives

$$\text{rms} = \left(\frac{3kT}{m}\right)^{1/2} \tag{1.25a}$$

which, because $k = R/L$ and $m = M/L$, can also be written as

$$\text{rms} = \left(\frac{3RT}{M}\right)^{1/2} \tag{1.25b}$$

EXAMPLE 1.21. Derive an expression for the most probable speed, α, by differentiating $(dN/L)/du$ with respect to u, setting the result equal to zero, and solving for u.

Performing the differentiation of (*1.24*) gives

$$\frac{d^2N/L}{du^2} = 4\pi\left(\frac{m}{2\pi kT}\right)^{3/2} e^{-\frac{1}{2}mu^2/kT}\left[2u - \frac{mu^3}{kT}\right]$$

The right-hand side vanishes at $u = 0$ (but this corresponds to a minimum) and at $u = \alpha$, where

$$2 - \frac{m\alpha^2}{kT} = 0$$

or

$$\alpha = \left(\frac{2kT}{m}\right)^{1/2} = \left(\frac{2RT}{M}\right)^{1/2} \tag{1.26}$$

EXAMPLE 1.22. Find the ratio rms / $\bar{u}$ / α, given that

$$\bar{u} = \left(\frac{8kT}{\pi m}\right)^{1/2} = \left(\frac{8RT}{\pi M}\right)^{1/2} \tag{1.27}$$

From (*1.25b*), (*1.27*) and (*1.26*),

$$\text{rms}\,/\,\bar{u}\,/\,\alpha = \left(\frac{3RT}{M}\right)^{1/2} \bigg/ \left(\frac{8RT}{\pi M}\right)^{1/2} \bigg/ \left(\frac{2RT}{M}\right)^{1/2}$$

$$= 3^{1/2}\,/\,(8/\pi)^{1/2}\,/\,2^{1/2} = 1.0000\,/\,0.9213\,/\,0.8165$$

Collision Parameters

1.17 VISCOSITY

The viscosity of a fluid is related to its resistance to flow. If flow is considered to be the movement of one layer of fluid with respect to another layer, the force necessary for movement is given by

$$f = \frac{\eta A u}{d} \tag{1.28}$$

where f is the force, A is the area of the layers, u is the difference in velocity of the layers, d is the distance between the layers, and η is the coefficient of viscosity for the fluid.

If the molecules of a gas are considered to be hard spheres with a collision diameter σ traveling at an average speed $\bar{u}$ as calculated from (*1.27*), η is given by

$$\eta = \frac{\bar{u}m}{2^{3/2}\pi\sigma^2} \tag{1.29}$$

The cgs unit for viscosity is the *poise*, which is equal to $0.1 \text{ N s m}^{-2} = 0.1 \text{ Pl}$ (poiseuille).

EXAMPLE 1.23. The coefficient of viscosity for argon is 221.7 μpoise at 20 °C. Calculate σ using (*1.29*) and compare this value to 3.84 Å, the atomic diameter as determined from X-ray crystallographic measurements.

Using (*1.27*), the average speed is

$$\bar{u} = \left[\frac{8(8.314 \text{ J mol}^{-1}\text{ K}^{-1})(293 \text{ K})}{\pi(39.948 \times 10^{-3}\text{ kg mol}^{-1})}\right]^{1/2} = 3.94 \times 10^2 \text{ m s}^{-1}$$

Rearranging (*1.29*) gives the collision diameter as

$$\sigma = \left(\frac{\bar{u}m}{2^{3/2}\pi\eta}\right)^{1/2} = \left[\frac{(3.94 \times 10^2 \text{ m s}^{-1})(39.948 \times 10^{-3}\text{ kg mol}^{-1}/L \text{ mol}^{-1})}{2^{3/2}\pi(221.7 \times 10^{-7}\text{ N s m}^{-2})}\right]^{1/2}$$

$$= (1.327 \times 10^{-19})^{1/2}\text{ m} = 3.64 \times 10^{-10}\text{ m} = 3.64 \text{ Å}$$

which is about 5% lower than the atomic diameter.

1.18 MEAN FREE PATH

For a binary mixture of gases having collision diameters σ_1 and σ_2, the average distance traveled between collisions is given by

$$\ell = (\pi 2^{1/2}\sigma_{12}^2 N_{12}^*)^{-1} \tag{1.30}$$

where ℓ is known as the *mean free path*, N_{12}^* is the total number of molecules in 1 m³ and can be determined from

$$N_{12}^* = \frac{nL}{V} = \frac{LP}{RT} \tag{1.31}$$

and the average diameter σ_{12} is given by

$$\sigma_{12} = \tfrac{1}{2}(\sigma_1 + \sigma_2) \tag{1.32}$$

EXAMPLE 1.24. Derive an equation for the mean free path of a molecule in a pure gas. Using the results of Example 1.23, calculate ℓ for Ar at 20 °C and 1 atm.

For a pure gas, (*1.32*) becomes

$$\sigma_{12} = \tfrac{1}{2}(\sigma + \sigma) = \sigma$$

and $N_{12}^* = N^*$, which upon substitution into (*1.30*) gives

$$\ell = (\pi 2^{1/2}\sigma^2 N^*)^{-1} \tag{1.33}$$

For argon at 20 °C,

$$N^* = \frac{(6.022 \times 10^{23}\text{ mol}^{-1})(1 \text{ atm})}{(8.21 \times 10^{-5}\text{ m}^3\text{ atm K}^{-1}\text{ mol}^{-1})(293 \text{ K})} = 2.50 \times 10^{25}\text{ m}^{-3}$$

and (*1.33*) gives

$$\ell = [\pi 2^{1/2}(3.64 \times 10^{-10}\text{ m})^2(2.50 \times 10^{25}\text{ m}^{-3})]^{-1} = 6.80 \times 10^{-8}\text{ m}$$

1.19 COLLISION NUMBERS

In a pure gas the average number of collisions per second, z_1, experienced by a single molecule is given by $z_1 = \bar{u}/\ell$, or

$$z_1 = 2^{1/2}\pi\sigma^2\bar{u}N^* \tag{1.34}$$

If we multiply z_1 by the number of molecules in 1 m³, N^*, we get a total in which each collision has been counted twice (since each collision involves two molecules). Hence, the number of collisions per second in 1 m³ is given by $z_{11} = \frac{1}{2}N^*z_1$, or

$$z_{11} = 2^{-1/2}\pi\sigma^2\bar{u}N^{*2} \tag{1.35}$$

For a binary gaseous mixture, the total rate of collisions per unit volume between unlike molecules is given by

$$z_{12} = \pi\sigma_{12}^2 N_1^* N_2^* (\bar{u}_1^2 + \bar{u}_2^2)^{1/2} \tag{1.36}$$

EXAMPLE 1.25. Compute z_1 and z_{11} for argon at 20 °C both at $P = 1$ atm and at $P = 0.1$ atm.

Using the results of Examples 1.23 and 1.24, (*1.34*) gives, at 1 atm,

$$z_1 = 2^{1/2}\pi(3.64 \times 10^{-10}\ \text{m})^2(3.94 \times 10^2\ \text{m s}^{-1})(2.50 \times 10^{25}\ \text{m}^{-3}) = 5.80 \times 10^9\ \text{s}^{-1}$$

and (*1.35*) gives

$$z_{11} = 2^{-1/2}\pi(3.64 \times 10^{-10}\ \text{m})^2(3.94 \times 10^2\ \text{m s}^{-1})(2.50 \times 10^{25}\ \text{m}^{-3})^2 = 7.25 \times 10^{34}\ \text{m}^{-3}\ \text{s}^{-1}$$

At fixed temperature, $z_1 \propto N^* \propto P$ and $z_{11} \propto N^{*2} \propto P^2$. Therefore, at $P = 0.1$ atm

$$z_1 = \frac{1}{10}(5.80 \times 10^9\ \text{s}^{-1}) = 5.80 \times 10^8\ \text{s}^{-1}$$

$$z_{11} = \frac{1}{100}(7.25 \times 10^{34}\ \text{m}^{-3}\ \text{s}^{-1}) = 7.25 \times 10^{32}\ \text{m}^{-3}\ \text{s}^{-1}$$

1.20 DIFFUSION

Diffusion involves the mixing of the molecules of substances by the random thermal motions and collisions of the molecules until the mixture attains uniform composition. The rate of diffusion in the z-direction is related to the concentration gradient, $\partial C/\partial z$, by *Fick's first law*:

$$\frac{dN}{dt} = -DA\frac{\partial C}{\partial z} \tag{1.37}$$

where D is the diffusion coefficient and A is the area of the contact surface. The changes in concentration with time and with distance are related by *Fick's second law* (the *diffusion equation*):

$$\frac{\partial C}{\partial t} = D\frac{\partial^2 C}{\partial z^2} \tag{1.38}$$

For spherical gaseous molecules

$$D = 0.599\,\ell\bar{u} \tag{1.39}$$

and for a gaseous mixture of n components where the mole fractions are $x_1, x_2, \ldots, x_n$:

$$D = \frac{x_1D_1 + x_2D_2 + \cdots + x_nD_n}{n} \tag{1.40}$$

EXAMPLE 1.26. An indication of the distance that a single molecule travels in time t during diffusion is given by

$$(\overline{z^2})^{1/2} = (2Dt)^{1/2} \tag{1.41}$$

If $D = 1.78 \times 10^{-5}\ \text{m}^2\ \text{s}^{-1}$ for O_2 in air at 0 °C and if $t = 1$ min, find this distance.

Upon substitution of the data, (*1.41*) gives

$$(\overline{z^2})^{1/2} = [2(1.78 \times 10^{-5}\ \text{m}^2\ \text{s}^{-1})(60\ \text{s})]^{1/2} = 0.0462\ \text{m} = 4.62\ \text{cm}$$

Solved Problems

Temperature and Pressure

1.1. Combine (*1.1*) with (*1.2*) to define the *Rankine scale* (°R), which is the absolute Fahrenheit scale.

The general form of the desired equation is $T(°\text{R}) = T(°\text{F}) + k$. Substituting (*1.2*) gives

$$T(°\text{R}) = (1.800\ °\text{F}\ °\text{C}^{-1})T(°\text{C}) + 32\ °\text{F} + k$$

and substituting (*1.1*) after solving for $T(°\text{C})$ gives

$$T(°\text{R}) = (1.800)[T(\text{K}) - 273.15°] + 32\ °\text{F} + k$$

The value of k can be determined by recognizing $0\ °\text{R} = 0\ \text{K}$, giving

$$0 = (1.800)(0 - 273.15) + 32 + k \qquad \text{or} \qquad k = 459.67°$$

Hence

$$T(°\text{R}) = T(°\text{F}) + 459.67°$$

1.2. The *benzene temperature scale* (°B) is defined as 0 °B for the freezing point of C_6H_6 (5.5 °C) and 100 °B for the normal boiling point of C_6H_6 (80.1 °C). Calculate the normal boiling point of water in °B.

As in Example 1.1, the relative size of the respective degrees is

$$\frac{100\ °\text{B} - 0\ °\text{B}}{80.1\ °\text{C} - 5.5\ °\text{C}} = 1.34\ °\text{B}\ °\text{C}^{-1}$$

The general form of the equation relating the temperature scales is then

$$T(°\text{B}) = (1.34\ °\text{B}\ °\text{C}^{-1})T(°\text{C}) + k$$

where k is evaluated from the boiling point data as

$$100\ °\text{B} = (1.34\ °\text{B}\ °\text{C}^{-1})(80.1\ °\text{C}) + k \qquad \text{or} \qquad k = -7.33\ °\text{B}$$

Using the equation $T(°\text{B}) = (1.34\ °\text{B}\ °\text{C}^{-1})T(°\text{C}) - 7.33\ °\text{B}$, the normal boiling point of water is

$$T(°\text{B}) = (1.34)(100) - 7.33 = 126.7\ °\text{B}$$

1.3. A cylinder contains 75 dm^3 of N_2 at 215 psig and 25 °C. If the room pressure is 14.4 psi, what mass of N_2 could be transferred to the laboratory? Assume the ideal gas law to be valid.

The number of moles of gas in the cylinder is

$$n_1 = \frac{PV}{RT} = \frac{(215 + 14.4)\ \text{psi}\ (1\ \text{atm}/14.6960\ \text{psi})(75\ \text{dm}^3)}{(0.0821\ \text{dm}^3\ \text{atm}\ \text{K}^{-1}\ \text{mol}^{-1})(298\ \text{K})} = 47.8\ \text{mol}$$

The number of moles of gas remaining in the cylinder at 0 psig is

$$n_2 = \frac{(0 + 14.4)(1/14.6960)(75)}{(0.0821)(298)} = 3.0\ \text{mol}$$

The amount transferred is

$$(47.8 - 3.0)\ \text{mol} \times (28.0134 \times 10^{-3}\ \text{kg mol}^{-1}) = 1.255\ \text{kg}$$

Laws for Ideal Gases

1.4. A vacuum manifold was calibrated using Boyle's law. A 0.503-dm^3 flask containing dry nitrogen at 746 torr was attached to the manifold, which was at 13 mtorr. After the stopcock was opened and the system allowed to reach equilibrium, the pressure of the combined system was 373 torr. Assuming isothermal conditions, what is the volume of the manifold?

Before opening the stopcock, the original condition of the system was given by

$$P_1V_1 = (745 \text{ torr})(0.503 \text{ dm}^3) + (13 \times 10^{-3} \text{ torr})(V)$$

and after opening the stopcock, the condition of the system was given by

$$P_2V_2 = (373 \text{ torr})(0.503 + V)\text{dm}^3$$

Equating these PV-terms via (*1.3*) gives

$$(746)(0.503) + (13 \times 10^{-3})V = (373)(0.503 + V) \quad \text{or} \quad V = 0.503 \text{ dm}^3$$

1.5. Equation (*1.4*) can be used as the basis of a thermometer. If V_{tp} represents the volume of an ideal gas in a probe at the triple point of water, 273.1600 K, and if V_T represents the volume of the gas at any temperature T, then

$$T = (273.1600 \text{ K})\frac{V_T}{V_{\text{tp}}}$$

Calculate the ratio of V_T to V_{tp} if the probe were immersed in boiling water at 1 atm.

Rearranging the given equation for the desired ratio gives

$$\frac{V_T}{V_{\text{tp}}} = \frac{T}{273.1600} = \frac{100.00° + 273.15°}{273.1600 \text{ K}} = 1.366$$

1.6. Equation (*1.6*) can be used to calculate the value of R. Assuming that the molar volume of most gases is 22.4 dm³ at STP, calculate R in units of $\text{dm}^3 \text{ atm K}^{-1} \text{ mol}^{-1}$.

$$R = \frac{PV}{nT} = \frac{(1.00 \text{ atm})(22.4 \text{ dm}^3)}{(1.00 \text{ mol})(273 \text{ K})} = 0.0821 \text{ dm}^3 \text{ atm K}^{-1} \text{ mol}^{-1}$$

1.7. A 5-dm³ flask containing N_2 at 5 atm was connected to a 4-dm³ flask containing He at 4 atm and the gases were allowed to mix isothermally. Calculate the individual pressures and total pressure for the resulting mixture.

Using Boyle's law, (*1.3*), for each gas gives

$$P_{\text{He}} = (4 \text{ atm})\frac{4 \text{ dm}^3}{9 \text{ dm}^3} = 1.78 \text{ atm} \qquad P_{N_2} = (5)\frac{5}{9} = 2.78 \text{ atm}$$

and (*1.7*) gives the total pressure as $P_t = P_{\text{He}} + P_{N_2} = 4.56$ atm.

1.8. The occurrence of heavy water ($M = 20.0 \text{ g mol}^{-1}$) is about 1 part for 6900 parts of regular water ($M = 18.0 \text{ g mol}^{-1}$). Compare the initial rates of effusion during a concentration step for obtaining D_2O.

Assuming $P_{H_2O} = 6900P_{D_2O}$, (*1-10a*) gives

$$\frac{\text{rate}_{H_2O}}{\text{rate}_{D_2O}} = \frac{6900P_{D_2O}}{\sqrt{18.0}} \bigg/ \frac{P_{D_2O}}{\sqrt{20.0}} = 7300$$

Real Gases

1.9. Compare the pressures predicted for 1 mole of *n*-octane confined to 20.0 dm³ at 200 °C by the combined gas law and by the van der Waals equation with constants

$$a = 37.32 \text{ dm}^6 \text{ atm mol}^{-2} \quad \text{and} \quad b = 0.2368 \text{ dm}^3 \text{ mol}^{-1}$$

Assuming an ideal gas, (*1.6*) gives

$$P = \frac{(1 \text{ mol})(0.0821 \text{ dm}^3 \text{ atm K}^{-1} \text{ mol}^{-1})(473 \text{ K})}{20.0 \text{ dm}^3} = 1.94 \text{ atm}$$

Assuming a van der Waals gas, (*1.11*) gives

$$P = \frac{nRT}{V - nb} - \frac{an^2}{V^2}$$

$$= \frac{(1)(0.0821)(473)}{20.0 - (1)(0.2368)} - \frac{(37.32)(1)^2}{(20.0)^2} = 1.96 - 0.09 = 1.87 \text{ atm}$$

There is about a 3.2% difference.

1.10. Discuss how B_v and C_v in (*1.13*) could be evaluated from experimental PVT data.

Using the result of Example 1.11, we write (*1.13*) as

$$P\bar{V} - RT = B_v(1/\bar{V}) + C_v(1/\bar{V})^2 + \cdots$$

Multiplying by $\bar{V}$ gives

$$\bar{V}(P\bar{V} - RT) = B_v + C_v(1/\bar{V}) + \cdots$$

A plot of $\bar{V}(P\bar{V} - RT)$ against $1/\bar{V}$ will have a vertical intercept of B_v and an initial slope of C_v.

1.11. Evaluate the virial coefficient A_v for one mole of gas using the van der Waals equation.

For one mole, (*1.11*) becomes

$$\left(P + \frac{a}{\bar{V}^2}\right)(\bar{V} - b) = RT$$

which upon rearrangement gives

$$P\bar{V} = (RT + bP) + (-a)(1/\bar{V}) + (ab)(1/\bar{V})^2$$

Comparison with (*1.13*) now yields

$$A_v = RT + bP$$

1.12. Repeat Problem 1.9 for one mole of *n*-octane using (*1.15*), given that $P_c = 24.7$ atm and $T_c = 296.2\ °\text{C}$.

To determine z from Fig. 1-2, the values of both P_r and T_r must be known. Because the unknown in this problem is P, the exact value of P_r is not known at the beginning of the problem and an iterative method must be used. As shown in Problem 1.9, (*1.6*) gives $P = 1.94$ atm, which upon substitution into (*1.16*) gives

$$P_r = \frac{1.94 \text{ atm}}{24.7 \text{ atm}} = 0.079 \qquad T_r = \frac{473 \text{ K}}{569.4 \text{ K}} = 0.831$$

The first approximation of z from Fig. 1-2 for these values is 0.94, which upon substitution into (*1.15*) gives the second approximation for P as

$$P = \frac{(0.94)(1.00 \text{ mol})(0.0821 \text{ dm}^3 \text{ atm K}^{-1} \text{ mol}^{-1})(473 \text{ K})}{20.0 \text{ dm}^3} = 1.83 \text{ atm}$$

which upon substitution into (*1.16*) gives

$$P_r = \frac{1.83}{24.7} = 0.074$$

The second approximation of z is 0.95, which gives

$$P = \frac{(0.95)(1.00)(0.0821)(473)}{20.0} = 1.84 \text{ atm}$$

This process is continued until P changes insignificantly. To three significant figures, $P = 1.84$ atm.

1.13. Calculate the van der Waals constants a and b for $(C_2H_5)_2S$ from the critical-point data given in Example 1.12 and compare the values to those given in Example 1.10.

From Example 1.13

$$a = \frac{27R^2T_c^2}{64P_c} = \frac{(27)(0.0821\ \text{dm}^3\ \text{atm mol}^{-1}\ \text{K}^{-1})^2(557.0\ \text{K})^2}{64(39.1\ \text{atm})} = 22.6\ \text{dm}^6\ \text{atm mol}^{-2}$$

$$b = \frac{RT_c}{8P_c} = \frac{(0.0821\ \text{dm}^3\ \text{atm K}^{-1}\ \text{mol}^{-1})(557.0\ \text{K})}{8(39.1\ \text{atm})} = 0.146\ \text{dm}^3\ \text{mol}^{-1}$$

These results differ by about −20% from those given in Example 1.10.

Molecular Weights

1.14. Calculate the molecular weight of CO_2 if a 0.308-g sample (after buoyancy corrections) at 245 torr and 25 °C occupies a volume of 0.532 dm³.

Substituting into (*1.18*) gives

$$M = \frac{(0.308\ \text{g})(0.0821\ \text{dm}^3\ \text{atm K}^{-1}\ \text{mol}^{-1})(298\ \text{K})}{(245\ \text{torr})(1\ \text{atm}/760\ \text{torr})(0.532\ \text{dm}^3)} = 43.9\ \text{g mol}^{-1}$$

1.15. The limiting value of d/P as $P \to 0$ for SiF_4 at 0 °C is 4.643842 g dm⁻³ atm⁻¹, as reported by Moles. Calculate the molecular weight.

The intercept of (*1.20*) gives

$$M = (\text{intercept})(RT) = (4.643842\ \text{g dm}^{-3}\ \text{atm}^{-1})(0.0820568\ \text{dm}^3\ \text{atm K}^{-1}\ \text{mol}^{-1})(273.15\ \text{K})$$
$$= 104.0862\ \text{g mol}^{-1}$$

Kinetic-Molecular Theory

1.16. Assume an atom of neon to be 1.12 Å in radius and one mole of the gas to occupy 22.4 dm³. What fraction of the volume is occupied by the atoms?

Neon is a monatomic gas, so that the desired fraction is

$$\frac{(L)(\text{volume of one molecule})}{22.4\ \text{dm}^3} = \frac{(6.022 \times 10^{23})(4/3)\pi(1.12 \times 10^{-10}\ \text{m})^3}{(22.4\ \text{dm}^3)(10^{-1}\ \text{m dm}^{-1})^3} = 1.58 \times 10^{-4}$$

1.17. Calculate the ratio of $\overline{u^2}$ for Ne at 25 °C to that for Ar at 25 °C.

Taking a ratio of the second and fourth terms of (*1.21*) for the gases gives

$$\frac{(1/3)(M_{\text{Ne}})\overline{u^2_{\text{Ne}}}}{(1/3)(M_{\text{Ar}})\overline{u^2_{\text{Ar}}}} = \frac{RT}{RT} = 1$$

which upon rearranging gives

$$\frac{\overline{u^2_{\text{Ne}}}}{\overline{u^2_{\text{Ar}}}} = \frac{M_{\text{Ar}}}{M_{\text{Ne}}} = \frac{39.984}{20.183} = 1.9811$$

1.18. What is the average translational kinetic energy for a mole of an ideal gas at 25 °C?

Equation (*1.21*) gives

$$\overline{\text{KE}} = \frac{3}{2}RT = \frac{3}{2}(8.314\ \text{J K}^{-1}\ \text{mol}^{-1})(298\ \text{K}) = 3716\ \text{J mol}^{-1}$$

1.19. What is the average translational kinetic energy of a molecule of an ideal gas at 25 °C?

The molar energy was found in Problem 1.18. Hence

$$\overline{\text{ke}} = \frac{\overline{\text{KE}}}{L} = \frac{3716\ \text{J mol}^{-1}}{6.022\times 10^{23}\ \text{molecules mol}^{-1}} = 6.17\times 10^{-21}\ \text{J molecule}^{-1}$$

1.20. Prepare plots of $(dN/L)/du$ against u for N_2 at 100 °C and 1000 °C, for values of u between 10 and 10^4 m s^{-1}. Indicate on the plots the values of α, rms and $\bar{u}$. Describe the distributions.

In order to perform the calculations, it will be necessary to evaluate e^x, where x can range from a very small number to a very large number. For the small values of x, usually $x < 10^{-3}$, $e^{\pm x}$ is given to a good approximation by $1 \pm x$. For the large values of x, usually $x > 10^2$, $e^{\pm x}$ is given by antilog $(\pm x/2.303)$. For values of x between these ranges, $e^{\pm x}$ can be evaluated by using the natural logarithm scales found on most commercial slide rules, or by converting from natural logarithms to base-ten logarithms, where $\log x = (\ln x)/2.303$ and then using regular log tables. Sample calculations follow at 1000 °C using *(1.24)* in the form

$$\frac{dN/L}{du} = 4\pi u^2\left[\frac{28.01\times 10^{-3}/L}{2\pi(1.381\times 10^{-23})(1273)}\right]^{3/2} e^{-\frac{1}{2}(28.0\times 10^{-3}/L)u^2/(1.381\times 10^{-23})(1273)}$$

$$= (3.434\times 10^{-9})u^2\, e^{-1.323\times 10^{-6}u^2}$$

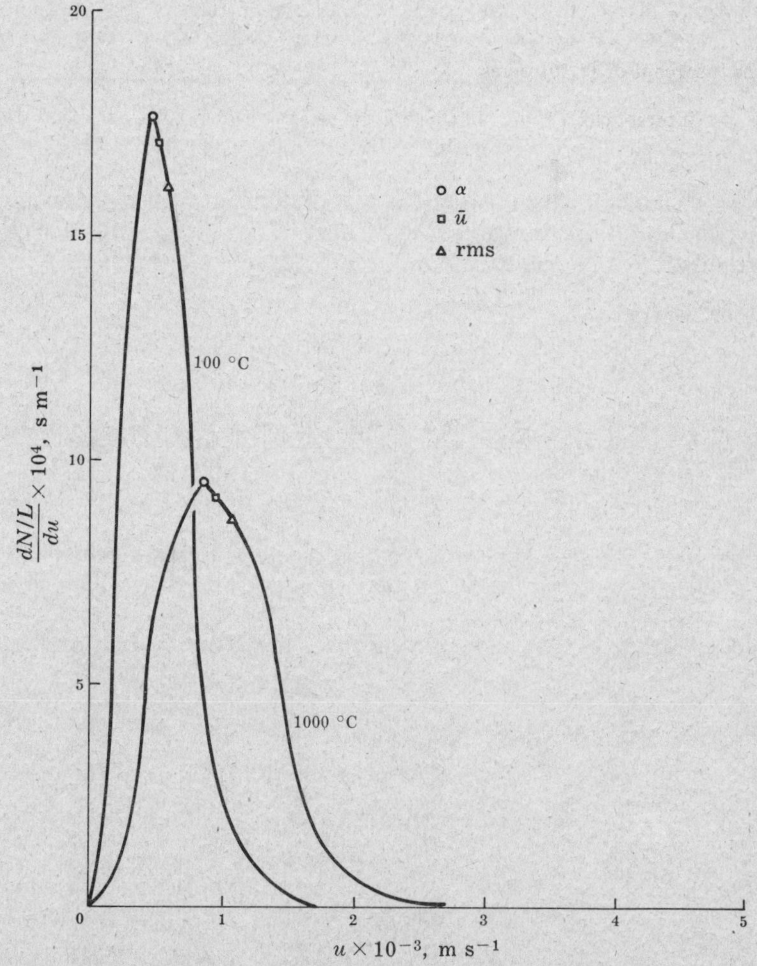

Fig. 1-3

For $u = 10$ m s^{-1}:

$$\frac{dN/L}{du} = (3.434\times10^{-9})(10)^2 e^{-1.323\times10^{-6}(10)^2}$$
$$= 3.434\times10^{-7} e^{-1.323\times10^{-4}}$$
$$= 3.434\times10^{-7}(1-0.000132)$$
$$= 3.434\times10^{-7}$$

For $u = 500$ m s^{-1}:

$$\frac{dN/L}{du} = (3.434\times10^{-9})(5\times10^2)^2 e^{-1.323\times10^{-6}(5\times10^2)^2}$$
$$= 85.84\times10^{-5} e^{-0.331}$$
$$= 8.584\times10^{-4}(0.718)$$
$$= 6.167\times10^{-4}$$

For $u = 10^4$ m s^{-1}:

$$\frac{dN/L}{du} = (3.434\times10^{-9})(10^4)^2 e^{-1.323\times10^{-6}(10^4)^2}$$
$$= 3.434\times10^{-1} e^{-132.3}$$
$$= 3.434\times10^{-1}(3.5\times10^{-58})$$
$$= 1.20\times10^{-58}$$

These data and others are shown in Fig. 1-3. The values for α, $\bar{u}$ and rms were calculated using (*1.25*) through (*1.27*). Both plots begin with very low fractions, increase to a maximum and decrease exponentially. Although the maximum of the curve at 1000 °C lies below the maximum of the curve at 100 °C, the plots cross and the curve at 1000 °C indicates the presence of a larger number of particles with high energy under this higher-temperature condition.

Collision Parameters

1.21. Calculate the mean free path and the collision number z_{12} of a molecule in air at 25 °C and 1 atm, assuming the presence of only N_2 and O_2. For these gases, the coefficients of viscosity are 175 and 209 μpoise, respectively.

Using (*1.31*) gives

$$N_{12}^* = \frac{(6.022\times10^{23}\ \text{mol}^{-1})(1\ \text{atm})}{(8.21\times10^{-5}\ \text{m}^3\ \text{atm K}^{-1}\ \text{mol}^{-1})(298\ \text{K})} = 2.46\times10^{25}\ \text{m}^{-3}$$

Using (*1.27*) gives $\bar{u} = 4.75\times10^2$ m s^{-1} for N_2 and 4.44×10^2 m s^{-1} for O_2, which upon substitution into (*1.29*) gives

$$\sigma_{N_2} = \left[\frac{(4.75\times10^2)(28.0\times10^{-3}/L)}{2^{3/2}\pi(175\times10^{-7})}\right]^{1/2} = 3.77\ \text{Å}$$

$$\sigma_{O_2} = \left[\frac{(4.44\times10^2)(32.0\times10^{-3}/L)}{2^{3/2}\pi(209\times10^{-7})}\right]^{1/2} = 3.56\ \text{Å}$$

Substituting these values of σ into (*1.32*) gives $\sigma_{12} = 3.66$ Å and using (*1.30*) gives

$$\ell = [\pi 2^{1/2}(3.66\times10^{-10}\ \text{m})^2(2.46\times10^{25}\ \text{m}^{-3})]^{-1} = 6.83\times10^{-8}\ \text{m}$$

Assuming that air is 80% N_2 and 20% O_2 gives

$$N_{N_2}^* = (0.80)(2.46\times10^{25}\ \text{m}^{-3}) = 1.97\times10^{25}\ \text{m}^{-3}$$

$$N_{O_2}^* = (0.20)(2.46\times10^{25}\ \text{m}^{-3}) = 0.49\times10^{25}\ \text{m}^{-3}$$

Using (*1.36*) gives

$$z_{12} = \pi(3.66\times10^{-10}\ \text{m})^2(1.97\times10^{25}\ \text{m}^{-3})(0.49\times10^{25}\ \text{m}^{-3}) \times [(4.75\times10^2\ \text{m s}^{-1})^2 + (4.44\times10^2\ \text{m s}^{-1})^2]^{1/2}$$
$$= 2.65\times10^{34}\ \text{m}^{-3}\ \text{s}^{-1}$$

Supplementary Problems

Temperature and Pressure

1.22. There is one temperature that is common to both the Celsius and Fahrenheit scales. What is this reading? *Ans.* $-40.0°$

1.23. Dibutyl phthalate is often used as a manometer fluid. If it has a density of 1.047×10^3 kg m^{-3}, how many torr are represented by one mm of this fluid? *Ans.* 0.077

Laws for Ideal Gases

1.24. Calculate the value of R in units of ft^3 psi °R^{-1} lbmole^{-1} using (*1.6*) and appropriate conversion factors. *Ans.* 10.73

1.25. Repeat Problem 1.7 assuming both flasks to contain N_2. *Ans.* $P_{N_2} = P_t = 4.56$ atm

1.26. Calculate the ratio of the rms of $^{238}UF_6$ to the rms of $^{235}UF_6$ at room temperature. *Ans.* 0.996

1.27. Show that for a fixed amount of gas at constant temperature (*1.21*) becomes Boyle's law, and for a fixed amount of gas at constant pressure (*1.21*) becomes Charles's law.

1.28. Based on the property of ideal gases that the temperature is directly proportional to the pressure at constant volume, an ideal-gas thermometer containing He was standardized at an internal pressure of 305 torr at the melting point of ice. If the pressure decreased to 85 torr when the probe was placed in a Dewar flask containing boiling liquid N_2, what is the boiling point of N_2? *Ans.* -197 °C

1.29. What is the difference in the density of dry air at 1 atm and 25 °C and moist air with 50% relative humidity under the same conditions? The vapor pressure of water at 25 °C is 23.7 torr. See Example 1.15 for additional data.

Ans. 1.185 kg m^{-3} for the dry air;
$P_{H_2O} = 11.8$ torr, 1.178 kg m^{-3} for the wet air; 0.007 kg m^{-3} difference

1.30. The probe of the gas thermometer described in Problem 1.28 is an active volume, V_a, and the manometer used for pressure readings is a dead volume, V_d. When the probe is placed at a low temperature T_1, a small amount of gas flows from the dead volume into the probe and the simple relationship $T_1 = T_0(P_1/P_0)$ is not valid because n has changed in the active volume. Using the relationships

$$P_0 = \frac{n_{0a}RT_0}{V_a} = \frac{n_{0d}RT_0}{V_d}$$

$$P_1 = \frac{n_{1a}RT_1}{V_a} = \frac{n_{1d}RT_0}{V_d}$$

$$n_{0a} + n_{0d} = n_{1a} + n_{1d}$$

show that

$$T_1 = T_0\frac{P_1}{P_0}\left[1 + \frac{V_d}{V_a}\frac{P_0 - P_1}{P_0}\right]^{-1}$$

Real Gases

1.31. The *Dieterici equation*

$$P = \frac{RT}{\bar{V} - b}e^{-a/\bar{V}RT} \tag{1.42}$$

may be expressed in a form similar to (*1.14*) by multiplying both sides of (*1.42*) by $\bar{V} - b$, solving for $P\bar{V}$, substituting $\bar{V} = RT/P$ in the correctional term, expanding the exponential as

$$e^x = 1 + x + \frac{x^2}{2} + \cdots$$

and collecting terms. Find A_p, B_p, and C_p.

Ans. $A_p = RT, \quad B_p = b - \dfrac{a}{RT}, \quad C_p = \dfrac{a^2}{2R^3T^3}$

1.32. Two molecules of a gas will collide when their centers are within a volume of $(4/3)\pi\sigma^3$. The excluded volume per molecule is $(2/3)\pi\sigma^3$; for a mole it is $b = (2/3)L\pi\sigma^3$. Using the diameter of argon as 3.84 Å, calculate b and compare the answer to the van der Waals value of 0.03219 dm³ mol⁻¹.

Ans. 0.0714 $dm^3\ mol^{-1}$, about 132% larger

1.33. Calculate the pressure for 1 mol of argon at 0 °C and 10.0 dm^3 using (*a*) the ideal gas law, (*b*) the van der Waals equation ($a = 1.345\ dm^6\ atm\ mol^{-2}$ and $b = 0.03219\ dm^3\ mol^{-1}$), and (*c*) the Dieterici equation ($a = 1.73\ dm^6\ atm\ mol^{-2}$ and $b = 0.035\ dm^3\ mol^{-1}$).

Ans. (*a*) 2.24 atm, (*b*) 2.24 atm, (*c*) 2.23 atm

1.34. Substitute $1/V = P/RT$ into the expression for PV derived in Problem 1.11 and rearrange the result into the form given by (*1.14*). Determine A_p, B_p, and C_p.

Ans. $A_p = RT,\ B_p = b - \dfrac{a}{RT},\ C_p = \dfrac{ab}{R^2T^2}$

1.35 Determine the value of B_p for SO_2 from the data in Example 1.16. Compare this value to that calculated from the expression for B_p given in Problem 1.34, where a and b are the van der Waals constants. *Ans.* slope = 0.0686, −0.538 $dm^3\ mol^{-1}$; −0.243 $dm^3\ mol^{-1}$; about 120% error

1.36. Evaluate the constants a and b in the Dieterici equation, (*1.42*), in terms of the critical point data. Determine the reduced form of this equation of state.

Ans. $a = \dfrac{4R^2T_c^2}{e^2P_c},\quad b = \dfrac{RT_c}{e^2P_c},\quad P_r = \dfrac{T_r}{2V_r - 1}e^{2-(2/T_rV_r)}$

Molecular Weight

1.37. The density of steam at 100 °C and 760.0 torr is 0.5974 kg m^{-3}. Calculate the molecular weight for water from these data. Explain any discrepancy from the value of 18.0152.

Ans. 18.3 g mol^{-1} (very near liquid state and gas shows deviation from ideal behavior)

1.38. The molecular weight of the vapor above NH_4Cl(s) is nearly 26.5 g mol^{-1}. Give an interpretation for this value.

Ans. The vapor consists of NH_3 and HCl, with an average M of 26.7 g mol^{-1}.

1.39. Moles reports the following values of d/P as a function of P for CO_2 at 0 °C:

P, atm	1.000	0.500	0.100	0.010	0.001	0.0001
d/P, g dm^{-3} atm^{-1}	1.997031	1.970233	1.964775	1.963544	1.963421	1.963409

From these data calculate the molecular weight of CO_2 and using the accepted value of 12.01115 for the atomic weight of C, find the atomic weight for O.

Ans. intercept = 1.963408, 44.00703 g mol^{-1}; 15.99794 g mol^{-1}

Kinetic-Molecular Theory

1.40. Prepare a plot of $(dN/L)/du_x$ against u_x for values from -10^4 to 10^4 m s^{-1} for u_x at 100 °C and 1000 °C. Describe the distributions.

Ans. Both curves are "bell-shaped" curves centered at $u_x = 0$. The plot at 100 °C falls more rapidly than the plot at 1000 °C, indicating there are fewer molecules with high energies at lower temperatures.

1.41. Beginning with $\bar{u} = \int_0^\infty u\,dN/L$, derive (*1.27*).

Collision Parameters

1.42. The coefficient of viscosity of water vapor at 150 °C and 1 atm is 144.5 μpoise. Calculate rms, $\bar{u}$, α, σ, ℓ, z_1 and z_{11} for these conditions.

Ans. 766 m s^{-1}; 705 m s^{-1}; 625 m s^{-1}; 4.06 Å; $N^* = 1.733 \times 10^{25}$ m^{-3}, 7.88×10^{-8} m; 8.95×10^{9} s^{-1}; 7.75×10^{34} s^{-1} m^{-3}

1.43. Using the data of Problem 1.21, compare the mean free path of a molecule in pure nitrogen at 25 °C and 1 atm to that in air under the same conditions. *Ans.* $\ell_{\text{pure}} = 6.44 \times 10^{-8}$ m, 94.2%

1.44. Most vacuum systems are capable of evacuating to 10^{-5} torr. Compare ℓ under these conditions to that at 1 atm. *Ans.* 8×10^{7} times greater

1.45. Find σ for O_2 and compare it to 3.56 Å as calculated from viscosity data in Problem 1.21, given that $D = 1.78 \times 10^{-5}$ m^2 s^{-1} at 0 °C.

Ans. $\bar{u} = 425$ m s^{-1}, $\ell = 6.99 \times 10^{-8}$ m, $N^* = 2.69 \times 10^{25}$ m^{-3}, $\sigma = 3.47$ Å; 3% lower

1.46. The rate that a gas collides with a unit area of the surface of its container is given by

$$\nu = N^*\left(\frac{RT}{2\pi M}\right)^{1/2} \qquad (1.43)$$

Find ν for O_2 at 25 °C and 1 atm. *Ans.* $N^* = 2.46 \times 10^{25}$ m^{-3}, $\nu = 2.73 \times 10^{27}$ m^{-2} s^{-1}

1.47. The ability of a gas to conduct heat is known as the *thermal conductivity*, k. For an ideal gas k is given by

$$k = \frac{5\eta C_V}{2M} \qquad (1.44)$$

where C_V is the molar heat capacity of the gas, see Section 2.7. Calculate k for water vapor if $\eta = 144.5$ μpoise and $C_V = 3R$. *Ans.* 5.01×10^{-2} J m^{-1} s^{-1} K^{-1}

Chapter 2

First Law of Thermodynamics

Internal Energy, Work, and Heat Flow

2.1 INTERNAL ENERGY, E

The internal energy of a system is the sum of the various kinetic and potential energy contributions. These include translational, rotational, vibrational, electronic, nuclear, positional, and mass contributions. Because the determination of an absolute value of E is difficult, most calculations and experimental measurements are concerned with the change in E, ΔE, where

$$\Delta E = E_{\text{final}} - E_{\text{initial}} \tag{2.1}$$

Equation (*2.1*) expresses the basic property of any *state* (or *point*) *function*: its increment is dependent only on the final and initial states of the system (and not on the path followed between these states).

For theoretical calculations involving ideal gases, ΔE can be equated to ΔE(thermal). The thermal energy represents the difference between the internal energy of the gas at some temperature T and the "rest" internal energy of the gas at 0 K:

$$E(\text{thermal}) = E_T - E_0 \tag{2.2}$$

The three major contributions to E(thermal) below 1000 K result from the translational, rotational and vibrational motions of the single molecules. For one mole of gas, each mode of molecular translational motion contributes

$$E(\text{thermal, trans}) = \tfrac{1}{2}RT \tag{2.3a}$$

each mode of rotational motion contributes

$$E(\text{thermal, rot}) = \tfrac{1}{2}RT \tag{2.3b}$$

and each mode of vibrational motion contributes

$$E(\text{thermal, vib}) = \frac{RTx}{e^x - 1} \tag{2.3c}$$

where

$$x \equiv \frac{h\nu}{kT} \tag{2.4}$$

The symbols h, ν, and k in (*2.4*) are Planck's constant, frequency of vibration and Boltzmann's constant, respectively. If the vibrational data are expressed in units of cm^{-1} via the wave number $\bar{\nu}$,

$$x = \frac{1.4388\,\bar{\nu}}{T} \tag{2.5}$$

EXAMPLE 2.1. Derive general expressions for E(thermal) for ideal monatomic, diatomic, linear polyatomic and nonlinear polyatomic gases.

If a molecule of the ideal gas contains Λ atoms, then the number of degrees of freedom is given by 3Λ. Three of these are assigned to the translational motion of the molecule, leaving $3\Lambda - 3$ degrees of freedom for rotational and vibrational motion. For an ideal monatomic gas, $3(1) - 3 = 0$; thus the entire contribution to E(thermal) is from translational motion, as given by (*2.3a*):

$$E(\text{thermal}) = 3\left(\frac{1}{2}RT\right) = \frac{3}{2}RT \tag{2.6a}$$

For a linear molecule there are two degrees of rotational motion, leaving $3\Lambda - 5$ degrees of freedom for vibrational motion. For an ideal diatomic gas, $3(2) - 5 = 1$; thus E(thermal) is given by (*2.3*) as

$$E(\text{thermal}) = 3\left(\frac{1}{2}RT\right) + 2\left(\frac{1}{2}RT\right) + \frac{RTx}{e^x - 1}$$

$$= \frac{5}{2}RT + \frac{RTx}{e^x - 1} \tag{2.6b}$$

and for an ideal linear polyatomic gas

$$E(\text{thermal}) = \frac{5}{2}RT + \sum_{i=1}^{3\Lambda-5} \frac{RTx_i}{e^{x_i} - 1} \tag{2.6c}$$

For a nonlinear molecule there are three degrees of rotational motion, leaving $3\Lambda - 6$ degrees of freedom for vibrational motion; thus

$$E(\text{thermal}) = 3\left(\frac{1}{2}RT\right) + 3\left(\frac{1}{2}RT\right) + \sum_{i=1}^{3\Lambda-6} \frac{RTx_i}{e^{x_i} - 1}$$

$$= 3RT + \sum_{i=1}^{3\Lambda-6} \frac{RTx_i}{e^{x_i} - 1} \tag{2.6d}$$

EXAMPLE 2.2. Compare the values of ΔE for heating an ideal monatomic gas and a nonlinear triatomic gas from 25 °C to 50 °C. Assume that the triatomic gas has three vibrational frequencies near 2000 cm^{-1}.

For the ideal monatomic gas (*2.6a*) gives

$$E(\text{thermal})_{298} = (3/2)(8.314\ \text{J mol}^{-1}\ \text{K}^{-1})(298\ \text{K}) = 3716\ \text{J mol}^{-1}$$

$$E(\text{thermal})_{323} = (3/2)(8.314)(323) = 4028\ \text{J mol}^{-1}$$

and (*2.1*) gives $\Delta E = 4028 - 3716 = 312\ \text{J mol}^{-1}$.

For the ideal nonlinear triatomic gas (*2.5*) gives

$$x_{298} = \frac{(1.4388)(2000)}{298} = 9.658 \qquad x_{323} = \frac{(1.4388)(2000)}{323} = 8.910$$

which upon substitution into (*2.6d*) gives

$$E(\text{thermal})_{298} = (3)(8.314)(298) + \frac{(3)(8.314)(298)(9.658)}{e^{9.658} - 1}$$

$$= 7433 + \frac{71{,}830}{1.57 \times 10^4} = 7438\ \text{J mol}^{-1}$$

$$E(\text{thermal})_{323} = 8056 + 10 = 8066\ \text{J mol}^{-1}$$

and (*2.1*) gives $\Delta E = 8066 - 7438 = 628\ \text{J mol}^{-1}$. The difference in the values is 316 J mol^{-1}, a factor of two.

2.2 WORK, W

Work can be defined as the product of an *intensity factor* (force, pressure, etc.) and a *capacity factor* (distance, electrical charge, etc.). The types of work given below are of interest in thermodynamics:

mechanical work	$đw = f\,dl$	(2.7a)
surface work	$đw = \gamma\,dA$	(2.7b)
electrical work	$đw = \mathcal{E}\,dq$	(2.7c)
gravitational work	$đw = mg\,dl$	(2.7d)
expansion work	$đw = P\,dV$	(2.7e)

where f is force, l is distance, γ is surface tension, $\mathcal{E}$ is potential difference, q is charge (current times time: $dq = I\,dt$), m is mass, g is the acceleration of gravity, P is the pressure exerted *on* a system by the surroundings, and V is the volume of the system.

The sign convention used in this book for work is that *a positive value means that the system under consideration has performed work on the surroundings and a negative value means that the surroundings have done work on the system.*

EXAMPLE 2.3. The symbol for the differential work, $đw$, used in (2.7) indicates that work is, in general, an inexact differential and the work involved in a process is path-dependent. To illustrate this, consider the expansion of one mole of an ideal gas from 0.0100 m^3 to 0.1000 m^3 at 25 °C by the following processes: (1) against a constant external pressure of 0.100 atm; (2) from 0.0100 m^3 to 0.0250 m^3 against a constant external pressure of 0.333 atm, followed by a second expansion from 0.0250 m^3 to 0.0500 m^3 against a constant pressure of 0.200 atm, followed by a third expansion from 0.0500 m^3 to 0.1000 m^3 against a constant pressure of 0.100 atm; (3) a reversible expansion.

For the first process (*2.7e*) gives

$$w = \int_{V_1}^{V_2} P\,dV = P\int_{V_1}^{V_2} dV = P\,\Delta V$$

$$= (0.100\ \text{atm})(0.1000\ \text{m}^3 - 0.0100\ \text{m}^3)(101{,}325\ \text{J m}^{-3}\ \text{atm}^{-1}) = 912\ \text{J}$$

For the second process, repeating the above calculation for each step gives

$$w = (0.333)(0.0250 - 0.0100) + (0.200)(0.0500 - 0.0250) + (0.100)(0.1000 - 0.0500)$$

$$= 0.0150\ \text{m}^3\ \text{atm} = 1519\ \text{J}$$

Under reversible conditions, the external pressure and the internal pressure differ only by dP, so substituting (*1.6*) into (*2.7e*) gives

$$w = \int_{V_1}^{V_2} \frac{nRT}{V}\,dV = nRT \ln\frac{V_2}{V_1}$$

$$= (1.00\ \text{mol})(8.314\ \text{J mol}^{-1}\ \text{K}^{-1})(298\ \text{K}) \ln 10 = 5705\ \text{J}$$

From the above calculations it can be seen that w is dependent on the process chosen and is greatest for a reversible process and smallest for the most irreversible process.

2.3 HEAT FLOW, q

The "zeroth law" of thermodynamics states that if the temperatures of systems A and B are the same and if the temperatures of systems B and C are the same, then no heat flow will occur if system A is placed in contact with system C. Unless work is done on the systems, heat flow will occur only if one system is at a higher temperature than the other and will be directed from the hotter to the colder system.

The sign convention for heat in this book is that *a negative value represents heat flow from a system to the surroundings* (an exothermic process) *and a positive value represents heat flow from the surroundings to the system* (an endothermic process).

Mathematical Statement of the First Law

2.4 STATEMENT

The first law can be written as

$$\Delta E = q - w \tag{2.8a}$$

or, in differential form, as

$$dE = đq - đw \tag{2.8b}$$

EXAMPLE 2.4. Consider a system consisting of one mole of a monatomic gas contained in a piston. What is the temperature change of the gas if $q = 50$ J and $w = 100$ J ?

From the first law

$$\Delta E = q - w = 50 - 100 = -50 \text{ J mol}^{-1}$$

For a monatomic ideal gas,

$$\Delta E = \Delta E(\text{thermal}) = \tfrac{3}{2}R\,\Delta T$$

hence

$$\Delta T = \frac{\Delta E}{\frac{3}{2}R} = \frac{-50 \text{ J mol}^{-1}}{\frac{3}{2}(8.314 \text{ J mol}^{-1}\text{ K}^{-1})} = -4.0\ ^\circ\text{C}$$

2.5 CONSTANT-VOLUME PROCESSES

For a system capable of performing only expansion work, if $dV = 0$ then $w = 0$, which upon substitution into (*2.8a*) gives

$$\Delta E = q_V \tag{2.9}$$

Thus the heat flow under constant-volume (*isochoric*) conditions is a direct measurement of ΔE. Heat of combustion measurements for substances are made under these conditions using a "bomb" calorimeter and hence are listed as ΔE(combustion).

2.6 ENTHALPY, H, AND CONSTANT-PRESSURE PROCESSES

The enthalpy of a system is defined as

$$H = E + PV \tag{2.10}$$

and the change in enthalpy is given by

$$\Delta H = \Delta E + \Delta(PV) \tag{2.11}$$

For a system operating under isobaric conditions, (*2.11*) becomes

$$\Delta H = \Delta E + P\,\Delta V$$

Since under these conditions $P\,\Delta V = w$ and $\Delta E = q_P - w$,

$$\Delta H = q_P \tag{2.12}$$

Thus the heat flow under constant-pressure conditions (such as the heat of reaction for a chemical reaction performed in a "solution" calorimeter, beaker, flask, etc.) is ΔH.

EXAMPLE 2.5. The ΔH for the formation of NOCl(g) from the gaseous elements is 12.57 kcal mol^{-1} at 25 °C. If the gases are ideal, calculate ΔE.

From the reaction

$$\tfrac{1}{2}N_2(g) + \tfrac{1}{2}O_2(g) + \tfrac{1}{2}Cl_2(g) = NOCl(g) \qquad \Delta H = 12.57 \text{ kcal}$$

it can be seen that $\Delta(PV)$ in (*2.11*) can be replaced by $RT\,\Delta n_g$, where

$$\Delta n_g = n_{\mathrm{NOCl}} - \tfrac{1}{2}n_{\mathrm{N}_2} - \tfrac{1}{2}n_{\mathrm{O}_2} - \tfrac{1}{2}n_{\mathrm{Cl}_2} = 1 - \tfrac{1}{2}(1) - \tfrac{1}{2}(1) - \tfrac{1}{2}(1) = -\tfrac{1}{2}\ \mathrm{mol}$$

because all substances are gases. Rearranging (*2.11*) gives

$$\begin{aligned}\Delta E &= \Delta H - \Delta(PV)\\ &= (12.57\ \mathrm{kcal})(4.184\ \mathrm{kJ\ kcal^{-1}}) - (8.314\times10^{-3}\ \mathrm{kJ\ mol^{-1}\ K^{-1}})(298\ \mathrm{K})(-\tfrac{1}{2}\ \mathrm{mol})\\ &= 52.59 + 1.24 = 53.83\ \mathrm{kJ}\end{aligned}$$

for the reaction, or $\Delta E = 53.83\ \mathrm{kJ\ mol^{-1}}$.

Heat Capacity

2.7 DEFINITIONS

The *molar heat capacity, C,* is defined as

$$C = \lim_{\Delta T\to 0}\frac{q}{\Delta T} \tag{2.13}$$

The *specific heat, c,* is related to C by

$$C = Mc \tag{2.14}$$

For constant-volume processes, $q = \Delta E$, and (*2.13*) gives

$$C_V = \lim_{\Delta T\to 0}\left(\frac{\Delta E}{\Delta T}\right)_V = \left(\frac{\partial E}{\partial T}\right)_V \tag{2.15}$$

and for constant-pressure processes, $q = \Delta H$, which gives

$$C_P = \lim_{\Delta T\to 0}\left(\frac{\Delta H}{\Delta T}\right)_P = \left(\frac{\partial H}{\partial T}\right)_P \tag{2.16}$$

For an ideal gas E and H are not dependent upon P or V; thus (*2.15*) and (*2.16*) become

$$dE = C_V\,dT \tag{2.17}$$

$$dH = C_P\,dT \tag{2.18}$$

EXAMPLE 2.6. Derive an equation for C_V for an ideal diatomic gas.

By (*2.17*), (*2.2*) and (*2.6b*),

$$C_V = \frac{d[E(\text{thermal}) + E_0]}{dT} = \frac{dE(\text{thermal})}{dT} = \frac{d}{dT}\left(\frac{5}{2}RT + \frac{RTx}{e^x - 1}\right)$$

in which x is given as a function of T by (*2.4*). Carrying out the differentiation, we find

$$C_V = \frac{5}{2}R + \frac{Rx^2e^x}{(e^x-1)^2}$$

2.8 HEAT-CAPACITY EXPRESSIONS

Example 2.6 illustrates the determination of theoretical values of C_V for ideal gases. For the condensed phases, the equations for C_V are much more complex, and empirical relations of the types

$$C_P = a + bT + cT^2 + dT^3 \tag{2.19a}$$

$$C_P = a + bT + c'T^{-2} \tag{2.19b}$$

are often used for these phases and to represent actual data for gases.

For metals at room temperature, C_P has an average value of 25.9 J mol^{-1} K^{-1}. Using this in combination with (*2.14*) generates the law of Dulong-Petit, which can be used to determine approximate atomic weights for metals from values of specific heat.

The Debye theory for metals gives as the atomic vibrational contribution to the heat capacity

$$C_V = \frac{9R}{(\Theta_D/T)^3}\int_0^{\Theta_D/T} \frac{x^4 e^x}{(e^x-1)^2}dx$$

where Θ_D is the *Debye temperature.* As $T \to \infty$, the vibrational contribution becomes

$$C_V = 3R\left[1 - \frac{(\Theta_D/T)^2}{20} + \frac{(\Theta_D/T)^4}{560} - \frac{(\Theta_D/T)^6}{18{,}144}\right]$$

and as $T \to 0$,

$$C_V \fallingdotseq 233.8(T/\Theta_D)^3 R$$

Combining the Debye result with a term for the electronic contribution as predicted by the free-electron model for metals gives

$$C_V = \frac{9R}{(\Theta_D/T)^3}\int_0^{\Theta_D/T} \frac{x^4 e^x}{(e^x-1)^2}dx + \eta T \tag{2.20}$$

where η is a constant which can be determined as $\pi^2 Rk/2E_f$, where E_f is the *Fermi energy* (see Section 18.3).

For liquids, exact values of heat capacity cannot be predicted. However, approximations include $3R$ for the vibrational modes of the centers of mass of the molecules, $Rx^2e^x/(e^x-1)^2$ for each intramolecular vibrational mode, and a contribution of from $\frac{1}{2}R$ to R for each mode of rotational motion.

EXAMPLE 2.7. The values of a and b in (*2.19a*) for aluminum are 4.94 cal mol^{-1} K^{-1} and 2.96×10^{-3} cal mol^{-1} K^{-2}, respectively. Calculate ΔH for heating one mole of Al from 25 °C to 100 °C.

Using (*2.18*) gives

$$\Delta H = \int_{T_1}^{T_2}(a+bT)\,dT = a(T_2 - T_1) + \frac{1}{2}b(T_2^2 - T_1^2)$$

$$= (4.94)(4.184)(373-298) + \frac{1}{2}(2.96\times10^{-3})(4.184)(373^2-298^2) = 1862 \text{ J mol}^{-1}$$

EXAMPLE 2.8. The low-temperature limit of (*2.20*) can be rearranged as

$$\frac{C_V}{T} = \frac{233.8}{\Theta_D^3}RT^2 + \eta$$

which is in the general form of a linear equation if C_V/T is plotted against T^2. (1) Prepare such a plot from the data given below for Al, assuming $C_V = C_P$ at these low temperatures, and determine the values of Θ_D and η. (2) Using these values of Θ_D and η, calculate C_V at 25 °C, assuming the high-temperature form of (*2.20*) to be valid. (3) Compare C_V to the value for C_P obtained from (*2.19a*) using the data of Example 2.7.

T, K	1	2	3	4	6	8	10
C_P, mJ mol^{-1} K^{-1}	1.38	2.91	4.75	7.04	13.49	23.74	37.77

The slope of the straight line through the first five data is 2.59×10^{-5} J mol^{-1} K^{-4}, which gives $\Theta_D = 422$ K, and the intercept is 1.36×10^{-3} J mol^{-1} K^{-2}, which is η. Using these values at 25 °C gives

$$C_V = 3(8.314)\left[1 - \frac{(422/298)^2}{20} + \frac{(422/298)^4}{560} - \frac{(422/298)^6}{18{,}144}\right] + (1.36\times10^{-3})(298)$$

$$= 3(8.314)(1 - 0.1003 + 0.0072 - 0.0004) + 0.41 = 23.01 \text{ J mol}^{-1}\text{ K}^{-1}$$

The value of C_P using (*2.19a*) is

$$C_P = (4.94)(4.184) + (2.96 \times 10^{-3})(4.184)(298) = 24.36 \text{ J mol}^{-1}\text{ K}^{-1}$$

Thus, if the high-temperature form of (*2.20*) is valid, there is a difference of about 1.35 J mol^{-1} K^{-1} between C_P and C_V (see Section 2.9). (The true value of the integral in (*2.20*) is 0.8581, which gives an exact value of $C_V = 23.02$ J mol^{-1} K^{-1}.)

2.9 RELATIONSHIP BETWEEN C_P AND C_V

The difference between the heat capacities can be shown to be

$$C_P - C_V = \left[P + \left(\frac{\partial E}{\partial V}\right)_T\right]\left(\frac{\partial V}{\partial T}\right)_P \tag{2.21}$$

For an ideal gas, $V = RT/P$ and $(\partial E/\partial V)_T = 0$, so (*2.21*) becomes

$$C_P - C_V = R \tag{2.22}$$

For solids and liquids, (*2.21*) yields

$$C_P - C_V = \frac{\alpha^2 VT}{\beta} \tag{2.23}$$

where α, the *coefficient of thermal expansion*, and β, the *isothermal compressibility factor*, are given by

$$\alpha = \frac{1}{V}\left(\frac{\partial V}{\partial T}\right)_P = \left(\frac{\partial \ln V}{\partial T}\right)_P$$

$$\beta = \frac{-1}{V}\left(\frac{\partial V}{\partial P}\right)_T = -\left(\frac{\partial \ln V}{\partial P}\right)_T$$

EXAMPLE 2.9. Assuming $\alpha = 69 \times 10^{-6}$ K^{-1}, $\beta = 1.34 \times 10^{-6}$ atm^{-1} and the density to be 2.702×10^3 kg m^{-3}, find the difference between C_P and C_V for Al at 25 °C.

Substituting these values into (*2.23*) gives

$$C_P - C_V = \frac{(69 \times 10^{-6}\text{ K}^{-1})^2(26.98 \times 10^{-3}\text{ kg mol}^{-1})(2.702 \times 10^3\text{ kg m}^{-3})^{-1}(298\text{ K})}{1.34 \times 10^{-6}\text{ atm}^{-1}}$$

$$= 10.57 \times 10^{-6}\text{ m}^3\text{ atm mol}^{-1}\text{ K}^{-1} = 1.07\text{ J mol}^{-1}\text{ K}^{-1}$$

Specific Applications of the First Law

2.10 REVERSIBLE ISOTHERMAL EXPANSION OF AN IDEAL GAS

Because the internal energy content of an ideal gas is a function only of temperature, under isothermal conditions

$$\Delta E = 0 \tag{2.24a}$$

$$\Delta H = \Delta E + \Delta(PV) = 0 + \Delta(nRT) = 0 \tag{2.24b}$$

Combining (*2.24a*), (*2.8a*) and (*2.7e*) with (*1.6*) gives

$$q = w = \int_{V_1}^{V_2} P\,dV = nRT \ln\frac{V_2}{V_1} \tag{2.24c}$$

EXAMPLE 2.10. Calculate ΔE, q, w, and ΔH for the compression of two moles of an ideal gas reversibly from 1.00 atm to 100.0 atm at 25 °C.

Equations (*2.24*) give

$$\Delta E = \Delta H = 0$$

$$q = w = nRT \ln \frac{V_2}{V_1} = nRT \ln \frac{P_1}{P_2}$$

$$= (2.00 \text{ mol})(8.314 \text{ J mol}^{-1} \text{ K}^{-1})(298 \text{ K}) \ln \frac{1.00}{100.0} = -22.8 \text{ kJ}$$

2.11 ISOTHERMAL ISOBARIC EXPANSION OF AN IDEAL GAS

For this process

$$\Delta E = \Delta H = 0 \qquad (2.25a)$$

$$q = w = \int_{V_1}^{V_2} P\,dV = P\,\Delta V \qquad (2.25b)$$

EXAMPLE 2.11. Calculate ΔE, q, w and ΔH for compressing two moles of an ideal gas from 1.00 atm to 100.0 atm at 25 °C, if the external pressure is 500.0 atm.

Using (*2.25a*) gives $\Delta E = \Delta H = 0$. Using (*1.6*) to determine the initial and final volumes gives

$$V_1 = \frac{nRT}{P_1} = \frac{(2.00 \text{ mol})(0.0821 \text{ dm}^3 \text{ atm K}^{-1} \text{ mol}^{-1})(298 \text{ K})}{1.00 \text{ atm}} = 48.9 \text{ dm}^3$$

$$V_2 = \frac{nRT}{100P_1} = 0.489 \text{ dm}^3$$

Now (*2.25b*) gives

$$q = w = P(V_2 - V_1) = (500.0 \text{ atm})(0.489 \text{ dm}^3 - 48.9 \text{ dm}^3)(101{,}325 \text{ J m}^{-3} \text{ atm}^{-1}) = -2.45 \text{ MJ}$$

2.12 ISOTHERMAL ISOBARIC PHASE CHANGE

For this process

$$q = \Delta H \qquad (2.26a)$$

$$w = \int_{V_1}^{V_2} P\,dV = P\,\Delta V \qquad (2.26b)$$

and ΔE is determined by the first law, (*2.8a*).

EXAMPLE 2.12. Calculate q, w and ΔE at 1 atm for the phase transitions

$$Li_2SO_4(\text{s-II}) = Li_2SO_4(\text{s-I})$$

$$Li_2SO_4(\text{s-I}) = Li_2SO_4(\text{liq})$$

the first of which takes place at 859 K and the second at 1132 K. The enthalpy changes are

$$\Delta H_{859}(\text{s-II} \rightarrow \text{s-I}) = 27.2 \text{ kJ mol}^{-1}$$

$$\Delta H_{1132}(\text{s-I} \rightarrow \text{liq}) = 7.5 \text{ kJ mol}^{-1}$$

and the densities of Li_2SO_4(s-II), Li_2SO_4(s-I) and Li_2SO_4(liq) are respectively 2.221×10^3, 2.07×10^3 and 2.004×10^3 kg m^{-3}.

For the solid-solid transition, (*2.26*) gives

$$q = \Delta H = 27.2 \text{ kJ}$$

$$w = P\,\Delta V = (1 \text{ mol})(1.00 \text{ atm})\left[(0.10994 \text{ kg mol}^{-1})\left(\frac{1}{2.07 \times 10^3 \text{ kg m}^{-3}} - \frac{1}{2.221 \times 10^3 \text{ kg m}^{-3}}\right)\right]$$

$$= (1.00)(53.1 \times 10^{-6} - 49.5 \times 10^{-6}) = 3.6 \times 10^{-6} \text{ m}^3 \text{ atm} = 0.365 \text{ J}$$

$$\Delta E = q - w = 27.2 \text{ kJ}$$

for the reaction, or $\Delta E = 27.2$ kJ mol^{-1}.

For the melting:

$$q = \Delta H = 7.5 \text{ kJ}$$

$$w = (1)(1.00)\left[(0.10994)\left(\frac{1}{2.004 \times 10^3} - \frac{1}{2.07 \times 10^3}\right)\right] = 0.177 \text{ J}$$

$$\Delta E = 7.5 \text{ kJ}$$

for the reaction, or $\Delta E = 7.5 \text{ kJ mol}^{-1}$.

2.13 REVERSIBLE ADIABATIC EXPANSION OF AN IDEAL GAS

For this process

$$q = 0 \tag{2.27a}$$

$$\Delta E = -w = \int_{T_1}^{T_2} nC_V \, dT \tag{2.27b}$$

$$\Delta H = \int_{T_1}^{T_2} nC_P \, dT \tag{2.27c}$$

To perform the calculations indicated by (*2.27*), both the initial and final temperatures must be known. Depending on the data, one of the following relationships may be used to determine the final temperature:

$$T_1^{C_V/R} V_1 = T_2^{C_V/R} V_2 \tag{2.28}$$

$$P_1 V_1^{\gamma} = P_2 V_2^{\gamma} \tag{2.29}$$

where

$$\gamma \equiv \frac{C_P}{C_V} \tag{2.30}$$

EXAMPLE 2.13. Calculate q, w, ΔH and ΔE for the adiabatic and reversible compression of one mole of a monatomic ideal gas from 0.1000 m^3 and 25 °C to 0.0100 m^3.

Using (*2.28*) to determine the final temperature gives

$$298^{C_V/R}(0.1000) = T_2^{C_V/R}(0.0100)$$

Substituting $C_V = (3/2)R$ and rearranging gives

$$T_2^{3/2} = (298)^{3/2}(10.0)$$

$$\frac{3}{2}\log T_2 = \frac{3}{2}\log 298 + \log 10.0 = \frac{3}{2}(2.474) + 1.000 = 4.711$$

from which $\log T_2 = 3.140$ and $T_2 = 1383$ K. Now (*2.27*) gives

$$q = 0$$

$$\Delta E = -w = \int_{298 \text{ K}}^{1383 \text{ K}} nC_V \, dT = n\left(\frac{3}{2}\right)R\,\Delta T$$

$$= (1.00 \text{ mol})\left(\frac{3}{2}\right)(8.314 \text{ J mol}^{-1} \text{ K}^{-1})(1383 \text{ K} - 298 \text{ K}) = 13.6 \text{ kJ}$$

$$\Delta H = \int_{298 \text{ K}}^{1383 \text{ K}} nC_P \, dT = n\left(\frac{5}{2}\right)R\,\Delta T = 22.6 \text{ kJ}$$

2.14 ISOBARIC ADIABATIC EXPANSION OF AN IDEAL GAS

For this process

$$q = 0 \tag{2.31a}$$

$$w = \int_{V_1}^{V_2} P \, dV = P\,\Delta V \tag{2.31b}$$

$$\Delta E = \int_{T_1}^{T_2} nC_V\,dT \qquad (2.31c)$$

$$\Delta H = \int_{T_1}^{T_2} nC_P\,dT \qquad (2.31d)$$

The final temperature can be determined by recognizing that the first law applies, giving

$$\int_{T_1}^{T_2} nC_V\,dT = -P\,\Delta V \qquad (2.32)$$

EXAMPLE 2.14. Calculate q, w, ΔH and ΔE for the isobaric adiabatic expansion of one mole of a monatomic ideal gas from 1.00 dm³ and 25 °C to 10.00 dm³ against an external pressure of 1.00 atm. (This is an irreversible expansion because of the finite difference between the applied and internal pressures.)

Using (*2.32*) to determine the final temperature gives

$$(1.00\text{ mol})\left(\frac{3}{2}\right)R(T_2 - 298) = -(1.00\text{ atm})(10.00\text{ dm}^3 - 1.00\text{ dm}^3)$$

$$T_2 = 298 - \frac{(1.00)(9.00)}{(3/2)(0.0821)(1.00)} = 298 - 73.1 = 225\text{ K}$$

Using (*2.31*) gives

$$q = 0$$

$$w = (1.00\text{ atm})(10.00\text{ dm}^3 - 1.00\text{ dm}^3)(101{,}325\text{ J m}^{-3}\text{ atm}^{-1}) = 912\text{ J}$$

$$\Delta E = -912\text{ J}$$

$$\Delta H = (1.00)\left(\frac{5}{2}\right)R(-73.1) = -1519\text{ J}$$

2.15 JOULE-THOMSON EFFECT

The *Joule-Thomson experiment* is a constant-enthalpy process which measures

$$(\partial T/\partial P)_H \equiv \mu_{jt}$$

as real gases undergo a throttled adiabatic expansion. A positive value of μ_{jt} indicates that a cooling will occur as the gas expands, because work is done at the expense of the internal energy of the gas.

EXAMPLE 2.15. The value of μ_{jt} for air at 0 °C is 0.249 K atm⁻¹ at 20 atm and 0.266 K atm⁻¹ at 1 atm. What is the approximate cooling observed as the gas undergoes this expansion?

Rearranging the definition of μ_{jt} gives

$$dT = \mu_{jt}\,dP \qquad (H = \text{constant})$$

$$\Delta T = \int_{P_1}^{P_2} \mu_{jt}\,dP$$

If μ_{jt} is assumed to be a linear function of pressure over this small pressure range, then the pressure-dependence can be expressed as

$$\mu_{jt} = 0.266 - 8.95 \times 10^{-4}\,P$$

using the data above. Substituting this relationship and integrating gives

$$\Delta T = \int_{20}^{1} (0.266 - 8.95 \times 10^{-4}\,P)\,dP$$

$$= (0.266)(1 - 20) - (4.93 \times 10^{-4})(1^2 - 20^2)$$

$$= -5.06 + 0.20 = -4.86\text{ K}$$

a cooling effect.

Solved Problems

Internal Energy, Work, and Heat Flow

2.1. Calculate the ratio of E(thermal) of a nonlinear polyatomic ideal gas to that of a linear polyatomic gas if only translational and rotational contributions are considered.

Taking a ratio of the nonvibrational terms of (*2.6d*) and (*2.6c*) gives

$$\frac{E(\text{thermal})_{\text{nonlinear}}}{E(\text{thermal})_{\text{linear}}} = \frac{3RT}{(5/2)RT} = 1.2$$

2.2. Consider a dry cell, $\mathcal{E} = 1.50$ V, large enough to deliver a constant current of exactly 0.01 A for an hour. If this cell powered a hoist able to lift a 200-lb man, how far off the ground would the man be at the end of the hour?

Assuming no loss of work, (*2.7c*) and (*2.7d*) give

$$\int_0^{1\,\text{hr}} \mathcal{E}I\,dt = \int_{l_1}^{l_2} mg\,dl$$

Solving for the change in distance gives

$$\Delta l = \frac{\mathcal{E}I\,\Delta t}{mg} = \frac{(1.50\text{ V})(0.0100\text{ A})(3600\text{ s})(\text{kg m}^2\text{ A}^{-1}\text{ s}^{-3}\text{ V}^{-1})}{(200\text{ lb})(0.454\text{ kg lb}^{-1})(9.80\text{ m s}^{-2})} = 6.07\text{ cm}$$

2.3. Consider a 1.00-kg block of iron at 99 °C placed in contact with a 1.00-kg block of iron at 25 °C. If the heat flow between these blocks is given by

$$q = mc_P\,\Delta T$$

where $c_P = 444\text{ J kg}^{-1}\text{ K}^{-1}$, find the final temperature of the system and the amount of heat that was transferred.

The "zeroth law" states that heat will be transferred from the hotter block to the cooler one until both have reached the same temperature, or

$$q_h = -q_c$$

$$m_h c_P(T_f - T_h) = -m_c c_P(T_f - T_c)$$

$$T_f = 0.5(T_h + T_c) = 0.5(99° + 25°) = 62\text{ °C}$$

Using this final temperature gives

$$q_h = -q_c = (1.00\text{ kg})(444\text{ J kg}^{-1}\text{ K}^{-1})(62° - 99°) = -16.4\text{ kJ}$$

Mathematical Statement of the First Law

2.4. Under isothermal conditions, $\Delta E = 0$ for the expansion of an ideal gas. If 100 J of work is done on the system consisting of one mole of an ideal gas, what amount of heat must be transferred?

The first law, (*2.8a*), gives

$$\Delta E = 0 = q - w \quad \text{or} \quad q = w = -100\text{ J}$$

Thus 100 J must be transferred from the system to maintain the constant temperature.

2.5. The heat of combustion of $H_2(g)$ to form $H_2O(liq)$ under constant-pressure conditions is -68.32 kcal mol^{-1} at 25 °C. If the water is formed at 1 atm and has a density of 1.00×10^3 kg m^{-3}, calculate ΔE for this reaction.

For the reaction

$$H_2(g) + \tfrac{1}{2}O_2(g) = H_2O(liq) \qquad \Delta H = -68.32 \text{ kcal}$$

the term $\Delta(PV)$ in (*2.11*) can be replaced by

$$\begin{aligned}\Delta(PV) &= (1 \text{ mol})(1 \text{ atm})(18.0 \times 10^{-3} \text{ kg mol}^{-1})(1.00 \times 10^3 \text{ kg m}^{-3})^{-1}(101{,}325 \text{ J m}^{-3} \text{ atm}^{-1}) \\ &\quad - (1 \text{ mol } H_2)RT - (\tfrac{1}{2} \text{ mol } O_2)RT \\ &= 1.82 \text{ J} - (\tfrac{3}{2} \text{ mol})RT\end{aligned}$$

Rearranging (*2.11*) gives

$$\begin{aligned}\Delta E &= \Delta H - \Delta(PV) \\ &= (-68.32 \text{ kcal})(4.184 \text{ kJ kcal}^{-1}) \\ &\qquad - [1.82 \times 10^{-3} \text{ kJ} - (\tfrac{3}{2} \text{ mol})(8.314 \times 10^{-3} \text{ kJ mol}^{-1} \text{ K}^{-1})(298 \text{ K})] \\ &= -285.9 - (-3.7) = -282.2 \text{ kJ}\end{aligned}$$

for the reaction, or $\Delta E = -282.2$ kJ mol^{-1}. Note that the PV-contribution of the liquid phase is negligible to that of the gaseous components of the reaction.

Heat Capacity

2.6. The heat capacity ratio C_P/C_V for a gas was experimentally measured as 1.38. If the empirical formula is ABA, what conclusions can be made concerning the structure?

Assuming the gas to be nearly ideal, (*2.22*) gives

$$C_P = C_V + R$$

which upon substitution into the desired ratio gives

$$\frac{C_V + R}{C_V} = 1.38 \qquad \text{or} \qquad C_V = 2.63\,R$$

If vibrational contributions are neglected, $C_V = 2.5\,R$ for a linear triatomic gas and $C_V = 3.0\,R$ for a nonlinear triatomic gas. Assuming the difference of $0.13\,R$ to be from vibrational contributions, the gas is linear.

2.7. Find ΔH for heating a mole of $H_2(g)$ from 0 °C to 100 °C if

$$C_P = 6.9469 - 0.1999 \times 10^{-3}\,T + 4.808 \times 10^{-7}\,T^2$$

in cal K^{-1} mol^{-1}.

Using (*2.18*) gives

$$\begin{aligned}\Delta H &= \int_{273\text{ K}}^{373\text{ K}} (4.184)(6.9469 - 0.1999 \times 10^{-3}T + 4.808 \times 10^{-7}T^2)\,dT \\ &= (4.184)\left[(6.9469)(373 - 273) - \left(\frac{0.1999 \times 10^{-3}}{2}\right)(373^2 - 273^2)\right. \\ &\qquad \left. + \left(\frac{4.808 \times 10^{-7}}{3}\right)(373^3 - 273^3)\right] \\ &= (4.184)(694.69 - 6.46 + 5.06) = 2900.7 \text{ J mol}^{-1}\end{aligned}$$

2.8. Calculate ΔH for heating one mole of an ideal diatomic gas from 0 °C to 100 °C excluding vibrational contributions. Compare the value to that determined for H_2 in Problem 2.7.

For a diatomic ideal gas, $C_V = (5/2)R$, so $C_P = (7/2)R$ and (*2.18*) gives

$$\Delta H = \int_{T_1}^{T_2} C_P\,dT = \int_{273\text{ K}}^{373\text{ K}} \frac{7}{2}R\,dT = \frac{7}{2}R(T_2 - T_1) = 2909.9\text{ J mol}^{-1}$$

This answer agrees quite well with the calculated value of 2900.7 J mol^{-1} that was determined for heating a mole of H_2.

2.9. Predict C_V for H_2O(liq) at 25 °C.

The vibrational contribution would be $3R = 25$ J mol^{-1} K^{-1}. The three degrees of rotational freedom each contribute between $\frac{1}{2}R$ and R for a total of 12 to 25 J mol^{-1} K^{-1}. The intramolecular vibrational frequencies for water are 3657, 1595 and 3756 cm^{-1}, giving values of x equal to 17.66, 7.70 and 18.13, respectively. Substituting these values into $Rx^2e^x/(e^x-1)^2$ gives a total contribution of about 0.4 J mol^{-1} K^{-1}. Adding the contributions gives a prediction of between 37 and 50 J mol^{-1} K^{-1}.

2.10. The coefficient of thermal expansion of water at 25 °C is 257.05×10^{-6} K^{-1} and the compressibility is 45.24×10^{-6} bar^{-1} (1 bar = 0.987 atm). If the density of water is 0.997075×10^3 kg m^{-3}, calculate $C_P - C_V$.

For the liquid, (*2.23*) gives

$$C_P - C_V = \frac{\alpha^2 VT}{\beta}$$

$$= \frac{(257.05\times10^{-6}\text{ K}^{-1})^2(18.015\times10^{-3}\text{ kg mol}^{-1})(0.997075\times10^3\text{ kg m}^{-3})^{-1}(298\text{ K})}{(45.24\times10^{-6}\text{ bar}^{-1})(0.987\text{ atm bar}^{-1})^{-1}}$$

$$= 7.76\times10^{-6}\text{ m}^3\text{ atm mol}^{-1}\text{ K}^{-1} = 0.786\text{ J mol}^{-1}\text{ K}^{-1}$$

which is about 1% of C_P (75.291 J mol^{-1} K^{-1}).

Specific Applications of the First Law

2.11. What would be the final volume occupied by a mole of an ideal gas initially at 0 °C and 1 atm if $q = 1000$ cal during a reversible isothermal expansion?

For the reversible isothermal expansion (*2.24c*) gives

$$q = nRT\ln\frac{V_2}{V_1}$$

Assuming $V_1 = 22.4\text{ dm}^3$,

$$(4.184\text{ J cal}^{-1})(1000\text{ cal}) = (1.00\text{ mol})(8.314\text{ J mol}^{-1}\text{ K}^{-1})(298\text{ K})\ln\frac{V_2}{22.4}$$

$$\ln\frac{V_2}{22.4} = 1.689$$

$$V_2 = (22.4\text{ dm}^3)(5.41) = 121.2\text{ dm}^3$$

2.12. Repeat Problem 2.11 assuming an isothermal expansion against a constant pressure of 1 atm.

For the isobaric isothermal expansion, (*2.25b*) gives $q = P(V_2 - V_1)$. Assuming $V_1 = 22.4\text{ dm}^3$,

$$(4.184\text{ J cal}^{-1})(1000\text{ cal})(101{,}325\text{ J m}^{-3}\text{ atm}^{-1})^{-1} = (1.00\text{ atm})(V_2 - 22.4\text{ dm}^3)$$

$$V_2 = 41.3 + 22.4 = 63.7\text{ dm}^3$$

2.13. Repeat Example 2.13 for a diatomic ideal gas, excluding vibrational contributions.

Performing the same calculations using $C_V = (5/2)R$ gives

$$T_2^{5/2} = (298)^{5/2}(10.0) \qquad \text{or} \qquad T_2 = 748 \text{ K}$$

Hence

$$q = 0$$

$$\Delta E = -w = n\left(\frac{5}{2}\right)R(748 - 298) = 9.35 \text{ kJ}$$

$$\Delta H = n\left(\frac{7}{2}\right)R(450) = 13.09 \text{ kJ}$$

2.14. Repeat Example 2.14 for a diatomic ideal gas, excluding vibrational contributions.

Performing the same calculations using $C_V = (5/2)R$ gives

$$T_2 = 298 - \frac{(1.00)(9.00)}{(5/2)(0.0821)(1.00)} = 254 \text{ K}$$

Thus

$$q = 0$$

$$w = 912 \text{ J}$$

$$\Delta E = -912 \text{ J}$$

$$\Delta H = (1.00)\left(\frac{7}{2}\right)R(-44.0) = -1280 \text{ J}$$

2.15. Calculate q, w and ΔE for the conversion of one mole of water at 100 °C and 1.00 atm to steam. Pertinent data are: $\Delta H = 970.3$ Btu lb^{-1}, 1 lb of liquid occupies 0.016719 ft^3, and 1 lb of gas occupies 26.799 ft^3.

Using (*2.26*) gives

$$\Delta H = q = (970.3 \text{ Btu lb}^{-1})(1054.35 \text{ J Btu}^{-1})(\text{lb}/0.45359 \text{ kg})(18.015 \times 10^{-3} \text{ kg mol}^{-1})$$

$$= 40.63 \text{ kJ mol}^{-1}$$

$$w = (1.00 \text{ atm})(26.799 \text{ ft}^3 - 0.016719 \text{ ft}^3)(28.316 \text{ dm}^3 \text{ ft}^{-3})$$
$$(101{,}325 \text{ J m}^{-3} \text{ atm}^{-1})(\text{lb}/0.45359 \text{ kg})(18.015 \times 10^{-3} \text{ kg mol}^{-1})$$

$$= 3.05 \text{ kJ mol}^{-1}$$

$$\Delta E = 40.63 - 3.05 = 37.58 \text{ kJ mol}^{-1}$$

Supplementary Problems

Internal Energy, Work, and Heat Flow

2.16. To illustrate the path-dependence of w and q, consider the initial state of a system to be an ideal gas confined to one half of a container and the final state to be the gas confined to the entire container. Qualitatively discuss the values of q and w if the process is performed (*a*) irreversibly, similar to the Joule-Thomson experiment; (*b*) reversibly, using a piston to change the external pressure as needed.

Ans. (*a*) $q = w = 0$, (*b*) $q = w > 0$

2.17. If the surface tension of water is 73.05×10^{-3} N m^{-1} at 18 °C, how much of a change in area could the dry cell described in Problem 2.2 produce in one hour? *Ans.* 739 m^2

2.18. Repeat the calculations of Problem 2.3 if the cooler block is 1.50 kg of Ag (c_P = 235 J K^{-1} kg^{-1}).

Ans. 66.3 °C, $q_h = -q_c = -14.5$ kJ

Mathematical Statement of the First Law

2.19. The heat of formation of FeS(α-s) is −22.72 kcal mol^{-1} at 25 °C under isobaric conditions. What is the value of ΔE? The densities of Fe, S and FeS(α-s) at 25 °C are 7.86×10^3, 2.07×10^3 and 4.74×10^3 kg m^{-3}, respectively. Assume all reactants and products to be at 1.00 atm.

Ans. $\Delta H = -95.06$ kJ mol^{-1}, $\Delta V = -4.05 \times 10^{-6}$ m^3 mol^{-1},
$\Delta(PV) = -0.41$ J, $\Delta E = -95.06$ kJ mol^{-1}

Heat Capacity

2.20. A 52.5-g sample of a yellowish metal at 99.8 °C was added to a 100.0-g sample of water at 23.2 °C. If the final temperature of the mixture was 26.7 °C, identify the metal. *Hint*: First, calculate the heat gained by the water, assuming the specific heat to be 4.18×10^3 J kg^{-1} K^{-1}; second, calculate the specific heat of the metal, assuming that heat was conserved in the process; third, use (*2.14*) to find an approximate atomic weight, assuming $C = 25.9$ J mol^{-1}; and fourth, use a periodic table.

Ans. 1463 J; c = 381 J kg^{-1} K^{-1}; M = 0.680 kg mol^{-1}; yellow color indicates Cu

2.21. Predict C_V at 25 °C for CCl_4(liq) given that the intramolecular vibrational frequencies are 458, 218 (doubly degenerate), 776 (triply degenerate) and 314 cm^{-1} (triply degenerate).

Ans. Translational = 24.9, rotational = 12.5 to 24.9, vibrational = 50.2;
sum is between 87.6 and 100.0 J mol^{-1} K^{-1}

2.22. If $\alpha = 1.25 \times 10^{-3}$ K^{-1} and $\beta = 10.7 \times 10^{-5}$ atm^{-1}, calculate $C_P - C_V$ for CCl_4. The density of CCl_4 is 1.5940×10^3 kg m^{-3} at 25 °C. If $C_P = 131.8$ J K^{-1} mol^{-1}, calculate C_V and compare it to the value predicted in Problem 2.21.

Ans. 4.20×10^{-4} m^3 atm mol^{-1} = 42.6 J mol^{-1} K^{-1};
89.8 J mol^{-1} K^{-1}, within the range of values determined in Problem 2.21

2.23. Using the low-temperature limit of (*2.20*), find an expression for the temperature at which the electronic and vibrational contributions are equal. Using $\Theta_D = 426$ K and $\eta = 1.36 \times 10^{-3}$ J mol^{-1} K^{-2}, evaluate this temperature for Al. *Ans.* $T = (\eta\Theta_D^3/233.8\,R)^{1/2}$, 7.4 K

2.24. In many of the problems the vibrational contribution to E(thermal) and C_V has been neglected. If the vibrational frequencies for CH_4 are 2917, 1534 (doubly degenerate), 3019 (triply degenerate) and 1306 cm^{-1} (triply degenerate), calculate E(thermal) and C_V at 25 °C and 500 °C, assuming the gas to be ideal. What fraction of the total contributions is the vibrational? Compare the predicted value of C_V to that calculated from $C_P - C_V = R$ if $C_P = 35.309$ J mol^{-1} K^{-1} at 298 K.

Ans. E(thermal) = 7540.4 and 26,570.7 J mol^{-1}, with vibrational contributions of 1.45% and 27.4% at 298 K and 773 K, respectively; $C_V = 27.311$ and 53.025 J mol^{-1} K^{-1}, with vibrational contributions of 8.67% and 53.0% at 298 K and 773 K, respectively; predicted $C_V = 26.995$ J mol^{-1} K^{-1}, which differs by 1.17% from the accepted value using (*2.22*).

2.25. An extension of the Dulong-Petit theory known as Kopp's rule can be used to estimate values of the heat capacity for a complex solid. If the formula of the compound contains Λ atoms, the high-temperature limit of C_V is given by

$$C_V = 3\Lambda R \tag{2.33}$$

Estimate C_V for $K_2B_8O_{13}$ at its melting point and compare your answer to $C_P = 134$ cal K^{-1} mol^{-1} assuming $C_P = C_V$.

Ans. 574 J mol^{-1} K^{-1}, 2.3% high

Specific Applications of the First Law

2.26. Five moles of a diatomic ideal gas is allowed to expand isothermally at 25 °C from 0.0200 to 0.1000 m^3. Calculate q, w, ΔE and ΔH if the expansion is performed (*a*) reversibly, and (*b*) isobarically against a constant pressure of 1.00 atm.

Ans. (*a*) $\Delta E = \Delta H = 0$, $q = w = 19.94$ kJ; (*b*) $\Delta E = \Delta H = 0$, $q = w = 8.11$ kJ

2.27. Calculate w for the expansion described in Problem 2.26 if it is performed isobarically in four steps: (1) against 4.00 atm until the volume is 0.0250 m^3, (2) 3.00 atm until 0.0300 m^3, (3) 2.00 atm until 0.0500 m^3, and (4) 1.00 atm until 0.1000 m^3. Comment on the values of w for the processes described.

Ans. $w = 12.67$ kJ; the reversible process described in Problem 2.26(*a*) generates the maximum amount of work, the pseudo-reversible process generates the secondmost amount of work, and the isobaric expansion described in Problem 2.26(*b*) generates the least amount of work.

2.28. At temperatures above the inversion temperature a gas heats upon expansion. What must be done to produce liquid H_2 by expansion-cooling if the inversion temperature is −80 °C?

Ans. The gas must be cooled below this temperature before cooling will occur upon expansion.

2.29. Consider the reversible isothermal expansion of a mole of steam from 1.00 dm^3 to 10.00 dm^3 at 500 °C. Calculate the work assuming (*a*) the gas to be ideal, (*b*) the gas to obey the van der Waals equation with $a = 5.464$ dm^6 atm mol^{-1} and $b = 0.03049$ dm^3 mol^{-1}, and (*c*) the gas to obey (*1.15*). A graphical integration of (*2.7e*) for the third case will be necessary because the value of z is a function of pressure. For simplicity, assume that the pressure of the steam for a given volume can be determined from the ideal gas law and that the corresponding value of z is correct. The critical data for water are 374.1 °C and 218.3 atm.

Ans. (*a*) 14.80 kJ, (*b*) 14.48 kJ, (*c*) 14.5 kJ

Chapter 3

Thermochemistry

Heat of Reaction

3.1 INTRODUCTION

The *heat of reaction* is the value of ΔH or ΔE which accompanies the isothermal chemical reaction

$$\text{reactants at } T = \text{products at } T$$

when carried out under constant-pressure or constant-volume conditions, respectively. Reactions with negative heats are known as *exothermic* and those with positive values as *endothermic*. In many cases, exothermic reactions will occur spontaneously while endothermic reactions will not. However, heat exchange is not the sole criterion for spontaneity (see Section 5.1). The value given for ΔE or ΔH beside a reaction represents the energy change for the reaction as written, and the units are simply the units of energy, e.g. kJ. Thermochemical data without an accompanying reaction apply to a mole of the substance in question, and the units are those of energy per mole, e.g. kJ mol^{-1}.

A complete thermochemical equation includes not only the stoichiometric and energy information, but also a description of the physical states of the substances involved. For example, (c) or (s) is used to represent the solid state, and if more information is necessary, symbols such as (α-s), (β), (rhombic), (solid-II), (dia) and (graph) are used to indicate which of the several possible solids is involved. Other notation includes (l) or (liq) for liquid, (g) for gas, ($C = 1$) or ($1M$) for a 1-molar solution, ($m = 2.5$) for a 2.5-molal solution, and (aq) for a very dilute aqueous solution. Throughout this book molarity will be expressed in mol dm^{-3} and molality in mol kg^{-1}. A superscript $^\circ$ indicates that the reaction was performed under standard pressure conditions (1 atm).

EXAMPLE 3.1. To a first approximation, a flame can be considered to be an adiabatic, isobaric process in which the heat of reaction is used to heat the product gases to the flame temperature. What would be the maximum temperature of a hydrogen-air flame?

For the reaction

$$H_2(g) + \tfrac{1}{2}O_2(g) = H_2O(g)$$

there is 241.82 kJ released at 25 °C for each mole of H_2 burned. In the gaseous mixture of products, for every mole of $H_2O(g)$ there are 2 moles of $N_2(g)$ from the air mixture, giving

$$\begin{aligned} C_P^\circ &= C_P^\circ(H_2O, g) + 2C_P^\circ(N_2, g) \\ &= (4.184)(7.256 + 2.298\times10^{-3}T + 2.83\times10^{-7}T^2) + 2(4.184)(6.524 + 1.250\times10^{-3}T - 0.01\times10^{-7}T^2) \\ &= 84.952 + 2.0075\times10^{-2}T + 1.176\times10^{-6}T^2 \end{aligned}$$

where the factor 4.184 converts the heat capacity from cal K^{-1} to J K^{-1}. The ΔH° of reaction would be equal to the heat released by the cooling of the product gases from the flame temperature, T_f, to 25 °C; so

$$\Delta H^\circ \quad = \quad \int_{T_f}^{298\,\mathrm{K}} C_P^\circ \, dT$$

$$-241{,}820 \quad = \quad 84.952(298 - T_f) + \frac{1}{2}(2.0075 \times 10^{-2})(298^2 - T_f^2) + \frac{1}{3}(1.176 \times 10^{-6})(298^3 - T_f^3)$$

Rearranging gives

$$3.93 \times 10^{-7} T_f^3 + 1.0037 \times 10^{-2} T_f^2 + 84.952\, T_f \quad = \quad 268{,}030$$

and solving by (*1.12*) gives $T_f = 2440$ K or 2170 °C. The actual temperature would be somewhat lower because the system is not truly adiabatic and because of incomplete combustion. Commercial torches are capable of reaching temperatures near 2000 °C.

3.2 CALORIMETRY

Measurements of ΔH are usually performed under constant-pressure conditions using a solution calorimeter such as an insulated flask or beaker, a "thermos" bottle or Dewar flask, a styrofoam cup, etc. Measurements of ΔE are usually performed under constant-volume conditions using a bomb calorimeter. For generality in this section, the measurement of ΔQ where $\Delta Q = \Delta E$ or ΔH, depending on the conditions of the experiment, will be considered.

Because ΔQ is a state function under conditions of constant pressure or volume, any path may be chosen to measure its value. Consider a two-step path consisting of an adiabatic process

$$\text{(reactants \& calorimeter) at } T \quad = \quad \text{(products \& calorimeter) at } T'$$

and a second process in which the products and calorimeter are restored to the original temperature:

$$\text{(products \& calorimeter) at } T' \quad = \quad \text{(products \& calorimeter) at } T$$

The sum of the two processes generates the definition of the heat of reaction as given in Section 3.1, and ΔQ equals the sum of the ΔQ's for the two processes. This particular two-step process is convenient because ΔQ for the first step is zero and ΔQ for the second step can be easily measured or else calculated as

$$\Delta Q \quad = \quad \int_{T'}^{T} C_i(\text{products \& calorimeter})\, dT \qquad (3.1)$$

where C_i denotes C_V or C_P. In many cases, calorimeters are designed such that C_i(products & calorimeter) is equal to C_i(calorimeter), and C_i(calorimeter) is constant over reasonable temperature changes.

EXAMPLE 3.2. For the reaction $A = B$, carried out under isobaric conditions, a temperature change of −2.7 °C was observed for the calorimeter and products. To determine C_P(products & calorimeter), the electrical heating circuit shown in Fig. 3-1 was used. If $\mathcal{E} = 1.09$ V, $R_{\mathrm{cal}} = 100.0\ \Omega$ and $R_{\mathrm{ref}} = 10.0\ \Omega$ for the circuit and if the calorimeter and products were heated 1.00 °C by the heater in sixty seconds, find ΔH for the reaction.

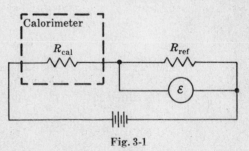

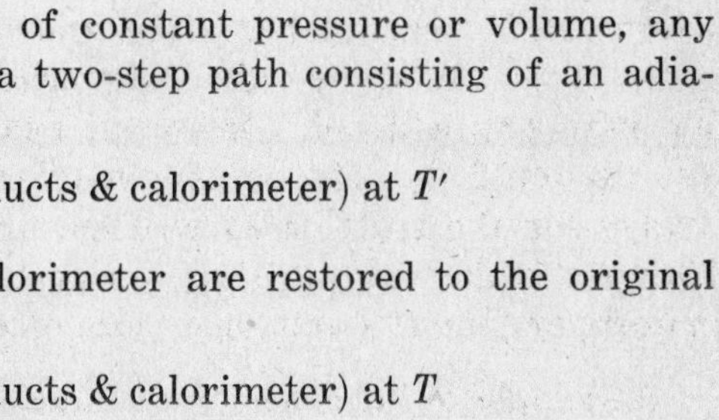

Fig. 3-1

The electrical work for the circuit is given by (*2.7c*) as

$$-w \quad = \quad \frac{R_{\mathrm{cal}}}{R_{\mathrm{ref}}^2} \int \mathcal{E}^2\, dt \quad = \quad \frac{100.0}{10.0^2}(1.09)^2(60.0) \quad = \quad 71.3 \text{ V s } \Omega^{-1} \quad = \quad 71.3 \text{ J}$$

The heat capacity of the system is given by

$$C_P(\text{products \& calorimeter}) = \frac{-w}{\Delta T} = \frac{71.3\ \text{J}}{1.00°} = 71.3\ \text{J K}^{-1}$$

Using (*3.1*) gives

$$\Delta H = \int (71.3\ \text{J K}^{-1})\, dT = (71.3)(2.7) = 192\ \text{J}$$

3.3 RELATION BETWEEN ΔE AND ΔH OF REACTION

As demonstrated in Problem 2.5 the term $\Delta(PV)$ in (*2.11*) can be neglected for condensed phases and, for gases, can be replaced by $RT\ \Delta n_g$, giving

$$\Delta H = \Delta E + RT\,\Delta n_g \tag{3.2}$$

where Δn_g is determined using the coefficients of the gaseous substances only.

EXAMPLE 3.3. What would be ΔH for the combustion of benzoic acid at 25 °C if $\Delta Q = -6316$ cal g^{-1} under isochoric conditions?

The value of ΔQ under isochoric conditions is ΔE, so for 1 mol of benzoic acid

$$\Delta E = (-6316\ \text{cal g}^{-1})(122.13\ \text{g mol}^{-1})(4.184\ \text{J cal}^{-1}) = -3.227\ \text{MJ mol}^{-1}$$

Thus, for the reaction

$$C_6H_5COOH(s) + \tfrac{15}{2}O_2(g) = 7CO_2(g) + 3H_2O(liq) \qquad \Delta E = -3.227\ \text{MJ}$$

the value of Δn_g is $7 - \frac{15}{2} = -\frac{1}{2}$ mol. Substituting into (*3.27*) gives

$$\Delta H = (-3.227\ \text{MJ}) + (8.314\ \text{J mol}^{-1}\ \text{K}^{-1})(298\ \text{K})(-\tfrac{1}{2}\ \text{mol})(10^{-6}\ \text{MJ J}^{-1}) = -3.228\ \text{MJ}$$

for the reaction, or $\Delta H(\text{combustion}) = -3.228$ MJ mol^{-1} for benzoic acid.

3.4 TEMPERATURE DEPENDENCE OF THE HEAT OF REACTION

The temperature dependence of ΔQ, where $\Delta Q = \Delta H$ or ΔE, is given by

$$d(\Delta Q) = (\Delta C_i)\, dT \tag{3.3}$$

where ΔC_i represents the sum of the heat capacities of the products less the sum of the heat capacities of the reactants.

If the heat capacity data are given in the form (*2.19*) and ΔH is known at 25 °C, then

$$\Delta H_T = \Delta H_{298} + (\Delta a)(T - 298) + \frac{1}{2}(\Delta b)(T^2 - 298^2) + \frac{1}{3}(\Delta c)(T^3 - 298^3) + \frac{1}{4}(\Delta d)(T^4 - 298^4) \tag{3.4a}$$

$$\Delta H_T = \Delta H_{298} + (\Delta a)(T - 298) + \frac{1}{2}(\Delta b)(T^2 - 298^2) - (\Delta c')(T^{-1} - 298^{-1}) \tag{3.4b}$$

If J and J' are defined as

$$J \equiv \Delta H_{298} - (\Delta a)(298) - \frac{1}{2}(\Delta b)(298^2) - \frac{1}{3}(\Delta c)(298^3) - \frac{1}{4}(\Delta d)(298^4) \tag{3.5a}$$

$$J' \equiv \Delta H_{298} - (\Delta a)(298) - \frac{1}{2}(\Delta b)(298^2) + (\Delta c')(298^{-1}) \tag{3.5b}$$

then (*3.4a*) and (*3.4b*) become

$$\Delta H_T = J + (\Delta a)T + \frac{1}{2}(\Delta b)T^2 + \frac{1}{3}(\Delta c)T^3 + \frac{1}{4}(\Delta d)T^4 \qquad (3.6a)$$

$$\Delta H_T = J' + (\Delta a)T + \frac{1}{2}(\Delta b)T^2 - (\Delta c')T^{-1} \qquad (3.6b)$$

The above equations are valid only for the temperature regions over which the heat capacity is correctly predicted by (*2.19*).

EXAMPLE 3.4. The heat of combustion of benzoic acid has been selected by the IUPAC as the standard for calibrating calorimeters. If the value of ΔH°_{273} is -771.2 kcal mol^{-1}, what is the value at 25 °C? For this small temperature interval, assume the heat capacities to be temperature-independent and equal to 8.87, 17.995 and 7.016 cal mol^{-1} K^{-1} for CO_2(g), H_2O(liq) and O_2(g), respectively, and equal to 0.287 cal g^{-1} K^{-1} for C_6H_5COOH(s).

For the reaction written in Example 3.3, ΔC°_P is given by

$$\Delta C^\circ_P = \Delta a = [7(8.87) + 3(17.995)] - [(0.287)(122.13) + \tfrac{15}{2}(7.016)]$$

$$= 28.4 \text{ cal K}^{-1} = 118.8 \text{ J K}^{-1}$$

Substituting into (*3.4*) gives

$$(-771.2 \text{ kcal})(4.184 \text{ kJ kcal}^{-1}) = \Delta H^\circ_{298} + (118.8 \text{ J K}^{-1})(293 \text{ K} - 298 \text{ K})$$

$$\Delta H^\circ_{298} = (-3226.7 + 0.6) \text{ kJ} = -3.2261 \text{ MJ}$$

for the reaction, or $\Delta H^\circ_{298} = -3.2261$ MJ mol^{-1}.

Calculations Involving Thermochemical Equations

3.5 LAW OF HESS

The law of Hess states that *the heat of reaction for a desired equation can be calculated by the algebraic combination of other thermochemical equations and their known heats of reaction.* Because the heat of reaction is a state function, the value calculated using the path consisting of the chosen series of thermochemical equations will be valid as long as the series of equations upon summation correctly predicts the reactants and products of the desired equation.

EXAMPLE 3.5. Combine the following thermochemical reactions

$$\text{S(rhombic)} + O_2(g) = SO_2(g) \qquad \Delta H^\circ_{298} = -70.944 \text{ kcal}$$

$$\text{S(monoclinic)} + O_2(g) = SO_2(g) \qquad \Delta H^\circ_{298} = -71.02 \text{ kcal}$$

to predict ΔH°_{298} for

$$\text{S(rhombic)} = \text{S(monoclinic)}$$

Subtracting the second equation from the first gives

$$[\text{S(rhombic)} + O_2(g)] - [\text{S(monoclinic)} + O_2(g)] = SO_2(g) - SO_2(g)$$

which can be rearranged to give the desired reaction, and so

$$\Delta H^\circ_{298} = -70.944 - (-71.02) = 80 \text{ cal} = 330 \text{ J}$$

3.6 HEAT OF FORMATION

The heat of reaction for the production of one mole of a compound from the elements in their naturally-occurring physical states is known as the *heat of formation* for the compound. The heat of formation for an element in its naturally-occurring physical state is zero.

If all thermochemical data to be used in predicting a heat of reaction for a desired equation are heats of formation, the law of Hess can be expressed as

$$\Delta H_T^\circ(\text{reaction}) = \sum_i^{\text{products}} n_i \Delta H_T^\circ(\text{formation}, i) - \sum_j^{\text{reactants}} n_j \Delta H_T^\circ(\text{formation}, j) \tag{3.7}$$

where n_i and n_j, the stoichiometric coefficients in the desired equation, have the units of mol.

EXAMPLE 3.6. One of the first steps in the refining of sulfide ores is the process of roasting, in which the ore is heated with oxygen to form the metal oxide and $SO_2(g)$. Calculate ΔH_{298}° for the roasting of sphalerite, ZnS, if the heats of formation of sphalerite, ZnO(s) and $SO_2(g)$ are −49.23, −83.24 and −70.994 kcal mol^{-1}, respectively, at 25 °C.

The desired equation is

$$\text{ZnS(sphalerite)} + \tfrac{3}{2}O_2(g) = \text{ZnO(s)} + SO_2(g)$$

and substituting the data into (*3.7*) gives

$$\begin{aligned}\Delta H_{298}^\circ &= [(1)\Delta H_{298}^\circ(\text{formation, ZnO}) + (1)\Delta H_{298}^\circ(\text{formation}, SO_2)] \\ &\qquad - [(1)\Delta H_{298}^\circ(\text{formation, ZnS}) + \tfrac{3}{2}\Delta H_{298}^\circ(\text{formation}, O_2)] \\ &= [(1)(-83.24) + (1)(-70.994)] - [(1)(-49.23) + \tfrac{3}{2}(0)] \\ &= (-105.00\ \text{kcal})(4.184\ \text{kJ kcal}^{-1}) = -439.32\ \text{kJ}\end{aligned}$$

3.7 HEAT OF COMBUSTION

The heat of reaction for the oxidation of one mole of a compound is known as the *heat of combustion.* If the substance contains C, H, O and/or N, the products of the oxidation at 25 °C are $CO_2(g)$, $H_2O(liq)$ and/or $N_2(g)$. Writing balanced equations for substances containing other elements, such as the halogens or sulfur, is difficult because a mixture of products usually occurs.

If all thermochemical data to be used in predicting a heat of reaction for a desired equation are heats of combustion, the law of Hess can be expressed as

$$\Delta H_T^\circ(\text{reaction}) = -\sum_i^{\text{products}} n_i \Delta H_T^\circ(\text{combustion}, i) + \sum_j^{\text{reactants}} n_j \Delta H_T^\circ(\text{combustion}, j) \tag{3.8}$$

where n_i and n_j, the stoichiometric coefficients in the desired equation, have the units of mol.

EXAMPLE 3.7. Predict ΔH_{298}° for the reaction

$$n\text{-}C_6H_{14}(liq) + CH_4(g) = n\text{-}C_7H_{16}(liq) + H_2(g)$$

if the heats of combustion are −989.8, −210.8, −1149.9 and −68.38 kcal mol^{-1} for n-C_6H_{14}, CH_4, n-C_7H_{16} and H_2, respectively, at 25 °C.

Applying (*3.8*) to the desired reaction gives

$$\begin{aligned}\Delta H_{298}^\circ &= -[(1)\Delta H_{298}^\circ(\text{combustion}, n\text{-}C_7H_{16}) + (1)\Delta H_{298}^\circ(\text{combustion}, H_2)] \\ &\qquad + [(1)\Delta H_{298}^\circ(\text{combustion}, n\text{-}C_6H_{14}) + (1)\Delta H_{298}^\circ(\text{combustion}, CH_4)] \\ &= -[(1)(-1149.9) + (1)(-68.38)] + [(1)(-989.8) + (1)(-210.8)] \\ &= (17.7\ \text{kcal})(4.184\ \text{kJ kcal}^{-1}) = 74.1\ \text{kJ}\end{aligned}$$

3.8 HEAT OF NEUTRALIZATION

The heat of reaction for the neutralization of an acid by a base is known as the *heat of neutralization.*

EXAMPLE 3.8. For the reaction between a strong acid and a strong base, i.e. those that are essentially 100% ionized or dissociated, the neutralization equation is essentially

$$H^+(aq) + OH^-(aq) = H_2O(liq)$$

If the heats of formation at 25 °C are −68.3171, 0 and −54.957 kcal mol^{-1} for H_2O, H^+ and OH^-, respectively, calculate the heat of neutralization for strong acids with strong bases.

Using (*3.7*) gives

$$\begin{aligned}\Delta H^\circ_{298}(\text{neutralization}) &= [(1)(-68.3171)] - [(1)(0) + (1)(-54.957)] \\ &= (-13.360\ \text{kcal})(4.184\ \text{kJ kcal}^{-1}) = -55.898\ \text{kJ}\end{aligned}$$

EXAMPLE 3.9. Consider the titration of a weak acid, such as HCN, with a strong base, such as NaOH:

$$HCN(aq) + NaOH(aq) = NaCN(aq) + H_2O(liq)$$

If the heats of formation are −68.3174, −21.2, −112.236 and 25.2 kcal mol^{-1} at 25 °C for H_2O, NaCN, NaOH and HCN, respectively, calculate ΔH°_{298}(neutralization). Account for the difference from −55.898 kJ mol^{-1} as found for the strong acid-strong base case.

Substituting the data into (*3.7*) gives

$$\begin{aligned}\Delta H^\circ_{298}(\text{neutralization}) &= [(1)(-68.3174) + (1)(-21.2)] - [(1)(-112.236) + (1)(25.2)] \\ &= (-2.5\ \text{kcal})(4.184\ \text{kJ kcal}^{-1}) = -10.5\ \text{kJ}\end{aligned}$$

Because HCN is a weak acid, the titration reaction may be considered to be the sum of two steps:

$$HCN(aq) = H^+(aq) + CN^-(aq) \qquad \Delta H^\circ_{298}(\text{ionization})$$

$$H^+(aq) + CN^-(aq) + NaOH(aq) = NaCN(aq) + H_2O(liq) \qquad \Delta H^\circ_{298} = -55.898\ \text{kJ}$$

where the ionization process required

$$\Delta H^\circ_{298}(\text{ionization}) = (-10.5) - (-55.898) = 45.4\ \text{kJ}$$

3.9 HEAT OF SOLUTION

The heat of reaction for dissolving one mole of solute in n moles of solvent is known as the (*integral*) *heat of solution.* For a gaseous solute, ΔH°(solution) is the result of the solvation of the solute molecules. For a solid molecular solute, the solution process can be considered to be the sum of two processes:

$$\text{solute(s)} = \text{solute(molecules)} \qquad \Delta H^\circ_T(\text{sublimation})$$

$$\text{solute(molecules)} + \text{solvent} = \text{solution} \qquad \Delta H^\circ_T(\text{solvation})$$

giving

$$\text{solute(s)} + \text{solvent} = \text{solution} \qquad \Delta H^\circ_T(\text{solution}) = \Delta H^\circ_T(\text{sublimation}) + \Delta H^\circ_T(\text{solvation})$$

For a solid ionic solute, similar equations can be written involving lattice energy, Coulombic attractions, etc.

For solutions that are very dilute, heats of formation of the aqueous ions can be used to predict heats of reaction. The ΔH°_{298}(formation) of H^+(aq) is assumed to be zero so that individual ionic values may be defined relative to it.

EXAMPLE 3.10. From the following set of ΔH°_{298}(formation, HNO_3 in n H_2O) data, calculate the values of ΔH°_{298}(solution) for HNO_3(liq) as a function of concentration and determine ΔH°_{298}(formation) for the nitrate ion at infinite dilution.

moles H_2O	pure HNO_3(liq)	1	2	3	4	5	7
ΔH°_{298}(formation), kcal mol^{-1}	−41.61	−44.845	−46.500	−47.459	−48.065	−48.462	−48.899
moles H_2O	10	15	25	50	100	500	1000
ΔH°_{298}(formation)	−49.192	−49.357	−49.430	−49.439	−49.440	−49.468	−49.484
moles H_2O	2000	5000	10,000	50,000	∞		
ΔH°_{298}(formation)	−49.501	−49.518	−49.529	−49.545	−49.56		

The values of ΔH°_{298}(solution) corresponding to the equation

$$HNO_3(\text{liq}) + nH_2O(\text{solvent}) = HNO_3(\text{in } n\ H_2O)$$

can be calculated by substituting the above data into (*3.7*), e.g.

$$\begin{aligned}\Delta H^\circ_{298}(\text{solution, } HNO_3 \text{ in } 100\ H_2O) &= [(1)\Delta H^\circ_{298}(\text{formation, } HNO_3 \text{ in } 100\ H_2O)] \\ &\quad - [(1)\Delta H^\circ_{298}(\text{formation, } HNO_3)] \\ &= (-49.440) - (-41.61) = -7.83 \text{ kcal}\end{aligned}$$

A plot of these values, Fig. 3-2, shows the trend of ΔH°_{298}(solution) with concentration. The ΔH°_{298}(formation, NO_3^-, ∞ dil) is

$$\begin{aligned}\Delta H^\circ_{298}(\text{solution, } HNO_3 \text{ in } \infty\ H_2O) &= (1)\Delta H^\circ_{298}(\text{formation, } H^+, \infty \text{ dil}) + (1)\Delta H^\circ_{298}(\text{formation, } NO_3^-, \infty \text{ dil}) \\ -49.56 &= (1)(0) + (1)\Delta H^\circ_{298}(\text{formation, } NO_3^-, \infty \text{ dil}) \\ \Delta H^\circ_{298}(\text{formation, } NO_3^-, \infty \text{ dil}) &= -49.56 \text{ kcal mol}^{-1} = -207.36 \text{ kJ mol}^{-1}\end{aligned}$$

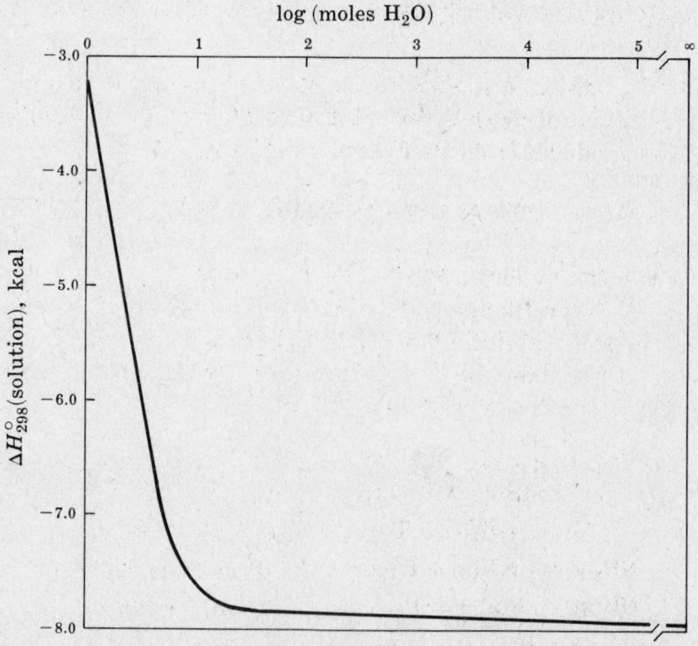

Fig. 3-2

EXAMPLE 3.11. If the heats of formation at 25 °C are 25.23, −49.56, −39.952 and −30.370 kcal mol^{-1} for Ag^+(∞ dil), NO_3^-(∞ dil), Cl^-(∞ dil) and AgCl(s), respectively, calculate the heat of reaction for

$$AgNO_3(aq) + HCl(aq) = AgCl(s) + HNO_3(aq)$$

Substituting the data into (*3.7*) gives

$$\begin{aligned}\Delta H^\circ_{298}(\text{reaction}) &= [(1)\Delta H^\circ_{298}(\text{formation, AgCl, s}) + (1)\Delta H^\circ_{298}(\text{formation, } H^+, \infty \text{ dil}) \\ &\quad + (1)\Delta H^\circ_{298}(\text{formation, } NO_3^-, \infty \text{ dil})] - [(1)\Delta H^\circ_{298}(\text{formation, } Ag^+, \infty \text{ dil}) \\ &\quad + (1)\Delta H^\circ_{298}(\text{formation, } NO_3^-, \infty \text{ dil}) + (1)\Delta H^\circ_{298}(\text{formation, } H^+, \infty \text{ dil}) \\ &\quad + (1)\Delta H^\circ_{298}(\text{formation, } Cl^-, \infty \text{ dil})] \\ &= (-30.370) - [(1)(25.23) + (1)(-39.952)] \\ &= -15.65 \text{ kcal} = -65.48 \text{ kJ}\end{aligned}$$

3.10 HEAT OF DILUTION

The heat of reaction for diluting one mole of solute in a solution of given concentration, by adding solvent to produce a solution of different concentration, is known as the (*integral*) *heat of dilution.*

EXAMPLE 3.12. What is ΔH°_{298}(dilution) for diluting a solution containing one mole of $AgNO_3$ in 100 moles of water by adding 400 moles of water? The heats of formation are −24.637 and −24.362 kcal mol^{-1} for the solutions consisting of 100 and 500 moles of water, respectively, added to one mole of $AgNO_3$ at 25 °C.

Using (*3.7*) gives

$$\begin{aligned}\Delta H^\circ_{298}(\text{dilution}) &= (1)\Delta H^\circ_{298}(\text{solution, } AgNO_3 \text{ in 500 } H_2O) - (1)\Delta H^\circ_{298}(\text{solution, } AgNO_3 \text{ in 100 } H_2O) \\ &= (1)(-24.362) - (1)(-24.637) = 275 \text{ cal} = 1.15 \text{ kJ}\end{aligned}$$

3.11 BOND ENERGY

The heat of reaction resulting from the breaking of a chemical bond in a gaseous molecule to form the respective gaseous molecular fragments is known as the *bond* (*dissociation*) *energy* (more correctly, *enthalpy*). The chemical environment of a given atom will influence the value of the bond energy, so values found in tables usually represent averages over several compounds.

Bond energies can be used to calculate the heats of reaction by assuming the reaction to consist of two steps: (1) the decomposition of the reactants into molecular fragments and (2) the formation of the products from the fragments. Thus

$$\Delta H^\circ_T(\text{reaction}) = -\sum_i^{\text{products}} n_i \,\text{BE}_i + \sum_j^{\text{reactants}} n_j \,\text{BE}_j \tag{3.9}$$

where BE represents the bond energy and n_i and n_j represent the number of moles of bonds involved in the reaction. Even though bond energies pertain to gaseous reactions, they are often used to predict heats of reaction for condensed reactions by combining heats of vaporization, sublimation, etc., or without further corrections if a cruder approximation will suffice or if the vaporization, etc., data are unknown.

EXAMPLE 3.13. The stepwise decomposition of NH_3(g) and the heats of reaction are given below. From these data, calculate the average bond energy, $\overline{\text{BE}}_{\text{N-H}}$.

$$\begin{aligned} NH_3(g) &= NH_2(g) + H(g) \qquad & \Delta H^\circ_{298} &= 104 \text{ kcal} \\ NH_2(g) &= NH(g) + H(g) & \Delta H^\circ_{298} &= 90 \text{ kcal} \\ NH(g) &= N(g) + H(g) & \Delta H^\circ_{298} &= 85 \text{ kcal}\end{aligned}$$

Adding the three reactions and enthalpies gives

$$NH_3(g) = N(g) + 3H(g) \qquad \Delta H^\circ_{298} = 279 \text{ kcal} = 1167 \text{ kJ}$$

so the average value for one bond would be

$$\overline{\text{BE}}_{\text{N-H}} = \frac{\Delta H^\circ_{298}}{3\ \text{mol}} = 389\ \text{kJ mol}^{-1}$$

EXAMPLE 3.14. Predict the heat of reaction for the oxidation of CH_3OH(liq) if the average bond energy at 25 °C for C—H is 415.9 kJ mol^{-1}, 463.6 for O—H, 327.2 for C—O, 804.2 for C═O and 498.3 for O═O and if the enthalpy of vaporization at 25 °C is 37.99 kJ mol^{-1} for CH_3OH and 44.011 for H_2O.

The desired reaction is

$$CH_3OH(\text{liq}) + \tfrac{3}{2}O_2(g) = CO_2(g) + 2H_2O(\text{liq})$$

which can be obtained from the following reactions:

$$CH_3OH(\text{liq}) = CH_3OH(g) \qquad \Delta H^\circ_{298} = 37.99\ \text{kJ}$$

$$H_2O(\text{liq}) = H_2O(g) \qquad \Delta H^\circ_{298} = 44.011\ \text{kJ}$$

$$CH_3OH(g) + \tfrac{3}{2}O_2(g) = CO_2(g) + 2H_2O(g)$$

where ΔH°_{298}(reaction) for the third reaction is calculated from (*3.9*) as

$$\Delta H^\circ_{298}(\text{reaction}) = -[(2)(804.2) + (4)(463.6)] + [(3)(415.9) + (1)(327.2) + (1)(463.6) + \tfrac{3}{2}(498.3)] = -676.9\ \text{kJ}$$

Applying the law of Hess,

$$\Delta H^\circ_{298}(\text{combustion}) = (-676.9) - 2(44.011) + (37.99) = -726.9\ \text{kJ}$$

This value differs from the actual value at 25 °C, −726.47 kJ, by 0.06%.

Physical Changes

3.12 STATES OF MATTER

Figure 3-3 is a diagram of the various states of matter and the corresponding phase changes. For clarity, not all the phase changes involving the lower-energy crystalline forms are shown, e.g. β-solid to liquid, α-solid to gas, α-solid to γ-solid. Because the glassy state is not a true equilibrium thermodynamic state, it has been represented by a dashed box.

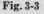

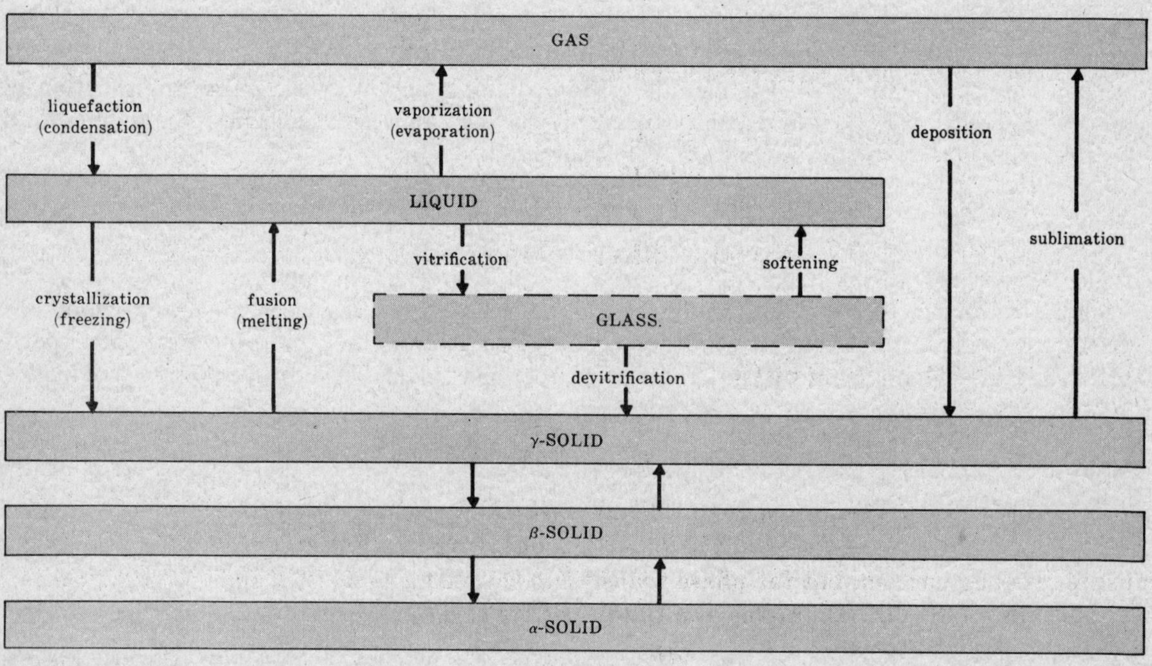

Fig. 3-3

To each phase transition there corresponds an energy change, e.g. s → liq, ΔH_T°(fusion); liq → s, ΔH_T°(crystallization); s → gas, ΔH_T°(sublimation); liq → gas, ΔH_T°(vaporization). Because of the conservation of energy, $\Delta H_T^\circ(\text{fusion}) = -\Delta H_T^\circ(\text{crystallization})$, etc.

3.13 APPROXIMATE VALUES OF HEATS OF TRANSITION

For substances which are not highly associated in the liquid state, e.g. H-bonding or dimer formation is not present, the following approximate relationship has been observed:

$$\Delta H_T^\circ(\text{vaporization}) \cong (88\ \text{J K}^{-1}\ \text{mol}^{-1})T_{bp} \qquad (3.10)$$

where T_{bp} is the normal boiling point of the liquid. For elements,

$$\Delta H_T^\circ(\text{fusion}) \cong (9.2\ \text{J K}^{-1}\ \text{mol}^{-1})T_{mp} \qquad (3.11)$$

where T_{mp} is the melting point of the solid.

EXAMPLE 3.15. If the boiling point of CCl_4 is 76.7 °C, give an estimate for the heat of vaporization.

Trouton's rule, (*3.10*), gives

$$\Delta H_{349.9}^\circ(\text{vaporization}) = 88T_{bp} = (88\ \text{J K}^{-1}\ \text{mol}^{-1})(349.9\ \text{K}) = 30.8\ \text{kJ mol}^{-1}$$

The accepted value is 30.00 kJ mol^{-1}.

3.14 ENTHALPY OF HEATING

The enthalpy change in changing the temperature of a substance is given by

$$\Delta H^\circ = \sum_i^{\text{phases}} \int C_{P,i}^\circ\, dT + \sum_j^{\text{transitions}} \Delta H_T^\circ(\text{transition}, j) \qquad (3.12)$$

EXAMPLE 3.16. What is the enthalpy change for heating one mole of ice from −5 °C to steam at 105 °C? Assume $C_P = 37.7\ \text{J mol}^{-1}\ \text{K}^{-1}$ for ice and steam, $C_P = 75.3\ \text{mol}^{-1}\ \text{K}^{-1}$ for water, $\Delta H^\circ(\text{vaporization}) = 9.717\ \text{kcal mol}^{-1}$ at 100 °C and $\Delta H^\circ(\text{fusion}) = 1.436\ \text{kcal mol}^{-1}$ at 0 °C.

The desired process can be represented as a series of five steps, as illustrated in Fig. 3-4, for which (*3.12*) becomes

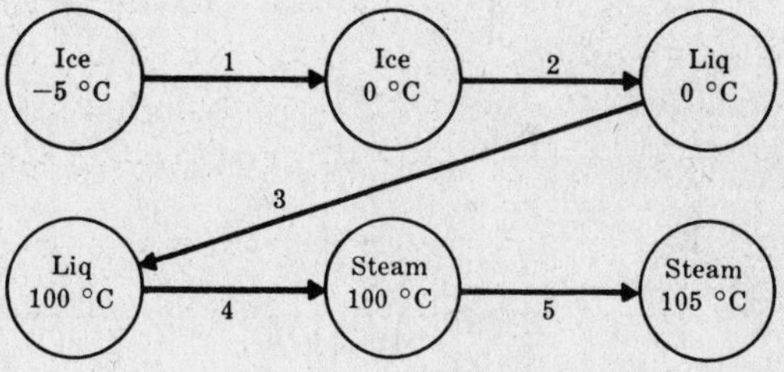

Fig. 3-4

$$\begin{aligned}\Delta H^\circ &= \Delta H^\circ(1) + \Delta H^\circ(2) + \Delta H^\circ(3) + \Delta H^\circ(4) + \Delta H^\circ(5)\\ &= \int_{268\,\text{K}}^{273\,\text{K}} C_P^\circ\, dT + \Delta H_{273}^\circ(\text{fusion}) + \int_{273\,\text{K}}^{373\,\text{K}} C_P^\circ\, dT + \Delta H_{373}^\circ(\text{vaporization}) + \int_{373\,\text{K}}^{378\,\text{K}} C_P^\circ\, dT\\ &= (37.7)(273-268) + (1436)(4.184) + (75.3)(373-273) + (9717)(4.184) + (37.7)(378-373)\\ &= 54.57\ \text{kJ mol}^{-1}\end{aligned}$$

3.15 CLAPEYRON EQUATION

For a phase change

$$\frac{dP}{dT} = \frac{\Delta H}{T\Delta V} \qquad (3.13)$$

where ΔH is the enthalpy change for the transition and ΔV is the corresponding volume change. If the phase change involves only condensed phases, (*3.13*), the *Clapeyron equation*, must be used as written; but for phase transitions between a condensed phase and a gas, ΔV is essentially $V_{gas} = RT/P$, giving the *Clausius-Clapeyron equation*

$$\frac{dP}{dT} = (\Delta H)\frac{P}{RT^2} \qquad (3.14)$$

EXAMPLE 3.17. Determine the heat of vaporization at 25 °C for water from the following vapor pressure data:

T, °C	20	21	22	23	24	25	26	27	28	29	30
P, torr	17.535	18.650	19.827	21.068	22.377	23.756	25.209	26.739	28.349	30.043	31.824

For small temperature intervals ΔH is temperature-independent and (*3.14*) can be written as

$$\frac{dP}{P} = \left(\frac{\Delta H}{R}\right)\frac{dT}{T^2}$$

which upon integration gives

$$\ln P = \left(\frac{-\Delta H}{R}\right)\frac{1}{T} + k \tag{3.15a}$$

Evaluation of the constant in (*3.15a*) for two sets of pressure-temperature data gives

$$\ln\frac{P_2}{P_1} = \left(\frac{-\Delta H}{R}\right)\left(\frac{1}{T_2} - \frac{1}{T_1}\right) \tag{3.15b}$$

The form of (*3.15a*) is such as to suggest that a plot of $\ln P$ against $1/T$ will give a straight line whose slope will be $-\Delta H/R$, see Fig. 3-5. From Fig. 3-5 the slope at 25 °C is -5.26×10^3 K, so

$$\Delta H^\circ_{298}(\text{vaporization}) = -(8.314 \text{ J mol}^{-1} \text{ K}^{-1})(-5.26 \times 10^3 \text{ K}) = 43.73 \text{ kJ mol}^{-1}$$

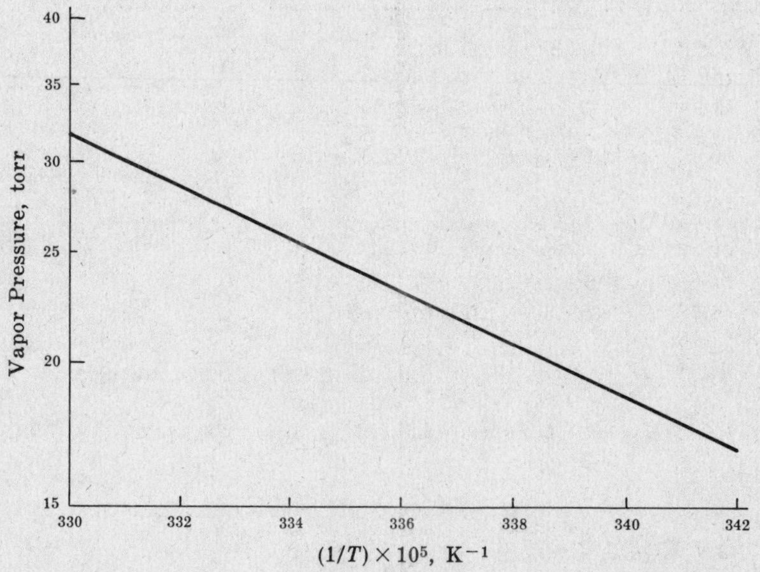

Fig. 3-5

EXAMPLE 3.18. If the density of ice is 0.917×10^3 kg m^{-3} and of water is 0.9998×10^3 kg m^{-3}, express the dependence of the melting point on the pressure. Assume ΔH°(fusion) to be pressure-independent and equal to 6.0095 kJ mol^{-1}. At what pressure will ice melt at -1.0 °C?

Rearranging (*3.13*) gives

$$\frac{dT}{T} = \left(\frac{\Delta V}{\Delta H}\right) dP$$

and integration gives

$$\ln \frac{T_2}{T_1} = \left(\frac{\Delta V}{\Delta H}\right)(P_2 - P_1)$$

Substituting the data gives

$$\ln \frac{272.15}{273.15} = \frac{\left(\dfrac{18.015 \times 10^{-3}}{0.9998 \times 10^{3}} - \dfrac{18.015 \times 10^{-3}}{0.917 \times 10^{3}}\right) \text{m}^3\ \text{mol}^{-1}\ (P_2 - 1)\ \text{atm}}{(6009.5\ \text{J mol}^{-1})(101{,}325\ \text{J m}^{-3}\ \text{atm}^{-1})^{-1}}$$

$$-0.0037 = -2.74 \times 10^{-5}(P_2 - 1)$$

$$P_2 = 135\ \text{atm}$$

3.16 HEAT OF FORMATION DIAGRAM

If the heats of formation for a compound in its various physical states are plotted as a function of temperature, a heat of formation diagram is generated from which it is possible to graphically determine various thermal properties.

EXAMPLE 3.19. Prepare a heat of formation diagram for LiI using the data below (JANAF Thermochemical Tables):

normal melting point: 742 K

normal boiling point: 1449 K

T, K	ΔH_T°(formation, s), kcal mol^{-1}	ΔH_T°(formation, liq), kcal mol^{-1}	ΔH_T°(formation, g), kcal mol^{-1}
0			−21.290
100			−21.077
200			−21.368
298	−64.550	−61.749	−21.750
300	−64.551	−61.744	−21.758
400	−66.527	−63.441	−24.122
500	−72.399	−69.111	−30.437
600	−72.192	−68.762	−30.721
700	−71.898	−68.402	−30.984
800	−71.508	−68.034	−31.234
900	−71.028	−67.667	−31.480
1000	−70.478	−67.300	−31.721
1100	−69.880	−66.931	−31.958
1200	−69.252	−66.564	−32.194
1300	−68.600	−66.194	−32.424
1400	−67.934	−65.825	−32.653
1500	−67.255	−65.455	−32.877

Find the heat of sublimation at 298 K if a vertical line between the solid and gas lines represents this quantity. Account for the three discontinuities at about 450 K.

The data are plotted in Fig. 3-6. The dashed vertical line at 298 K intersects the solid and gas curves at −64.55 and −21.75 kcal, giving ΔH_{298}°(sublimation) $= 42.80$ kcal mol^{-1} $= 179.08$ kJ mol^{-1}. At 450 K, the reactant Li undergoes a phase change from the solid to the liquid state and the discontinuity corresponds to the heat of fusion (about 750 cal mol^{-1} $= 3100$ J mol^{-1}).

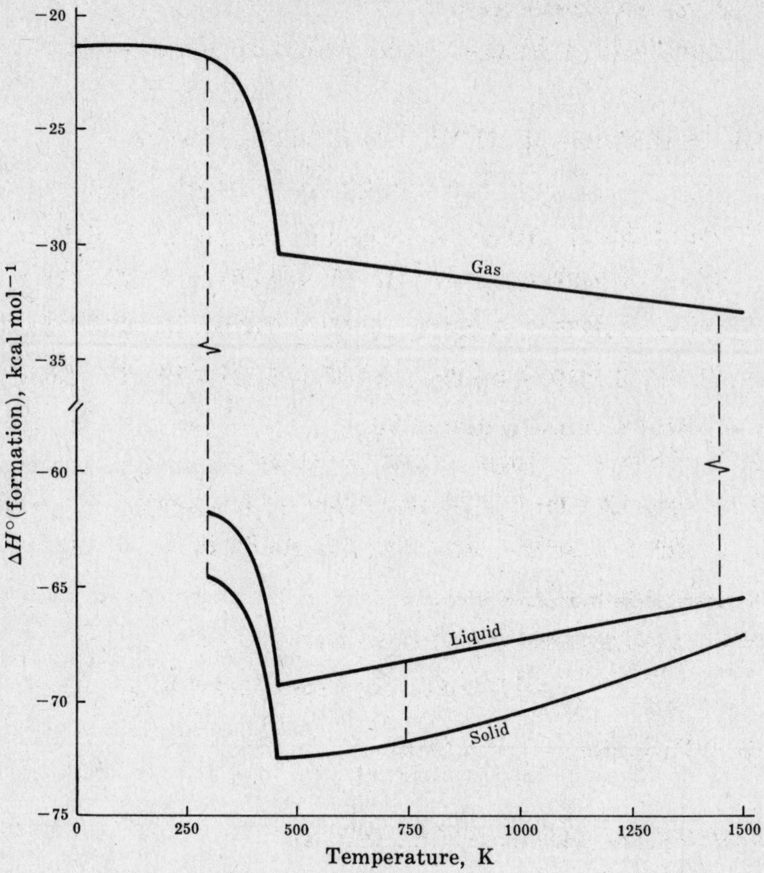

Fig. 3-6

Solved Problems

Heat of Reaction

3.1. A bomb calorimeter was constructed so that the contribution of the reaction products to the heat capacity is negligible. To calibrate this calorimeter, a 1.320-g sample of benzoic acid was oxidized, giving a temperature change of 5.88 °C. If ΔE°_{298} for the oxidation of benzoic acid is −6316 cal g^{-1}, calculate C_V(calorimeter).

For the combustion,

$$\Delta E^\circ_{298} = (1.320 \text{ g})(-6316 \text{ cal g}^{-1})(4.184 \text{ J cal}^{-1}) = -34.88 \text{ kJ}$$

Assuming the calorimeter constant to be temperature-independent, (*3.1*) becomes

$$34.88 \text{ kJ} = \int C_V(\text{calorimeter})\, dT = C_V(\text{calorimeter})\, \Delta T$$

whence

$$C_V(\text{calorimeter}) = \frac{34.88 \text{ kJ}}{5.88^\circ} = 5932 \text{ J K}^{-1}$$

3.2. Calculate $(\Delta H^\circ - \Delta E^\circ)$ for the reaction between glycine and nitrous acid:

$$NH_2\text{—}CH_2\text{—}COOH(aq) + HONO(aq) \overset{25\,^\circ C}{=} HO\text{—}CH_2\text{—}COOH(aq) + N_2(g) + H_2O(liq)$$

Using (*3.2*) for this reaction gives

$$\Delta H^\circ - \Delta E^\circ = RT\,\Delta n_g = (8.314\ \text{J mol}^{-1}\ \text{K}^{-1})(298\ \text{K})(1\ \text{mol}) = 2478\ \text{J}$$

3.3. What would be the value of ΔH° at 1000 K for the reaction

$$H_2(g) + Cl_2(g) = 2HCl(g)$$

if $\Delta H^\circ_{298} = -44.124$ kcal? Assume that the heat capacities are given in cal mol^{-1} K^{-1} by

$$C^\circ_P = 6.9469 - 0.1999\times10^{-3}T + 4.808\times10^{-7}T^2 \quad \text{for } H_2(g)$$

$$C^\circ_P = 7.5755 + 2.4244\times10^{-3}T - 9.650\times10^{-7}T^2 \quad \text{for } Cl_2(g)$$

$$C^\circ_P = 6.7319 + 0.4325\times10^{-3}T + 3.697\times10^{-7}T^2 \quad \text{for } HCl(g)$$

Using the given heat-capacity information,

$$\Delta a = 2(6.7319) - [6.9469 + 7.5755] = 1.0586$$

$$\Delta b = 2(0.4325\times10^{-3}) - [-0.1999\times10^{-3} + 2.4244\times10^{-3}] = -1.3595\times10^{-3}$$

$$\Delta c = 2(3.697\times10^{-7}) - [4.808\times10^{-7} + -9.650\times10^{-7}] = 12.236\times10^{-7}$$

which upon substitution into (*3.4a*) gives

$$\Delta H^\circ_{1000} = -44.124 + (1.0586\times10^{-3})(1000-298) + \frac{1}{2}(-1.3595\times10^{-6})(1000^2-298^2) + \frac{1}{3}(12.236\times10^{-10})(1000^3-298^3)$$

$$= -43.603\ \text{kcal} = -182.435\ \text{kJ}$$

Calculations Involving Thermochemical Equations

3.4. Using the following data

$$Fe(s) + \tfrac{1}{2}O_2(g) = FeO(s) \qquad \Delta H^\circ_{298} = -65.0\ \text{kcal}$$

$$2Fe(s) + \tfrac{3}{2}O_2(g) = Fe_2O_3(\text{hematite}) \qquad \Delta H^\circ_{298} = -197.0\ \text{kcal}$$

predict ΔH°_{298} for the reaction

$$2FeO(s) + \tfrac{1}{2}O_2(g) = Fe_2O_3(\text{hematite})$$

Subtracting two-times the first equation from the second gives

$$[2Fe(s) + \tfrac{3}{2}O_2(g)] - 2[Fe(s) + \tfrac{1}{2}O_2(g)] = Fe_2O_3(\text{hematite}) - 2FeO(s)$$

which upon combining terms and rearranging generates the desired reaction. Therefore

$$\Delta H^\circ_{298} = -197.0 - 2(-65.0) = -67.0\ \text{kcal} = -280.3\ \text{kJ}$$

3.5. Using the following data

$$Li(liq) + \tfrac{1}{2}Cl_2(g) = LiCl(liq) \qquad \Delta H^\circ_{883} = -92.374\ \text{kcal}$$

$$Li(liq) + \tfrac{1}{2}Cl_2(g) = LiCl(s) \qquad \Delta H^\circ_{883} = -97.105\ \text{kcal}$$

predict the heat of fusion for LiCl at 883 K.

For the reaction $LiCl(s) = LiCl(liq)$, (*3.7*) gives

$$\Delta H^\circ_{883} = (1)(-92.374) - (1)(-97.105) = 4.731\ \text{kcal} = 19.795\ \text{kJ}$$

3.6. Calculate the heat of reaction for the process

$$C_2H_4(g) + HCl(g) = C_2H_5Cl(g)$$

given that the heats of formation of C_2H_5Cl, HCl and C_2H_4 are −26.81, −22.062 and 12.49 kcal mol^{-1}, respectively, at 25 °C.

For the reaction written above, (*3.7*) gives

$$\Delta H^\circ_{298} = (1)(-26.81) - [(1)(12.49) + (1)(-22.062)] = -17.24 \text{ kcal} = -72.13 \text{ kJ}$$

3.7. In the formation of stalagmites and stalactites, aragonite undergoes the following reaction with a very dilute solution of carbonic acid (carbon dioxide dissolved in water):

$$CaCO_3(\text{aragonite}) + H_2CO_3(\text{aq}) = Ca(HCO_3)_2(\text{aq})$$

If the heats of formation at 25 °C are −288.49, −167.0, −129.77 and −165.18 kcal mol^{-1} for $CaCO_3$, H_2CO_3, Ca^{++} and HCO_3^-, respectively, calculate ΔH°_{298}(reaction).

Applying (*3.7*) to the reaction gives

$$\Delta H^\circ_{298} = [(1)(-129.77) + (2)(-165.18)] - [(1)(-288.49) + (1)(-167.0)]$$

$$= -4.6 \text{ kcal} = -19.2 \text{ kJ}$$

3.8. Commercial concentrated sulfuric acid is 17.8 *M*, or 0.287 moles H_2O for each mole of H_2SO_4. If this acid is diluted to 6*N* (16.3 moles H_2O for each mole of H_2SO_4), what is ΔH°_{298}(dilution), if the heats of formation of the dilute and concentrated solutions are −211 and −195 kcal mol^{-1} at 25 °C, respectively? Assuming the dilution to be an adiabatic process such that the heat of dilution raises the final solution from 25 °C to a higher temperature, find this final temperature if one mole of H_2SO_4 is contained in 400 g of final solution and the specific heat is assumed to be 4.2 kJ kg^{-1} K^{-1}.

The heat of dilution is

$$\Delta H^\circ_{298}(\text{dilution}) = (1)(-211) - (1)(-195) = -16 \text{ kcal} = -67 \text{ kJ}$$

which upon changing sign and substitution into (*2.18*) gives

$$67 \text{ kJ} = (0.400 \text{ kg})(4.2 \text{ kJ kg}^{-1}\text{ K}^{-1})(T_f - 25\ ^\circ\text{C}) \quad \text{or} \quad T_f = 65\ ^\circ\text{C}$$

3.9. Consider the formation of gaseous methanol from the gaseous molecular fragments:

$$C(g) + 4H(g) + O(g) = CH_3OH(g)$$

If the enthalpy of formation at 25 °C for $CH_3OH(g)$ is −47.96 kcal mol^{-1}, 171.291 for C(g), 52.095 for H and 59.553 for O(g), and if the average bond energy at 25 °C for C—H is 415.9 kJ mol^{-1} and 463.6 for O—H, calculate the bond energy for C—O.

Substituting the data into (*3.7*) and (*3.9*) gives

$$\Delta H^\circ_{298}(\text{reaction}) = [(1)(-47.96)] - [(1)(171.291) + (4)(52.095) + (1)(59.553)]$$

$$= -487.18 \text{ kcal} = -2038.36 \text{ kJ}$$

and

$$-2038.36 = -[(3)(415.9) + (1)(463.6) + (1)BE_{C-O}] + [0]$$

$$BE_{C-O} = 327.1 \text{ kJ mol}^{-1}$$

3.10. Predict the heat of reaction for

$$CH_4(g) + 4F_2(g) = CF_4(g) + 4HF(g)$$

from the bond energies 415.9 kJ mol^{-1} for C—H, 159.0 for F—F, 566.1 for H—F and 490.0 for C—F at 25 °C.

Application of (*3.9*) to the desired reaction gives

$$\Delta H^\circ_{298} = -[(4)(490.0) + (4)(566.1)] + [(4)(415.9) + (4)(159.0)] = -1925 \text{ kJ}$$

Physical Changes

3.11. From the following set of data, calculate ΔH° for heating one mole of Fe from 298 K to 3200 K:

$$\Delta H^\circ(\alpha\text{-solid} \rightarrow \beta\text{-solid}) = 0.0 \text{ kcal mol}^{-1} \text{ at } 1033 \text{ K}$$

$$\Delta H^\circ(\beta\text{-solid} \rightarrow \gamma\text{-solid}) = 0.215 \text{ kcal mol}^{-1} \text{ at } 1183 \text{ K}$$

$$\Delta H^\circ(\gamma\text{-solid} \rightarrow \delta\text{-solid}) = 0.165 \text{ kcal mol}^{-1} \text{ at } 1673 \text{ K}$$

$$\Delta H^\circ(\delta\text{-solid} \rightarrow \text{liq}) = 3.67 \text{ kcal mol}^{-1} \text{ at } 1812 \text{ K}$$

$$\Delta H^\circ(\text{vaporization}) = 83.90 \text{ kcal mol}^{-1} \text{ at } 3160 \text{ K}$$

$$C_P^\circ = 8.0 \text{ cal mol}^{-1} \text{ K}^{-1} \text{ for } \alpha\text{-solid, } 10.8 \text{ for } \beta\text{-solid, } 8.5 \text{ for } \gamma\text{-solid,}$$
$$9.5 \text{ for } \delta\text{-solid, } 10.7 \text{ for liq and } 6.0 \text{ for gas}$$

For this heating process, (*3.12*) gives

$$\begin{aligned}\Delta H^\circ = {} & (8.0 \times 10^{-3})(1033-298) + (0.0) + (10.8 \times 10^{-3})(1183-1033) + (0.215) \\ & + (8.5 \times 10^{-3})(1673-1183) + (0.165) + (9.5 \times 10^{-3})(1812-1673) \\ & + (3.67) + (10.7 \times 10^{-3})(3160-1812) + (83.90) + (6.0 \times 10^{-3})(3200-3160) \\ = {} & 115.60 \text{ kcal mol}^{-1} = 483.67 \text{ kJ mol}^{-1}\end{aligned}$$

3.12. The sublimation pressure of $CO_2(s)$ is 1008.9 torr at −75 °C and 438.6 torr at −85 °C. Calculate ΔH°(sublimation) and the normal sublimation point.

Substituting the data into (3.15*b*) gives

$$\Delta H^\circ(\text{sublimation}) = -\frac{R \ln(1008.9/438.6)}{(198^{-1} - 188^{-1})\text{K}^{-1}}$$

$$= -\frac{(8.314 \text{ J mol}^{-1} \text{ K}^{-1})(0.833)}{(5.05 \times 10^{-3} - 5.32 \times 10^{-3})\text{K}^{-1}} = 25.65 \text{ kJ mol}^{-1}$$

Using this value and one set of the given pressure-temperature information, the predicted sublimation temperature at 1 atm is given by (*3.15b*) as

$$\frac{1}{T_2} = -\frac{(8.314)\ln(760.0/438.6)}{25.65 \times 10^3} + \frac{1}{188}$$

$$= -\frac{(8.314)(0.549)}{25.65 \times 10^3} + 5.32 \times 10^{-3} = 5.14 \times 10^{-3}$$

$$T_2 = 194 \text{ K} = -78 \text{ °C}$$

3.13. Evaluate the heats of fusion and vaporization at the melting and boiling points, respectively, for LiI using Fig. 3-6. At what temperature will the next discontinuity occur?

The vertical differences shown on the diagram give ΔH°(fusion) = 3.50 kcal mol^{-1} = 14.64 kJ mol^{-1} at 742 K and ΔH°(vaporization) = 32.90 kcal mol^{-1} = 137.65 kJ mol^{-1} at 1499 K. The curves should remain continuous until 1590 K, at which point Li boils giving a discontinuity of about 35 kcal mol^{-1} = 146 kJ mol^{-1} (the heat of vaporization of Li).

Supplementary Problems

Heat of Reaction

3.14. Consider an adiabatic calorimeter in which 1.000 kg of water at 98.3 °C is mixed with 0.100 kg of water at 0.0 °C. What is the final temperature of the 1.100 kg of water? If the 0.100 kg of water were originally ice at 0.0 °C, what would be the final temperature of the mixture? Assume the specific heat of water to be constant at 4.18 kJ kg^{-1} K^{-1} and the heat of fusion to be 1.436 kcal mol^{-1}.

Ans. 89.4 °C; 82.1 °C

3.15. An oxygen bomb calorimeter was calibrated using a 0.325-g sample of benzoic acid,

$$\Delta E^\circ(\text{combustion}) = -6316 \text{ cal g}^{-1}$$

which gave a change in temperature of 1.48 °C. What is the calorimeter constant? A 0.69-g sample of gasoline was oxidized in the calorimeter, resulting in a temperature change of 4.89 °C. What is the heat of combustion for a gram of the gasoline?

Ans. $q = 8588$ J, 5803 J K^{-1}; $q = 28.4$ kJ, -41.1 kJ g^{-1}

3.16. Consider a calorimeter which measures the heat of reaction by the amount of ice that is melted at 0 °C, $\Delta H^\circ_{273}(\text{fusion}) = 1436.3$ cal mol^{-1}. After corrections for heat loss of the calorimeter, 0.251 g of ice melted when the following reaction was performed in the calorimeter:

$$NaNO_3(\text{in } 200\ H_2O) + KCl(\text{in } 200\ H_2O) = KNO_3(\text{in } 400\ H_2O) + NaCl(\text{in } 400\ H_2O)$$

Calculate the heat of reaction. *Ans.* -20.01 cal $= -83.72$ J

3.17. Calculate $(\Delta H - \Delta E)$ for the explosion of TNT at 25 °C:

$$C_6H_2CH_3(NO_2)_3(s) + \tfrac{33}{4}O_2(g) = 7CO_2(g) + \tfrac{5}{2}H_2O(g) + 3NO_2(g)$$

Ans. $\Delta n_g = 4.25$, 10.535 kJ

3.18. For the gaseous reaction

$$CO(g) + \tfrac{1}{2}O_2(g) = CO_2(g)$$

$\Delta H^\circ_{298} = -67.635$ kcal mol^{-1}. Find ΔH°_{1000} if the heat capacities, in cal mol^{-1} K^{-1}, are given by

$$C_P^\circ = 6.420 + 1.665 \times 10^{-3}T - 1.96 \times 10^{-7}T^2 \quad \text{for } CO(g)$$

$$C_P^\circ = 6.214 + 10.396 \times 10^{-3}T - 35.45 \times 10^{-7}T^2 \quad \text{for } CO_2(g)$$

$$C_P^\circ = 6.148 + 3.102 \times 10^{-3}T - 9.23 \times 10^{-7}T^2 \quad \text{for } O_2(g)$$

Ans. $\Delta a = -3.280$, $\Delta b = 7.180 \times 10^{-3}$, $\Delta c = -28.88 \times 10^{-7}$; $-67{,}604$ cal $= -282.855$ kJ

3.19. Repeat the calculations of Example 3.1, assuming 10% heat loss to the surroundings and 10% incomplete combustion of the hydrogen. Additional heat capacity data (in cal mol^{-1} K^{-1}) are

$$C_P^\circ = 6.148 + 3.102 \times 10^{-3}T - 9.23 \times 10^{-7}T^2 \quad \text{for } O_2(g)$$

$$C_P^\circ = 6.9469 - 0.1999 \times 10^{-3}T + 4.808 \times 10^{-7}T^2 \quad \text{for } H_2(g)$$

Ans. gas mixture is 0.9 mol H_2O, 0.05 mol O_2, 0.10 mol H_2 and 2.0 mol N_2;
$\Delta a = 20.573$, $\Delta b = 4.703 \times 10^{-3}$, $\Delta c = 2.55 \times 10^{-7}$; 2043 K

Calculations Involving Thermochemical Equations

3.20. Consider the combustion of one mole of $CH_4(g)$ with $O_2(g)$, giving $CO_2(g)$ and H_2O at 25 °C. If the product is $H_2O(liq)$, $\Delta H^\circ_{298} = -212.80$ kcal, and if $H_2O(g)$, $\Delta H^\circ_{298} = -191.76$ kcal. Calculate $\Delta H^\circ(\text{vaporization})$ for water at 25 °C. *Ans.* 44.02 kJ mol^{-1}

3.21. Calculate ΔH°_{298}(solution) for the reactions

$$KCl(g) + \infty H_2O(liq) = KCl(aq)$$

$$KCl(s) + \infty H_2O(liq) = KCl(aq)$$

given that the heats of formation at 25 °C are −51.6 kcal mol^{-1} for KCl(g), −104.175 for KCl(s), −60.04 for K^+(aq) and −40.023 for Cl^-(aq). What is the heat of sublimation for KCl at this temperature?

Ans. −48.5 kcal mol^{-1} = −202.9 kJ mol^{-1}, 4.12 kcal mol^{-1} = 17.24 kJ mol^{-1}, 52.6 kcal mol^{-1} = 220.1 kJ mol^{-1}

3.22. (*a*) Calculate ΔH°_{298}(reaction) for the deamination of L-aspartic acid to fumaric acid:

$$\text{HOOC—}\underset{\substack{|\\ NH_2}}{\text{CH}}\text{—}\overset{\substack{H\\ |}}{\text{CH}}\text{—COOH} = \text{HOOC—CH=CH—COOH} + NH_3$$

given that the heats of formation at 25 °C for the acids, as reported by Burton and Krebs, are −233.75 kcal mol^{-1} for L-aspartic acid and −194.13 kcal mol^{-1} for fumaric acid, while for NH_3, ΔH°_{298}(formation) = −11.02 kcal mol^{-1}. (*b*) Bond energies are sometimes used to estimate heats of reaction for condensed-phase reactions when other thermodynamic data are not available. Repeat the calculation in (*a*) using average bond energies at 25 °C of 330.5 kJ mol^{-1} for C—C, 300.4 for C—N, 415.9 for C—H, 589.5 for C=C and 389.1 for N—H, and compare results. (In the bond energy calculation, it is not necessary to break the reactant completely down to fragments, but only to consider the parts of the molecule that are changing.)

Ans. (*a*) 28.60 kcal = 119.66 kJ

(*b*) 68.2 kJ, about 43% low but of correct sign and order of magnitude

3.23. Combine the following thermochemical equations

$$CHCl_3(liq) + \tfrac{5}{4}O_2(g) = CO_2(g) + \tfrac{1}{2}H_2O(liq) + \tfrac{3}{2}Cl_2(g) \qquad \Delta H^\circ_{298} = -89.2 \text{ kcal}$$

$$C(graph) + 2H_2(g) = CH_4(g) \qquad \Delta H^\circ_{298} = -17.88 \text{ kcal}$$

$$C(graph) + O_2(g) = CO_2(g) \qquad \Delta H^\circ_{298} = -94.051 \text{ kcal}$$

$$H_2(g) + \tfrac{1}{2}O_2(g) = H_2O(liq) \qquad \Delta H^\circ_{298} = -68.315 \text{ kcal}$$

to predict ΔH°_{298} for

$$CH_4(g) + \tfrac{3}{2}Cl_2(g) = CHCl_3(liq) + \tfrac{3}{2}H_2(g)$$

Ans. −21.1 kcal = −88.4 kJ

3.24. The heat of formation of calcite, one form of $CaCO_3$(s), is −288.45 kcal mol^{-1} at 25 °C and the heat of formation of aragonite, another form of $CaCO_3$(s), is −288.49 kcal mol^{-1}. Calculate ΔH°_{298} for the reaction

$$CaCO_3(calcite) = CaCO_3(aragonite)$$

Ans. −40 cal = −170 J

3.25. Calculate ΔH°_{293} for the hydrogenation of benzene to cyclohexane:

$$C_6H_6(liq) + 3H_2(g) = C_6H_{12}(liq)$$

if the heats of combustion at 20 °C are −782.3, −68.38 and −937.8 kcal mol^{-1} for C_6H_6, H_2 and C_6H_{12}, respectively. *Ans.* −49.6 kcal = −207.5 kJ

3.26. Calculate ΔH°_{298}(neutralization) for the reaction between HCl(aq) and NaOH(aq) if the heats of formation are −40.023, −112.236, −97.302 and −68.3174 kcal mol^{-1} at 25 °C for HCl, NaOH, NaCl and H_2O, respectively, in very dilute solutions. *Ans.* −13.360 kcal = −55.898 kJ

3.27. Prepare a graph of the calculated values of ΔH°_{298}(solution) for $AgNO_3$(s) against the number of moles of water, using the following heat of formation data:

moles H_2O	pure $AgNO_3$(s)	50	100	200	400	500	1000
ΔH°_{298}(formation), kcal mol^{-1}	−29.73	−24.915	−24.637	−24.467	−24.379	−24.362	−24.328
moles H_2O	2000	5000	10,000	50,000	∞		
ΔH°_{298}(formation)	−24.314	−24.309	−24.311	−24.318	−24.33		

Using these data and the result of Example 3.10, calculate ΔH°_{298}(formation) for Ag^+(∞ dil).

Ans. The plot will have heat of solution values ranging from 4.81 kcal mol^{-1} at 50 moles H_2O to 5.42 kcal mol^{-1} at 5000 moles H_2O, a maximum, and an infinite-dilution value of 5.40 kcal mol^{-1}. The value of the ionic heat of formation is 105.56 kJ mol^{-1}.

3.28. Saturated solutions of ammonium chloride are often used in sports to reduce the swelling of a sprained ankle. Calculate the temperature drop for

$$NH_4Cl(s) + 10H_2O(liq) = NH_4Cl(\text{in } 10\ H_2O)$$

if the heat of formation of NH_4Cl(in 10 H_2O) is −71.567 kcal mol^{-1} and that of NH_4Cl(s) is −75.15 kcal mol^{-1}. The specific heat of the solution is 3.77 kJ kg^{-1} K^{-1}.

Ans. $\Delta H = 14.99$ kJ, $C = 0.881$ kJ mol^{-1} K^{-1}; 17 °C

3.29. From the following data for the stepwise decomposition of CH_4(g), calculate $\overline{BE}_{C-H}$.

$$CH_4(g) = CH_3(g) + H(g) \qquad \Delta H^\circ_{298} = 102.7 \text{ kcal}$$

$$CH_3(g) = CH_2(g) + H(g) \qquad \Delta H^\circ_{298} = 113.1 \text{ kcal}$$

$$CH_2(g) = CH(g) + H(g) \qquad \Delta H^\circ_{298} = 100.8 \text{ kcal}$$

$$CH(g) = C(g) + H(g) \qquad \Delta H^\circ_{298} = 81 \text{ kcal}$$

Ans. 99.4 kcal mol^{-1} = 415.9 kJ mol^{-1}

3.30. Calculate the bond energy for C—I if the enthalpy of formation for CH_3I(g) is 3.1 kcal mol^{-1}, 52.095 for H(g), 171.291 for C(g) and 25.535 for I(g), and if the average bond energy for the C—H bond is 415.9 kJ mol^{-1}. *Ans.* 216.7 kJ mol^{-1} (measured value is 232.2 ± 12.6 kJ mol^{-1})

3.31. (*a*) Assuming benzene to consist of six C—H bonds, three C—C bonds and three C═C bonds, what would be the value of ΔH°_{298}(formation) of gaseous C_6H_6 if the bond energies at 25 °C are 415.9, 330.5 and 631.4 kJ mol^{-1}, respectively? (*b*) The heats of formation at 25 °C of C(g), H(g) and C_6H_6(g) are 171.291, 52.095 and 19.820 kcal mol^{-1}, respectively. Calculate ΔH°_{298} for the reaction

$$6C(g) + 6H(g) = C_6H_6(g)$$

The difference between this value for the heat of formation and that found in (*a*) is known as the *resonance energy* of the molecule; it is due to the delocalized pi bonding in the ring. Find the resonance energy. *Ans.* (*a*) −5381.1 kJ; (*b*) −5524.955 kJ, −143.9 kJ

Physical Changes

3.32. Krypton melts at −157.21 °C. Give an estimate of $\Delta H^\circ_{115.94}$(fusion) for this element and compare it to 1636 J mol^{-1}. *Ans.* 1100 J mol^{-1}, 33% low

3.33. Lozana reported a 1.57% volume increase at 1 atm upon melting for lithium metal at 180.54 °C. If the density of the liquid is 0.515×10^3 kg m^{-3} and the heat of fusion is 722.8 cal mol^{-1}, what will be the melting point at 1000 atm?

Ans. $\Delta H^\circ = 29.85 \times 10^{-3}$ m^3 atm mol^{-1}, $\Delta V = 0.211 \times 10^{-6}$ m^3 mol^{-1}, $dT = \Delta T = 3.20$ K mol^{-1}; 183.74 °C

3.34. From the following vapor pressure data for Hg, calculate the heat of vaporization and the normal boiling point.

T, °C	300	320	340	350	352	354	356
P, torr	246.80	376.33	577.90	672.69	697.83	723.73	750.43

Ans. slope $= -7.20 \times 10^3$; 59.86 kJ mol^{-1}; 629.3 K

3.35. One of the major components of mothballs, naphthalene, has a sublimation pressure of 1.09×10^{-2} torr at 6 °C and 5.37×10^{-2} torr at 21 °C. Using these data, calculate the heat of sublimation and the sublimation pressure in a warm closet at 78 °F. If the closet is 11 ft × $3\frac{1}{2}$ ft × 9 ft, calculate the mass of naphthalene, $C_{10}H_8$, in the gaseous state, assuming an ambient room pressure of 747 torr.

Ans. 72.4 kJ mol^{-1}; 8.47×10^{-2} torr; 0.0446 mol = 5.72 g (ambient room pressure is irrelevant)

3.36. Prepare a graph of ΔH_T°(formation) for $AlCl_3$ as a function of temperature from the following data (JANAF Thermochemical Tables):

T, K	ΔH_T°(formation, s), kcal mol^{-1}	ΔH_T°(formation, liq), kcal mol^{-1}	ΔH_T°(formation, g), kcal mol^{-1}
0	−168.323		−139.274
100	−169.004		−139.468
200	−168.961		−139.604
298	−168.650	−161.280	−139.700
300	−168.643	−161.258	−139.702
400	−168.200	−160.102	−139.773
500	−167.614	−159.013	−139.837
600	−166.869	−157.975	−139.911
700	−165.954	−156.977	−139.998
800	−164.873	−156.023	−140.113
900	−163.633	−155.120	−140.266
1000	−164.760	−156.794	−142.988
1100	−163.108	−155.899	−143.135
1200	−161.250	−155.008	−143.281
1300	−159.184	−154.119	−143.425
1400	−156.912	−153.234	−143.571
1500	−154.433	−152.352	−143.717

From the graph, determine ΔH°(fusion) at 465.7 K and ΔH°(sublimation) at 298 K.

Ans. 8.45 kcal mol^{-1} = 35.35 kJ mol^{-1}, 28.95 kcal mol^{-1} = 121.13 kJ mol^{-1}

Chapter 4

Entropy

The Second Law of Thermodynamics

4.1 STATEMENTS

Unlike the first law of thermodynamics, the second law does not have just one statement, but several: (1) a cyclic process must transfer heat from a hot to a cold reservoir if it is to convert heat into work; (2) work must be done to transfer heat from a cold to a hot reservoir; (3) no engine can operate more efficiently than a Carnot engine; (4) a perpetual-motion machine of the second kind (one that extracts heat from surroundings at T, does work on surroundings, and returns to initial state without transferring heat to another system at a temperature lower than T) cannot exist; (5) the entropy, or randomness, of the universe is increasing; etc. Most of these statements can be reduced to the assertion that all real processes are irreversible, i.e. the system and the surroundings cannot both be restored to their original states.

Entropy changes can be used to predict the spontaneity of constant-energy processes. At fixed energy, only those processes will occur spontaneously for which there is an increase in entropy. Predicting the spontaneity of a process under combined changes of energy and entropy will be considered in Section 5.1.

4.2 THE CARNOT CYCLE

The operation of an arbitrary heat engine is represented in Fig. 4-1. A *Carnot engine* is an (idealized) heat engine that follows the cyclic process indicated in Fig. 4-2. This *Carnot cycle* consists of four steps performed on an ideal gas: (1) a reversible isothermal expansion from V_1 to V_2 at T_h, (2) a reversible adiabatic expansion from V_2 to V_3 with a temperature change from T_h to T_c, (3) a reversible isothermal compression from V_3 to V_4 at T_c, and (4) a reversible adiabatic compression from V_4 to V_1 with a temperature change from T_c to T_h.

For a Carnot engine, $q_h = q_1$ and $q_c = q_3$.

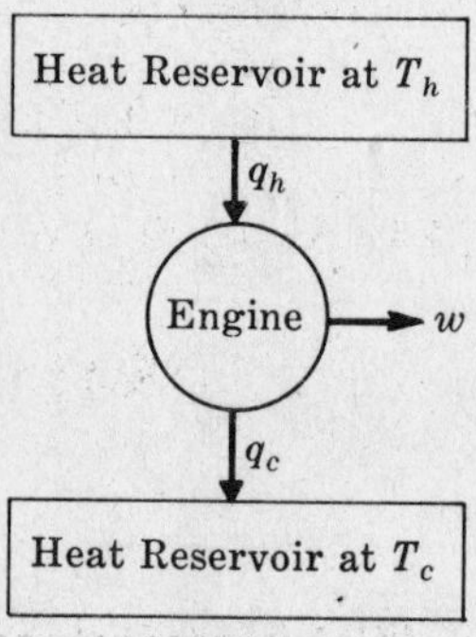

Fig. 4-1

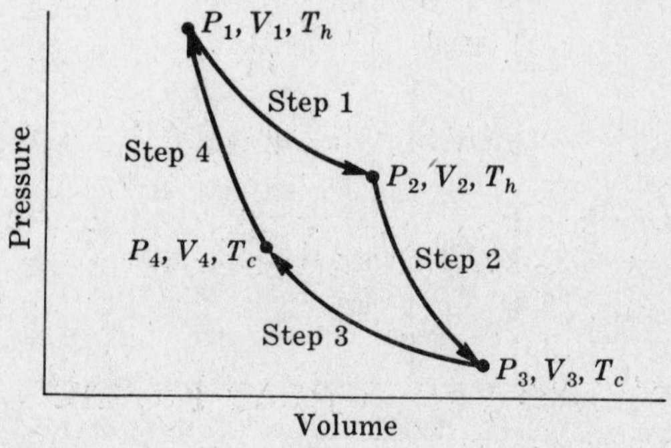

Fig. 4-2

EXAMPLE 4.1. Consider a Carnot engine operating between 500 °C and 0 °C using one mole of an ideal monatomic gas. If $V_1 = 0.0100\ \text{m}^3$ and $V_2 = 0.1000\ \text{m}^3$, calculate V_3 and V_4; q, w and ΔE for each step; and q, w and ΔE for the overall process. Prepare a sketch similar to Fig. 4-1 for this engine.

The relationship between the temperatures is given by (*2.28*) as

$$T_h^{C_V/R}V_2 = T_c^{C_V/R}V_3 \qquad T_h^{C_V/R}V_1 = T_c^{C_V/R}V_4$$

Since $C_V = (3/2)R$ for an ideal monatomic gas,

$$V_3 = V_2\left(\frac{T_h}{T_c}\right)^{C_V/R} = (0.1000\ \text{m}^3)\left(\frac{773\ \text{K}}{273\ \text{K}}\right)^{3/2} = 0.477\ \text{m}^3$$

Dividing the two volume-temperature equations written above, we obtain

$$V_4 = V_3\frac{V_1}{V_2} = (0.477\ \text{m}^3)\frac{0.0100\ \text{m}^3}{0.1000\ \text{m}^3} = 0.0477\ \text{m}^3$$

The values of ΔE, q and w for each step can be determined by using (*2.24*) and (*2.27*). For the first step:

$$\Delta E_{(1)} = 0$$

$$q_1 = w_1 = nRT_h \ln\frac{V_2}{V_1} = (1.00\ \text{mol})(8.314\ \text{J mol}^{-1}\ \text{K}^{-1})(773\ \text{K}) \ln\frac{0.1000}{0.0100} = 14.80\ \text{kJ}$$

For the second step:

$$q_2 = 0$$

$$\Delta E_{(2)} = -w_2 = n\int_{T_h}^{T_c} C_V\,dT = n\int_{T_h}^{T_c}\frac{3}{2}R\,dT = (1.00\ \text{mol})\left(\frac{3}{2}\right)(8.314\ \text{J mol}^{-1}\ \text{K}^{-1})(273\ \text{K} - 773\ \text{K})$$

$$= -6.24\ \text{kJ}$$

For the third step:

$$\Delta E_{(3)} = 0$$

$$q_3 = w_3 = nRT_c \ln\frac{V_4}{V_3} = (1.00)(8.314)(273) \ln\frac{0.0477}{0.477} = -5.23\ \text{kJ}$$

For the fourth step:

$$q_4 = 0$$

$$\Delta E_{(4)} = -w_4 = n\int_{T_c}^{T_h} C_V\,dT = 6.24\ \text{kJ}$$

For the overall cycle it can be shown that

$$\Delta E = 0$$

$$q = w = nR(T_h - T_c)\ln\frac{V_2}{V_1}$$

$$= (1.00)(8.314)(733 - 273)\ln\frac{0.1000}{0.0100} = 9.57\ \text{kJ}$$

The work is equivalent to the area enclosed by the cycle shown in Fig. 4-2. The diagram for this engine is Fig. 4-3.

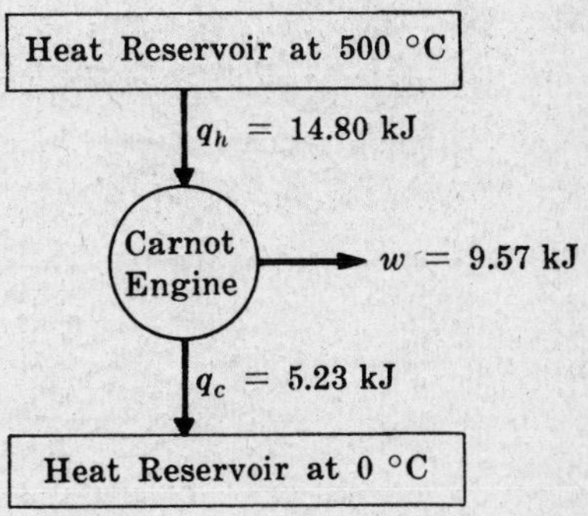

Fig. 4-3

4.3 EFFICIENCY OF A HEAT ENGINE

For an engine that operates between two heat reservoirs, the *efficiency* (expressed in %) is

$$\varepsilon \equiv 100\frac{w}{q_h} \tag{4.1}$$

EXAMPLE 4.2. Substitute the expressions for w and q_1 found in Example 4.1 into (*4.1*) to derive a general expression for the efficiency of a Carnot engine. Calculate the efficiency of the engine described in Example 4.1.

Using the expressions for w and $q_1 = q_h$ gives

$$\varepsilon_{\text{carnot}} = 100\frac{T_h - T_c}{T_h} \tag{4.2}$$

Substituting the numerical values into (*4.1*) gives

$$\varepsilon_{\text{carnot}} = 100\frac{9.57\text{ kJ}}{14.80\text{ kJ}} = 64.7\%$$

or substituting the temperatures into (*4.2*) gives

$$\varepsilon_{\text{carnot}} = 100\frac{773\text{ K} - 273\text{ K}}{773\text{ K}} = 64.7\%$$

4.4 REFRIGERATORS

An engine can be used as a refrigerator to pump heat from a cold to a hot reservoir, see Fig. 4-4. The efficiency of a refrigerator, expressed in %, is

$$\varepsilon_{\text{ref}} \equiv 100\frac{w}{q_c} \tag{4.3a}$$

For a Carnot refrigerator,

$$\varepsilon_{\text{ref}} = 100\frac{T_h - T_c}{T_c} \tag{4.3b}$$

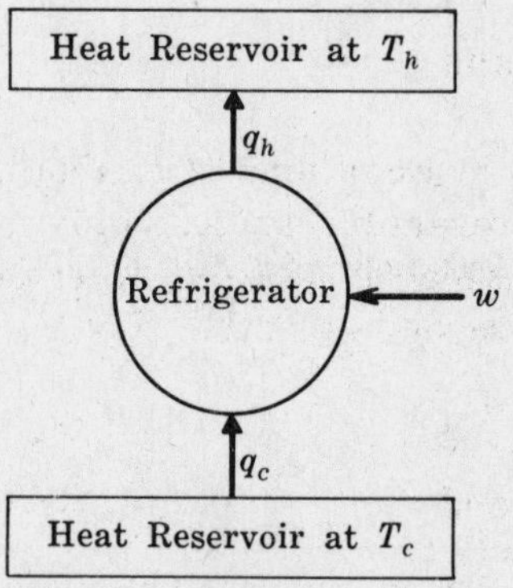

Fig. 4-4

EXAMPLE 4.3. Calculate the maximum efficiency of a commercial refrigerator operating between the temperatures of −10 °C (inside temperature) and 25 °C (room temperature). What minimum amount of work must be done to remove 100 J of heat from the inside of the refrigerator?

According to one of the statements of the second law, the maximum efficiency occurs in a Carnot engine. Thus (*4.3b*) gives

$$\varepsilon_{\text{ref}} = 100\frac{298\text{ K} - 263\text{ K}}{263\text{ K}} = 13.3\%$$

The minimum amount of work required to remove the heat is found using (*4.3a*) as

$$0.133 = \frac{w}{100\text{ J}} \qquad \text{or} \qquad w = 13.3\text{ J}$$

Entropy Calculations

4.5 DEFINITION OF ENTROPY

For the Carnot cycle, it can be shown that

$$\varepsilon_{\text{carnot}} = 100\frac{q_h + q_c}{q_h} = 100\frac{T_h - T_c}{T_h}$$

which can be rearranged to give

$$\frac{q_c}{T_c} + \frac{q_h}{T_h} = 0$$

Any reversible cyclic process can be considered to be the sum of a large number of smaller Carnot cycles, giving

$$\sum \frac{q_{\text{rev}}}{T} = 0$$

or, as the number of subcycles becomes very large,

$$\oint \frac{đq_{\text{rev}}}{T} = 0$$

The above condition—that the integral over a cycle is zero—is the general definition of a state or point function. Calling this particular function the *entropy*, S, we have

$$dS = \frac{đq_{\text{rev}}}{T} \tag{4.4a}$$

and

$$\Delta S = \int \frac{đq_{\text{rev}}}{T} \tag{4.4b}$$

Equations (*4.4*) require that the entropy change for the system be calculated using a reversible process only. For an irreversible process, a reversible path must be defined which has the same endstates as the actual process, and (*4.4*) must be applied along this reversible path. For a reversible process,

$$\Delta S(\text{system}) = -\Delta S(\text{surroundings})$$

and

$$\Delta S(\text{universe}) = \Delta S(\text{system}) + \Delta S(\text{surroundings}) = 0$$

For an irreversible process, $\Delta S(\text{universe}) > 0$.

The units of entropy in the older physical system are cal K^{-1} (or gibbs), which have been represented by eu; in the SI system the units are J K^{-1}, which are represented by EU (1 eu = 4.184 EU).

4.6 ΔS FOR ISOTHERMAL EXPANSIONS

For an ideal gas

$$\Delta S(\text{system}) = nR \ln \frac{V_2}{V_1} = nR \ln \frac{P_1}{P_2} \tag{4.5}$$

and for a condensed system

$$\Delta S(\text{system}) = -\int \left(\frac{\partial V}{\partial T}\right)_P dP \tag{4.6}$$

For the surroundings, it is assumed that the heat can be transferred reversibly and isothermally, so that

$$\Delta S(\text{surroundings}) = \frac{q}{T} \tag{4.7}$$

EXAMPLE 4.4. Compare the entropy changes for the system, surroundings and universe for the reversible isothermal expansion of one mole of an ideal gas from 0.010 m^3 to 0.1000 m^3 at 298 K to the entropy changes for the same expansion performed irreversibly against a constant external pressure of 0.100 atm.

For the reversible expansion (*4.5*) gives

$$\Delta S(\text{system}) = (1.00\text{ mol})(8.314\text{ J mol}^{-1}\text{ K}^{-1}) \ln \frac{0.1000}{0.0100} = 19.14\text{ EU}$$

For the surroundings, $q = -nRT \ln (V_2/V_1)$, which upon substitution into (4.7) gives

$$\Delta S(\text{surroundings}) = -nR \ln \frac{V_2}{V_1} = -19.14 \text{ EU}$$

For the universe

$$\Delta S(\text{universe}) = 19.14 + (-19.14) = 0$$

For the irreversible process, ΔS(system) must be calculated using a reversible path, so

$$\Delta S(\text{system}) = 19.14 \text{ EU}$$

as in the reversible case. For the surroundings, (2.25b) gives $q = P\,\Delta V$, so (4.7) becomes

$$\Delta S(\text{surroundings}) = \frac{P\,\Delta V}{T} = \frac{(0.100 \text{ atm})(-0.0900 \text{ m}^3)(101{,}325 \text{ J m}^{-3} \text{ atm}^{-1})}{298 \text{ K}} = -3.06 \text{ EU}$$

a smaller magnitude than in the reversible case. For the universe

$$\Delta S(\text{universe}) = 19.14 + (-3.06) = 16.08 \text{ EU}$$

a positive value, implying that the entropy content of the universe is increasing for a real process.

4.7 ΔS FOR PHASE TRANSITIONS

For a system undergoing a phase transition

$$\Delta S(\text{system}) = \frac{\Delta H}{T} \tag{4.8}$$

For the surroundings, a similar equation may be derived.

EXAMPLE 4.5. What are the entropy changes for the reversible vaporization and fusion of one mole of water at 100 °C and 0 °C, respectively? Assume ΔH(vaporization) = 9.7171 kcal mol^{-1} and ΔH(fusion) = 1.4363 kcal mol^{-1}. Qualitatively compare the entropy changes for the system.

For both processes

$$\Delta S(\text{system}) = -\Delta S(\text{surroundings}) \quad \text{and} \quad \Delta S(\text{universe}) = 0$$

For the vaporization, (4.8) gives

$$\Delta S(\text{system}) = \frac{(1.00 \text{ mol})(9717.1 \text{ cal mol}^{-1})}{373.15 \text{ K}} = 26.04 \text{ eu} = 108.95 \text{ EU}$$

and for the fusion

$$\Delta S(\text{system}) = \frac{(1.00)(1436.3)}{273.15} = 5.258 \text{ eu} = 21.999 \text{ EU}$$

The values of ΔS(system) indicate that there is a larger increase in randomness in going from the liquid state to the gaseous state than from the solid state to the liquid state.

4.8 ΔS FOR TEMPERATURE CHANGES

For a system undergoing a temperature change

$$\Delta S(\text{system}) = \int \frac{C_i}{T}\,dT \tag{4.9}$$

where C_i is C_V or C_P depending on the process being considered. For the surroundings, (4.9) is valid for a reversible process and (4.7) is used for an irreversible process.

EXAMPLE 4.6. Compare the entropy changes for heating one mole of ethane from 298 K to 1500 K at constant pressure if the process is done: (1) reversibly; (2) irreversibly by placing the gas in an oven at 1500 K. Assume

$$C_P = 1.279 + 42.464 \times 10^{-3} T - 164.20 \times 10^{-7} T^2 + 2.035 \times 10^{-9} T^3$$

in cal mol^{-1} K^{-1}.

For both processes, (*4.9*) gives

$$\Delta S(\text{system}) = (1 \text{ mol}) \int_{298\text{ K}}^{1500\text{ K}} \frac{C_P}{T}\, dT = 1.279 \ln \frac{1500}{298} + (42.464 \times 10^{-3})(1500 - 298)$$

$$- \left(\frac{164.20 \times 10^{-7}}{2}\right)(1500^2 - 298^2)$$

$$+ \left(\frac{2.035 \times 10^{-9}}{3}\right)(1500^3 - 298^3)$$

$$= 2.07 + 51.04 - 17.74 + 2.27 = 37.64 \text{ eu} = 157.49 \text{ EU}$$

For the reversible process, (*4.9*) will be valid for the surroundings, giving

$$\Delta S(\text{surroundings}) = -157.49 \text{ EU} \quad \text{and} \quad \Delta S(\text{universe}) = 157.49 + (-157.49) = 0$$

For the irreversible process, the heat transferred from the oven is given by

$$q = -(1 \text{ mol}) \int_{298\text{ K}}^{1500\text{ K}} C_P\, dT = -(1.279)(1500 - 298) - \left(\frac{42.464 \times 10^{-3}}{2}\right)(1500^2 - 298^2)$$

$$+ \left(\frac{164.20 \times 10^{-7}}{3}\right)(1500^3 - 298^3) - \left(\frac{2.035 \times 10^{-9}}{4}\right)(1500^4 - 298^4)$$

$$= -31{,}668 \text{ cal} = -132{,}499 \text{ J}$$

and applying (*4.7*) gives

$$\Delta S(\text{surroundings}) = \frac{-132{,}499}{1500} = -88.33 \text{ EU}$$

For the universe

$$\Delta S(\text{universe}) = 157.49 + (-88.33) = 69.16 \text{ EU}$$

4.9 ΔS FOR ADIABATIC PROCESSES

For a reversible adiabatic process

$$\Delta S(\text{system}) = 0 \qquad (4.10)$$

4.10 ΔS FOR ISOTHERMAL MIXING

For a mixture

$$\Delta S(\text{system}) = -R \sum_i n_i \ln x_i \qquad (4.11a)$$

where n_i is the number of moles, and x_i is the mole fraction, of component i in the mixture. For one mole of solution (*4.11a*) becomes

$$\Delta S(\text{system}) = -R \sum_i x_i \ln x_i \qquad (4.11b)$$

EXAMPLE 4.7. What is the entropy change for preparing a mixture containing one mole of O_2(g) and two moles of H_2(g), assuming no chemical reaction and isothermal mixing?

For the binary mixture, (*4.11a*) gives

$$\Delta S(\text{system}) = -(8.314 \text{ J mol}^{-1} \text{ K}^{-1})[(1.00 \text{ mol})(\ln 0.333) + (2.00 \text{ mol})(\ln 0.667)]$$

$$= 15.88 \text{ EU}$$

4.11 GENERAL ENTROPY CALCULATIONS

To calculate the entropy changes for processes more complex than those described in Sections 4.6 through 4.10, the complex process is described as a series of steps corresponding to those processes and (*4.5*) through (*4.11*) applied to the respective steps.

EXAMPLE 4.8. What are the entropy changes for heating 1 mole of $H_2(g)$ from 0.0100 m^3 at 100 K to 0.1000 m^3 at 600 K if the process is done: (1) reversibly; (2) irreversibly by placing it in an oven at 750 K and allowing it to expand against a constant external pressure of 1.00 atm? Assume that for H_2

$$C_V = 4.960 - 0.19999 \times 10^{-3}T + 4.808 \times 10^{-7}T^2$$

in cal mol^{-1} K^{-1}.

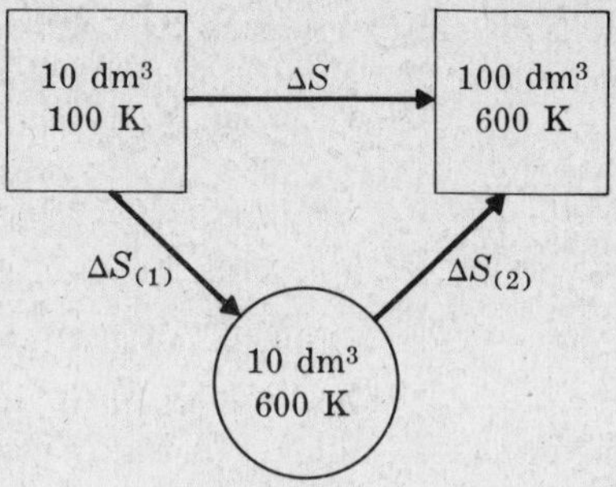

Fig. 4-5

The heating and expansion can be considered to be a two-step process, see Fig. 4-5, where $\Delta S_{(1)}$, corresponding to a reversible constant-volume heating, is given by (*4.9*) and $\Delta S_{(2)}$, corresponding to a reversible isothermal expansion, is given by (*4.5*).

For the reversible process, the overall ΔS(system) is given by

$$\begin{aligned}\Delta S(\text{system}) &= \Delta S_{(1)}(\text{system}) + \Delta S_{(2)}(\text{system}) \\ &= (1\text{ mol})\int_{100\text{ K}}^{600\text{ K}} \frac{C_V}{T}\,dT + nR\ln\frac{V_2}{V_1} \\ &= (4.184)\left[(4.960)\ln\frac{600}{100} - (0.19999\times 10^{-3})(600-100) + \left(\frac{4.808\times 10^{-7}}{2}\right)(600^2 - 100^2)\right] \\ &\quad + (1.00)(8.314)\ln\frac{0.1000}{0.0100} \\ &= (4.184)(8.89 - 0.10 + 0.084) + 19.14 = 56.26\text{ EU}\end{aligned}$$

For the surroundings and universe,

$$\Delta S(\text{surroundings}) = -56.26\text{ EU} \quad \text{and} \quad \Delta S(\text{universe}) = 0$$

For the irreversible process, ΔS(system) will be the same. For the surroundings, the heat required for the two steps is

$$\begin{aligned} q = -(1\text{ mol})\int_{100\text{ K}}^{600\text{ K}} C_V\,dT + w &= (4.184)\left[-(4.960)(600-100) + \left(\frac{0.19999\times 10^{-3}}{2}\right)(600^2-100^2)\right. \\ &\quad \left. - \left(\frac{4.808\times 10^{-7}}{3}\right)(600^3 - 100^3)\right] \\ &\quad + (1.00\text{ atm})(-0.090\text{ m}^3)(101{,}325\text{ J m}^{-3}\text{ atm}^{-1}) \\ &= -10{,}374 - 9119 = -19{,}493\text{ J}\end{aligned}$$

giving

$$\Delta S(\text{surroundings}) = \frac{-19{,}493\text{ J}}{750\text{ K}} = 25.99\text{ EU}$$

$$\Delta S(\text{universe}) = 56.26 + (-25.99) = 30.27\text{ EU}$$

The Third Law of Thermodynamics

4.12 STATEMENT

The third law of thermodynamics can be stated as "the entropy content of all perfect crystalline materials is the same at 0 K." For these materials, the value of S_0° is chosen as zero. For nonperfect crystalline materials, S_0° is greater than zero and must be determined using theoretical considerations.

The value of S_0° for crystals in which unsymmetrical molecules may orient themselves in Ω ways is given by

$$S_0^\circ = nR\ln\Omega \tag{4.12}$$

Because the molecules in a real crystal are not completely random in their orientation, owing to weak intermolecular forces, size considerations, etc., the value of S_0° predicted by (*4.12*) is often slightly too large.

For a glassy material, the value of S_0° depends on the actual processes used in the production of the glass. In general, the value will lie between S_0° for the solid state and S_0° for the liquid state.

For a polymorphic material, the third law holds only for the stable crystalline state of the substance. Even though a perfect crystal is formed by a metastable polymorph at 0 K, S_0° will be positive.

For ideal solid solutions, the entropy of mixing given by (*4.11*) is still present at 0 K and so $S_0^\circ = \Delta S^\circ(\text{mixing})$.

EXAMPLE 4.9. What is the value of S_0° for 1 mol of water?

A portion of an ice crystal is shown in Fig. 4-6. Each oxygen is in the center of a tetrahedron of hydrogens and a larger tetrahedron of oxygens. A given water molecule can be oriented in any of six positions if all positions are open. Because the adjacent water molecules can also be oriented in six positions, there is a chance of one in two that a given position is filled; and because this can happen twice, the number of random orientations for the given molecule is cut down by a factor of $\frac{1}{2} \times \frac{1}{2} = \frac{1}{4}$. Thus $\Omega = 6/4$ and (*4.12*) gives

$$S_0^\circ = (1\ \text{mol})R \ln\frac{6}{4} = 3.371\ \text{EU}$$

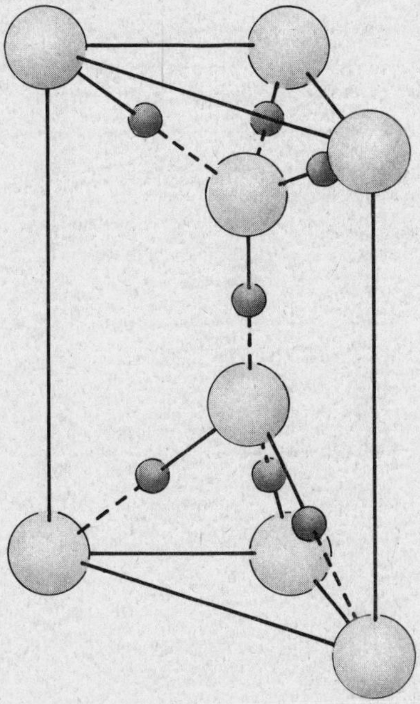

Fig. 4-6

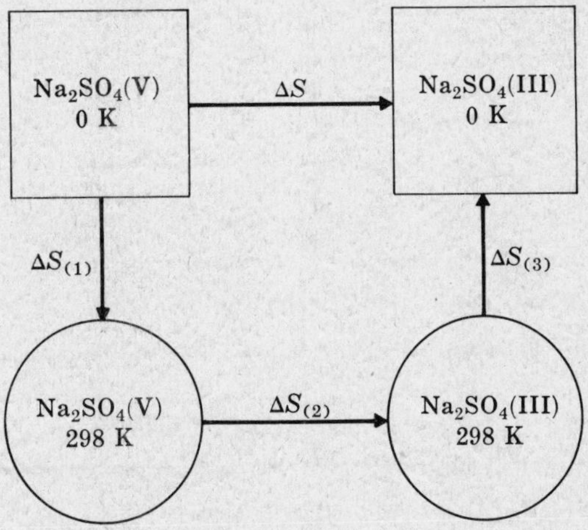

Fig. 4-7

EXAMPLE 4.10. The stable form of Na_2SO_4 at 0 K is Na_2SO_4(V). What is S_0° for Na_2SO_4(III), a metastable form, if $\Delta H^\circ(\text{V} \rightarrow \text{III}) = 716\ \text{cal mol}^{-1}$ at 298 K, $S_{298}^\circ - S_0^\circ = 37.027\ \text{eu mol}^{-1}$ for (III) and $S_{298}^\circ - S_0^\circ = 35.751\ \text{eu mol}^{-1}$ for (V)?

The value of S_0°(III) can be calculated using the series of steps shown in Fig. 4-7, where

$$\Delta S = S_0^\circ(\text{III}) - S_0^\circ(\text{V}) = S_0^\circ(\text{III})$$

because $S_0^\circ(\text{V})$ is zero. Recognizing that

$$\Delta S = \Delta S_{(1)} + \Delta S_{(2)} + \Delta S_{(3)}$$

$$= [S_{298}^\circ(\text{V}) - S_0^\circ(\text{V})] + \left[\frac{\Delta H^\circ}{T}\right] + [S_0^\circ(\text{III}) - S_{298}^\circ(\text{III})]$$

gives

$$S_0^\circ(\text{III}) = 35.751 + \frac{716}{298} + (-37.027) = 1.127 \text{ eu mol}^{-1} = 4.715 \text{ EU mol}^{-1}$$

4.13 VALUES OF S_T°

The contributions to S_T° for a material are given by (*4.8*) and (*4.9*):

$$S_T^\circ = S_0^\circ + \sum_i^{\text{phases}} \int \frac{C_P^\circ}{T} dT + \sum_j^{\text{transitions}} \frac{\Delta H_j^\circ}{T_j} \qquad (4.13a)$$

$$= S_0^\circ + \sum_i^{\text{phases}} \int C_P^\circ \, d(\ln T) + \sum_j^{\text{transitions}} \frac{\Delta H_j^\circ}{T_j} \qquad (4.13b)$$

In (*4.13*) the value of S_0° is determined as in Section 4.12. The numerical value of the heat-capacity contribution is usually determined from graphical integration of a plot of C_P°/T against T or a plot of C_P° against ln T, for all stable phases that the material exists in from 0 K to T.

EXAMPLE 4.11. Calculate S_{1500}° for liquid Na_2SO_4 from the following data:

$S_0^\circ(\text{V}) = 0$

$C_P^\circ(\text{V})$, cal mol^{-1} K^{-1}	0.222	0.581	1.213	2.026	2.981	4.054	5.206	6.402	7.595
T, K	15	20	25	30	35	40	45	50	55
$C_P^\circ(\text{V})$	8.746	10.851	12.754	14.439	15.941	17.258	18.441	20.502	22.232
T	60	70	80	90	100	110	120	140	160
$C_P^\circ(\text{V})$	23.793	25.217	27.656	29.744	30.603	32.819	34.710	36.672	
T	180	200	240	280	298.15	350	400	458	

$\Delta H^\circ(\text{V} \rightarrow \text{IV}) = 75$ cal mol^{-1} at 458 K

$C_P^\circ(\text{IV})$, cal mol^{-1} K^{-1}	36.672	37.055	37.989	38.417
T, K	458	470	500	514

$\Delta H^\circ(\text{IV} \rightarrow \text{I}) = 2611$ cal mol^{-1} at 514 K

$C_P^\circ(\text{I})$, cal mol^{-1} K^{-1}	40.889	41.358	43.940	45.611	48.101
T, K	514	550	750	850	950

$\Delta H^\circ(\text{I} \rightarrow \delta) = 80$ cal mol^{-1} at 980 K

$C_P^\circ(\delta)$, cal mol^{-1} K^{-1}	48.254	50.000
T, K	1000	1100

$$\Delta H^\circ(\delta \to \text{liq}) = 5500 \text{ cal mol}^{-1} \text{ at } 1157 \text{ K}$$

$$C_P^\circ(\text{liq}) = 47.180 \text{ cal mol}^{-1} \text{ K}^{-1} \text{ from } 1157 \text{ K to } 1500 \text{ K}$$

The contribution from 0 K to 15 K is found by assuming that $C_P^\circ = kT^3$, where

$$k = \frac{0.222}{15^3} = 6.58 \times 10^{-5}$$

Then (*4.9*) gives, since $S_0^\circ = 0$,

$$S_{15}^\circ = \int_{0\,\text{K}}^{15\,\text{K}} 6.58 \times 10^{-5} T^2\, dT = 0.074 \text{ eu mol}^{-1}$$

The remaining contribution of the heat capacities is found by graphical integration of Fig. 4-8 or Fig. 4-9, giving 103.16 eu mol^{-1}. The contributions from the phase changes are

$$S^\circ(\text{V} \to \text{IV}) = \frac{75}{458} = 0.164 \text{ eu mol}^{-1}$$

$$S^\circ(\text{IV} \to \text{I}) = \frac{2611}{514} = 5.080 \text{ eu mol}^{-1}$$

$$S^\circ(\text{I} \to \delta) = \frac{80}{980} = 0.082 \text{ eu mol}^{-1}$$

$$S^\circ(\delta \to \text{liq}) = \frac{5500}{1157} = 4.754 \text{ eu mol}^{-1}$$

Summing these values gives $S_{1500}^\circ = 113.31 \text{ eu mol}^{-1} = 474.09 \text{ EU mol}^{-1}$. The value reported in the JANAF tables is 112.973 eu mol^{-1}.

4.14 ΔS_T° FOR A CHEMICAL REACTION

The value of ΔS_T° for a chemical reaction is given by

$$\Delta S_T^\circ(\text{reaction}) = \sum_i^{\text{products}} n_i S_{T,i}^\circ - \sum_j^{\text{reactants}} n_j S_{T,j}^\circ \tag{4.14}$$

where n_i and n_j are the stoichiometric coefficients of the balanced equation.

Because the entropy content of a material reflects the amount of randomness in the material, the values of $\Delta S_T^\circ(\text{reaction})$ can be checked qualitatively by observing whether any transitions between the condensed phases and the gaseous state have occurred, whether a change in the number of gaseous moles has occurred, etc.

EXAMPLE 4.12. Calculate ΔS_{298}°(formation) for CH_3OH(liq) if the molar values of S_{298}° are 30.3 eu mol^{-1} for CH_3OH(liq), 1.372 eu mol^{-1} for C(graph), 31.208 eu mol^{-1} for H_2(g) and 49.003 eu mol^{-1} for O_2(g).

For the reaction

$$\text{C(graph)} + 2\text{H}_2\text{(g)} + \tfrac{1}{2}\text{O}_2\text{(g)} = \text{CH}_3\text{OH(liq)}$$

(*4.14*) gives

$$\begin{aligned}\Delta S_{298}^\circ &= [(1)S_{298,\,\text{CH}_3\text{OH}}^\circ] - [(1)S_{298,\,\text{C}}^\circ + (2)S_{298,\,\text{H}_2}^\circ + (\tfrac{1}{2})S_{298,\,\text{O}_2}^\circ] \\ &= [(1)(30.3)] - [(1)(1.372) + (2)(31.208) + (\tfrac{1}{2})(49.003)] \\ &= -58.0 \text{ eu} = -242.7 \text{ EU}\end{aligned}$$

or ΔS_{298}°(formation) $= -242.7$ EU mol^{-1}. As a qualitative check, there are 2.5 moles of a gas reacting with 1 mole of a solid to give 1 mole of a liquid, so a large decrease in randomness would be expected.

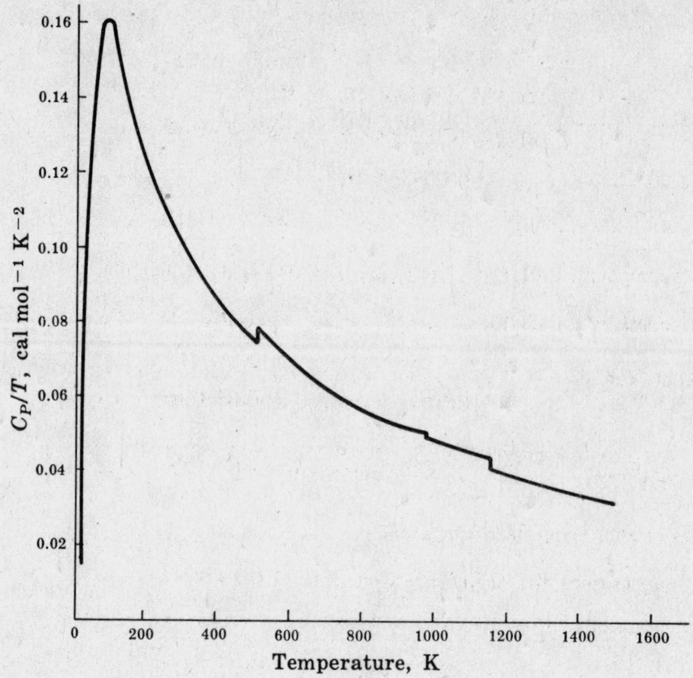
0.16
0.14
0.12
0.10
0.08
0.06
0.04
0.02
C_P/T, cal mol^{-1} K^{-2}
0
200
400
600
800
1000
1200
1400
1600
Temperature, K

Fig. 4-8

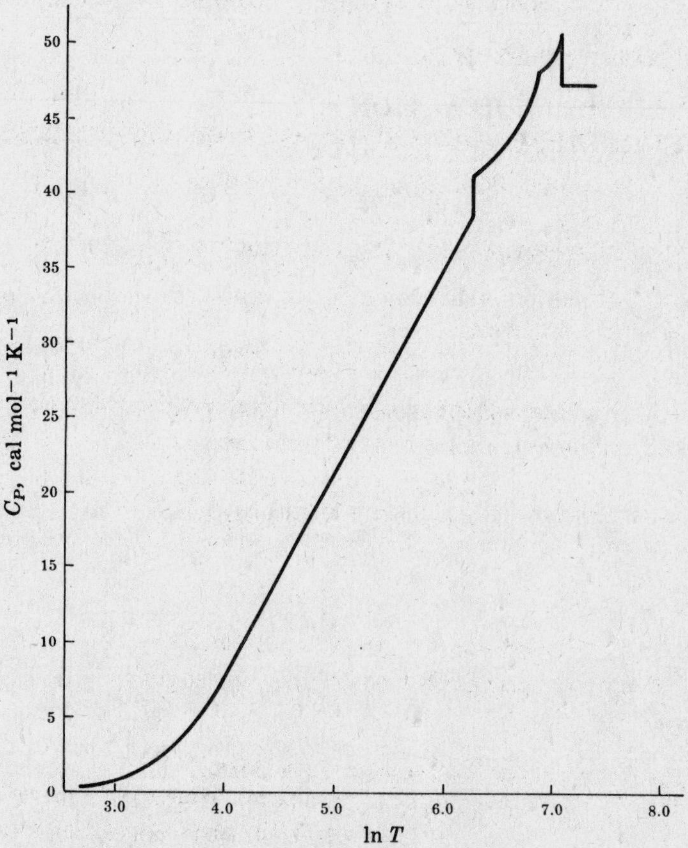
50
45
40
35
30
25
20
15
10
5
0
C_P, cal mol^{-1} K^{-1}
3.0
4.0
5.0
6.0
7.0
8.0
ln T

Fig. 4-9

EXAMPLE 4.13. Consider the reactions

$$\tfrac{1}{2}H_2(g) + \tfrac{1}{2}Cl_2(g) = HCl(g)$$
$$2C(graph) + 2H_2(g) = C_2H_4(g)$$
$$2C(graph) + \tfrac{5}{2}H_2(g) + \tfrac{1}{2}Cl_2(g) = C_2H_5Cl(g)$$

and the corresponding expressions for ΔS°_T(formation)

$$\Delta S^\circ_T(\text{formation, HCl}) = [(1)S^\circ_{T,\text{HCl}}] - [(\tfrac{1}{2})S^\circ_{T,\text{H}_2} + (\tfrac{1}{2})S^\circ_{T,\text{Cl}_2}]$$
$$\Delta S^\circ_T(\text{formation, C}_2\text{H}_4) = [(1)S^\circ_{T,\text{C}_2\text{H}_4}] - [(2)S^\circ_{T,\text{C}} + (2)S^\circ_{T,\text{H}_2}]$$
$$\Delta S^\circ_T(\text{formation, C}_2\text{H}_5\text{Cl}) = [(1)S^\circ_{T,\text{C}_2\text{H}_5\text{Cl}}] - [(2)S^\circ_{T,\text{C}} + (\tfrac{5}{2})S^\circ_{T,\text{H}_2} + (\tfrac{1}{2})S^\circ_{T,\text{Cl}_2}]$$

Show that ΔS°_T(reaction) for

$$HCl(g) + C_2H_4(g) = C_2H_5Cl(g)$$

is given by

$$\Delta S^\circ_T(\text{reaction}) = \sum_i^{\text{products}} n_i\,\Delta S^\circ_T(\text{formation}, i) - \sum_j^{\text{reactants}} n_j\,\Delta S^\circ_T(\text{formation}, j) \tag{4.15}$$

where n_i and n_j are the stoichiometric coefficients.

Substituting the expressions for ΔS°_T(formation) into (*4.15*) gives

$$\begin{aligned}\Delta S^\circ_T(\text{reaction}) = {} & [(1)S^\circ_{T,\text{C}_2\text{H}_5\text{Cl}} - (2)S^\circ_{T,\text{C}} - (\tfrac{5}{2})S^\circ_{T,\text{H}_2} - (\tfrac{1}{2})S^\circ_{T,\text{Cl}_2}] \\ & - [(1)S^\circ_{T,\text{HCl}} - (\tfrac{1}{2})S^\circ_{T,\text{H}_2} - (\tfrac{1}{2})S^\circ_{T,\text{Cl}_2} + (1)S^\circ_{T,\text{C}_2\text{H}_4} \\ & - (2)S^\circ_{T,\text{C}} - (2)S^\circ_{T,\text{H}_2}]\end{aligned}$$

Upon cancellation of common terms and rearrangment,

$$\Delta S^\circ_T(\text{reaction}) = [(1)S^\circ_{T,\text{C}_2\text{H}_5\text{Cl}}] - [(1)S^\circ_{T,\text{HCl}} + (1)S^\circ_{T,\text{C}_2\text{H}_4}]$$

which is identical to the equation predicted by (*4.14*).

4.15 TEMPERATURE DEPENDENCE OF ΔS°_T FOR A CHEMICAL REACTION

If ΔS°_{298}(reaction) is known, then ΔS°_T(reaction) is given by

$$\Delta S^\circ_T(\text{reaction}) = \Delta S^\circ_{298}(\text{reaction}) + \int_{298\,\text{K}}^{T} \frac{\Delta C^\circ_P}{T}\,dT \tag{4.16}$$

EXAMPLE 4.14. Calculate ΔS°_{1000}(reaction) for

$$H_2(g) + Cl_2(g) = 2HCl(g)$$

if $S^\circ_{298} = 31.208$ eu mol^{-1} for $H_2(g)$, 53.288 eu mol^{-1} for $Cl_2(g)$ and 44.646 eu mol^{-1} for HCl(g), and if

$$C^\circ_P = 6.9469 - 0.1999\times10^{-3}T + 4.808\times10^{-7}T^2 \quad \text{for } H_2(g)$$
$$C^\circ_P = 7.5755 + 2.4244\times10^{-3}T - 9.650\times10^{-7}T^2 \quad \text{for } Cl_2(g)$$
$$C^\circ_P = 6.7319 + 0.4325\times10^{-3}T + 3.697\times10^{-7}T^2 \quad \text{for } HCl(g)$$

all in cal mol^{-1} K^{-1}.

For the reaction, (*4.14*) gives

$$\begin{aligned}\Delta S^\circ_{298} &= [(2)S^\circ_{298,\text{HCl}}] - [(1)S^\circ_{298,\text{H}_2} + (1)S^\circ_{298,\text{Cl}_2}] \\ &= [(2)(44.646)] - [(1)(31.208) + (1)(53.288)] = 4.796 \text{ eu}\end{aligned}$$

The value of ΔC°_P is

$$\begin{aligned}\Delta C^\circ_P = {} & [(2)(6.7319) - (1)(6.9469) - (1)(7.5755)] \\ & + [(2)(0.4325) - (1)(-0.1999) - (1)(2.4244)]\times10^{-3}T \\ & + [(2)(3.697) - (1)(4.808) - (1)(-9.650)]\times10^{-7}T^2 \\ = {} & -1.0586 - 1.3595\times10^{-3}T + 12.236\times10^{-7}T^2\end{aligned}$$

giving

$$\Delta S^\circ_{1000} = 4.796 + \int_{298\text{ K}}^{1000\text{ K}} (-1.0586T^{-1} - 1.3595\times 10^{-3} + 12.236\times 10^{-7}T)\,dT$$

$$= 4.796 - (1.0586)\ln\frac{1000}{298} - (1.3595\times 10^{-3})(1000-298)$$

$$+ \left(\frac{12.236\times 10^{-7}}{2}\right)(1000^2 - 298^2)$$

$$= 4.796 - 1.282 - 0.954 + 0.557 = 3.117\text{ eu} = 13.042\text{ EU}$$

Solved Problems

The Second Law of Thermodynamics

4.1. Repeat the calculations of Example 4.1, using an ideal diatomic gas instead of the monatomic gas. Compare the results.

Assuming $C_V = (5/2)R$ for the diatomic gas,

$$V_3 = (0.1000\text{ m}^3)\left(\frac{773\text{ K}}{273\text{ K}}\right)^{5/2} = 1.349\text{ m}^3 \qquad V_4 = (1.349\text{ m}^3)\frac{0.0100}{0.1000} = 0.1349\text{ m}^3$$

The volume required for the cycle is much larger for the diatomic gas than for the monatomic gas.

For the first step:

$$\Delta E_{(1)} = 0$$

$$q_1 = w_1 = (1.00\text{ mol})(8.314\text{ J mol}^{-1}\text{ K}^{-1})(773\text{ K})\ln\frac{0.1000}{0.0100} = 14.80\text{ kJ}$$

for the second step:

$$q_2 = 0$$

$$\Delta E_{(2)} = -w_2 = (1.00\text{ mol})\left(\frac{5}{2}\right)(8.314\text{ J mol}^{-1}\text{ K}^{-1})(273\text{ K} - 773\text{ K}) = -10.39\text{ kJ}$$

for the third step:

$$\Delta E_{(3)} = 0$$

$$q_3 = w_3 = (1.00)(8.314)(273)\ln\frac{0.1345}{1.345} = -5.23\text{ kJ}$$

for the fourth step:

$$q_4 = 0$$

$$\Delta E_{(4)} = -w_4 = 10.39\text{ kJ}$$

and overall:

$$\Delta E = 0 + (-10.39) + 0 + 10.39 = 0$$

$$q = w = 14.80 + 0 + (-5.23) + 0 = 9.57\text{ kJ}$$

The values determined for the individual steps 2 and 4 differ because of the difference in heat capacities between the diatomic and monatomic gases, but the values determined for the individual steps 1 and 3, as well as the overall values, do not differ. The engine diagram is Fig. 4-3, as in the monatomic case.

4.2. What are the efficiencies of a Carnot engine operating as a heat engine between two reservoirs at 500 K and 100 K and as a refrigerator between the same reservoirs?

For the heat engine, (*4.2*) gives

$$\varepsilon_{\text{carnot}} = 100\,\frac{500\text{ K} - 100\text{ K}}{500\text{ K}} = 80\%$$

and (*4.3b*) gives for the refrigerator

$$\varepsilon_{\text{ref}} = 100\,\frac{500\text{ K} - 100\text{ K}}{100\text{ K}} = 400\%$$

4.3. Figure 4-10 shows a Carnot heat engine driving a Carnot refrigerator. Determine the value of q_h'.

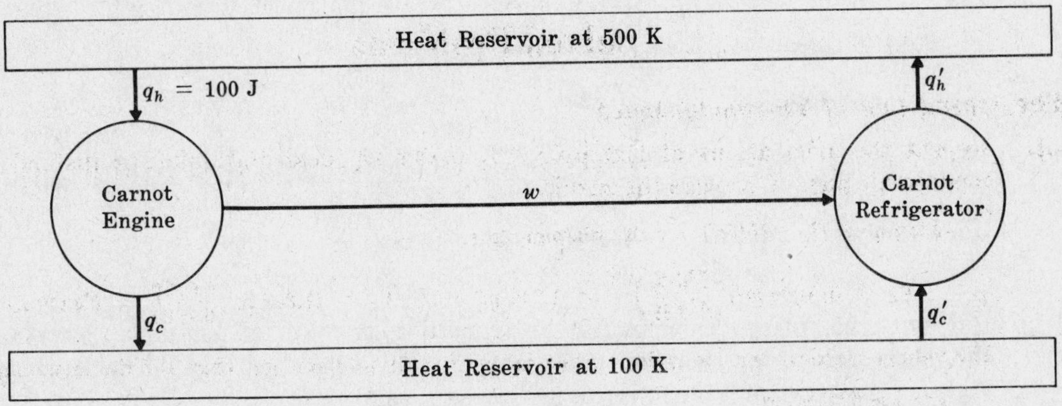

Fig. 4-10

The efficiencies of the Carnot engines are 80% and 400%, as calculated in Problem 4.2. If $q_h =$ 100 J, then from (*4.1*)

$$w = \varepsilon q_h = (0.80)(100\text{ J}) = 80\text{ J}$$

and

$$q_c = 100 - 80 = 20\text{ J}$$

If $w = 80$ J, then from (*4.3a*),

$$q_c' = \frac{w}{\varepsilon_{\text{ref}}} = \frac{80\text{ J}}{400/100} = 20\text{ J}$$

and

$$q_h' = 20 + 80 = 100\text{ J}$$

Entropy Calculations

4.4. Calculate ΔS(system) for the isothermal expansion of one mole of solid aluminum from 100.0 atm to 1.0 atm if $\alpha \equiv (1/V)(\partial V/\partial T)_P = 69 \times 10^{-6}\text{ K}^{-1}$ and $d = 2.702 \times 10^3\text{ kg m}^{-3}$.

Assuming that the pressure change can be performed reversibly, (*4.6*) gives

ΔS(system)

$$= -\int_{P_1}^{P_2}\left(\frac{\partial V}{\partial T}\right)_P dP = -\alpha V \int_{100.0}^{1.0} dP$$

$$= -(69 \times 10^{-6}\text{ K}^{-1})(1\text{ mol})\left(\frac{26.9815 \times 10^{-3}\text{ kg mol}^{-1}}{2.702 \times 10^3\text{ kg m}^{-3}}\right)(1.0 - 100.0)\text{ atm }(101{,}325\text{ J m}^{-3}\text{ atm}^{-1})$$

$$= 6.91 \times 10^{-3}\text{ EU}$$

4.5. What are the entropy changes for the isothermal compression of one mole of an ideal gas from 1.00 atm to 5.00 atm at 25 °C if the compression is performed (1) reversibly? (2) irreversibly using an external pressure of 100.0 atm?

For both processes (*1.6*) gives

$$V_1 = \frac{(1.00 \text{ mol})(0.0821 \text{ dm}^3 \text{ atm K}^{-1} \text{ mol}^{-1})(298 \text{ K})}{1.00 \text{ atm}} = 24.5 \text{ dm}^3$$

$$V_2 = \frac{(1.00)(0.0821)(298)}{5.00} = 4.9 \text{ dm}^3$$

which upon substitution into (*4.5*) gives

$$\Delta S(\text{system}) = (1.00 \text{ mol})(8.314 \text{ J mol}^{-1} \text{ K}^{-1}) \ln \frac{4.9}{24.5} = -13.38 \text{ EU}$$

For the reversible process,

$$\Delta S(\text{surroundings}) = 13.38 \text{ EU} \quad \text{and} \quad \Delta S(\text{universe}) = 0$$

For the irreversible process, (*2.25b*) gives

$$\Delta S(\text{surroundings}) = \frac{q}{T} = \frac{P\,\Delta V}{T}$$

$$= \frac{(100.0 \text{ atm})(24.5 \text{ dm}^3 - 4.9 \text{ dm}^3)(101{,}325 \text{ J m}^{-3} \text{ atm}^{-1})}{298 \text{ K}} = 666 \text{ EU}$$

and

$$\Delta S(\text{universe}) = 666 + (-13.38) = 653 \text{ EU}$$

4.6. Calculate the entropy changes for the transition at 368 K of one mole of sulfur from the monoclinic to the rhombic solid state, if $\Delta H = -96.01$ cal mol^{-1} for the transition. Assume the surroundings to be an ice-water bath at 0 °C.

Assuming the phase transition at 368 K to occur reversibly, (*4.8*) gives

$$\Delta S(\text{system}) = \frac{(1.00 \text{ mol})(-96.01 \text{ cal mol}^{-1})(4.184 \text{ J cal}^{-1})}{368 \text{ K}} = -1.092 \text{ EU}$$

The ice-water bath absorbs the 96.01 cal mol^{-1} = 401.71 J mol^{-1} at a temperature of 0 °C, so for the surroundings

$$\Delta S(\text{surroundings}) = \frac{(1.00 \text{ mol})(401.71 \text{ J mol}^{-1})}{273 \text{ K}} = 1.471 \text{ EU}$$

Summing these gives

$$\Delta S(\text{universe}) = (-1.092) + 1.471 = 0.379 \text{ EU}$$

4.7. Calculate the entropy changes for heating one mole of silver from 298 K to 1500 K at constant pressure if the process is performed (1) reversibly; (2) irreversibly by placing the silver in an oven at 1500 K. The average value of C_P for silver is 25.9 J mol^{-1} K^{-1}.

For both processes, (*4.9*) gives

$$\Delta S(\text{system}) = (1 \text{ mol}) \int_{T_1}^{T_2} \frac{25.9}{T}\, dT = (25.9) \ln \frac{1500}{298} = 41.9 \text{ EU}$$

For the reversible process,

$$\Delta S(\text{surroundings}) = -41.9 \text{ EU} \quad \text{and} \quad \Delta S(\text{universe}) = 0$$

For the irreversible process, q for the surroundings is

$$q = -(1 \text{ mol}) \int_{T_1}^{T_2} C_P\, dT = -(25.9)(T_2 - T_1) = -(25.9)(1500 - 298) = -31.13 \text{ kJ}$$

and (*4.7*) gives

$$\Delta S(\text{surroundings}) = -\frac{31{,}130}{1500} = -20.75 \text{ EU}$$

For the universe,

$$\Delta S(\text{universe}) = 41.9 + (-20.75) = 21.2 \text{ EU}$$

4.8. What are the values of the entropy changes for the cooling of one mole of O_2(g) from 298 K to O_2(liq) at 90.19 K if the process is done (1) reversibly? (2) irreversibly by placing the sample in liquid hydrogen at 13.96 K? Assume ΔH(vaporization) = 1630 cal mol^{-1} at 90.19 K and $C_P = (7/2)R$ for the gas.

Considering the process to be a combination of a reversible cooling at constant pressure and a reversible phase transition, (*4.9*) and (*4.8*) give for both processes

$$\begin{aligned}\Delta S(\text{system}) &= \int_{298\,\text{K}}^{90.19\,\text{K}} \frac{C_P}{T}\,dT + \frac{-\Delta H(\text{vaporization})}{T_{bp}} \\ &= (1.00\text{ mol})\left(\frac{7}{2}\right)(8.314\text{ J mol}^{-1}\text{ K}^{-1})\ln\frac{90.19\text{ K}}{298\text{ K}} \\ &\quad + \frac{(1.00\text{ mol})(-1630\text{ cal mol}^{-1})(4.184\text{ J cal}^{-1})}{90.19\text{ K}} \\ &= (-34. \quad + (-75.62) = -110.40\text{ EU}\end{aligned}$$

For the reversible process,

$$\Delta S(\text{surroundings}) = 110.40\text{ EU} \quad \text{and} \quad \Delta S(\text{universe}) = 0$$

For the irreversible process, q for the surroundings is

$$\begin{aligned} q &= -\int_{298\,\text{K}}^{90.19\,\text{K}} C_P\,dT + \Delta H(\text{vaporization}) \\ &= -(1.00\text{ mol})\left(\frac{7}{2}\right)(8.314\text{ J mol}^{-1}\text{ K}^{-1})(90.19\text{ K} - 298\text{ K}) \\ &\quad + (1.00\text{ mol})(1630\text{ cal mol}^{-1})(4.184\text{ J cal}^{-1}) = 12.87\text{ kJ}\end{aligned}$$

and (*4.7*) gives

$$\Delta S(\text{surroundings}) = \frac{12{,}870}{13.96} = 922\text{ EU} \quad \text{and} \quad \Delta S(\text{universe}) = 922 + (-110.40) = 812\text{ EU}$$

The Third Law of Thermodynamics

4.9. What is the value of S_0° for a mole of CO or NO?

In the solid state there are two possible orientations of the molecule. Using (*4.12*) gives

$$S_0^\circ = (1\text{ mol})(8.314\text{ J mol}^{-1}\text{ K}^{-1})\ln 2 = 5.763\text{ EU}$$

4.10. Compare the ΔS_{298}°(formation) of H_2O(g) and H_2O(liq) if $S_{298}^\circ = 31.208$ eu mol^{-1} for H_2(g), 49.003 eu mol^{-1} for O_2(g), 16.71 eu mol^{-1} for H_2O(liq) and 45.104 eu mol^{-1} for H_2O(g).

Applying (*4.14*) to the reaction

$$H_2(g) + \tfrac{1}{2}O_2(g) = H_2O$$

gives

$$\Delta S_{298}^\circ = [(1)S_{298,\,H_2O}^\circ] - [(1)S_{298,\,H_2(g)}^\circ + (\tfrac{1}{2})S_{298,\,O_2(g)}^\circ]$$

For the gaseous water

$$\begin{aligned}\Delta S_{298}^\circ &= [(1)(45.104)] - [(1)(31.208) + (\tfrac{1}{2})(49.003)] \\ &= -10.606\text{ eu} = -44.376\text{ EU}\end{aligned}$$

or ΔS_{298}°(formation) = -44.376 EU mol^{-1}, indicating a slight decrease in randomness as 1.5 moles of gaseous reactants form 1 mole of gaseous products.

For forming water in the liquid state

$$\begin{aligned}\Delta S_{298}^\circ &= [(1)(16.71)] - [(1)(31.208) + (\tfrac{1}{2})(49.003)] \\ &= -39.00\text{ eu} = -163.18\text{ EU}\end{aligned}$$

or ΔS_{298}°(formation) = -163.18 EU mol^{-1}, indicating a large decrease in randomness as 1.5 moles of gaseous reactants form 1 mole of products in the liquid state.

4.11. The reaction

$$C_2H_5OH(liq) + HI(g) = C_2H_5I(liq) + H_2O(liq)$$

was run at 60 °C in order to change the rate of reaction. If $S^\circ_{298} = 38.4$ eu mol^{-1} for $C_2H_5OH(liq)$, 49.351 eu mol^{-1} for HI(g), 50.6 eu mol^{-1} for $C_2H_5I(liq)$ and 16.71 eu mol^{-1} for $H_2O(liq)$, and if $C^\circ_P = 26.64$ cal mol^{-1} K^{-1} for $C_2H_5OH(liq)$, 6.969 for HI(g), 27.5 for $C_2H_5I(liq)$ and 17.995 for $H_2O(liq)$, calculate ΔS°_{333} for the reaction.

Applying (*4.14*) to the reaction gives

$$\Delta S^\circ_{298}(\text{reaction}) = [(1)S^\circ_{298,\,C_2H_5I} + (1)S^\circ_{298,\,H_2O}] - [(1)S^\circ_{298,\,C_2H_5OH} + (1)S^\circ_{298,\,HI}]$$

$$= [(1)(50.6) + (1)(16.71)] - [(1)(38.4) + (1)(49.351)] = -20.4 \text{ eu}$$

The value of ΔC°_P is

$$\Delta C^\circ_P = [(1)(27.5) + (1)(17.995)] - [(1)(26.64) + (1)(6.969)] = 11.9 \text{ cal K}^{-1}$$

and (*4.16*) gives

$$\Delta S^\circ_{333}(\text{reaction}) = -20.4 + \int_{298\text{ K}}^{333\text{ K}} \frac{11.9}{T}\,dT$$

$$= -20.4 + (11.9)\ln\frac{333}{298} = -19.1 \text{ eu} = -79.9 \text{ EU}$$

4.12. The voltage of the electrochemical cell for the reaction

$$Ag(s) + \tfrac{1}{2}Cl_2(g) = AgCl(liq)$$

as reported by Metz and Seifert is given by $\mathcal{E}^\circ = 0.9081 - 0.280\,X + 0.110\,X^2$ where $X = (T - 728.2)10^{-3}$ K. If

$$\Delta S^\circ = n\mathcal{F}\frac{d\mathcal{E}^\circ}{dT}$$

where $n = 1$ mol and $\mathcal{F} = 9.648456 \times 10^4$ C mol^{-1} find an expression for ΔS° and determine its value at 1000 K.

The chain rule of differentiation,

$$\frac{dx}{dy} = \frac{dx}{dz}\frac{dz}{dy} \qquad (4.17)$$

gives

$$\Delta S^\circ_T = n\mathcal{F}\frac{d\mathcal{E}^\circ}{dT} = n\mathcal{F}\frac{d\mathcal{E}^\circ}{dX}\frac{dX}{dT}$$

$$= (1\text{ mol})(9.648456 \times 10^4 \text{ C mol}^{-1})(\text{s A/C})(\text{J/s A V})[(-0.280) + (0.110)(2)X](10^{-3})(\text{V/K})$$

$$= (-27.02 + 21.23\,X) \text{ J K}^{-1}$$

At 1000 K,

$$\Delta S^\circ_{1000}(\text{reaction}) = -27.02 + (21.23)(1000 - 728.2)10^{-3} = -27.02 + 5.77 = -21.25 \text{ EU}$$

Supplementary Problems

The Second Law of Thermodynamics

4.13. What is the maximum efficiency of a steam engine operating between 120 °C and 20 °C?

Ans. $\varepsilon_{carnot} = 25.4\%$

4.14. Equation (4.4a) can be rearranged into

$$đq_{rev} = T\,dS$$

which upon integration gives

$$q_{rev} = \int T\,dS$$

A graphical integration of a plot of T against S will thus give the value of q_{rev}. Prepare a plot for the Carnot cycle described in Example 4.1 and perform the graphical integration to evaluate q_{rev}, which is equal to w. For this calculation it is not necessary to know the original value of S for the gas, so assume a value of zero to make the graphing and calculations easier.

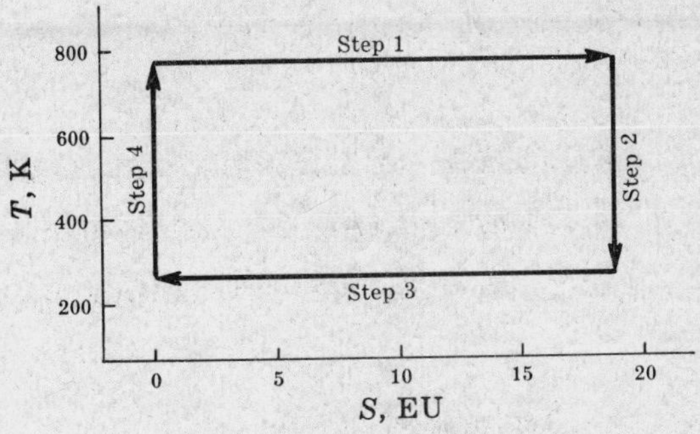

Fig. 4-11

Ans. $\Delta S_{(1)} = 14{,}800/773 = 19.15$, $\Delta S_{(2)} = 0$, $\Delta S_{(3)} = -19.15$, $\Delta S_{(4)} = 0$ (see Fig. 4-11); $q_{rev} = w = 9.59$ kJ

4.15. Prepare a plot of P against V for the Carnot engine described in Example 4.1 and perform the graphical integration to evaluate w. Assume a linear plot between V_2 and V_3 and between V_3 and V_4.

Ans. See Fig. 4-12; 9.75 kJ.

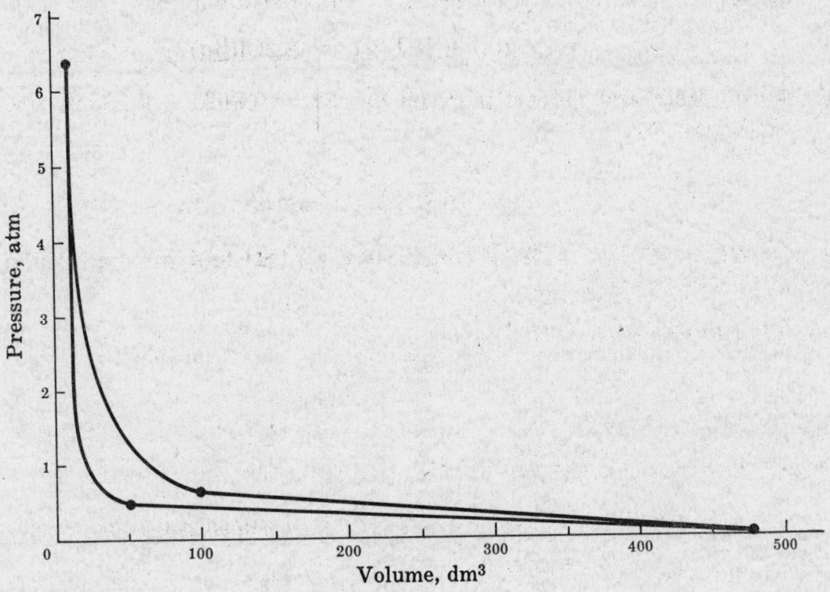

Fig. 4-12

4.16. Repeat the calculations of Example 4.1 using an ideal nonlinear triatomic gas instead of the monatomic gas.

Ans. $C_V = 3R$, $V_3 = 2.270\ \text{m}^3$, $V_4 = 0.227\ \text{m}^3$, $\Delta E_{(1)} = 0$, $q_1 = w_1 = 14.80$ kJ, $q_2 = 0$, $\Delta E_{(2)} = -w_2 = -12.47$ kJ, $\Delta E_{(3)} = 0$, $q_3 = w_3 = -5.23$ kJ, $q_4 = 0$, $\Delta E_{(4)} = -w_4 = -12.47$ kJ, $\Delta E = 0$, $q = w = 9.57$ kJ

Entropy Calculations

4.17. Calculate ΔS(system) for the isothermal expansion of one mole of CCl_4(liq) from 100.0 atm to 1.0 atm if $\alpha = 1.25 \times 10^{-3}\ \text{K}^{-1}$ and $d = 1.5940 \times 10^3\ \text{kg m}^{-3}$. *Ans.* 1.210 EU

4.18. Calculate the entropy changes for melting one mole of sulfur from the monoclinic state at 388 K if ΔH(fusion) = 410 cal mol^{-1}. Assume the sulfur is placed in a burner flame at 1400 °C.

Ans. ΔH = 1715 J mol^{-1}, ΔS(system) = 4.42 EU, ΔS(surroundings) = −1.03 EU, ΔS(universe) = 3.39 EU

4.19. Calculate the entropy changes for evaporating one mole of superheated water at 110 °C and 1 atm, given ΔH(vaporization) = 9596 cal mol^{-1} at 1.414 atm and 110 °C and $(\partial V/\partial T)_P = -0.15 \times 10^{-6}$ m^3 K^{-1} for water. *Hint*: Use cycle of pressure increase, evaporation and pressure decrease.

Ans. ΔS(system) = 107.72 EU, ΔS(surroundings) = −104.83 EU, ΔS(universe) = 2.89 EU

4.20. Calculate ΔS(system) for isothermally preparing a mixture containing 99 moles of O_2(g) and 1 mole of N_2(g). *Ans.* 46.60 EU

4.21. What is the value of ΔS(system) if 0.5 mole of CCl_4(liq) is mixed with 0.5 mole of CH_2Cl_2(liq) at 25 °C and the final temperature of the solution was 27 °C? Assume C_P = 31.49 cal mol^{-1} K^{-1} for CCl_4(liq) and 23.9 for CH_2Cl_2(liq).

Ans. ΔS(mixing) = 5.762 EU, ΔS(heating) = 0.440 EU for CCl_4 and 0.334 EU for CH_2Cl_2; 6.536 EU

The Third Law of Thermodynamics

4.22. Calculate ΔS(mixing) for preparing one mole of an ideal solid solution having the composition $x_{AgBr(s)} = 0.728$ and $x_{AgCl(s)} = 0.272$. The value of $S^\circ_{298} - S^\circ_{15}$ for the solution was determined as 0.0 ± 0.1 eu mol^{-1} by Eastman and Milner. Determine S°_0 for this mixture assuming that $S^\circ_{15} - S^\circ_0 = 0$.

Ans. 4.86 EU, 4.86 EU

4.23. Calculate ΔS°_{298} for the reaction

$$CaCO_3(\text{calcite}) = CaCO_3(\text{aragonite})$$

if S°_{298} = 22.2 eu mol^{-1} for calcite and 21.2 eu mol^{-1} for aragonite. Qualitatively interpret the results.

Ans. −1.0 eu = −4.2 EU, a small change in randomness resulting from one mole of a condensed phase being transformed into one mole of a condensed phase.

4.24. Calculate ΔS°_{298}(reaction) for the deamination of L-aspartic acid to fumaric acid:

$$\text{HOOC—}\underset{\text{NH}_2}{\underset{|}{\text{CH}}}\text{—CH}_2\text{—COOH} = \text{HOOC—CH=CH—COOH} + \text{NH}_3$$

given that the entropies of formation for the acids, as reported by Burton and Krebs, are −194.1 eu mol^{-1} for L-aspartic acid and −126.2 eu mol^{-1} for fumaric acid, and ΔS°_{298}(formation, NH_3) = −23.72 eu mol^{-1}.

Ans. 44.2 eu = 184.9 EU, a large increase in randomness resulting from the production of 1 mol of gas and 1 mol of condensed phase from 1 mol of condensed phase.

4.25. The transition between monoclinic and rhombic sulfur is quite slow and it is possible to supercool the monoclinic form to 0 K. Find S°_0 for the metastable monoclinic form if $S^\circ_0 = 0$ for the rhombic form, $S^\circ_{298} - S^\circ_0$ = 7.62 eu mol^{-1} for the rhombic form and $S^\circ_{298} - S^\circ_0$ = 7.78 eu mol^{-1} for the monoclinic form. Assume C°_P = 5.40 cal mol^{-1} K^{-1} for the rhombic form and 5.65 cal mol^{-1} K^{-1} for the monoclinic form, between 298 K and 368.54 K. ΔH°(rhombic → monoclinic) = 96.01 cal mol^{-1} at 368.54 K.

Ans. Use the process rhombic(0 K) → rhombic(298 K) → rhombic(368.54 K) → monoclinic(368.54 K) → monoclinic(298 K) → monoclinic(0 K) to obtain $S^\circ_{0,\text{monoclinic}}$ = 0.05 eu mol^{-1} = 0.21 EU mol^{-1}.

4.26. Calculate S°_{298} and S°_{1500} for Cu from the following data:

C°_P, cal mol^{-1} K^{-1}	T, K	C°_P, cal mol^{-1} K^{-1}	T, K	C°_P, cal mol^{-1} K^{-1}	T, K
0.00018	1	0.41	30	6.16	500
0.00042	2	0.89	40	6.31	600
0.00081	3	1.47	50	6.46	700
0.0014	4	2.84	75	6.61	800
0.0023	5	3.83	100	6.76	900
0.0072	8	4.90	150	6.91	1000
0.013	10	5.41	200	7.06	1100
0.044	15	5.68	250	7.21	1200
0.11	20	5.85	298	7.36	1300
0.23	25	6.01	400		

$$\Delta H^\circ(\text{fusion}) = 3120 \text{ cal mol}^{-1} \text{ at } 1356 \text{ K}$$

$$C^\circ_P = 7.50 \text{ cal mol}^{-1}\text{ K}^{-1} \text{ for the liquid from 1356 K to 1500 K}$$

Ans. 7.97 eu mol^{-1} = 33.35 EU mol^{-1}, 20.81 eu mol^{-1} = 87.07 EU mol^{-1}

4.27. For the reaction

$$Ag(s) + \tfrac{1}{2}Cl_2(g) = AgCl(liq)$$

Metz and Seifert reported $\Delta C^\circ_P = 3.70 + 5.08\,X$ in cal mol^{-1} K^{-1}, where $X = (T - 728.2)10^{-3}$. If $\Delta S^\circ_{728} = -6.47$ eu, find ΔS°_{1000}. *Ans.* -5.09 eu = -21.30 EU

4.28. Calculate ΔS for the flame reaction described in Example 3.1. Assume $S^\circ_{298} = 49.003$ eu mol^{-1} for $O_2(g)$, 31.208 eu mol^{-1} for $H_2(g)$ and 45.104 eu mol^{-1} for $H_2O(g)$.

Ans. $\Delta S^\circ_{298}(\text{reaction}) = -44.376$ EU, $\Delta S = 201.0$ EU for heating; 156.6 EU

Chapter 5

Free Energy and Chemical Equilibrium

Free Energy

5.1 DEFINITION AND SIGNIFICANCE

The *Gibbs free energy* (or just *free energy*), G, is defined as

$$G \equiv H - TS \tag{5.1}$$

and the *Helmholtz free energy, A*, is defined as

$$A \equiv E - TS \tag{5.2}$$

Because absolute values for H and E are difficult to calculate, absolute values of G and A are not used. Instead, processes are analyzed in terms of changes in free energies, where

$$\Delta G = \Delta H - \Delta(TS) \tag{5.3}$$

$$\Delta A = \Delta E - \Delta(TS) \tag{5.4}$$

Under constant pressure and temperature conditions, ΔG will be negative for a spontaneous process, positive for a nonspontaneous process, and zero for a state of equilibrium. Similar statements hold true for the values of ΔA for processes performed under constant volume and temperature conditions.

A superscript $^\circ$ attached to the symbol for the free energy implies standard pressure conditions (1 atm) for the substances involved in the process.

EXAMPLE 5.1. What is the value of $\Delta G^\circ - \Delta A^\circ$ for the combustion of benzoic acid at 25 °C?

Subtracting (*5.4*) from (*5.3*) and substituting (*2.11*) gives

$$\Delta G - \Delta A = \Delta(PV) \tag{5.5}$$

For the reaction

$$C_6H_5COOH(s) + \tfrac{15}{2}O_2(g) = 7CO_2(g) + 3H_2O(liq)$$

the contribution of the condensed phases to $\Delta(PV)$ in (*5.5*) is negligible (see Section 3.3), giving

$$\Delta G^\circ - \Delta A^\circ = RT\,\Delta n_g = (8.314\ \mathrm{J\ mol^{-1}\ K^{-1}})(298\ \mathrm{K})(-\tfrac{1}{2}\ \mathrm{mol}) = -1239\ \mathrm{J}$$

EXAMPLE 5.2. The standard-state emf for the Daniell-cell reaction

$$Zn(s) + Cu^{2+}(1M) = Zn^{2+}(1M) + Cu(s)$$

at 25 °C was reported by Buckbee, Surdzial and Metz as 1.0913 V. What is ΔG°_{298}(reaction)? Is this reaction spontaneous?

Values of ΔG can be calculated from experimental electrochemical measurements using the relationship

$$\Delta G = -n\mathcal{F}\mathcal{E} \tag{5.6}$$

where n is the number of moles of electrons (equivalents) in the balanced reaction, $\mathcal{F}$ is the Faraday constant (9.648456×10^4 C mol^{-1} = 9.648456×10^4 J mol^{-1} V^{-1}) and $\mathcal{E}$ is the cell potential. Substituting into (*5.6*) gives

$$\Delta G^\circ_{298}(\text{reaction}) = -(2\text{ mol})(96.485\text{ kJ mol}^{-1}\text{ V}^{-1})(1.0913\text{ V}) = -210.59\text{ kJ}$$

Because the reaction takes place under standard conditions, $\Delta G^\circ = \Delta G$ and the large negative value for ΔG indicates a spontaneous reaction.

EXAMPLE 5.3. The differential of (*5.1*) is

$$dG = dE + P\,dV + V\,dP - T\,dS - S\,dT \tag{5.7}$$

What is the significance of dG for a reversible isobaric and isothermal process? Qualitatively discuss this interpretation for the reaction considered in Example 5.2, where $\Delta H^\circ_{298}(\text{reaction}) = -228.53$ kJ.

Under reversible constant pressure and temperature conditions, (*5.7*) becomes

$$dG = P\,dV - đw_{\text{rev}} \tag{5.8}$$

Equation (*5.8*) implies that the free energy is the net useful work that may be obtained from a reversible process performed under these restraints.

For the Daniell cell, of the 228.53 kJ of heat released by the chemical reaction, only 210.59 kJ was available for doing useful work. The remainder of the energy was lost to PV-expansion of the system, etc.

5.2 FREE ENERGY CALCULATIONS

For the large number of processes of chemical interest that occur at constant temperature, (*5.3*) can be simplified to

$$\Delta G = \Delta H - T\,\Delta S \tag{5.9}$$

EXAMPLE 5.4. For any phase transition, (*4.8*) gives $T\,\Delta S = \Delta H$, and so $\Delta G = 0$.

EXAMPLE 5.5. What is $G - G^\circ$ for one mole of an ideal gas at 1.00×10^{-3} torr and 25 °C?

For an isothermal expansion from P_1 to P_2 (*2.24b*), (*4.5*) and (*5.9*) give

$$\Delta G = nRT \ln \frac{P_2}{P_1} = nRT \ln \frac{V_1}{V_2} \tag{5.10}$$

Here $P_1 = 1$ atm $= 760$ torr and $P_2 = 1.00 \times 10^{-3}$ torr, so that

$$\Delta G = G - G^\circ = (1.00\text{ mol})(8.314\text{ J mol}^{-1}\text{ K}^{-1})(298\text{ K}) \ln \frac{1.00 \times 10^{-3}}{760}$$

$$= (1.00)(8.314)(298)(-13.542) = -33.55\text{ kJ}$$

The logarithm term was evaluated using the techniques presented in Problem 1.20.

EXAMPLE 5.6. Calculate $\Delta G^\circ_{298}(\text{formation})$ for gaseous and liquid H_2O if $\Delta H^\circ_{298}(\text{formation}) = -57.796$ and -68.315 kcal mol^{-1} and $S^\circ_{298} = 45.104$ and 16.71 eu mol^{-1}, respectively. Assume $S^\circ_{298} = 31.208$ eu mol^{-1} for H_2(g) and 49.003 eu mol^{-1} for O_2(g). Use (*5.10*) to predict the vapor pressure above the liquid at equilibrium.

For the reaction

$$H_2(g) + \tfrac{1}{2}O_2(g) = H_2O$$

the values of ΔS°_{298} are given by (*4.14*) as

$$\begin{aligned}\Delta S^\circ_{298}(\text{liq}) &= [(1)S^\circ_{298}(\text{liq})] - [(1)S^\circ_{298}(H_2) + (\tfrac{1}{2})S^\circ_{298}(O_2)]\\ &= [(1)(16.71)] - [(1)(31.208) + (\tfrac{1}{2})(49.003)]\\ &= -39.00\text{ eu} = -163.2\text{ EU}\end{aligned}$$

or ΔS°_{298}(formation, liq) $= -163.2$ EU mol^{-1}, and

$$\Delta S^\circ_{298}(g) = [(1)(45.104)] - [(1)(31.208) + (\tfrac{1}{2})(49.003)]$$
$$= -10.606 \text{ eu} = -44.38 \text{ EU}$$

or ΔS°_{298}(formation, g) $= -44.38$ EU mol^{-1}. Then (*5.9*) gives

$$\Delta G^\circ_{298}(\text{formation, liq}) = (-68.315 \text{ kcal mol}^{-1})(4.184 \text{ kJ kcal}^{-1}) - (298 \text{ K})(-163.2 \times 10^{-3} \text{ kJ K}^{-1} \text{ mol}^{-1})$$
$$= -237.20 \text{ kJ mol}^{-1}$$

$$\Delta G^\circ_{298}(\text{formation, g}) = (-57.796)(4.184) - (298)(-44.38 \times 10^{-3}) = -228.59 \text{ kJ mol}^{-1}$$

Under standard conditions at 25 °C, hydrogen will react with oxygen to produce liquid water having some gaseous water, at vapor pressure P, in equilibrium with it. To predict P, consider the following reactions

$$H_2O(\text{liq}) = H_2O(g, P)$$
$$H_2O(g, P) = H_2O(g, 1.00 \text{ atm})$$

For the first reaction $\Delta G^\circ_{(1)} = 0$ (see Example 5.4) and for the second reaction (*5.10*) gives

$$\Delta G^\circ_{(2)} = nRT \ln \frac{1.00 \text{ atm}}{P}$$

For the overall process $H_2O(\text{liq}) = H_2O(g, 1.00 \text{ atm})$,

$$\Delta G^\circ = \Delta G^\circ_{(1)} + \Delta G^\circ_{(2)}$$

where ΔG° for the reaction is given by

$$\Delta G^\circ(\text{reaction}) = \sum_i^{\text{products}} n_i \, \Delta G^\circ(\text{formation}, i) - \sum_j^{\text{reactants}} n_j \Delta G^\circ(\text{formation}, j) \tag{5.11}$$

Substituting values gives

$$(1)\Delta G(\text{formation, g}) - (1)\Delta G^\circ(\text{formation, liq}) = \Delta G^\circ_{(1)} + \Delta G^\circ_{(2)}$$
$$(1)(-228.59 \times 10^3) - (1)(-237.20 \times 10^3) = 0 + (1.00)(8.314)(298) \ln \frac{1.00}{P}$$
$$\ln \frac{1.00}{P} = 3.475$$
$$P = 0.0310 \text{ atm} = 3140 \text{ N m}^{-2}$$

5.3 PRESSURE AND TEMPERATURE DEPENDENCE OF G

For reversible processes having only expansion work, (*5.7*) becomes

$$dG = V\,dP - S\,dT$$

which implies that

$$\left(\frac{\partial G}{\partial P}\right)_T = V \tag{5.12}$$

$$\left(\frac{\partial G}{\partial T}\right)_P = -S \tag{5.13}$$

The temperature dependence of ΔG is given by

$$\frac{1}{T_2}\Delta G_{T_2} = \frac{1}{T_1}\Delta G_{T_1} - \int_{T_1}^{T_2} \frac{\Delta H}{T^2}\,dT \tag{5.14}$$

If the temperature dependence of ΔH is described by (*3.6*), then

$$\Delta G_T = J + KT - \Delta a\, T \ln T - \frac{\Delta b}{2}T^2 - \frac{\Delta c}{6}T^3 - \frac{\Delta d}{12}T^4 \qquad (5.15a)$$

$$\Delta G_T = J' + K'T - \Delta a\, T \ln T - \frac{\Delta b}{2}T^2 - \frac{\Delta c'}{2}T^{-1} \qquad (5.15b)$$

where

$$K \equiv \frac{\Delta G_{298} - J}{298} + \Delta a \ln 298 + \frac{\Delta b}{2}(298) + \frac{\Delta c}{6}(298^2) + \frac{\Delta d}{12}(298^3) \qquad (5.16a)$$

$$K' \equiv \frac{\Delta G_{298} - J'}{298} + \Delta a \ln 298 + \frac{\Delta b}{2}(298) + \frac{\Delta c'}{2}(298^{-2}) \qquad (5.16b)$$

Tabulated values of the free energy function $(G_T^\circ - H_0^\circ)/T$ are convenient for determining ΔG_T°(reaction). The change in this free energy function for a reaction is given by

$$\frac{\Delta(G_T^\circ - H_0^\circ)}{T} = \sum_i^{\text{products}} n_i \left\{\frac{G_T^\circ - H_0^\circ}{T}\right\}_i - \sum_j^{\text{reactants}} n_j \left\{\frac{G_T^\circ - H_0^\circ}{T}\right\}_j \qquad (5.17a)$$

and the temperature dependence of ΔG°(reaction) by

$$\Delta G_T^\circ(\text{reaction}) = T\left[\frac{\Delta(G_T^\circ - H_0^\circ)}{T}\right] + \Delta H_0^\circ(\text{reaction}) \qquad (5.18a)$$

EXAMPLE 5.7. For many years the standard room temperature was 20 °C instead of 25 °C. What value of ΔG° would a worker report at 20 °C for the reaction

$$\text{S(monoclinic)} = \text{S(rhombic)}$$

if ΔH_{298}°(formation) = 71 and 0 cal mol^{-1}, ΔG_{298}°(formation) = 23 and 0 cal mol^{-1}, and C_P° = 5.65 and 5.40 cal mol^{-1} K^{-1} for the monoclinic and rhombic forms, respectively?

At 298 K

$$\Delta H^\circ(\text{reaction}) = (1)(0) - (1)(71) = -71 \text{ cal} = -297 \text{ J}$$

$$\Delta G^\circ(\text{reaction}) = (1)(0) - (1)(23) = -23 \text{ cal} = -96 \text{ J}$$

$$\Delta C_P^\circ = (1)(5.40) - (1)(5.65) = -0.25 \text{ cal K}^{-1} = -1.05 \text{ J K}^{-1}$$

Supposing C_P° temperature-independent, we have $\Delta b = \Delta c = \Delta d = 0$ and $\Delta a = \Delta C_P^\circ$ in (*3.5a*) and (*5.16a*). Hence

$$J = -297 - (-1.05)(298) = -297 - (-313) = 16 \text{ J}$$

and
$$K = \frac{-96 - 16}{298} + (-1.05)\ln 298 = -0.376 + (-5.98) = -6.36 \text{ J K}^{-1}$$

Now (*5.15a*) gives

$$\Delta G_{293}^\circ(\text{reaction}) = 16 + (-6.36)(293) - (-1.05)(293)\ln 293$$
$$= 16 - 1866 + 1748 = -102 \text{ J}$$

EXAMPLE 5.8. Because of the availability of ΔH_{298}°(formation) data, it is convenient to use a free energy function based on 298 K instead of 0 K. Find the relation between $(G_T^\circ - H_{298}^\circ)/T$ and $(G_T^\circ - H_0^\circ)/T$, and rewrite (*5.17a*) and (*5.18a*) for the function based on 298 K.

By adding and subtracting H_0° in the numerator of the function based on 298 K, we obtain

$$\frac{G_T^\circ - H_{298}^\circ}{T} = \frac{G_T^\circ - H_{298}^\circ + H_0^\circ - H_0^\circ}{T} = \frac{G_T^\circ - H_0^\circ}{T} - \frac{H_{298}^\circ - H_0^\circ}{T} \qquad (5.19)$$

In terms of the function based on 298 K, (*5.17a*) and (*5.18a*) become

$$\frac{\Delta(G_T^\circ - H_{298}^\circ)}{T} = \sum_i^{\text{products}} n_i \left\{\frac{G_T^\circ - H_{298}^\circ}{T}\right\}_i - \sum_j^{\text{reactants}} n_j \left\{\frac{G_T^\circ - H_{298}^\circ}{T}\right\}_j \qquad (5.17b)$$

$$\Delta G_T^\circ(\text{reaction}) = T\left[\frac{\Delta(G_T^\circ - H_{298}^\circ)}{T}\right] + \Delta H_{298}^\circ(\text{reaction}) \qquad (5.18b)$$

Activities

5.4 INTRODUCTION

For a substance undergoing an isothermal change from state 1 to state 2,

$$G_2 - G_1 = nRT \ln\frac{a_2}{a_1} \qquad (5.20)$$

where a_i is the *activity* of the substance in state *i*. If state 1 is the standard state where $a_1 = a^\circ = 1.00$ atm, then

$$G - G^\circ = nRT \ln a \qquad (5.21)$$

provided that a is expressed in atm. Sections 5.5 through 5.8 consider the determination of the activities for ideal and real gases, liquids, solids, and the solutes in electrolytic solutions. Activities of solvents and nonelectrolytic solutions are considered in Section 9.9.

5.5 ACTIVITIES FOR IDEAL GASES

Integration of (*5.12*) gives (*5.21*) if

$$a = P \qquad (5.22)$$

where P is expressed in atmospheres.

EXAMPLE 5.9. What is $G - G^\circ$ for one mole of an ideal gas at 5.00 atm and 25 °C?

Using (*5.21*) and (*5.22*) gives

$$G - G^\circ = (1.00\text{ mol})(8.314\text{ J mol}^{-1}\text{ K}^{-1})(298\text{ K}) \ln 5.00 = 3987\text{ J}$$

5.6 ACTIVITIES FOR REAL GASES

For real gases some appropriate equation of state may be solved for V, and the result substituted into (*5.12*) and integrated, giving a complicated expression for the activity. Rather than doing this, we retain the simple form of (*5.21*) by letting

$$a = f \qquad (5.23)$$

where the *fugacity*, f, is given by

$$f = \gamma P \qquad (5.24)$$

The *activity coefficient*, γ, contains the corrections for the nonideal behavior of the gas. Note that the standard state is now taken as $f^\circ = 1$ (not $P^\circ = 1$). Values of the activity coefficient may be determined by a graphical integration of $\overline{V} - (RT/P)$, where $\overline{V}$ is the molar volume, against P to give $RT \ln \gamma$; or $z - 1$ against $\ln P_r$ to give $\ln \gamma$; or from Fig. 5-1. Each curve in Fig. 5-1 corresponds to a fixed value of T_r. The value of γ in a gaseous mixture is assumed to be the same as the value for the pure gas under the same conditions.

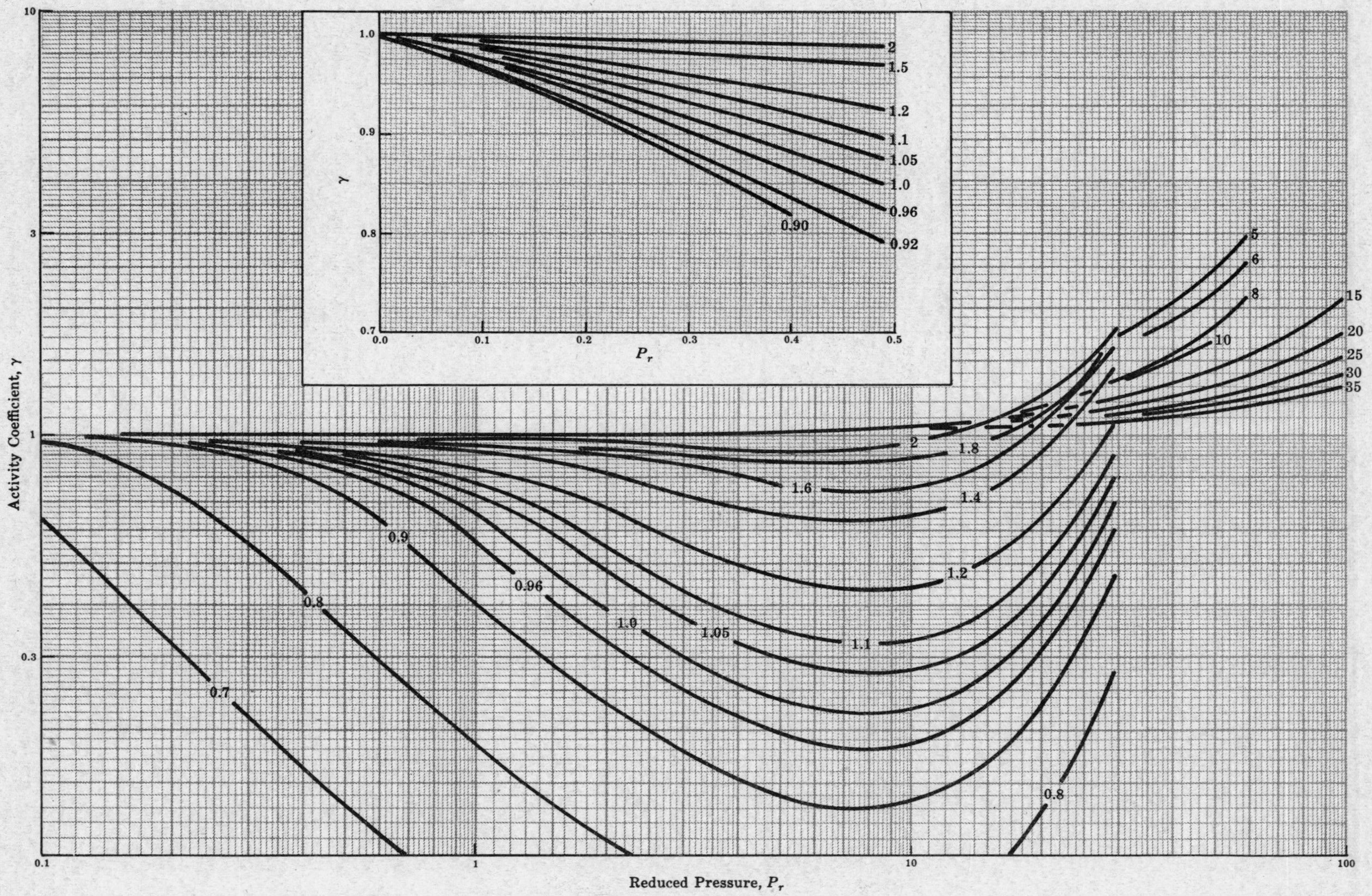

Activity Coefficient, γ
Reduced Pressure, P_r
10
3
1
0.3
0.1
1
10
100
0.7
0.8
0.9
0.96
1.0
1.05
1.1
1.2
1.4
1.6
1.8
2
5
6
8
10
15
20
25
30
35
γ
P_r
1.0
0.9
0.8
0.7
0.0
0.1
0.2
0.3
0.4
0.5
2
1.5
1.2
1.1
1.05
1.0
0.96
0.92
0.90

Fig. 5-1

EXAMPLE 5.10. Determine γ and a for CO at 250 atm and 0 °C from Fig. 5-1 if $T_c = -140.2$ °C and $P_c = 35.68$ atm.

Using Fig. 5-1 for $P_r = 250 \text{ atm}/35.68 \text{ atm} = 7.0$ and $T_r = 273 \text{ K}/133 \text{ K} = 2.05$ gives $\gamma = 0.95$. Substituting into (*5.23*) and (*5.24*) gives

$$a = f = \gamma P = (0.95)(250 \text{ atm}) = 238 \text{ atm}$$

EXAMPLE 5.11. Using the following data, determine γ and a for CO at 250 atm and 0 °C by performing a graphical integration of a plot of $\overline{V} - (RT/P)$ against P:

P, atm	1	20	40	50	60	80	100
$\overline{V}$, dm³ mol⁻¹	22.4	1.11	0.551	0.438	0.364	0.272	0.218
P	120	140	160	180	200	250	
$\overline{V}$	0.182	0.157	0.139	0.126	0.114	0.096	

Sample calculations for the data plotted in Fig. 5-2 follow for 60 atm and 250 atm:

$$\overline{V} - \frac{RT}{P} = 0.364 \text{ dm}^3 \text{ mol}^{-1} - \frac{(0.0821 \text{ dm}^3 \text{ atm K}^{-1} \text{ mol}^{-1})(273 \text{ K})}{60 \text{ atm}} = -0.010 \text{ dm}^3 \text{ mol}^{-1}$$

$$\overline{V} - \frac{RT}{P} = 0.096 - \frac{(0.0821)(273)}{250} = 0.006$$

Graphical integration of Fig. 5-2 gives $RT \ln \gamma = -1.171$ or $\gamma = 0.949$. From (*5.23*) and (*5.24*), $a = 237$ atm.

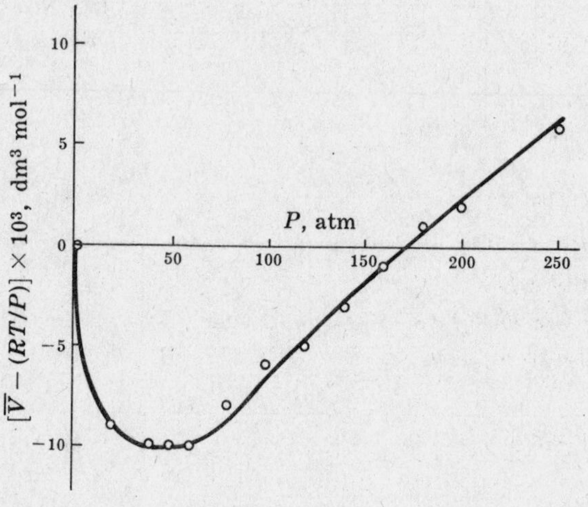

Fig. 5-2

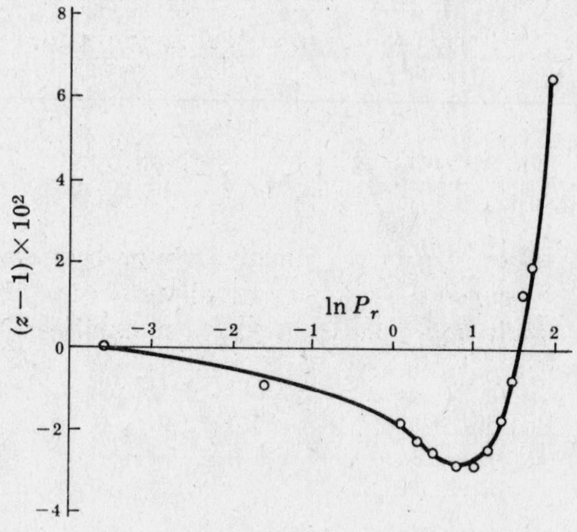

Fig. 5-3

EXAMPLE 5.12. The area under the curve of a plot of $z - 1$ against $\ln P_r$ is equal to $\ln \gamma$. Prepare such a plot for CO at 273 K by choosing several pressures up to 250 atm, calculating P_r and $\ln P_r$, and finding values of z from Fig. 1-2 along the $T_r = 2.05$ isotherm. Calculate γ and a.

As a sample calculation, for $P = 50$ atm

$$P_r = \frac{50 \text{ atm}}{35.68 \text{ atm}} = 1.40$$

and $\ln P_r = 0.336$. From Fig. 1-2 the value of z is 0.97, giving $z - 1 = -0.03$. Similar calculations yield Fig. 5-3. The graphical integration gives $\ln \gamma = -0.0466$ or $\gamma = 0.954$, and (*5.23*) and (*5.24*) give

$$a = \gamma P = (0.954)(250 \text{ atm}) = 239 \text{ atm}$$

5.7 ACTIVITIES FOR LIQUIDS AND SOLIDS

For a condensed phase under isothermal conditions

$$\ln a = \frac{1}{RT}\int_{1\,\text{atm}}^{P} \bar{V}\,dP \tag{5.25}$$

Because the molar volume $\bar{V}$ is essentially a constant and much less than RT, $\ln a$ is quite small and a is usually assumed to be unity for processes involving moderate changes in pressure.

EXAMPLE 5.13. Calculate a for water at 10 atm and 25 °C if

$$\beta = 45.8 \times 10^{-6}\ \text{atm}^{-1} \qquad \text{and} \qquad d = 0.99707 \times 10^{3}\ \text{kg m}^{-3}$$

Assuming that $\bar{V} = \bar{V}_{298}(1 - \beta P)$, (5.25) gives

$$\ln a = \frac{\bar{V}_{298}}{RT}\left[(P-1) - \frac{\beta}{2}(P^2 - 1^2)\right]$$

$$= \frac{(18.01 \times 10^{-3}\ \text{kg mol}^{-1})/(0.99707 \times 10^{3}\ \text{kg m}^{-3})}{(8.21 \times 10^{-5}\ \text{m}^3\ \text{atm mol}^{-1}\ \text{K}^{-1})(298\ \text{K})}\left[(9\ \text{atm}) - \frac{45.8 \times 10^{-6}\ \text{atm}^{-1}}{2}(99\ \text{atm}^2)\right]$$

$$= 0.00664$$

Taking the exponential gives $a = 1.00666$ atm.

5.8 ACTIVITIES FOR ELECTROLYTIC SOLUTIONS

For a solute undergoing ionization or dissociation in solution according to the reaction

$$A_mB_n = mA^{+z_+} + nB^{-z_-}$$

the mean activity, $a_\pm$, is given by

$$a_\pm = \gamma_\pm C_\pm \tag{5.26}$$

where $\gamma_\pm$ is the mean activity coefficient and $C_\pm$ is the mean ionic molar concentration. Observe that the standard state 1 in (5.20) is now a $1M$ solution. In terms of the individual ionic activities a_+ and a_-, molarities C_+ and C_-, and activity coefficients γ_+ and γ_-,

$$a_\pm = (a_+^m a_-^n)^{1/\nu} \tag{5.27}$$

$$\gamma_\pm = (\gamma_+^m \gamma_-^n)^{1/\nu} \tag{5.28}$$

$$C_\pm = (C_+^m C_-^n)^{1/\nu} \tag{5.29}$$

where

$$\nu = m + n \tag{5.30}$$

For concentrations of the electrolyte in mole fraction, x, or molarity, m, we may rewrite (5.26) as $a_\pm = \gamma_x x$ or $a_\pm = \gamma_m m$, where

$$\gamma_x = \gamma_\pm\left[\frac{d(\text{solution}) - M(\text{solute})\,C + M(\text{solvent})\,C\nu}{d(\text{solvent})}\right] \tag{5.31}$$

$$\gamma_m = \gamma_\pm\left[\frac{C}{d(\text{solvent})m10^{-3}}\right] \tag{5.32}$$

Here d is the density (kg m^{-3}), M is the molecular weight (g mol^{-1}) and C is the molarity (mol dm^{-3}).

EXAMPLE 5.14. The Debye-Hückel theory allows the calculation of the mean activity coefficient by

$$\log \gamma_\pm = -\frac{z_+ z_- A I^{1/2}}{1 + aBI^{1/2}} + bI \tag{5.33}$$

where A, a, B and b are various parameters, and the ionic strength, I, is given by

$$I = \frac{1}{2} \sum_i^{\text{ions}} C_i z_i^2 \tag{5.34}$$

In (*5.34*) z_i is the absolute value of the ionic valence and the sum is performed over *all* ions in solution (if there are others present besides A^{+z_+} and B^{-z_-}). Calculate $\gamma_\pm$ for $1.0 \times 10^{-4}M$ $Al_2(SO_4)_3$ at 25 °C.

Since one mole of $Al_2(SO_4)_3$ yields two moles of Al^{3+} and three moles of SO_4^{2-}, the ionic strength of the solution is given by (*5.34*) as

$$I = \frac{1}{2}[(2.0 \times 10^{-4})(3)^2 + (3.0 \times 10^{-4})(2)^2] = 15.0 \times 10^{-4}M$$

For aqueous solutions at 25 °C with concentrations of $I = 10^{-2}M$ or less, (*5.33*) reduces to the *Debye-Hückel limiting law*:

$$\log \gamma_\pm = -z_+ z_- (0.5116) I^{1/2} \tag{5.35}$$

which upon substitution of $I = 15.0 \times 10^{-4}$ gives

$$\log \gamma_\pm = -(3)(2)(0.5116)(15.0 \times 10^{-4})^{1/2} = -0.119 = 0.881 - 1$$

$$\gamma_\pm = 0.760$$

EXAMPLE 5.15. Although γ_+ and γ_- cannot be experimentally measured, the Debye-Hückel limiting law allows their calculation by

$$\log \gamma_i = -z_i^2 (0.5116) I^{1/2} \tag{5.36}$$

Calculate γ_+ and γ_- for the $Al_2(SO_4)_3$ solution described in Example 5.14.

Substituting $I = 15.0 \times 10^{-4}$ and the appropriate valences into (*5.36*) gives

$$\log \gamma_+ = -(3)^2(0.5116)(15.0 \times 10^{-4})^{1/2} = -0.178 = 0.822 - 1$$

$$\gamma_+ = 0.663$$

$$\log \gamma_- = -(2)^2(0.5116)(15.0 \times 10^{-4})^{1/2} = -0.079 = 0.921 - 1$$

$$\gamma_- = 0.833$$

As a check, substituting these ionic activity coefficients into (*5.28*) gives

$$\gamma_\pm = [(0.663)^2(0.833)^3]^{1/5} = (0.254)^{1/5} = 0.760$$

the same value as determined in Example 5.14.

Equilibrium Constants

5.9 INTRODUCTION

For the general reaction

$$lL + mM + \cdots = rR + sS + \cdots$$

the change in the free energy is given by

$$\Delta G = \Delta G^\circ + RT \ln Q \tag{5.37}$$

where Q, the *reaction quotient*, is given by

$$Q = \frac{a_R^r a_S^s \cdots}{a_L^l a_M^m \cdots} \tag{5.38}$$

At equilibrium, $\Delta G = 0$ and Q becomes the *thermodynamic equilibrium constant, K,* giving

$$\ln K = \frac{-\Delta G^\circ}{RT} \tag{5.39a}$$

$$K = e^{-\Delta G^\circ/RT} \tag{5.39b}$$

Note: In applying (*5.37*) and (*5.39*) the gas constant R must be multiplied by the factor (mol) in order to make the results dimensionally correct. The same holds true for (*5.40*) through (*5.43*), as well as (*5.48*). See Section 6.17 for a discussion of this point.

EXAMPLE 5.16. For the chemical reaction

$$Ag(s) + \tfrac{1}{2}Cl_2(g) = AgCl(liq)$$

Metz and Seifert reported $\mathcal{E}^\circ = 0.8401$ V at 1000 K. If $a_{Ag} = a_{AgCl} = 1.00$ and $a_{Cl_2} = 0.76$ atm, find $\mathcal{E}$. What is the value of K for the reaction at this temperature?

If electrochemical measurements are used to determine ΔG°, (*5.37*) becomes the *Nernst equation* upon substitution of (*5.6*):

$$\mathcal{E} = \mathcal{E}^\circ - \frac{RT}{n\mathcal{F}} \ln Q \tag{5.40}$$

and (*5.39a*) can be written as

$$\ln K = \frac{n\mathcal{F}\mathcal{E}^\circ}{RT} \tag{5.41}$$

For the given nonstandard conditions (*5.40*) and (*5.38*) give

$$\mathcal{E} = \mathcal{E}^\circ - \frac{RT}{n\mathcal{F}} \ln \frac{a_{AgCl}}{a_{Ag}(a_{Cl_2})^{1/2}}$$

$$= 0.8401 - \frac{(8.314\ \text{J mol}^{-1}\ \text{K}^{-1})(\text{mol})(1000\ \text{K})}{(1\ \text{mol})(9.6485 \times 10^4\ \text{J mol}^{-1}\ \text{V}^{-1})} \ln \frac{1.00}{(1.00)(0.76)^{1/2}}$$

$$= 0.8401 - (0.0862) \ln \frac{1}{0.872} = 0.8401 - 0.0119 = 0.8283\ \text{V}$$

The reaction under these nonstandard conditions is less favored than under standard conditions.

Using (*5.41*) gives

$$\ln K = \frac{(1\ \text{mol})(9.6485 \times 10^4\ \text{J mol}^{-1}\ \text{V}^{-1})(0.8401\ \text{V})}{(8.314\ \text{J mol}^{-1}\ \text{K}^{-1})(\text{mol})(1000\ \text{K})} = 9.75$$

and taking the antilog gives $K = 1.7 \times 10^4$.

5.10 TEMPERATURE DEPENDENCE OF K

From (*5.14*) and (*5.39a*)

$$\ln (K_{T_2}/K_{T_1}) = \frac{1}{R}\int_{T_1}^{T_2} \frac{\Delta H^\circ}{T^2}\,dT \tag{5.42}$$

which simplifies to

$$\ln (K_{T_2}/K_{T_1}) = \frac{\Delta H^\circ}{R}\left(\frac{1}{T_1} - \frac{1}{T_2}\right) \tag{5.43}$$

for small temperature intervals where ΔH° is essentially constant. Equation (*5.43*) states that a plot of $\ln K$ against $1/T$ will be linear with a slope of $-\Delta H^\circ/R$.

EXAMPLE 5.17. Stern and Weise give $K = 3.87 \times 10^{-16}$ at 400 K and 1.67×10^{-8} at 600 K for the reaction

$$BeSO_4(s) = BeO(s) + SO_3(g)$$

Assuming (*5.43*) to be valid over this somewhat large temperature interval, estimate ΔH°_{500}(reaction).

Rearranging (*5.43*) gives

$$\Delta H^\circ = R \frac{\ln (K_{T_2}/K_{T_1})}{\dfrac{1}{T_1} - \dfrac{1}{T_2}}$$

$$= (8.314 \text{ J mol}^{-1} \text{ K}^{-1})(\text{mol}) \frac{\ln [(1.67 \times 10^{-8})/(3.87 \times 10^{-16})]}{\left(\dfrac{1}{400} - \dfrac{1}{600}\right)\text{K}^{-1}} = 175 \text{ kJ}$$

5.11 GASEOUS EQUILIBRIUM CONSTANTS

Several different equilibrium constants are encountered when dealing with gaseous reactions. These are related to K by

$$K = K_\gamma K_p \tag{5.44}$$

$$K_p = (RT)^{\Delta n} K_c \tag{5.45}$$

$$K_p = P^{\Delta n} K_x \tag{5.46}$$

where K_γ is defined as

$$K_\gamma \equiv \frac{\gamma_R^r \gamma_S^s \cdots}{\gamma_L^l \gamma_M^m \cdots} \tag{5.47}$$

K_p is similarly defined in terms of partial pressures (atm), K_c in terms of molarities (mol dm^{-3}), and K_x in terms of mole fractions. Note that P in (*5.46*) is the *total* pressure of the gases, including any inert gases that may be present. If the experimental conditions are not too severe, K_γ in (*5.44*) is often set equal to unity to simplify the calculations.

EXAMPLE 5.18. Calculate K, K_γ, K_p, K_c and K_x at 25 °C and 1.00 atm total pressure for the reaction

$$H_2(g) + \tfrac{1}{2}O_2(g) = H_2O(g)$$

if $\Delta G^\circ_{298}(\text{reaction}) = -54.634$ kcal. Assume that $T_c = 374.2$ °C and $P_c = 218.3$ atm for H_2O, -240 °C and 13 atm for H_2, and -118 °C and 50.2 atm for O_2.

As mentioned in Section 2.6, the value of γ for a gas in a mixture is assumed to be the same as the value for the pure gas under the same conditions. Thus, calculating the reduced pressures using 1.00 atm and the reduced temperatures for the gases gives $P_r = 4.6 \times 10^{-3}$ and $T_r = 0.797$ for H_2O, 7.7×10^{-2} and 9.04 for H_2, and 2.0×10^{-2} and 1.92 for O_2. From Fig. 5-1, $\gamma_{H_2O} = 0.98$, $\gamma_{H_2} = 1.00$ and $\gamma_{O_2} = 1.00$, giving

$$K_\gamma = \frac{\gamma_{H_2O}}{\gamma_{H_2}(\gamma_{O_2})^{1/2}} = \frac{0.98}{(1.00)(1.00)^{1/2}} = 0.98$$

Equation (*5.39b*) gives

$$K = e^{-(-54{,}634)(4.184)/(8.314)(298)} = e^{92.26} = 1.17 \times 10^{40}$$

and (*5.44*) gives

$$K_p = \frac{K}{K_\gamma} = \frac{1.17 \times 10^{40}}{0.98} = 1.20 \times 10^{40}$$

Because molarities are expressed in mol dm^{-3} and pressures are in atm, we have from (*5.45*)

$$K_c = K_p(RT)^{-\Delta n} = (1.20 \times 10^{40})[(0.0821 \text{ dm}^3 \text{ atm K}^{-1} \text{ mol}^{-1})(298)]^{-(-1/2)} = 5.82 \times 10^{40}$$

and from (*5.46*)

$$K_x = K_p P^{-\Delta n} = (1.20 \times 10^{40})(1)^{-(-1/2)} = 1.20 \times 10^{40}$$

5.12 LE CHATELIER'S PRINCIPLE

If a stress is imposed upon a system at equilibrium, the system will change concentrations of the products and reactants in such a way as to relieve the stress. The mathematical description of the change in the system is given by combining (*5.9*), (*5.39b*), (*5.44*) and (*5.46*), and solving for the mole fraction of one of the products to give

$$x_R^r = \frac{x_L^l x_M^m \cdots}{x_S^s \cdots} K_\gamma^{-1} P^{-\Delta n} e^{-\Delta H^\circ/RT} e^{\Delta S^\circ/R} \tag{5.48}$$

Even though a change in P will change γ, and hence K_γ, the change in K_γ will be not nearly as important as the change in P for most cases.

EXAMPLE 5.19. Determine the effect on the equilibrium at 25 °C for the reaction

$$H_2(g) + \tfrac{1}{2}O_2(g) = H_2O(g)$$

of (1) an increase in x_{H_2}, (2) a decrease in x_{O_2}, (3) an increase in total pressure, (4) an increase in temperature given that ΔH° is negative, and (5) forming liquid water instead of gaseous water.

According to (*5.48*), (1) for an increase in x_{H_2}, the value of x_{H_2O} increases; (2) for a decrease in x_{O_2}, the value of x_{H_2O} decreases; (3) for an increase in P, the term $P^{-(-1/2)}$ becomes larger, resulting in a larger value for x_{H_2O}; (4) for an increase in T, even though ΔH° becomes slightly more negative, the exponent becomes less positive, resulting in a decrease in x_{H_2O}; and (5) in forming liquid water, the changes in ΔS° and ΔH° are such that ΔG° is more negative, giving an increase in x_{H_2O}.

Equilibrium Calculations

5.13 CALCULATIONS FOR IDEAL GASES

The necessary background material for these calculations has been presented in Sections 5.5, 5.9, 5.11 and 1.6.

EXAMPLE 5.20. Calculate the percent conversion to PCl_5 and the partial pressure of PCl_5 at 1.00 atm total pressure and 400 K for the reaction

$$PCl_3(g) + Cl_2(g) = PCl_5(g)$$

if the original reaction mixture contained 1.00 mole of PCl_3 and 2.00 moles of Cl_2. For this reaction, $\Delta G^\circ_{400} = -855$ cal.

Using (*5.39b*) gives

$$K = e^{-(-855)(4.184)/(8.314)(400)} = e^{1.076} = 2.93$$

Because the bases are assumed to be ideal, (*5.44*) gives $K = K_p = 2.93$. Letting x be the number of moles of $PCl_5(g)$ at equilibrium, the number of moles of $PCl_3(g)$ is $1.00 - x$, and of $Cl_2(g)$ is $2.00 - x$. The total number of moles is

$$x + (1.00 - x) + (2.00 - x) = 3.00 - x$$

The partial pressures are given by (*1.8*) as

$$P_{PCl_5} = \frac{xP}{3.00 - x} \qquad P_{Cl_2} = \frac{(2.00 - x)P}{3.00 - x} \qquad P_{PCl_3} = \frac{(1.00 - x)P}{3.00 - x}$$

and substituting into (*5.38*) gives

$$2.93 = \left[\frac{xP}{3.00 - x}\right]^1 \Big/ \left[\frac{(2.00 - x)P}{3.00 - x}\right]^1 \left[\frac{(1.00 - x)P}{3.00 - x}\right]^1$$

Solving for x with $P = 1.00$ atm gives $x = 0.628$ and $P_{PCl_5} = 0.265$ atm.

5.14 CALCULATIONS FOR REAL GASES

The necessary background material for these calculations has been presented in Sections 5.6, 5.9, 5.11 and 1.6.

EXAMPLE 5.21. Find K_γ for the reaction mixture described in Example 5.20 if the actual value of x is 0.600 for the real gases.

The value of K_p for the real gases is

$$K_p = \left[\frac{(0.600)(1.00)}{2.40}\right]^1 \Big/ \left[\frac{(1.40)(1.00)}{2.40}\right]^1 \left[\frac{(0.40)(1.00)}{2.40}\right]^1 = 2.57$$

and (*5.44*) gives

$$K_\gamma = \frac{K}{K_p} = \frac{2.93}{2.57} = 1.14$$

5.15 CALCULATIONS FOR HETEROGENEOUS SYSTEMS

Although the equilibrium constants are written as in (*5.38*), they are simplified by choosing the activities of the condensed phases as unity (unless large pressure changes are involved) and assuming the gases to be ideal (unless they are significantly nonideal). A special type of calculation involves the solubility of a highly insoluble ionic substance, where the equilibrium constant is known as the *solubility product*, K_{sp}.

EXAMPLE 5.22. Calculate the pressure of oxygen over a sample of NiO(s) at 25 °C if $\Delta G° = 211.7$ kJ for the reaction

$$\mathrm{NiO(s)} = \mathrm{Ni(s)} + \tfrac{1}{2}\mathrm{O_2(g)}$$

The equilibrium constant for the reaction is

$$K = (a_{\mathrm{Ni}})^1(a_{\mathrm{O_2}})^{1/2}/(a_{\mathrm{NiO}})^1$$

which simplifies to

$$K = (a_{\mathrm{O_2}})^{1/2} = (P_{\mathrm{O_2}})^{1/2}$$

The value of K using (*5.39b*) is

$$K = e^{-(211{,}700)/(8.314)(298)} = e^{-85.5} = 7.8 \times 10^{-38}$$

Solving for the pressure gives

$$P_{\mathrm{O_2}} = K^2 = (7.8 \times 10^{-38})^2 = 6 \times 10^{-75} \text{ atm}$$

The assumption of ideal behavior for O_2 is valid at this very low pressure.

EXAMPLE 5.23. Find the concentration of Ag^+ in a solution which (1) is saturated with AgBr, (2) contains 0.01 M NaBr, and (3) contains 0.01 M HNO_3. ΔG°_{298}(reaction) = 70.04 kJ for

$$\mathrm{AgBr(s)} = \mathrm{Ag^+(aq)} + \mathrm{Br^-(aq)}$$

For the reaction, (*5.39b*) gives

$$K = K_{sp} = e^{-(70{,}040)/(8.314)(298)} = e^{-28.3} = 5.3 \times 10^{-13}$$

where

$$K_{sp} = a_{\mathrm{Ag^+}} a_{\mathrm{Br^-}}$$

For the first solution (*5.26*) gives

$$K_{sp} = a_\pm^2 = \gamma_\pm^2 C_\pm^2 = \gamma_\pm^2 C^2$$

where C is the concentration of either ion. Assuming $\gamma_\pm$ to be near unity for the solution,

$$C = K_{sp}^{1/2} = (5.3 \times 10^{-13})^{1/2} = 7.3 \times 10^{-7} M$$

As a check on the assumption concerning $\gamma_\pm$, for a 1 : 1 electrolyte (*5.34*) gives

$$I = C = 7.3 \times 10^{-7} M$$

and (*5.35*) gives

$$\log \gamma_\pm = -(1)(1)(0.5116)(7.3 \times 10^{-7})^{1/2} = -4.4 \times 10^{-4}$$

Taking the antilog gives $\gamma_\pm = 0.999$, which is very close to unity. Thus the Ag^+ concentration is $7.3 \times 10^{-7} M$.

The effect of the common ion in the second solution will be to decrease the concentration of the AgBr. Because the total ionic strength is now appreciable, $\gamma_\pm$ must be calculated. By (*5.34*),

$$I = \frac{1}{2}[(C_{Na^+})(z_{Na^+})^2 + (C_{Br^-})(z_{Br^-})^2 + (C_{Ag^+})(z_{Ag^+})^2]$$

$$= \frac{1}{2}[(0.01)1^2 + (0.01 + C)1^2 + (C)1^2] \approx \frac{1}{2}[(0.01)1^2 + (0.01)1^2] = 0.01\,M$$

and (*5.35*) gives

$$\log \gamma_\pm = -(1)(1)(0.5116)(0.01)^{1/2} = -0.05116$$

and taking the antilog gives $\gamma_\pm = 0.888$. The equilibrium expression becomes

$$K_{sp} = 5.3 \times 10^{-13} = (0.889)^2(C)(0.01 + C)$$

and solving for C gives $6.7 \times 10^{-11} M$. Thus the Ag^+ concentration has decreased to $6.7 \times 10^{-11} M$.

For the third solution, the total ionic strength will be nearly 0.01 M, giving $\gamma_\pm = 0.888$. The equilibrium expression in this case is

$$5.3 \times 10^{-13} = (0.889)^2 C^2$$

and solving for C gives $8.2 \times 10^{-7} M$, a slight increase in the solubility.

5.16 CALCULATIONS FOR AQUEOUS SOLUTIONS

Very often the activity coefficients in aqueous solutions are neglected because there is no simple way to calculate them. In most expressions for K_a, the *acid ionization constant*; K_b, the *base ionization constant*; and K_w, the *water ionization constant*, concentrations are used directly for activities.

In aqueous media, C_{H^+} is often expressed as pH, where

$$pH = -\log C_{H^+} \tag{5.49}$$

and C_{OH^-} as pOH, where

$$pOH = -\log C_{OH^-} \tag{5.50}$$

In (*5.49*) and (*5.50*) the concentrations are, as usual, in mol dm^{-3}. Note that

$$pH + pOH = pK_w = 14.000 \tag{5.51}$$

If an ionic salt dissolves in water, the concentration of the various species in solution can be determined by using the equilibrium expressions for hydrolysis, where K_h, the *hydrolysis constant*, is given by

$$K_h = \frac{K_w}{K_a} \tag{5.52}$$

for the salt of a strong base and a weak acid, by

$$K_h = \frac{K_w}{K_b} \tag{5.53}$$

for the salt of a weak base and a strong acid, and by

$$K_h = \frac{K_w}{K_a K_b} \tag{5.54}$$

for the salt of a weak base and a weak acid.

EXAMPLE 5.24. Compare the pH values of the following solutions: (1) 0.100 *M* $HC_2H_3O_2$, (2) 0.100 *M* $NaC_2H_3O_2$, (3) a buffer solution prepared by adding 0.500 mol of $NaC_2H_3O_2$ to 1 dm³ of 0.100 *M* $HC_2H_3O_2$, and (4) the buffer solution after the addition of 0.001 mol of NaOH. $K_a = 1.76 \times 10^{-5}$ for the reaction

$$HC_2H_3O_2(aq) = H^+(aq) + C_2H_3O_2^-(aq)$$

For the first solution the equilibrium expression is

$$K_a = \frac{(x)(x)}{0.100 - x} = 1.76 \times 10^{-5}$$

where $x = C_{H^+} = C_{C_2H_3O_2^-}$. Solving gives $x = 1.32 \times 10^{-3}M$ and (*5.49*) gives

$$pH = -\log(1.32 \times 10^{-3}) = -(0.121 - 3) = 2.879$$

For the $NaC_2H_3O_2$ solution, the acetate ion undergoes hydrolysis according to the reaction

$$C_2H_3O_2^-(aq) + H_2O = HC_2H_3O_2(aq) + OH^-(aq)$$

where the hydrolysis equilibrium constant is given by (*5.52*) as

$$K_h = \frac{1.00 \times 10^{-14}}{1.76 \times 10^{-5}} = 5.68 \times 10^{-10}$$

Letting $x = C_{OH^-}$, the equlibrium expression becomes

$$K_h = \frac{(x)(x)}{0.100 - x} = 5.68 \times 10^{-10}$$

and solving gives $x = 7.54 \times 10^{-6}M$. Using (*5.50*) and (*5.51*) gives

$$pOH = -\log(7.54 \times 10^{-6}) = 5.123 \qquad pH = 8.877$$

For the original buffer, letting $x = C_{H^+}$,

$$K_a = \frac{x(0.500 + x)}{0.100 - x} = 1.76 \times 10^{-5}$$

and solving gives $x = 3.52 \times 10^{-6}M$, which upon substitution into (*5.49*) gives

$$pH = -\log(3.52 \times 10^{-6}) = 5.453$$

After the addition of the NaOH, the concentrations become

$$C_{H^+} = x, \quad C_{C_2H_3O_2^-} = 0.500 + x + 0.001, \quad C_{HC_2H_3O_2} = 0.100 - x - 0.001$$

which upon substitution into the equilibrium expression give

$$K_a = \frac{x(0.500 + x + 0.001)}{0.100 - x - 0.001} = 1.76 \times 10^{-5}$$

and solving gives $x = 3.47 \times 10^{-6}M$. Equation (*5.49*) gives

$$pH = -\log(3.47 \times 10^{-6}) = 5.459$$

Thermodynamic Relations

5.17 MAXWELL RELATIONS

The *Maxwell relations* for closed reversible systems in which only PV-work is considered can be derived from the following set of differential energy expressions:

$$dE = T\,dS - P\,dV \tag{5.55}$$

$$dH = T\,dS + V\,dP \tag{5.56}$$

$$dG = -S\,dT + V\,dP \tag{5.57}$$

$$dA = -S\,dT - P\,dV \tag{5.58}$$

There are several Maxwell relations because of the number of ways that the four variables—T, S, P and V—can be distributed in the following format

$$\left(\frac{\partial W}{\partial X}\right)_Z = \pm\left(\frac{\partial Y}{\partial Z}\right)_X \tag{5.59}$$

It is possible to construct any one of the relations from (5.59) if the following rules are used: (1) the cross products XY and WZ must be work terms, i.e. PV and ST; (2) the negative sign is chosen if W and X or Z and Y are T and V.

EXAMPLE 5.25. From (5.58) derive the Maxwell relation $(\partial S/\partial V)_T = (\partial P/\partial T)_V$. Compare this result to that predicted by (5.59).

At constant V, (5.58) becomes

$$\left(\frac{\partial A}{\partial T}\right)_V = -S$$

while at constant T it becomes

$$\left(\frac{\partial A}{\partial V}\right)_T = -P$$

Differentiating the first equation with respect to V at constant T, and the second equation with respect to T at constant V, gives

$$\frac{\partial}{\partial V}\left(\left(\frac{\partial A}{\partial T}\right)_V\right)_T = -\left(\frac{\partial S}{\partial V}\right)_T \qquad \text{and} \qquad \frac{\partial}{\partial T}\left(\left(\frac{\partial A}{\partial V}\right)_T\right)_V = -\left(\frac{\partial P}{\partial T}\right)_V$$

But A is a point function and one of the properties of such a function is that the order of differentiation is not important. Hence, the above second derivatives are equal, which gives the desired result.

If $W = S$ and $X = V$ in (5.59), the first rule requires that $Y = P$ and $Z = T$, giving

$$\left(\frac{\partial S}{\partial V}\right)_T = \pm\left(\frac{\partial P}{\partial T}\right)_V$$

By the second rule the plus sign is chosen, so the final result is the same as derived above.

5.18 TRANSFORMATIONS

The physical properties P, V, T, C_V and C_P are experimentally measurable for a system. When other properties such as H, E, G, or S appear in an equation, the equation is usually transformed from those variables to the measurable variety. To make these transformations, the Maxwell relations are used, as well as the following properties of partial derivatives:

$$\left(\frac{\partial x}{\partial y}\right)_w = \left(\frac{\partial x}{\partial z}\right)_w \left(\frac{\partial z}{\partial y}\right)_w \tag{4.17}$$

$$\left(\frac{\partial x}{\partial y}\right)_z \left(\frac{\partial y}{\partial z}\right)_x \left(\frac{\partial z}{\partial x}\right)_y = -1 \tag{5.60}$$

$$\left(\frac{\partial z}{\partial x}\right)_y = \left[\left(\frac{\partial x}{\partial z}\right)_y\right]^{-1} \tag{5.61}$$

EXAMPLE 5.26. Evaluate $(\partial P/\partial S)_V$.

The transformation involves three steps: (1) inversion, (5.61); (2) chain rule, (4.17); and (3) substitution of the result for $(\partial S/\partial T)_V$ which is derived in Problem 5.20.

$$\left(\frac{\partial P}{\partial S}\right)_V = \frac{1}{\left(\frac{\partial S}{\partial P}\right)_V} = \frac{1}{\left(\frac{\partial S}{\partial T}\right)_V \left(\frac{\partial T}{\partial P}\right)_V} = \frac{T}{C_V\left(\frac{\partial T}{\partial P}\right)_V}$$

5.19 FREE ENERGY CURVES

The signs of the various thermodynamic properties at a given temperature can be determined from a plot of ΔG° against temperature. (1) For ΔG°, the sign corresponds to the value of ΔG° on the plot; (2) for $(\partial \Delta G^\circ/\partial T)_P$, the sign corresponds to the slope of the curve at that temperature; (3) for ΔS°, (*5.13*) gives $\Delta S^\circ = -(\partial \Delta G^\circ/\partial T)_P$ and the sign will be opposite that of the slope; (4) for ΔH°, (*5.9*) gives $\Delta H^\circ = \Delta G^\circ + T\,\Delta S^\circ$ and the sign will be that of the numerically larger quantity, ΔG° or $T\,\Delta S^\circ$; (5) for $(\partial \Delta S^\circ/\partial T)_P$, if $\Delta S^\circ = -(\partial \Delta G^\circ/\partial T)_P$, then $(\partial \Delta S^\circ/\partial T)_P = -(\partial^2 \Delta G^\circ/\partial T^2)_P$ and the sign will be opposite that of the second derivative of ΔG° (which is usually zero at a point of inflection, positive at a minimum and negative at a maximum); (6) for $(\partial \Delta H^\circ/\partial T)_P$, taking the derivative of (*5.9*) gives $(\partial \Delta H^\circ/\partial T)_P = T(\partial \Delta S^\circ/\partial T)_P$ and the sign will be that of $(\partial \Delta S^\circ/\partial T)_P$; (7) for ΔC_P°, (*4.9*) gives $\Delta C_P^\circ = T(\partial \Delta S^\circ/\partial T)_P$ and the sign will be that of $(\partial \Delta S^\circ/\partial T)_P$; (8) for $(\partial \Delta C_P^\circ/\partial T)_P$, taking the derivative of (*3.3*) gives $(\partial \Delta C_P^\circ/\partial T)_P = (\partial^2 \Delta H^\circ/\partial T^2)_P$ and the sign will be that of the second derivative of ΔH° (which will be very difficult to estimate qualitatively); (9) for $\ln K$, (*5.39a*) gives $\ln K = -\Delta G^\circ/RT$ and the sign will be opposite that of ΔG°; and (10) for $(\partial \ln K/\partial T)_P$, (*5.42*) gives $(\partial \ln K/\partial T)_P = \Delta H^\circ/RT^2$ and the sign will be that of ΔH°.

Solved Problems

Free Energy Functions

5.1. Calculate $\Delta G^\circ - \Delta A^\circ$ for the reaction between glycine and nitrous acid at 25 °C:

$$NH_2{-}CH_2{-}COOH(aq) + HONO(aq) = HO{-}CH_2{-}COOH(aq) + N_2(g) + H_2O(liq)$$

Assuming $\Delta(PV)$ for the condensed phases to be negligible, we have from (*5.5*):

$$\Delta G^\circ - \Delta A^\circ = \Delta(PV) = RT\,\Delta n_g = (8.314\ \text{J mol}^{-1}\ \text{K}^{-1})(298\ \text{K})(1\ \text{mol}) = 2478\ \text{J}$$

5.2. For the reaction

$$Ag(s) + \tfrac{1}{2}Cl_2(g) = AgCl(liq)$$

Metz and Seifert reported

$$\mathcal{E}^\circ = 0.9081 - 0.280\,X + 0.110\,X^2$$

where $$X = (T - 728.2)10^{-3}\ \text{K}$$

If $n = 1$ mol, find ΔG° as a function of X and calculate ΔG°_{1000}. Is the reaction favored at this temperature?

Using (*5.6*) gives

$$\Delta G^\circ = -(1\ \text{mol})(96.485\ \text{kJ mol}^{-1}\ \text{V}^{-1})(0.9081 - 0.280\,X + 0.110\,X^2)\ \text{V}$$
$$= (-87.620 + 27.02\,X - 10.61\,X^2)\ \text{kJ}$$

Evaluating X at 1000 K gives $X = 0.2718$ K and

$$\Delta G^\circ_{1000} = -87.620 + (27.02)(0.2718) - (10.61)(0.2718)^2 = -81.060\ \text{kJ}$$

which is favorable under standard conditions.

5.3. In terms of ΔS, ΔH and ΔG discuss the spontaneity of the reaction $H_2O(s) = H_2O(liq)$ in an ice-water bath at 0 °C.

For the given reaction, ΔS is positive because of the increase in randomness in going from a solid to a liquid. Thus, for a constant-enthalpy system, the spontaneous change would be for all ice to melt. However, ΔH for the process is positive (because of overcoming the intermolecular attractions), which would indicate a nonspontaneous change. Thus, if only ΔH is considered, the spontaneous change would be for the water to freeze. ΔG for the process is zero, which predicts a state of equilibrium in which the entropy change is canceled by the enthalpy change.

5.4. Calculate ΔG for the isothermal expansion of one mole of an ideal gas from 0.0100 m^3 to 0.1000 m^3 at 25 °C.

Substituting the volumes into (*5.10*) gives

$$\Delta G = (1.00 \text{ mol})(8.314 \text{ J mol}^{-1} \text{ K}^{-1})(298 \text{ K}) \ln \frac{0.0100}{0.1000} = -5705 \text{ J}$$

5.5. Calculate ΔG°_{298}(reaction) for the roasting of sphalerite,

$$\text{ZnS(sphalerite)} + \tfrac{3}{2}\text{O}_2(\text{g}) = \text{ZnO(s)} + \text{SO}_2(\text{g})$$

if ΔG°_{298}(formation) $= -48.11$ kcal mol^{-1} for ZnS, -76.08 for ZnO and -71.748 for SO_2. Qualitatively describe the driving force of the reaction.

Equation (*5.11*) gives

$$\begin{aligned} \Delta G^\circ_{298}(\text{reaction}) &= [(1)\Delta G^\circ_{298}(\text{formation, ZnO}) + (1)\Delta G^\circ_{298}(\text{formation, SO}_2)] \\ &\quad - [(1)\Delta G^\circ_{298}(\text{formation, ZnS}) + (\tfrac{3}{2})\Delta G^\circ_{298}(\text{formation, O}_2)] \\ &= [(1)(-76.08) + (1)(-71.748)] - [(1)(-48.11) + (\tfrac{3}{2})(0)] \\ &= -99.72 \text{ kcal} = -417.2 \text{ kJ} \end{aligned}$$

The change in randomness is not very large, so the driving force of the reaction is the large enthalpy change.

5.6. Find the value of ΔG°_{1000} for the reaction

$$\text{H}_2(\text{g}) + \text{Cl}_2(\text{g}) = 2\text{HCl}(\text{g})$$

if $\Delta H^\circ_{298} = -44.124$ kcal, $\Delta G^\circ_{298} = -45.554$ kcal, and the heat capacities in cal mol^{-1} K^{-1} are:

$$\begin{aligned} C^\circ_P &= 6.9469 - 0.1999 \times 10^{-3}T + 4.808 \times 10^{-7}T^2 \quad \text{for H}_2(\text{g}) \\ C^\circ_P &= 7.5755 + 2.4244 \times 10^{-3}T - 9.650 \times 10^{-7}T^2 \quad \text{for Cl}_2(\text{g}) \\ C^\circ_P &= 6.7319 + 0.4325 \times 10^{-3}T + 3.697 \times 10^{-7}T^2 \quad \text{for HCl(g)} \end{aligned}$$

For this reaction

$$\begin{aligned} \Delta C^\circ_P &= [(2)(6.7319) - (1)(6.9469) - (1)(7.5755)] \\ &\quad + [(2)(0.4325) - (1)(-0.1999) - (1)(2.4244)] \times 10^{-3}T \\ &\quad + [(2)(3.697) - (1)(4.808) - (1)(-9.650)] \times 10^{-7}T^2 \\ &= -1.0586 - 1.3595 \times 10^{-3}T + 12.236 \times 10^{-7}T^2 \end{aligned}$$

Using (*3.5a*) gives

$$\begin{aligned} J &= -44{,}124 - (-1.0586)(298) - \frac{1}{2}(-1.3595 \times 10^{-3})(298^2) - \frac{1}{3}(12.236 \times 10^{-7})(298^3) \\ &= -44{,}124 + 315 + 60 - 11 = -43{,}760 \text{ cal} \end{aligned}$$

and using (*5.16a*) gives

$$\begin{aligned} K &= \frac{-45{,}554 - (-43{,}760)}{298} + (-1.0586)\ln(298) + \frac{-1.3595 \times 10^{-3}}{2}(298) + \frac{12.236 \times 10^{-7}}{6}(298^2) \\ &= -6.020 - 6.031 - 0.203 + 0.018 = -12.236 \text{ cal K}^{-1} \end{aligned}$$

Substituting into (*5.15a*) gives

$$\Delta G^\circ_{1000} = -43{,}760 + (-12.236)(1000) - (-1.0586)(1000)\ln 1000$$
$$- \frac{-1.3595\times 10^{-3}}{2}(1000^2) - \frac{12.236\times 10^{-7}}{6}(1000^3)$$
$$= -43{,}760 - 12{,}236 + 7313 + 680 - 204 = -48.206 \text{ kcal} = -201.694 \text{ kJ}$$

5.7. The values of $(G^\circ_T - H^\circ_0)/T$ at 298 K and 500 K are -45.27 and -50.77 cal K^{-1} mol^{-1} for C_2H_6(g), -43.98 and -48.74 cal K^{-1} mol^{-1} for C_2H_4(g), and -24.42 and -27.95 cal K^{-1} mol^{-1} for H_2(g). If $H^\circ_{298} - H^\circ_0 = 2.856$ kcal mol^{-1} for C_2H_6(g), 2.525 kcal mol^{-1} for C_2H_4(g), and 2.0238 kcal mol^{-1} for H_2(g), and if ΔH°_{298}(formation) = -20.24 kcal mol^{-1} for C_2H_6(g), 12.49 kcal mol^{-1} for C_2H_4(g), and 0 kcal mol^{-1} for H_2(g), calculate ΔG°_T(reaction) for

$$C_2H_6(g) = C_2H_4(g) + H_2(g)$$

at 298 K and 400 K and compare the spontaneity at these temperatures.

Converting the values of $(G^\circ_T - H^\circ_0)/T$ to $(G^\circ_T - H^\circ_{298})/T$ for C_2H_6(g) using (*5.19*) gives

$$\frac{G^\circ_{298} - H^\circ_{298}}{298} = -45.27 \text{ cal K}^{-1}\text{ mol}^{-1} - \frac{2856 \text{ cal mol}^{-1}}{298 \text{ K}} = -54.85 \text{ cal K}^{-1}\text{ mol}^{-1}$$

$$\frac{G^\circ_{500} - H^\circ_{298}}{500} = -50.77 - \frac{2856}{500} = -56.48 \text{ cal K}^{-1}\text{ mol}^{-1}$$

Likewise, $(G^\circ_T - H^\circ_{298})/T = -52.45$ and -53.79 cal K^{-1} mol^{-1} for C_2H_4(g), and -31.21 and -32.00 cal K^{-1} mol^{-1} for H_2(g), at 298 K and 500 K, respectively.

For the reaction at 298 K, ΔH°_{298}(reaction) is found by using (*3.7*):

$$\Delta H^\circ_{298}(\text{reaction}) = [(1 \text{ mol})(12.49 \text{ kcal mol}^{-1}) + (1 \text{ mol})(0 \text{ kcal mol}^{-1})]$$
$$- [(1 \text{ mol})(-20.24 \text{ kcal mol}^{-1})] = 32.73 \text{ kcal}$$

and the change in the free energy function at 298 K is given by (*5.17b*) as

$$\frac{\Delta(G^\circ_{298} - H^\circ_{298})}{298} = [(1 \text{ mol})(-52.45 \text{ cal K}^{-1}\text{ mol}^{-1}) + (1 \text{ mol})(-31.21 \text{ cal K}^{-1}\text{ mol}^{-1})]$$
$$- [(1 \text{ mol})(-54.85 \text{ cal K}^{-1}\text{ mol}^{-1})] = -28.81 \text{ cal K}^{-1}$$

which upon substitution into (*5.18b*) gives

$$\Delta G^\circ_{298}(\text{reaction}) = (298 \text{ K})(-28.81 \text{ cal K}^{-1})(10^{-3} \text{ kcal cal}^{-1}) + 32.73 \text{ kcal}$$
$$= 24.14 \text{ kcal} = 101.00 \text{ kJ}$$

One of the convenient features of the free energy function is that values between known values may be determined by linear interpolation. Thus, for C_2H_6(g) at 400 K,

$$\frac{G^\circ_{400} - H^\circ_{298}}{400} = -54.85 \text{ cal K}^{-1}\text{ mol}^{-1}$$
$$+ \frac{400 \text{ K} - 298 \text{ K}}{500 \text{ K} - 298 \text{ K}}[-56.48 \text{ cal K}^{-1}\text{ mol}^{-1} - (-54.85 \text{ cal K}^{-1}\text{ mol}^{-1})]$$
$$= -54.85 + (-0.82) \doteq -55.67 \text{ cal K}^{-1}\text{ mol}^{-1}$$

Likewise $(G^\circ_{400} - H^\circ_{298})/400 = -53.13$ cal K^{-1} mol^{-1} for C_2H_4(g) and -31.61 cal K^{-1} mol^{-1} for H_2(g). For the reaction at 400 K, (*5.17b*) gives

$$\frac{\Delta(G^\circ_{400} - H^\circ_{298})}{400} = [(1)(-53.13) + (1)(-31.61)] - [(1)(-55.67)] = -29.07 \text{ cal K}^{-1}$$

and (*5.18b*) gives

$$\Delta G^\circ_{400}(\text{reaction}) = (400)(-29.07)(10^{-3}) + 32.73 = 21.10 \text{ kcal} = 88.28 \text{ kJ}$$

The reaction is favored slightly more under standard conditions at 400 K than at 298 K because the value of ΔG_T°(reaction) is less positive.

Activities

5.8. As an indication of ideality, gases can be categorized according to molecular structure. Compare molar values at 25 °C and 1 atm of $G - G^\circ$ for (1) a nonpolar, slightly polarizable gas such as Ar ($T_c = -122.4$ °C, $P_c = 48.8$ atm); (2) a nonpolar, easily polarizable gas such as CF_4 ($T_c = -47.9$ °C, $P_c = 39.8$ atm); (3) a polar, slightly polarizable gas such as CO ($T_c = -140.2$ °C, $P_c = 35.68$ atm); (4) a polar, easily polarizable gas such as CH_3Cl ($T_c = 143.1$ °C, $P_c = 66.6$ atm); and (5) a gas having hydrogen bonding between the molecules such as CH_3OH ($T_c = 239.4$ °C, $P_c = 79.2$ atm).

Using (*1.16*) and (*1.17*) for the gases gives $T_r = 1.98, 1.32, 2.24, 0.72$ and 0.58 and $P_r = 0.0205$, $0.0251, 0.0280, 0.0150$ and 0.0126 for Ar, CF_4, CO, CH_3Cl and CH_3OH, respectively. Figure 5-1 gives $\gamma = 0.998, 0.997, 0.999, 0.99$ and 0.98, respectively. The values for CH_3Cl and CH_3OH are only approximate.

Using (*5.24*), (*5.23*) and (*5.21*) gives

$$G - G^\circ = (1.00 \text{ mol})(8.314 \text{ J mol}^{-1} \text{ K}^{-1})(298 \text{ K}) \ln (0.998)(1.00) = -5.0 \text{ J}$$

for Ar, -7.4 J for CF_4, -2.5 J for CO, -25 J for CH_3Cl and -50 J for CH_3OH. Since $G - G^\circ$ for an ideal gas is zero, these values indicate that gases that are easily polarizable or have hydrogen bonding within them deviate from ideality more than those that are slightly polarizable. For routine calculations where ΔG is of the order of several kJ, the assumption of ideality does not seem to present a significant problem.

5.9. Calculate γ_{Na^+} in a 0.01 *M* NaCl–0.01 *M* Na_2SO_4 mixture, assuming the Debye-Hückel limiting law to apply.

Using (*5.34*) gives

$$I = \frac{1}{2}[(C_{Na^+})(z_{Na^+})^2 + (C_{Cl^-})(z_{Cl^-})^2 + (C_{SO_4^{2-}})(z_{SO_4^{2-}})^2]$$

$$= \frac{1}{2}[(0.03)(1)^2 + (0.01)(1)^2 + (0.01)(2)^2] = 0.04\,M$$

Equation (*5.36*) gives

$$\log \gamma_{Na^+} = -(1)^2(0.5116)(0.04)^{1/2} = -0.102$$

and taking the antilog gives $\gamma_{Na^+} = 0.790$.

Equilibrium Constants

5.10. Express Q for the reactions

$$Ag(s) + \tfrac{1}{2}Cl_2(g) = AgCl(liq)$$

$$2Ag(s) + Cl_2(g) = 2AgCl(liq)$$

and find the relation between them.

Substituting into (*5.38*) gives for the first reaction

$$Q_1 = \frac{a_{AgCl}}{a_{Ag}(a_{Cl_2})^{1/2}}$$

and for the second reaction

$$Q_2 = \frac{(a_{AgCl})^2}{(a_{Ag})^2 a_{Cl_2}} = Q_1^2$$

5.11. Calculate ΔG_{298} for the reaction

$$H_2(g) + \tfrac{1}{2}O_2(g) = H_2O(liq)$$

if $\Delta G^\circ_{298} = -56.687$ kcal, $a_{H_2O} = 1.00$, $P_{H_2} = 10^{-3}$ atm and $P_{O_2} = 10^{-6}$ atm. Is the reaction favored under these reduced pressure conditions?

Equations (*5.37*) and (*5.38*) give

$$\Delta G = \Delta G^\circ + RT \ln \frac{a_{H_2O}}{P_{H_2}(P_{O_2})^{1/2}}$$

$$= (-56.687)(4.184) + (8.314 \times 10^{-3}\ \text{kJ mol}^{-1}\ \text{K}^{-1})(\text{mol})(298\ \text{K}) \ln \frac{1.00}{(10^{-3})(10^{-6})^{1/2}}$$

$$= -237.18 + 34.23 = -202.95\ \text{kJ}$$

The value of ΔG is negative, so the reaction is spontaneous as written, but less so than at standard conditions.

5.12. Using the data in Examples 5.2 and 5.3 for the Daniell cell, calculate K_{298} and estimate K_{303}.

At 25 °C, (*5.39b*) gives

$$K_{298} = e^{-(-210{,}590)/(8.314)(298)} = e^{85.00} = 8.2 \times 10^{36}$$

Assuming (*5.43*) to be valid,

$$\ln \frac{K_{303}}{8.2 \times 10^{36}} = \frac{-228{,}530}{8.314}\left(\frac{1}{298} - \frac{1}{303}\right) = -1.522$$

$$K_{303} = (0.218)(8.2 \times 10^{36}) = 1.8 \times 10^{36}$$

Equilibrium Calculations

5.13. Assuming real-gas behavior, what is K_x at 100 atm and 25 °C for the reaction

$$SO_2(g) + \tfrac{1}{2}O_2(g) = SO_3(g)$$

if $\Delta G^\circ_{298} = -70.88$ kJ and if $T_c = 157.4$ °C and $P_c = 78.6$ atm for SO_2, -118.5 °C and 50.5 atm for O_2, and 218.3 °C and 83.6 atm for SO_3? If the original reaction mixture contained 1.00 mol SO_2 and 0.50 mol O_2, find x_{SO_3}.

Reduced values are: $T_r = 0.693$ and $P_r = 1.27$ for SO_2, 1.93 and 1.98 for O_2, and 0.606 and 1.20 for SO_3. Figure 5-1 gives $\gamma = 0.059$(approximately), 0.95 and 0.022(approximately), respectively. Then

$$K_\gamma = \frac{\gamma_{SO_3}}{\gamma_{SO_2}(\gamma_{O_2})^{1/2}} = (0.022)/(0.059)(0.95)^{1/2} = 0.38$$

Using (*5.39b*) gives

$$K = e^{-(-70{,}880)/(8.314)(298)} = e^{28.6} = 2.7 \times 10^{12}$$

Using (*5.44*) gives

$$K_p = \frac{K}{K_\gamma} = \frac{2.7 \times 10^{12}}{0.38} = 7.1 \times 10^{12}$$

and using (*5.46*) gives

$$K_x = K_p P^{-\Delta n} = (7.1 \times 10^{12})(100)^{-(-1/2)} = 7.1 \times 10^{13}$$

If x represents the number of moles of SO_3 at equilibrium, then the number of moles of SO_2 is $1.00 - x$ and of O_2 is $0.50 - (x/2)$. The total number of moles is $1.50 - (x/2)$, giving the mole fractions as

$$x_{SO_2} = \frac{1.00 - x}{1.50 - (x/2)} \qquad x_{O_2} = \frac{0.50 - (x/2)}{1.50 - (x/2)} \qquad x_{SO_3} = \frac{x}{1.50 - (x/2)}$$

Substituting into (*5.38*) gives

$$K_x = 7.1 \times 10^{13} = \left[\frac{x}{1.50 - (x/2)}\right] \Big/ \left[\frac{1.00 - x}{1.50 - (x/2)}\right]\left[\frac{0.50 - (x/2)}{1.50 - (x/2)}\right]^{1/2}$$

Solving, we obtain $x = 1.00$ and $x_{SO_3} = 1.00$, to three significant figures.

5.14. What is the partial pressure of NH_3 above a sample of NH_4Cl as a result of decomposition at 25 °C if ΔG°_{298}(formation) = −48.51 kcal mol⁻¹ for $NH_4Cl(s)$, −3.94 kcal mol⁻¹ for $NH_3(g)$, and −22.777 kcal mol⁻¹ for $HCl(g)$?

For the reaction $NH_4Cl(s) = NH_3(g) + HCl(g)$, (*5.11*) gives

$$\Delta G^\circ_{298}(\text{reaction}) = [(1)(-3.94) + (1)(-22.777)] - [(1)(-48.51)] = 21.79 \text{ kcal} = 91.17 \text{ kJ}$$

and (*5.39b*) gives

$$K = e^{-(91,170)/(8.314)(298)} = e^{-36.80} = 1.04 \times 10^{-16}$$

Recognizing that $a_{NH_4Cl} = 1.00$ and $a_{NH_3} = a_{HCl} = P_{HCl}$, (*5.38*) gives

$$1.04 \times 10^{-16} = (P_{HCl})^2 \qquad \text{or} \qquad P_{HCl} = 1.02 \times 10^{-8} \text{ atm}$$

5.15. What is the concentration of Ca^{2+} in a solution which is saturated with calcite? For the reaction

$$CaCO_3(\text{calcite}) = Ca^{2+}(aq) + CO_3^{2-}(aq)$$

$\Delta G^\circ_{298} = 47.20$ kJ. Repeat the calculations if the solution is (1) 0.0100 *M* Na_2CO_3 and (2) 0.0100 *M* $NaNO_3$. Assume (*5.35*) to be valid for all solutions.

For the reaction, (*5.39b*) gives $K = e^{-(47,200)/(8.314)(298)} = e^{-19.05} = 5.32 \times 10^{-9}$. Assuming $\gamma_\pm$ to be unity, the first approximation of the concentration of either ion, *C*, can be found by substituting $a_{CaCO_3} = 1.00$ into (*5.38*), giving

$$5.32 \times 10^{-9} = \frac{(\gamma_\pm C)(\gamma_\pm C)}{1.00} \qquad \text{or} \qquad C = 7.30 \times 10^{-5} M$$

Using this value of *C*, (*5.34*) gives

$$I = \frac{1}{2}[(7.30 \times 10^{-5})(2)^2 + (7.30 \times 10^{-5})(2)^2] = 29.19 \times 10^{-5} M$$

and (*5.35*) gives

$$\log \gamma_\pm = -(2)(2)(0.5116)(29.19 \times 10^{-5})^{1/2} = -0.0350 \qquad \text{or} \qquad \gamma_\pm = 0.923$$

Equation (*5.38*) now gives the second approximation of *C* as

$$5.32 \times 10^{-9} = \frac{(0.923)C(0.923)C}{1.00} \qquad \text{or} \qquad C = 7.91 \times 10^{-5} M$$

which corresponds to $I = 31.64 \times 10^{-5} M$ and $\gamma_\pm = 0.920$. Using $\gamma_\pm = 0.920$ gives the third estimate of *C* as $7.93 \times 10^{-5} M$ and upon continuing this reiterative process, $C = 7.94 \times 10^{-5} M$.

For the solution containing 0.0100 *M* Na_2CO_3, we assume that the contribution to *I* by the $CaCO_3$ will be negligible, so (*5.34*) and (*5.35*) give

$$I = \frac{1}{2}[(0.0200)(1)^2 + (0.0100)(2)^2] = 0.0300 M$$

$$\log \gamma_\pm = -(2)(2)(0.5116)(0.0300)^{1/2} = -0.3544$$

$$\gamma_\pm = 0.442$$

Assuming $C_{Ca^{2+}} = C$, $C_{CO_3^{2-}} = 0.0100 + C$ and $a_{CaCO_3} = 1.00$, (*5.38*) gives

$$5.32 \times 10^{-9} = \frac{(0.442)C(0.442)(0.0100 + C)}{1.00} \qquad \text{or} \qquad C = 2.72 \times 10^{-6} M$$

In solving for *C*, the approximation $0.0100 + C \approx 0.0100$ was made. As a check, $C = 2.72 \times 10^{-6}$ is indeed negligible compared to 0.0100. Furthermore, it is negligible compared to $I = 0.0300 M$ and so the assumption made above is valid.

For the solution containing $0.0100\,M$ $NaNO_3$, $I = 0.0100\,M$ and $\gamma_\pm = 0.624$. Assuming that $C = C_{Ca^{2+}} = C_{CO_3^{2-}}$ and $a_{CaCO_3} = 1.00$, *(5.34)* gives $C = 1.17 \times 10^{-4} M$, a sizable increase over a pure solution of $CaCO_3$.

5.16. What is the pH of a $0.1\,M$ $NH_4C_2H_3O_2$ solution?

For the reaction

$$NH_4^+(aq) + C_2H_3O_2^-(aq) \;=\; NH_3(aq) + HC_2H_3O_2(aq)$$

the equilibrium constant is calculated from *(5.54)* as

$$K_h \;=\; \frac{K_w}{K_a K_b} \;=\; \frac{1.00 \times 10^{-14}}{(1.76 \times 10^{-5})(1.79 \times 10^{-5})} \;=\; 3.17 \times 10^{-5}$$

and the equilibrium expression is

$$K_h \;=\; \frac{C_{NH_3} C_{HC_2H_3O_2}}{C_{NH_4^+} C_{C_2H_3O_2^-}} \;=\; 3.17 \times 10^{-5}$$

Letting $x = C_{NH_3} = C_{HC_2H_3O_2}$ and $0.100 - x \;=\; C_{NH_4^+} = C_{C_2H_3O_2^-}$,

$$\frac{(x)(x)}{(0.100 - x)(0.100 - x)} \;=\; 3.17 \times 10^{-5}$$

and solving gives $x = 5.61 \times 10^{-4} M$. Letting $y = C_{H^+}$, $C_{HC_2H_3O_2} = 5.63 \times 10^{-4}$ and $C_{C_2H_3O_2^-} = 0.0994$, the expression for K_a gives

$$K_a \;=\; \frac{(y)(0.0994)}{5.63 \times 10^{-4}} \;=\; 1.76 \times 10^{-5}$$

Solving gives $y = 9.96 \times 10^{-8} M$ and

$$\mathrm{pH} \;=\; -\log\,(9.96 \times 10^{-8}) \;=\; 7.002$$

Thermodynamic Relations

5.17. Derive *(5.55)*.

Beginning with the first law of thermodynamics,

$$dE \;=\; đq - đw$$

substitute $đq = T\,dS$, which holds under reversible conditions, and $đw = P\,dV$ to obtain

$$dE \;=\; T\,dS - P\,dV$$

5.18. Derive *(5.56)*.

The differential of

$$H \;=\; E + PV$$

is

$$dH \;=\; dE + P\,dV + V\,dP$$

Substituting *(5.55)* for dE gives

$$dH \;=\; (T\,dS - P\,dV) + P\,dV + V\,dP \;=\; T\,dS + V\,dP$$

5.19. Using the format of *(5.59)*, express the Maxwell relation that begins $(\partial S/\partial P)_T$.

Letting $W = S$ and $X = P$, the first rule says that Y must be V and Z must be T, so that the cross products are PV and ST for XY and WZ, respectively. Thus

$$\left(\frac{\partial S}{\partial P}\right)_T \;=\; \pm\left(\frac{\partial V}{\partial T}\right)_P$$

and the negative sign is chosen in view of the second rule (Y and Z are T and V).

5.20. **Express $(\partial S/\partial T)_P$ and $(\partial S/\partial T)_V$ in terms of measurable properties.**

Beginning with the definition of dS,

$$dS = \frac{đq}{T}$$

we recognize that at constant pressure $đq = dH = C_P\,dT$, so that

$$\frac{dS}{dT} = \left(\frac{\partial S}{\partial T}\right)_P = \frac{C_P}{T}$$

Likewise, at constant volume,

$$\left(\frac{\partial S}{\partial T}\right)_V = \frac{C_V}{T}$$

5.21. **Express $(\partial P/\partial V)_S$ in terms of measurable properties.**

Applying (*5.60*), (*5.61*), (*4.17*) and the results of Problem 5.20 to the expression gives

$$\left(\frac{\partial P}{\partial V}\right)_S = -\left(\frac{\partial S}{\partial V}\right)_P\left(\frac{\partial P}{\partial S}\right)_V = -\left(\frac{\partial S}{\partial V}\right)_P \Big/ \left(\frac{\partial S}{\partial P}\right)_V$$

$$= -\left(\frac{\partial S}{\partial T}\right)_P\left(\frac{\partial T}{\partial V}\right)_P \Big/ \left(\frac{\partial S}{\partial T}\right)_V\left(\frac{\partial T}{\partial P}\right)_V$$

$$= -C_P\left(\frac{\partial T}{\partial V}\right)_P \Big/ C_V\left(\frac{\partial T}{\partial P}\right)_V$$

5.22. **Supposing that ΔG° varies with temperature as shown in Fig. 5-4, prepare a table of signs for the thermodynamic properties.**

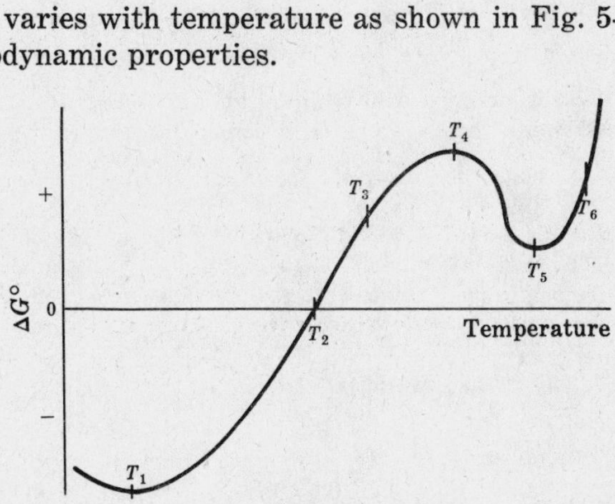

Fig. 5-4

Applying the rules outlined in Section 5.19 gives:

	ΔG°	$(\partial\Delta G^\circ/\partial T)_P$	ΔS°	ΔH°	$(\partial\Delta S^\circ/\partial T)_P$	$(\partial\Delta H^\circ/\partial T)_P$	ΔC_P°	$\ln K$	$(\partial \ln K/\partial T)_P$
T_1	−	0	0	−	−	−	−	+	−
T_2	0	+	−	−	0	0	0	0	−
T_3	+	+	−	+	+	+	+	−	+
T_4	+	0	0	+	+	+	+	−	+
T_5	+	0	0	+	−	−	−	−	+
T_6	+	+	−	+	−	−	−	−	+

For the ΔH° entries at T_3 and T_6, the + value resulted from assuming ΔG° to be numerically greater than $T\,\Delta S^\circ$.

Supplementary Problems

Free Energy Functions

5.23. For the reaction

$$Ag(s) + \tfrac{1}{2}Br_2(g) \;=\; AgBr(liq)$$

Metz and Seifert reported $\mathcal{E}^\circ = 0.7997 - 0.288\,Y + 0.097\,Y^2$ where $Y = (T - 705.2)10^{-3}$ K. Calculate ΔG°_{1000} and compare the value to ΔG° for the AgCl reaction considered in Problem 5.2.

Ans. $\mathcal{E}^\circ = 0.7232$ V, -69.779 kJ; less favorable

5.24. For the reaction

$$Ag(s) + \tfrac{1}{2}I_2(g) \;=\; AgI(liq)$$

Metz and Seifert reported $\mathcal{E}^\circ = (0.5720 - 0.227\,Z + 0.220\,Z^2)$ V where $Z = (T - 831.2)10^{-3}$ K. Find expressions for ΔG°, ΔS°, ΔH° and ΔC_P° in terms of Z.

Ans. $\Delta G^\circ = -n\mathcal{F}\mathcal{E}^\circ = (-55.191 + 21.90\,Z - 21.23\,Z^2)$ kJ,

$\Delta S^\circ = -(\partial \Delta G^\circ/\partial T)_P = (-21.90\,Z + 42.46)$ EU,

$\Delta H^\circ = \Delta G^\circ + T\Delta S^\circ = (-73.394 + 35.29\,Z + 21.23\,Z^2)$ kJ,

$\Delta C_P^\circ = (\partial \Delta H^\circ/\partial T)_P = (35.29 + 42.46\,Z)$ J K^{-1}

5.25. What is ΔG for the reversible isothermal compression of one mole of an ideal gas from 1.00 to 5.00 atm at 25° C? What is ΔG if the process were performed irreversibly?

Ans. 3989 J; 3989 J (ΔG is path-independent)

5.26. What is ΔG for the phase transition

$$H_2O(liq) \;=\; H_2O(s)$$

at -15 °C if the vapor pressure above water at this temperature is 191.5 N m^{-2} and above ice is 165.5 N m^{-2}? Assume a three-step process consisting of an evaporation, a pressure change and a deposition. *Ans.* $\Delta G_{(1)} = \Delta G_{(3)} = 0$, $\Delta G_{(2)} = -313$ J

5.27. Calculate q, w, ΔE, ΔH, ΔS, ΔG and ΔA for a reversible isothermal expansion of one mole of an ideal diatomic gas at 100 °C from 1.00 dm^3 to 10.00 dm^3. What would be the values of these parameters if the process were performed irreversibly against a constant external pressure of 1.00 atm?

Ans. $q = w = 7146$ J, $\Delta E = \Delta H = 0$, $\Delta S = 19.15$ EU, $\Delta G = \Delta A = -7146$ J;

$q = w = 912$ J, rest are unchanged

5.28. Calculate ΔG°_{298} for the reaction

$$CaCO_3(calcite) \;=\; CaCO_3(aragonite)$$

if ΔG_{298}(formation) $= -269.78$ kcal mol^{-1} for calcite and -269.53 kcal mol^{-1} for aragonite. Which crystal form is the more stable at 25 °C under standard conditions?

Ans. 0.25 kcal = 1.05 kJ; nonspontaneous, calcite more stable

5.29. Calculate ΔG°_{298}(reaction) for

$$C_2H_4(g) + HCl(g) \;=\; C_2H_5Cl(g)$$

if ΔG°_{298}(formation) $= 16.28$ kcal mol^{-1} for C_2H_4(g), -22.777 for HCl(g) and -14.45 for C_2H_5Cl(g). Why is ΔH° larger than ΔG°?

Ans. -7.95 kcal $= -33.26$ kJ; a decrease in entropy decreases the spontaneity

5.30. Calculate ΔG°_{298}(reaction) for the deamination of L-aspartic acid to fumaric acid:

$$\underset{\displaystyle NH_2}{HOOC{-}\underset{|}{C}H{-}CH_2{-}COOH} \;=\; HOOC{-}CH{=}CH{-}COOH + NH_3$$

given that the free energies of formation for the acids, as reported by Burton and Krebs, are −174.88 kcal mol^{-1} for L-aspartic acid and −156.49 kcal mol^{-1} for fumaric acid, and ΔG°_{298}(formation) = −3.94 kcal mol^{-1} for NH_3. Why does this reaction proceed?

Ans. 14.45 kcal = 60.46 kJ; the change from the standard state may make ΔG favorable or this reaction may be only one step in a series of reactions which the set of ΔG values for the various steps makes favorable

5.31. Find the temperature at which the spontaneity of the reaction

$$2CO(g) = C(graph) + CO_2(g)$$

reverses. ΔG°_{298}(formation) and ΔH°_{298}(formation) = −94.254 and −94.051 kcal mol^{-1} for CO_2(g), and −32.780 and −26.416 kcal mol^{-1} for CO(g). In cal mol^{-1} K^{-1},

$$C_P = 5.152 + 15.224 \times 10^{-3}T - 96.81 \times 10^{-7}T^2 + 2.313 \times 10^{-9}T^3 \quad \text{for } CO_2(g)$$

$$C_P = 6.420 + 1.665 \times 10^{-3}T - 1.96 \times 10^{-7}T^2 \quad \text{for } CO(g)$$

$$C_P = 2.673 + 2.617 \times 10^{-3}T - 1.169 \times 10^{5}T^{-2} \quad \text{for graphite}$$

Ans. $\Delta C_P^\circ = (-5.015 + 14.511 \times 10^{-3}T - 92.89 \times 10^{-7}T^2 + 2.313 \times 10^{-9}T^3 - 1.169 \times 10^5 T^{-2})$ cal mol^{-1} K^{-1},

$\Delta H^\circ_{298} = -41.219$ kcal, $\Delta G^\circ_{298} = -28.694$ kcal, $J = -40.684$ kcal, $K = 13.02$ cal,

$\Delta G = (-40{,}684 + 13.02\,T + 5.015\,T \ln T - 7.256 \times 10^{-3}T^2 + 15.48 \times 10^{-7}T^3 - 0.193 \times 10^{9}T^4 + 0.585 \times 10^5 T^{-1})$ cal; $T = 937$ K

5.32. The tabulated values of $(G^\circ_T - H^\circ_{298})/T$ for F_2(g) are −48.447 and −60.427 cal K^{-1} mol^{-1}, for Cl_2(g) are −53.289 and −65.617 cal K^{-1} mol^{-1}, and for ClF(g) are −52.064 and −64.091 cal K^{-1} mol^{-1}, at 298 K and 3000 K, respectively. If ΔG°_{298}(formation) = −12.497 kcal mol^{-1} for ClF(g), find ΔH°_{298}(reaction) and ΔG°_{3000}(reaction) for

$$F_2(g) + Cl_2(g) = 2ClF(g)$$

Ans. ΔH°_{298}(reaction) = −24.281 kcal, ΔG°_{3000}(reaction) = −30.695 kcal = −128.428 kJ

5.33. If $(G^\circ_{800} - H^\circ_{298})/800$ = −113.048 cal K^{-1} mol^{-1} for WCl_6(g), −33.715 cal K^{-1} mol^{-1} for H_2(g), −9.959 cal K^{-1} mol^{-1} for W(s), and −47.163 cal K^{-1} mol^{-1} for HCl(g), could the reaction

$$WCl_6(g) + 3H_2(g) = W(s) + 6HCl(g)$$

be used at 800 K to prepare W(s)? Assume ΔH°_{298}(formation) = −118.000 kcal mol^{-1} for WCl_6(g) and −22.063 kcal mol^{-1} for HCl(g).

Ans. Yes: ΔG°_{800}(reaction) = −77.373 kcal = −323.729 kJ, which is favorable.

5.34. The formation of ozone in the upper atmosphere (25–30 km, 230 K) takes place as an O_2 molecule is dissociated by ultraviolet radiation and the atomic O formed reacts with a second O_2 molecule according to the reactions

$$O_2(g) + h\nu = 2O(g)$$

$$O(g) + O_2(g) = O_3(g)$$

If $(G^\circ_T - H^\circ_{298})/T$ = −38.468 and −38.953 cal K^{-1} mol^{-1} for O(g), −49.004 and −49.643 cal K^{-1} mol^{-1} for O_2(g), and −57.080 and −57.909 cal K^{-1} mol^{-1} for O_3(g), at 298 K and 200 K, respectively, find ΔG°_{230}(reaction) for the second reaction. Use the values ΔH°_{298}(formation) = 59.559 kcal mol^{-1} for O(g) and 34.100 kcal mol^{-1} for O_3(g). *Ans.* −18.422 kcal = −77.078 kJ

Activities

5.35. At what pressure will $G - G^\circ$ be 100 J mol^{-1} for an ideal gas at 25 °C? *Ans.* 1.041 atm

5.36. What is the value of $G - G^\circ$ for ethane at 100 atm and 100 °C assuming ideal-gas behavior? If T_c = 32.2 °C and P_c = 48.3 atm, find γ from Fig. 5-1 and calculate $G - G^\circ$ for the real gas. From the following data, confirm the value of γ:

d, mol dm^{-3}	0.5	1.0	1.5	2.0	2.5	3.0	3.5	4.0	4.5	5.0	5.5
P, atm	14.43	27.28	38.79	49.03	58.29	66.68	74.36	81.50	88.25	94.73	101.36

Ans. 14.29 kJ; $T_r = 1.22$, $P_r = 2.07$ giving $\gamma = 0.69$, 13.12 kJ;
$\overline{V} = 1/d$, plot of $\overline{V} - (RT/P)$ against P gives $RT \ln \gamma = -10.0$ or $\gamma = 0.72$

5.37. Express I in terms of C for a 2:2 electrolyte and calculate I for a 0.0025 M solution of $CuSO_4$.

Ans. $I = 4C = 0.01\,M$

5.38. Calculate $\gamma_{Cu^{2+}}$, γ_{Cl^-}, $\gamma_\pm$ and $a_\pm$ for a solution of $CuCl_2$ having $I = 0.01\,M$.

Ans. 0.624, 0.889, 0.790, 0.00790

Equilibrium Constants

5.39. Calculate ΔG_{298} for the reaction

$$Cu^{2+}(aq) + 4NH_3(aq) = Cu(NH_3)_4{}^{2+}(aq)$$

if $\Delta G^\circ_{298} = -70.54$ kJ, $a_{Cu^{2+}} = 0.01$, $a_{NH_3} = 0.01$ and $a_{complex} = 0.01$. *Ans.* -24.89 kJ

5.40. If $\Delta G^\circ_{298} = -237.178$ kJ for the reaction

$$H_2(g) + \tfrac{1}{2}O_2(g) = H_2O(liq)$$

what is K? *Ans.* 3.7×10^{41}

5.41. Find K, ΔH° and ΔS° at 25 °C for the reaction

$$\text{glycerol} + HPO_4{}^{2-} = \text{DL-glycerol-1-phosphate}^{2-} + H_2O$$

if $K = 0.0122$ at 37 °C and $\Delta G^\circ_{298} = 2.24$ kcal (= 9.37 kJ), as reported by Burton and Krebs.

Ans. $K = 0.0228$, $\Delta H^\circ = -40.07$ kJ, $\Delta S^\circ = -165.9$ EU

5.42. Calculate the various equilibrium constants at 1000 K and 100 atm total pressure for the reaction

$$\tfrac{3}{2}H_2(g) + \tfrac{1}{2}N_2(g) = NH_3(g)$$

if $\Delta G^\circ = 61.890$ kJ. Assume that $\gamma = 1.04$ for H_2, 1.02 for N_2 and 1.00 for NH_3.

Ans. $K_\gamma = 0.93$, $K = 5.85 \times 10^{-4}$, $K_p = 6.29 \times 10^{-4}$, $K_c = 5.16 \times 10^{-2}$, $K_x = 6.29 \times 10^{-2}$

5.43. Determine the effect on the equilibrium at 25 °C for the endothermic reaction

$$CH_4(g) + HCl(g) = CH_3Cl(g) + H_2(g)$$

of (1) an increase in x_{HCl}, (2) a decrease in x_{H_2}, (3) an increase in pressure, and (4) an increase in temperature.

Ans. x_{CH_3Cl} will (1) increase, (2) increase, (3) not change, and (4) increase.

Equilibrium Calculations

5.44. What is the percent dissociation of NOCl(g) into NO(g) and Cl_2(g) at 1.00 atm and 10^{-3} atm if ΔG°_{298}(formation) = 15.79 kcal mol^{-1} for NOCl(g) and 20.69 kcal mol^{-1} for NO(g)? Assume ideal gas behavior.

Ans. ΔG°_{298}(reaction) = 20.50 kJ for 1 mol NOCl(g), $K = K_p = 2.55 \times 10^{-4}$; 0.51% and 4.93%

5.45. Assuming real-gas behavior for the reaction

$$\tfrac{3}{2}H_2(g) + \tfrac{1}{2}N_2(g) = NH_3(g)$$

at 25 °C and 100.0 atm, calculate the mole fraction of NH_3 at equilibrium, if $\gamma_{H_2} = 1.10$, $\gamma_{N_2} = 1.00$, $\gamma_{NH_3} = 0.40$ and $\Delta G^\circ_{298}(\text{reaction}) = -16.38$ kJ.

Ans. $K = 7.43 \times 10^2$, $K_\gamma = 0.345$, $K_p = 2.15 \times 10^3$; 0.9981

5.46. Calculate the pressure of $CO_2(g)$ over a sample of $CaCO_3(s)$ at 1000 K if $\Delta G^\circ_{1000} = 22.90$ kJ for the reaction

$$CaCO_3(s) = CaO(s) + CO_2(g)$$

Ans. $K = K_p = a_{CO_2} = P_{CO_2} = 6.39 \times 10^{-2}$ atm

5.47. What is the concentration of Hg_2^{2+} in a saturated solution of Hg_2Cl_2 if $K_{sp} = 2 \times 10^{-18}$? What is the concentration of Hg_2^{2+} in a 0.500 *M* solution of NaCl assuming the Debye-Hückel limiting law to be valid? What is the solubility of Hg_2^{2+} in surface seawater (10,500 ppm Na^+, 1350 ppm Mg^{2+}, 400 ppm Ca^{2+}, 380 ppm K^+, 19,000 ppm Cl^- and 2700 ppm SO_4^{2-}, with $d = 1.02 \times 10^3$ kg m^{-3}) assuming the Debye-Hückel limiting law to be valid?

Ans. $8 \times 10^{-7} M$; $I = 0.500$, $\gamma_\pm = 0.189$, 1.2×10^{-15};
$C = 0.46\,M$ for Na^+, 0.06 for Mg^{2+}, 0.01 for Ca^{2+} and K^+,
0.55 for Cl^- and 0.03 for SO_4^{2-}, $I = 0.71\,M$, $\gamma_\pm = 0.137$; $2.6 \times 10^{-15} M$

5.48. What are the pOH and pH of a 0.100 *M* solution of NH_3 if the weak base establishes the following equilibrium

$$NH_3(0.1\,M) = NH_4^+(aq) + OH^-(aq)$$

where $K_b = 1.79 \times 10^{-5}$?

Ans. $C = 1.33 \times 10^{-3} M$ for OH^-; pOH = 2.876, pH = 11.124

5.49. What is the pH of a 0.100 *M* NH_4Cl solution? $K_b = 1.79 \times 10^{-5}$ for NH_3.

Ans. $K_h = 5.59 \times 10^{-10}$, $C = 7.48 \times 10^{-6} M$ for H^+ and NH_3 (or NH_4OH),
$C = 0.100\,M$ for NH_4^+; pH = 5.126

5.50. Calculate the pH of a buffer solution prepared by adding 0.500 mol of NH_4Cl to 1 dm³ of 0.100 *M* NH_3. What is the pH after the addition of 0.001 mol of HCl to the buffer? $K_b = 1.79 \times 10^{-5}$ for NH_3.

Ans. $C_{OH^-} = 3.58 \times 10^{-6}$, pOH = 5.446, pH = 8.554;
$C_{OH^-} = 3.54 \times 10^{-6}$, pOH = 5.451, pH = 8.549

5.51. Calculate the pH of a 0.0100 *M* solution of α-alanine benzoate if $K_a = 6.46 \times 10^{-5}$ and $K_b = 4.52 \times 10^{-3}$.

Ans. $K_h = 3.42 \times 10^{-8}$, $C = x$ for base and acid and $0.0100 - x$ for α-alanine and benzoate ions, $x = 1.85 \times 10^{-6}$, $C = y$ for H^+, $0.0100 - x + y$ for benzoate ion and $x - y$ for benzoic acid, $y = 1.195 \times 10^{-8}$; pH = 7.922

5.52. For the reaction

$$2CrO_4^{2-} + 2H^+ = Cr_2O_7^{2-} + H_2O$$

the concentration equilbrium constant was determined by Smith and Metz as 1.3×10^{16} in solutions with I = 0.375 *M*. If $\Delta G^\circ_{298}(\text{formation}) = -173.96$ kcal mol^{-1} for CrO_4^{2-}, -311.0 kcal mol^{-1} for $Cr_2O_7^{2-}$ and -56.687 kcal mol^{-1} for H_2O, calculate *K*. What is the value of K_γ?

Ans. $\Delta G^\circ_{298}(\text{reaction}) = -19.8$ kcal $= -82.7$ kJ; $K = 3.3 \times 10^{14}$, $K_\gamma = 2.5 \times 10^{-2}$

5.53. The *buffer capacity* is the number of moles of strong acid or base required to change the pH of 1 dm³ of solution by one pH unit. To calculate the buffer capacity, the amount of strong acid or base added is divided by the resulting pH change of the solution. Calculate the capacity for adding

0.0010 mol of NaOH (*a*) to 1 dm^3 of pure water, (*b*) to a buffer prepared by adding 0.0100 mol of $NaC_2H_3O_2$ to 1 dm^3 of 0.0100 *M* $HC_2H_3O_2$ and (*c*) to a buffer prepared by adding 0.500 mol of $NaC_2H_3O_2$ to 1 dm^3 of 0.100 *M* $HC_2H_3O_2$. $K_a = 1.76 \times 10^{-5}$ for $HC_2H_3O_2$.

Ans. (*a*) pH = 7.00 for water, 11.00 for solution, 2.5×10^{-4};

(*b*) pH = 4.754 for buffer, 4.741 after, 0.077;

(*c*) pH = 5.453 for buffer, 5.458 after, 0.20

5.54. When distilled water is stored in a tank that is open to the air, the dissolved gases—mainly CO_2—change the pH from 7.00. (*a*) What is the pH of a saturated CO_2 solution if the solubility of CO_2 is 0.145 g in 100 g of water at 25 °C and 1.00 atm CO_2? Assume only the following reaction occurs:

$$CO_2(aq) + H_2O = H^+(aq) + HCO_3^-(aq)$$

where ΔG°_{298}(formation) = −92.26 kcal mol^{-1} for CO_2(aq), −56.687 kcal mol^{-1} for H_2O and −140.26 kcal mol^{-1} for HCO_3^-(aq). (*b*) If the actual concentration of CO_2 in a solution having air over it is given by

$$C_{CO_2} = kP_{CO_2}$$

where *k* is a constant, determine the pH of water in contact with air if $P_{CO_2} = 4 \times 10^{-2}$ atm.

Ans. (*a*) ΔG°_{298} = 8.69 kcal = 36.36 kJ, $K = 4.25 \times 10^{-7}$, $C = 0.0329$ *M* CO_2, pH = 3.93;

(*b*) $k = 0.145$ g (100 g $H_2O)^{-1}$ atm^{-1}, $C = 0.00132$ *M* CO_2, pH = 4.63

Thermodynamic Relations

5.55. Beginning with the definitions of *G* and *A*, show that (*5.57*) and (*5.58*) are valid.

5.56. Beginning with (*5.55*), show that

$$\left(\frac{\partial T}{\partial V}\right)_S = -\left(\frac{\partial P}{\partial S}\right)_V$$

5.57. Using the format of (*5.59*), express the Maxwell relation that begins $(\partial T/\partial P)_S$.

Ans. $\left(\frac{\partial T}{\partial P}\right)_S = \left(\frac{\partial V}{\partial S}\right)_P$

5.58. Show that

(*a*) $\left(\frac{\partial H}{\partial P}\right)_T = -T\left(\frac{\partial V}{\partial T}\right)_P + V$ (*c*) $\left(\frac{\partial G}{\partial V}\right)_T = V\left(\frac{\partial P}{\partial V}\right)_T$

(*b*) $\left(\frac{\partial H}{\partial G}\right)_T = \frac{1}{V}\left[-T\left(\frac{\partial V}{\partial T}\right)_P + V\right]$ (*d*) $\left(\frac{\partial P}{\partial T}\right)_G = \frac{S}{V}$

5.59. From the plot of ΔG°(formation) against temperature shown in Fig. 5-5 for the reaction

$$Pb + Br_2 = PbBr_2(g)$$

complete the following table of signs of the thermodynamic properties:

	ΔG°	$(\partial \Delta G^\circ/\partial T)_P$	ΔS°	ΔH°	$(\partial \Delta S^\circ/\partial T)_P$	$(\partial \Delta H^\circ/\partial T)_P$	ΔC_P°	ln *K*	$(\partial \ln K/\partial T)_P$
100 K				−					
1000 K				−					
2000 K		−		−					
4000 K									
5000 K				−					

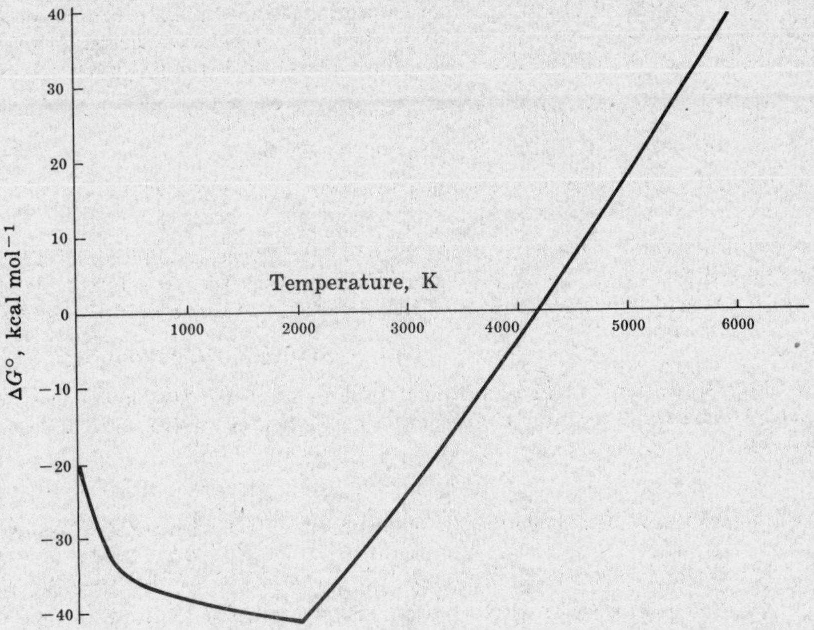

Fig. 5-5

Ans.

	$\Delta G°$	$(\partial \Delta G°/\partial T)_P$	$\Delta S°$	$\Delta H°$	$(\partial \Delta S°/\partial T)_P$	$(\partial \Delta H°/\partial T)_P$	$\Delta C_P°$	$\ln K$	$(\partial \ln K/\partial T)_P$
100 K	−	−	+	−	−	−	−	+	−
1000 K	−	−	+	−	−	−	−	+	−
2000 K	−	−	+	−	−	−	−	+	−
4000 K	−	+	−	−	−	−	−	+	−
5000 K	+	+	−	−	−	−	−	−	−

Chapter 6

Statistical Thermodynamics

Ensembles

6.1 INTRODUCTION

A *canonical ensemble* consists of N_s distinguishable systems which are identical in that they have the same number of molecules, N; volume, V; and thermodynamic state. As N_s becomes large, the time (or observable) average of any mechanical property of a system, such as P or E, becomes equal to the instantaneous ensemble average value for the property. Nonmechanical properties, such as T and S, must be calculated using known thermodynamic relationships. The ensemble acts as a single supersystem having a volume of N_sV, number of molecules equal to N_sN, and a total energy of E_t.

The *Boltzmann statistics* used in this chapter is obtained as the limiting case of *Fermi-Dirac statistics* (systems described by antisymmetric wave functions) and *Bose-Einstein statistics* (systems described by symmetric wave functions) when it is assumed that there are many more energy states available than molecules, so that there is a very low probability of two molecules being in the same energy state. The results of Boltzmann statistics often fail for certain systems at low temperatures.

EXAMPLE 6.1. Even though the systems in a canonical ensemble are macroscopically indistinguishable, they are not necessarily in the same microscopic state. Because each system in the ensemble has the same volume, each system has the same available energy states. However, a given system may be found in any quantum state consistent with the given values of N, V and E. Determine the possible distributions among energy states of three simple harmonic oscillators (SHO) such that $E_t = 9E_0$, if the quantum mechanical solution for energy is

$$E_v = \left(v + \frac{1}{2}\right)h\nu \qquad (6.1)$$

where E_v is the energy of the state corresponding to the integer v ($v = 0, 1, 2, \ldots$), h is Planck's constant, and ν is the frequency of oscillation. Is $(1, 0, 1, 1, 0, \ldots)$ an acceptable answer?

The energies of the first few states are $E_0 = (1/2)h\nu$, $E_1 = (3/2)h\nu = 3E_0$, $E_2 = (5/2)h\nu = 5E_0$, etc. The distribution $(1, 0, 1, 1, 0, \ldots)$ means that there is one oscillator in state 0, contributing E_0 to the total energy; none in state 1; one in state 2, contributing $5E_0$; one in state 3, contributing $7E_0$; and none above state 3. The total energy would be $13E_0$, and so the proposed distribution is not acceptable. The distributions $(1, 1, 1, 0, 0, \ldots)$, $(2, 0, 0, 1, 0, \ldots)$ and $(0, 3, 0, 0, 0, \ldots)$ are the only ones that give $E_t = 9E_0$.

6.2 COMBINATORIAL THEOREMS

If the first step in a process can be performed in n_1 ways, the second step in n_2 ways, ..., then the whole process can be performed in t ways, where

$$t = n_1 n_2 \cdots \qquad (6.2)$$

The number of permutations of N distinguishable objects is

$$t = N! \qquad (6.3)$$

where
$$N! = N(N-1)(N-2)\cdots(2)(1) \tag{6.4}$$

Note that
$$1! = 0! = 1 \tag{6.5}$$

The number of ways of grouping N distinguishable objects into r groups such that N_i are in group i is

$$t = \frac{N!}{\prod_{i=1}^{r} N_i!} \tag{6.6}$$

The number of ways of selecting n distinguishable objects from a set of $N \geq n$ distinguishable objects is

$$t = \frac{N!}{(N-n)!\,n!} \tag{6.7}$$

The number of ways of putting N indistinguishable objects into $g \geq N$ distinguishable locations with no more than one object to a location is

$$t = \frac{g!}{(g-N)!\,N!} \tag{6.8}$$

The number of ways of putting N indistinguishable objects into g distinguishable locations with no restrictions on occupation is

$$t = \frac{(N+g-1)!}{N!\,(g-1)!} \tag{6.9}$$

The number of ways of putting N distinguishable objects into g locations with no restrictions is

$$t = g^N \tag{6.10}$$

EXAMPLE 6.2. In many problems, $N!$ or $\ln N!$ must be evaluated where N is a large number. Using *Stirling's approximation,*

$$\ln N! \approx N \ln N - N \tag{6.11}$$

evaluate $\ln L!$.

From (*6.11*),

$$\begin{aligned} \ln L! &\approx L \ln L - L \\ &= (6.022 \times 10^{23})(2.303) \log (6.022 \times 10^{23}) - (6.022 \times 10^{23}) \\ &= (6.022 \times 10^{23})[(2.303)(23.780) - 1] = 323.77 \times 10^{23} \end{aligned}$$

6.3 ENSEMBLE ENERGY STATES AND PROBABILITIES

From (*6.6*), the number of ensemble states corresponding to a given $(N_1, N_2, \ldots)$ is

$$\Omega = \frac{N_s!}{\prod_i N_i!} \tag{6.12a}$$

in terms of energy states, or

$$\Omega = \frac{N_s!\,(\prod_j \omega_j)}{\prod_j N_j!} \tag{6.12b}$$

in terms of energy levels, where ω_j is the degeneracy of level j.

The conditional probability of finding a chosen system in the ith quantum state, E_i, given that the distribution is $(N_1, N_2 \ldots)$ is

$$P_i(N_1, N_2, \ldots) = \frac{N_i}{N_s} \tag{6.13}$$

where N_i represents the number of systems in the ith quantum state under the given distribution and N_s is the total number of systems. Therefore, considering all distributions, the overall probability of finding a chosen system in state E_i is

$$P_i = \sum \left(\frac{N_i}{N_s}\right)\left(\frac{\Omega}{\Sigma\Omega}\right) = \frac{\Sigma N_i \Omega}{N_s \Sigma \Omega} \tag{6.14}$$

In (*6.14*) the summations are extended over all distributions.

EXAMPLE 6.3. Find Ω for each of the three acceptable distributions described in Example 6.1. Prepare a table showing how these distributions are realized for three distinguishable SHO's A, B and C.

For $(1,1,1,0,0,\ldots)$ (*6.12a*) gives

$$\Omega(1,1,1,0,0,\ldots) = \frac{3!}{1!\,1!\,1!\,0!\,0!\cdots} = 6$$

Similarly, $\Omega(2,0,0,1,0,\ldots) = 3$ and $\Omega(0,3,0,0,0,\ldots) = 1$. The various assignments of the SHO's are:

Energy state:	0	1	2	3	4	5	...
Energy:	E_0	$3E_0$	$5E_0$	$7E_0$	$9E_0$	$11E_0$	...
$(1,1,1,0,0,\ldots)$:	A	B	C				
	A	C	B				
	B	A	C				
	B	C	A				
	C	A	B				
	C	B	A				
$(2,0,0,1,0,\ldots)$:	AB			C			
	AC			B			
	BC			A			
$(0,3,0,0,0,\ldots)$:		ABC					

EXAMPLE 6.4. What is the probability of finding system B in E_0 for the acceptable SHO distribution $(1,1,1,0,0,\ldots)$? Compare the numerical answer to the actual count of the number of times system B appears in the E_0-column of the table prepared in Example 6.3 for this distribution.

Using (*6.13*) with $N_s = 3$ and $N_0 = 1$ gives $P_0(1,1,1,0,0,\ldots) = 1/3$. In Example 6.3, system B appears twice in the column labeled E_0 out of six entries, making the conditional probability of finding B in E_0 to be 2/6, or 1/3.

EXAMPLE 6.5. What is the overall probability of finding system B in E_0 for the acceptable SHO distributions given in Example 6.3? Compare the numerical answer to that predicted by actual count of the number of times system B appears in the entire E_0-column.

Substituting $\Omega(1,1,1,0,0,\ldots) = 6$, $\Omega(2,0,0,1,0,\ldots) = 3$ and $\Omega(0,3,0,0,0,\ldots) = 1$ into (*6.14*) gives

$$P_0 = \frac{(1)(6) + (2)(3) + (0)(1)}{3(6+3+1)} = 0.400$$

Among the ten entries in the E_0-column of Example 6.3, system B appears four times, giving a probability of 4/10 or 0.400.

6.4 MOST PROBABLE DISTRIBUTION

As N_s becomes large, $\overline{N}_i$, the average of N_i, approaches N_i^*, the *most probable distribution*, which is given by

$$N_i^* = \frac{N_s e^{-E_i/kT}}{Q} \tag{6.15}$$

where k is Boltzmann's constant ($k = 1.380662 \times 10^{-23}$ J K^{-1}) and the *partition function*, Q, is defined as

$$Q = \sum_i e^{-E_i/kT} = \sum_j \omega_j e^{-E_j/kT} \tag{6.16}$$

In this limiting case, (*6.14*) becomes

$$P_i = \frac{e^{-E_i/kT}}{Q} \tag{6.17}$$

EXAMPLE 6.6. The ratio of the most probable numbers of systems at two different energies in the ensemble can be computed from

$$\frac{N_b^*}{N_a^*} = e^{-(E_b - E_a)/kT} \tag{6.18}$$

Find this ratio if $E_b - E_a = kT$. If E_b and E_a represent energy levels, (*6.18*) is multiplied by the ratio of the degeneracies, ω_b/ω_a. Repeat the calculations for $\omega_b = 3$ and $\omega_a = 1$.

Substituting into (*6.18*) gives

$$\frac{N_b^*}{N_a^*} = e^{-kT/kT} = 0.367$$

assuming singly-degenerate energy states, and after multiplying by 3/1 gives $N_b^*/N_a^* = 1.101$ for the levels.

Ideal-Gas Partition Functions

6.5 INTRODUCTION

Assume the system under consideration to consist of a large number, N, of molecules, each of which may occupy a number of quantum states. The energy of the system is

$$E_i = \varepsilon_1 + \varepsilon_2 + \cdots + \varepsilon_N$$

where ε_1 is the energy of molecule 1, ε_2 is the energy of molecule 2, etc. Equation (*6.16*) becomes

$$Q = q_1 q_2 \cdots q_N$$

in which q_α, the *molecular partition function* for molecule α, is given by

$$q_\alpha = \sum e^{-\varepsilon_\alpha/kT} \tag{6.19}$$

The summation in (*6.19*) is over all the values of ε_α which correspond to the quantum states of molecule α. Because the molecules are all the same, $q_1 = q_2 = \cdots = q_N = q$ and $Q = q^N$. Correcting for the indistinguishability of the molecules, we obtain

$$Q = \frac{q^N}{N!} \tag{6.20}$$

The contributions to ε_α for an ideal gas are nuclear, electronic, vibrational, rotational and translational (see Sections 6.10, ..., 6.6) giving

$$\varepsilon_\alpha = \varepsilon_{\text{nuc}} + \varepsilon_{\text{elec}} + \varepsilon_{\text{vib}} + \varepsilon_{\text{rot}} + \varepsilon_{\text{trans}}$$

$$q = q_{\text{nuc}} q_{\text{elec}} q_{\text{vib}} q_{\text{rot}} q_{\text{trans}}$$

$$Q = (q_{\text{nuc}} q_{\text{elec}} q_{\text{vib}} q_{\text{rot}})^N \frac{q_{\text{trans}}^N}{N!} \tag{6.21}$$

The $N!$ correction term is traditionally associated with the translational partition function because not all gases have vibrational and rotational contributions, and the nuclear and electronic contributions are negligible for most gases. Equation (6.21) does not contain minor contributions for rotational-vibrational interactions or for intramolecular rotation energy levels.

6.6 MOLECULAR TRANSLATIONAL PARTITION FUNCTION

For an ideal gas with Λ atoms in the molecule, of the total of 3Λ degrees of freedom, three are attributed to translational motion of the molecule as a whole. The quantum mechanical solution for a particle of mass m in a three-dimensional box of side a, see Problem 11.20, gives the energy as

$$\varepsilon_{\text{trans}} = (n_x^2 + n_y^2 + n_z^2)\frac{h^2}{8ma^2} \tag{6.22}$$

where the n_i are integers and h is Planck's constant ($h = 6.626176 \times 10^{-34}$ J s).

EXAMPLE 6.7. The values of $\varepsilon_{\text{trans}}$ are of the order of 10^{-42} J apart and at room temperature a large number of states are occupied by the molecules (because $kT \approx 4 \times 10^{-21}$ J). Using the above expression for $\varepsilon_{\text{trans}}$, show that

$$q_{\text{trans}} = (2\pi mkT)^{3/2}\frac{V}{h^3} \tag{6.23}$$

where V is the volume of the box.

Substituting (6.22) into (6.19) gives

$$q_{\text{trans}} = \sum_{n_x, n_y, n_z} e^{-(n_x^2+n_y^2+n_z^2)h^2/8ma^2kT}$$

$$= \left[\sum_{n_x=0}^{\infty} e^{-n_x^2h^2/8ma^2kT}\right]\left[\sum_{n_y=0}^{\infty} e^{-n_y^2h^2/8ma^2kT}\right]\left[\sum_{n_z=0}^{\infty} e^{-n_z^2h^2/8ma^2kT}\right]$$

Replacing the summations by integration because of the large number of states occupied gives

$$q_{\text{trans}} = \left[\int_0^{\infty} e^{-n^2h^2/8ma^2kT}\,dn\right]^3 = \left[(2\pi mkT)^{1/2}\frac{a}{h}\right]^3 = (2\pi mkT)^{3/2}\frac{V}{h^3}$$

6.7 MOLECULAR ROTATIONAL PARTITION FUNCTION

A diatomic or linear polyatomic molecule has two rotational degrees of freedom. For the diatomic molecule, these are described by the quantum mechanical solution for the rigid rotator (see Problem 11.22), giving

$$\varepsilon_{\text{rot}} = J(J+1)\frac{h^2}{8\pi^2 I} \tag{6.24}$$

where $J = 0, 1, 2, \ldots$; each level has a degeneracy of $2J+1$; and the moment of inertia, I, is given by

$$I = \mu r^2 \tag{6.25}$$

where r is the distance between the atoms in the diatomic molecule and the *reduced mass*, μ, is given by

$$\mu = \frac{m_1 m_2}{m_1 + m_2} \tag{6.26}$$

The values of ε_{rot} are of the order of 10^{-23} J apart and at room temperature a large number of levels are occupied by the molecules.

Substituting the above expression for ε_{rot} for a diatomic or linear polyatomic molecule into (*6.19*) and integrating over J gives

$$q_{rot} = \frac{8\pi^2 IkT}{h^2\sigma} \tag{6.27}$$

The symmetry number, σ, of the molecule represents the number of indistinguishable positions into which the molecule can be placed by simple rigid rotations, e.g. $\sigma = 1$ for asymmetric linear molecules such as CO and HCN and $\sigma = 2$ for symmetric linear molecules such as O_2 and CO_2. For nonlinear polyatomic molecules having three rotational degrees of freedom,

$$q_{rot} = \frac{8\pi^2(8\pi^3 I_x I_y I_z)^{1/2}(kT)^{3/2}}{h^3\sigma} \tag{6.28}$$

where I_x, I_y and I_z represent the moments of inertia around three mutually perpendicular axes through the molecule and $\sigma = 2$ for C_2H_2, 3 for NH_3, 4 for C_2H_4, 12 for CH_4, etc.

6.8 MOLECULAR VIBRATIONAL PARTITION FUNCTION

The remaining degrees of freedom, $3\Lambda - 5$ for diatomic or linear polyatomic molecules or $3\Lambda - 6$ for nonlinear polyatomic molecules, are attributed to vibrational motion within the molecule. The energy is described by the quantum mechanical solution for the SHO problem (see Problem 11.5):

$$\varepsilon_{vib} = \sum_{i=1}^{3\Lambda-5 \text{ or } 3\Lambda-6} \left(v_i + \frac{1}{2}\right)h\nu_i \tag{6.29}$$

Here v_i and ν_i are the quantum number and fundamental frequency associated with the ith mode of vibration. The values of ε_{vib} are of the order of 10^{-20} J mol^{-1} apart and at room temperature most of the molecules are in the lower states.

Inserting (*6.29*) into (*6.19*) and summing over $0 \leq v_1 \leq \infty$, $0 \leq v_2 \leq \infty$, ...,

$$q_{vib} = \prod_{i=1}^{3\Lambda-5 \text{ or } 3\Lambda-6} \frac{1}{1-e^{-x_i}} \tag{6.30}$$

where x_i is given in terms of ν_i or $\bar{\nu}_i = \nu_i/c$ by (*2.4*) or (*2.5*), if the energy levels are measured with respect to the zero vibrational state of the molecule. If the energy levels are measured with respect to the hypothetical minimum of the potential energy well, $e^{-x_i/2}$ appears in the numerator of (*6.30*).

The number of molecules in a given vibrational state compared to that in the ground state is given by

$$N_v = N_0 e^{-vx} \tag{6.31}$$

and the number in the ground state compared to the total number present is given by

$$N_0 = N(1 - e^{-x}) \tag{6.32}$$

6.9 MOLECULAR ELECTRONIC PARTITION FUNCTION

Because the electronic energy states are of the order of 10^{-19} J apart, at room temperature most of the molecules are in the ground state. The partition function for such a system (see Problem 6.24) is

$$q_{elec} = \omega_0 \tag{6.33}$$

where ω_0 is the degeneracy of the ground level.

6.10 MOLECULAR NUCLEAR PARTITION FUNCTION

Because the nuclear energy states are spaced very far apart, only a negligible number of atoms in the molecule are not in the ground state at room temperature. The partition function becomes

$$q_{\text{nuc}} = \omega_{n,0} \tag{6.34}$$

where $\omega_{n,0}$ is the degeneracy of the nuclear ground state.

Application to Thermodynamics Involving Ideal Gases

6.11 GENERAL THERMODYNAMIC FUNCTIONS

In terms of the partition function,

$$A = -kT \ln Q \tag{6.35}$$

$$S = kT\left(\frac{\partial \ln Q}{\partial T}\right)_{V,N} + k \ln Q \tag{6.36}$$

$$P = kT\left(\frac{\partial \ln Q}{\partial V}\right)_{T,N} \tag{6.37}$$

$$E = kT^2\left(\frac{\partial \ln Q}{\partial T}\right)_{V,N} \tag{6.38}$$

The following sections describe the calculation of various thermodynamic properties of one mole of ideal gas, i.e. $N = L$. In general, the partition function is pressure-dependent, so we shall assume standard pressure conditions (denoted, as usual, by °).

6.12 MOLAR THERMAL ENERGY

The energy content of a mole of ideal gas can be considered to be the sum of the energy contributed by the molecular ground states, E_0°, and any additional thermal energy, E°(thermal), resulting from occupation of higher energy levels by the molecules when $T > 0$. Thus

$$E^\circ = E_0^\circ + E^\circ(\text{thermal}) \tag{6.39}$$

Note that $E_0^\circ = H_0^\circ = A_0^\circ = G_0^\circ$ for ideal gases because H°, A° and G° differ from E° either by RT or ST, which vanish at 0 K.

EXAMPLE 6.8. Derive expressions for E°(thermal) for ideal gases.

Applying (*6.38*) and (*6.21*) to (*6.23*), (*6.27*) or (*6.28*), (*6.30*), (*6.33*) and (*6.34*) gives

$$E^\circ(\text{thermal, trans}) = \frac{3}{2}RT \tag{6.40a}$$

$$E^\circ(\text{thermal, rot}) = \begin{cases} RT & \text{for a diatomic or linear polyatomic molecule} \\ \frac{3}{2}RT & \text{for a nonlinear polyatomic molecule} \end{cases} \tag{6.40b}$$

$$E^\circ(\text{thermal, vib}) = \sum_{i=1}^{3\Lambda-5 \text{ or } 3\Lambda-6} \frac{RTx_i}{e^{x_i}-1} \tag{6.40c}$$

$$E^\circ(\text{thermal, elec}) = 0 \tag{6.40d}$$

$$E^\circ(\text{thermal, nuc}) = 0 \tag{6.40e}$$

EXAMPLE 6.9. Evaluate E°(thermal) for $H_2O(g)$ at 373.12 K. The vibrational frequencies are $\bar{\nu}_1 = 3656.7$, $\bar{\nu}_2 = 1594.6$ and $\bar{\nu}_3 = 3755.8\ \text{cm}^{-1}$.

Substituting the values of $\bar{\nu}$ into *(2.5)* gives $x_1 = 14.101$, $x_2 = 6.149$ and $x_3 = 14.483$. Using *(6.40)* gives

$$E^\circ(\text{thermal, trans}) = \frac{3}{2}(8.314\ \text{J mol}^{-1}\ \text{K}^{-1})(373.12\ \text{K}) = 4653\ \text{J mol}^{-1}$$

$$E^\circ(\text{thermal, rot}) = \frac{3}{2}(8.314)(373.12) = 4653\ \text{J mol}^{-1}$$

$$E^\circ(\text{thermal, vib}) = (8.314)(373.12)\left(\frac{14.101}{e^{14.101}-1} + \frac{6.149}{e^{6.149}-1} + \frac{14.483}{e^{14.483}-1}\right)$$

$$= 0.033 + 40.6 + 0.023 = 40.7\ \text{J mol}^{-1}$$

$$E^\circ(\text{thermal, elec}) = E^\circ(\text{thermal, nuc}) = 0$$

Summing these contributions gives $E^\circ(\text{thermal}) = 9347\ \text{J mol}^{-1}$.

6.13 MOLAR THERMAL ENTHALPY

The molar thermal enthalpy, H°(thermal), is defined as

$$H^\circ = E_0^\circ + H^\circ(\text{thermal}) \qquad (6.41)$$

where

$$H^\circ(\text{thermal}) = E^\circ(\text{thermal}) + RT \qquad (6.42)$$

EXAMPLE 6.10. Evaluate H°(thermal) for $H_2O(g)$ at 373.12 K.

Substituting the result of Example 6.9 into *(6.42)* gives

$$H^\circ(\text{thermal}) = 9347 + (8.314)(373.12) = 12.449\ \text{kJ mol}^{-1}$$

6.14 MOLAR HEAT CAPACITY

In view of *(2.22)*, only one heat capacity must be calculated from statistical mechanics.

EXAMPLE 6.11. From the definition of C_V given in Example 2.6, derive the contributions to C_V° for an ideal gas.

Taking the derivatives of *(6.40)* gives the contributions as

$$C_V^\circ(\text{trans}) = \frac{3}{2}R \qquad (6.43a)$$

$$C_V^\circ(\text{rot}) = \begin{cases} R \text{ for a diatomic or linear polyatomic molecule} \\ \frac{3}{2}R \text{ for a nonlinear polyatomic molecule} \end{cases} \qquad (6.43b)$$

$$C_V^\circ(\text{vib}) = \sum_{i=1}^{3\Lambda-5 \text{ or } 3\Lambda-6} \frac{Rx_i^2 e^{x_i}}{(e^{x_i}-1)^2} \qquad (6.43c)$$

$$C_V^\circ(\text{elec}) = 0 \qquad (6.43d)$$

$$C_V^\circ(\text{nuc}) = 0 \qquad (6.43e)$$

EXAMPLE 6.12. Find C_V° and C_P° for $H_2O(g)$ at 373.12 K.

Using the results of Example 6.9 and (*6.43*) gives

$$C_V^\circ(\text{trans}) = \frac{3}{2}(8.314\ \text{J mol}^{-1}\ \text{K}^{-1}) = 12.471\ \text{J mol}^{-1}\ \text{K}^{-1}$$

$$C_V^\circ(\text{rot}) = \frac{3}{2}(8.314) = 12.471\ \text{J mol}^{-1}\ \text{K}^{-1}$$

$$C_V^\circ(\text{vib}) = (8.314)\left[\frac{(14.101)^2 e^{14.101}}{(e^{14.101}-1)^2} + \frac{(6.149)^2 e^{6.149}}{(e^{6.149}-1)^2} + \frac{(14.483)^2 e^{14.483}}{(e^{14.483}-1)^2}\right]$$

$$= 0.0012 + 0.673 + 0.0009 = 0.675\ \text{J mol}^{-1}\ \text{K}^{-1}$$

$$C_V^\circ(\text{elec}) = C_V^\circ(\text{nuc}) = 0$$

Summing these contributions gives $C_V^\circ = 25.617\ \text{J mol}^{-1}\ \text{K}^{-1}$ and (*2.22*) gives

$$C_P^\circ = C_V^\circ + R = 25.617 + 8.314 = 33.931\ \text{J mol}^{-1}\ \text{K}^{-1}$$

6.15 MOLAR ENTROPY

Applying (*6.36*) and (*6.21*) to (*6.23*), (*6.27*) or (*6.28*), (*6.30*), (*6.33*) and (*6.34*) gives

$$S^\circ(\text{trans}) = \frac{E^\circ(\text{thermal, trans})}{T} + R\ln\frac{q_{\text{trans}}}{L} + R$$

$$= R\left[\frac{5}{2} + \ln\frac{(2\pi mkT)^{3/2}V^\circ}{h^3L}\right] \tag{6.44a}$$

$$S^\circ(\text{rot}) = \frac{E^\circ(\text{thermal, rot})}{T} + R\ln\frac{q_{\text{rot}}}{L}$$

$$= \begin{cases} R\left(1 + \ln\dfrac{8\pi^2 IkT}{h^2\sigma}\right) & \text{for a diatomic or linear polyatomic molecule} \\ R\left[\dfrac{3}{2} + \ln\dfrac{8\pi^2(8\pi^3 I_xI_yI_z)^{1/2}(kT)^{3/2}}{h^3\sigma}\right] & \text{for a nonlinear polyatomic molecule} \end{cases} \tag{6.44b}$$

$$S^\circ(\text{vib}) = \frac{E^\circ(\text{thermal, vib})}{T} + R\ln\frac{q_{\text{vib}}}{L}$$

$$= R\sum_{i=1}^{3\Lambda-5\text{ or }3\Lambda-6}\left[\frac{x_i}{e^{x_i}-1} - \ln(1-e^{-x_i})\right] \tag{6-44c}$$

$$S^\circ(\text{elec}) = R\ln\omega_0 \tag{6.44d}$$

$$S^\circ(\text{nuc}) = R\ln\omega_{n,0} \tag{6.44e}$$

For most chemical reactions, $S^\circ(\text{nuc})$ is neglected.

EXAMPLE 6.13. Calculate S° for $H_2O(g)$ at 373.12 K and 1.00 atm. The moments of inertia for the molecule are such that $I_xI_yI_z = 5.7658\times10^{-141}\ \text{kg}^3\ \text{m}^6$. The ground-state degeneracy for the electronic contribution is 1 and $\sigma = 2$.

Assuming ideality, (*1.6*) gives

$$V^\circ = \frac{(8.21\times10^{-5}\ \text{m}^3\ \text{atm mol}^{-1}\ \text{K}^{-1})(373.12\ \text{K})}{1.00\ \text{atm}} = 3.06\times10^{-2}\ \text{m}^3\ \text{mol}^{-1}$$

and the mass of one molecule is $m = (0.01801\ \text{kg mol}^{-1})/L = 2.991\times10^{-26}\ \text{kg}$.

Using (*6.44*) and the results of Example 6.9 gives

$$S°(\text{trans}) = (8.314)\left\{\frac{5}{2} + \ln\frac{[(2\pi)(2.991\times10^{-26})(1.3806\times10^{-23})(373.12)]^{3/2}(3.06\times10^{-2})}{(6.626\times10^{-34})^3(6.022\times10^{23})}\right\}$$

$$= (8.314)\left[\frac{5}{2} + \ln\frac{(30.1\times10^{-69})(3.06\times10^{-2})}{(6.626\times10^{-34})^3(6.022\times10^{23})}\right]$$

$$= (8.314)\left[\frac{5}{2} + \ln(5.26\times10^{6})\right] = 149.47\ \text{EU mol}^{-1}$$

$$S°(\text{rot}) = (8.314)\left\{\frac{3}{2} + \ln\frac{(8\pi^2)[8\pi^3(5.7658\times10^{-141})]^{1/2}[(1.3806\times10^{-23})(373.12)]^{3/2}}{(6.626\times10^{-34})^3(2)}\right\}$$

$$= (8.314)\left(\frac{3}{2} + \ln 60.3\right) = 46.64\ \text{EU mol}^{-1}$$

$$S°(\text{vib}) = (8.314)\left[\frac{14.101}{e^{14.101}-1} - \ln(1-e^{-14.101}) + \frac{6.149}{e^{6.149}-1}\right.$$

$$\left. - \ln(1-e^{-6.149}) + \frac{14.483}{e^{14.483}-1} - \ln(1-e^{-14.483})\right]$$

$$= (8.314)[1\times10^{-5} - \ln(1-7.52\times10^{-7}) + 0.013 - \ln(1-2.14\times10^{-3})$$
$$+ 7\times10^{-6} - \ln(1-5.13\times10^{-7})] = 0.13\ \text{EU mol}^{-1}$$

$$S°(\text{elec}) = R\ln 1 = 0\ \text{EU mol}^{-1}$$

$$S°(\text{nuc}) = 0\ \text{EU mol}^{-1}$$

The total of the contributions is $S° = 196.24$ EU mol^{-1}.

6.16 HEATS OF REACTION

The change in thermal enthalpy or thermal energy for a chemical reaction, represented in (*6.45*) by $\Delta Z°$(thermal), can be calculated by

$$\Delta Z°(\text{thermal}) = \sum_i^{\text{products}} n_i Z°(\text{thermal}, i) - \sum_j^{\text{reactants}} n_j Z°(\text{thermal}, j) \qquad (6.45)$$

where n_i and n_j are the stoichiometric coefficients of the balanced equation. The total change in enthalpy or energy for a reaction is given by

$$\Delta Z°(\text{reaction}) = \Delta E_0°(\text{reaction}) + \Delta Z°(\text{thermal}) \qquad (6.46)$$

EXAMPLE 6.14. Calculate $\Delta H_{373.12}°$(reaction) for

$$2H(g) + O(g) = H_2O(g)$$

if $\Delta H_{298}°$(reaction) = −221.5 kcal. The values of $H°$(thermal) at 298 K and 373.12 K are 2370 and 2975 cal mol^{-1} for H_2O(g) and 1480 and 1853 cal mol^{-1} for both H(g) and O(g), respectively.

For the reaction, (*6.45*) gives

$$\Delta H_{298}°(\text{thermal}) = [(1)(2370)] - [(2)(1480) + (1)(1480)] = -2070\ \text{cal} = -8.7\ \text{kJ}$$

The value of $\Delta E_0°$(reaction) is determined by rearranging (*6.46*) and substituting values of $\Delta H_{298}°$(reaction) and $\Delta H_{298}°$(thermal) giving

$$\Delta E_0°(\text{reaction}) = (-221.5)(4.184) - (-8.7) = -918.1\ \text{kJ}$$

At the higher temperature, (*6.45*) gives

$$\Delta H^\circ_{373.12}(\text{thermal}) = [(1)(2975)] - [(2)(1853) + (1)(1853)] = -2584 \text{ cal} = -10.8 \text{ kJ}$$

and (*6.46*) gives

$$\Delta H^\circ_{373.12}(\text{reaction}) = (-918.1) + (-10.8) = -928.9 \text{ kJ}$$

6.17 FREE ENERGY AND EQUILIBRIUM CONSTANTS

The free energy is related to the partition functions by

$$G^\circ = E_0^\circ - kT \ln\left[\left(\frac{q^\circ_{\text{trans}}}{N}\right)^N (q^\circ_{\text{rot}} q^\circ_{\text{vib}} q^\circ_{\text{elec}} q^\circ_{\text{nuc}})^N\right] \qquad (6.47a)$$

or

$$\frac{G^\circ - E_0^\circ}{T} = -k \ln\left[\left(\frac{q^\circ_{\text{trans}}}{N}\right)^N (q^\circ_{\text{rot}} q^\circ_{\text{vib}} q^\circ_{\text{elec}} q^\circ_{\text{nuc}})^N\right] \qquad (6.47b)$$

For a chemical reaction

$$\Delta G^\circ(\text{reaction}) = \Delta E_0^\circ(\text{reaction}) + T\,\Delta\left(\frac{G^\circ - E_0^\circ}{T}\right) \qquad (6.48)$$

and the equilibrium constant can be calculated using (*5.39b*).

EXAMPLE 6.15. Predict K for the isotopic exchange reaction

$$^{35}\text{Cl}_2(\text{g}) + {}^{37}\text{Cl}_2(\text{g}) = 2\,{}^{35}\text{Cl}\,{}^{37}\text{Cl}(\text{g})$$

assuming that any differences in the translational, vibrational, electronic and nuclear contributions are negligible and that the rotational contributions differ only with respect to σ.

For the reaction, (*6.47b*) gives

$$\begin{aligned}\Delta\left(\frac{G^\circ - E_0^\circ}{T}\right) &= 2\left\{-k \ln\left[\left(\frac{q^\circ_{\text{trans}}}{N}\right)^N (q^\circ_{\text{rot}} q^\circ_{\text{vib}} q^\circ_{\text{elec}} q^\circ_{\text{nuc}})^N\right]_{35\text{-}37}\right\}\\ &\quad -1\left\{-k \ln\left[\left(\frac{q^\circ_{\text{trans}}}{N}\right)^N (q^\circ_{\text{rot}} q^\circ_{\text{vib}} q^\circ_{\text{elec}} q^\circ_{\text{nuc}})^N\right]_{35\text{-}35}\right\}\\ &\quad -1\left\{-k \ln\left[\left(\frac{q^\circ_{\text{trans}}}{N}\right)^N (q^\circ_{\text{rot}} q^\circ_{\text{vib}} q^\circ_{\text{elec}} q^\circ_{\text{nuc}})^N\right]_{37\text{-}37}\right\}\\ &= -k \ln\left[\frac{(q^\circ_{\text{trans}}/N)^{2N} (q^\circ_{\text{vib}} q^\circ_{\text{elec}} q^\circ_{\text{nuc}})^{2N} (q^\circ_{\text{rot},\,35\text{-}37})^{2N}}{(q^\circ_{\text{trans}}/N)^{2N} (q^\circ_{\text{vib}} q^\circ_{\text{elec}} q^\circ_{\text{nuc}})^{2N} (q^\circ_{\text{rot},\,35\text{-}35})^N (q^\circ_{\text{rot},\,37\text{-}37})^N}\right]\\ &= -Nk \ln \frac{(q^\circ_{\text{rot},\,35\text{-}37})^2}{(q^\circ_{\text{rot},\,35\text{-}35})(q^\circ_{\text{rot},\,37\text{-}37})}\end{aligned}$$

Now, by (*6.27*) and our assumption regarding the rotational contributions, q°_{rot} is proportional to $1/\sigma$. Hence,

$$\Delta\left(\frac{G^\circ - E_0^\circ}{T}\right) = -Nk \ln \frac{(\sigma_{35\text{-}35})(\sigma_{37\text{-}37})}{(\sigma_{35\text{-}37})^2} = -Nk \ln \frac{(2)(2)}{(1)^2} = -Nk \ln 4$$

In accordance with our convention of normalizing all reaction energies to a unit stoichiometric coefficient, we set $N = L$ and obtain

$$\Delta\left(\frac{G^\circ - E_0^\circ}{T}\right) = -R \ln 4$$

with the understanding that this result has to be multiplied by the factor (mol) to achieve consistency of units.

Because the bond energies of the molecules are assumed the same, $\Delta E_0^\circ = 0$ and (*6.48*) gives

$$\Delta G^\circ(\text{reaction}) = -R\,(\text{mol})T \ln 4$$

and then (*5.39b*) gives $K = e^{\ln 4} = 4$.

Monatomic Crystals

6.18 PARTITION FUNCTIONS AND MOLAR HEAT CAPACITIES

The atoms in a crystal are localized at definite lattice points rather than being able to move freely as in a gas. Einstein assumed the vibrational motion of the atoms located at these lattice points to be given by the solution to the SHO problem; the corresponding partition function for each of the three directions is then given by a term similar to those found in *(6.30)*.

The expressions for C_V as derived from the Debye theory were presented in Section 2.8. See Example 2.8 and Problem 2.23 for related calculations.

6.19 OTHER THERMODYNAMIC PROPERTIES

In terms of the Debye theory for solids,

$$\frac{E^\circ - E_0^\circ}{3RT} = 3\left(\frac{T}{\Theta_D}\right)^3 \int_0^{\Theta_D/T} \frac{x^4\,dx}{e^x - 1} \tag{6.49}$$

$$-\frac{A^\circ - E_0^\circ}{3RT} = 3\left(\frac{T}{\Theta_D}\right)^3 \int_0^{\Theta_D/T} x^2 \ln(1 - e^{-x})\,dx \tag{6.50}$$

$$\frac{S^\circ}{3R} = 3\left(\frac{T}{\Theta_D}\right)^3 \int_0^{\Theta_D/T} \left[\frac{x^4}{e^x - 1} - x^2 \ln(1 - e^{-x})\right] dx \tag{6.51}$$

The right-hand sides of *(6.49)* through *(6.51)*, as well as that of *(2.20)* exclusive of the electronic term, have been tabulated as functions of Θ_D/T.

Solved Problems

Ensembles

6.1. How many ways can two indistinguishable balls be placed in three boxes? How many if the balls are distinguishable?

For the indistinguishable balls *(6.9)* gives

$$t = \frac{(3+2-1)!}{(3-1)!\,2!} = 6$$

and for the distinguishable balls *(6.10)* gives

$$t = (3)^2 = 9$$

6.2. The quantum mechanical solution for a particle in a one-dimensional box is

$$E_n = n^2 \frac{h^2}{8ma^2}$$

where E_n is the energy of the state corresponding to the integer n, $n = 1, 2, 3, \ldots$; h is Planck's constant; m is the mass of the particle; and a is the length of the box. (*a*) What are the energies of the first four states expressed in terms of E_1? (*b*) What are the possible distributions of three particles such that $E_t = 81E_1$?

Is (0, 0, 0, 0, 0, 0, 0, 0, 1, 0, . . .) an acceptable answer? (*c*) Find Ω for each of the acceptable distributions. (*d*) What is the probability of finding particle *A* in E_1 for the distribution (1, 0, 0, 1, 0, 0, 0, 1, 0, . . .)? (*e*) What is the overall probability of finding particle *A* in E_1 for the acceptable distributions?

(*a*)
$$E_1, \quad E_2 = 4E_1, \quad E_3 = 9E_1, \quad E_4 = 16E_1$$

(*b*) The distributions

$$(1,0,0,1,0,0,0,1,0,\ldots), \quad (0,0,0,2,0,0,1,0,0,\ldots), \quad (0,0,1,0,0,2,0,0,0,\ldots)$$

have $E_t = 81E_1$. The energy of (0, 0, 0, 0, 0, 0, 0, 0, 1, 0, . . .) is $E_t = 9^2E_1 = 81E_1$, but because only one particle is present, it does not satisfy the requirements.

(*c*) Applying (*6.12a*) to the distributions gives

$$\Omega(1,0,0,1,0,0,0,1,0,\ldots) = \frac{3!}{1!\,0!\,0!\,1!\,0!\,0!\,0!\,1!\,0!\cdots} = 6$$

$$\Omega(0,0,0,2,0,0,1,0,0,\ldots) = \frac{3!}{0!\,0!\,0!\,2!\,0!\,0!\,1!\,0!\,0!\cdots} = 3$$

$$\Omega(0,0,1,0,0,2,0,0,0,\ldots) = \frac{3!}{0!\,0!\,1!\,0!\,0!\,2!\,0!\,0!\,0!\cdots} = 3$$

(*d*) Using (*6.13*) with $N_s = 3$ and $N_1 = 1$ gives

$$P_1(1,0,0,1,0,0,0,1,0,\ldots) = \frac{1}{3}$$

(*e*) Equation (*6.14*) gives

$$P_1 = \frac{(1)(6) + (0)(3) + (0)(3)}{(3)(6+3+3)} = \frac{1}{6}$$

6.3. The energy difference between the ground state and first vibrational state for O_2 is 3.1391×10^{-20} J. Compare the ratios of molecules in these states at 750 K (a typical atmospheric nighttime temperature at 400 km) and 2000 K (a typical daytime temperature).

Using (*6.18*) gives

$$\frac{N_b^*}{N_a^*} = e^{-(3.1391\times10^{-20}\text{ J})/(1.3807\times10^{-23}\text{ J K}^{-1})(750\text{ K})} = 0.0482$$

at night and, similarly, $N_b^*/N_a^* = 0.3209$ during the day, an increase by a factor of about 6.7.

Ideal-Gas Partition Functions

6.4. Calculate $\varepsilon_{\text{trans}}(1,1,2)$ for an oxygen molecule in a container of side $a = 1.00$ m.

The molecular mass is given by

$$m = \frac{32.0\times10^{-3}\text{ kg mol}^{-1}}{6.022\times10^{23}\text{ mol}^{-1}} = 5.31\times10^{-26}\text{ kg}$$

Equation (*6.22*) gives

$$\varepsilon_{\text{trans}} = (1^2+1^2+2^2)\frac{(6.626\times10^{-34}\text{ J s})^2}{8(5.31\times10^{-26}\text{ kg})(1.00\text{ m})^2} = 6.20\times10^{-42}\text{ J}$$

6.5. Calculate $\varepsilon_{\text{rot}}(J=1)$ for an oxygen molecule if $r = 1.2074$ Å.

Using (*6.26*) gives

$$\mu = \frac{(16.00 \times 10^{-3}/L)(16.00 \times 10^{-3}/L)}{(16.00 \times 10^{-3}/L) + (16.00 \times 10^{-3}/L)} = 1.328 \times 10^{-26}\ \text{kg}$$

and (*6.25*) gives

$$I = (1.328 \times 10^{-26}\ \text{kg})(1.2074 \times 10^{-10}\ \text{m})^2 = 1.936 \times 10^{-46}\ \text{kg m}^2$$

which upon substitution into (*6.24*) gives

$$\varepsilon_{\text{rot}} = (1)(1+1)\frac{(6.626 \times 10^{-34}\ \text{J s})^2}{8\pi^2(1.936 \times 10^{-46}\ \text{kg m}^2)} = 5.74 \times 10^{-23}\ \text{J}$$

6.6 Calculate ε_{vib} for an oxygen molecule if $v = 0$ and $\bar{\nu} = 1580.246\ \text{cm}^{-1}$.

Here there is a single vibrational mode with $v_1 = v$ and $\nu_1 = c\bar{\nu}$. Thus (*6.29*) gives

$$\begin{aligned}\varepsilon_{\text{vib}} &= (0 + \tfrac{1}{2})(6.6262 \times 10^{-34}\ \text{J s})(2.9979 \times 10^{10}\ \text{cm s}^{-1})(1580.246\ \text{cm}^{-1})\\ &= 1.5696 \times 10^{-20}\ \text{J}\end{aligned}$$

Application to Thermodynamics Involving Ideal Gases

6.7. Calculate $E°$(thermal) and $H°$(thermal) for CH_4(g) at 25° C if $\nu = 2917.0\ \text{cm}^{-1}$, $1533.6\ \text{cm}^{-1}$ (doubly degenerate), $3018.9\ \text{cm}^{-1}$ (triply degenerate) and $1306.2\ \text{cm}^{-1}$ (triply degenerate).

Using (*6.40*) gives

$$E°(\text{thermal, trans}) = \frac{3}{2}(8.314\ \text{J mol}^{-1}\ \text{K}^{-1})(298\ \text{K}) = 3716\ \text{J mol}^{-1}$$

$$E°(\text{thermal, rot}) = \frac{3}{2}(8.314)(298) = 3716\ \text{J mol}^{-1}$$

For the $3\Lambda - 6 = 9$ vibrational modes, (*2.5*) gives

$$x_1 = \frac{(1.4388)(2917.0)}{298} = 14.08$$

$x_2 = x_3 = 7.404$, $x_4 = x_5 = x_6 = 14.58$ and $x_7 = x_8 = x_9 = 6.307$. Then,

$$\begin{aligned}E°(\text{thermal, vib}) &= RT\left[\frac{14.08}{e^{14.08}-1} + \frac{(2)(7.404)}{e^{7.404}-1} + \frac{(3)(14.58)}{e^{14.58}-1} + \frac{(3)(6.307)}{e^{6.307}-1}\right]\\ &= (8.314)(298)(1.1 \times 10^{-5} + 9.03 \times 10^{-3} + 2.0 \times 10^{-5} + 3.46 \times 10^{-2})\\ &= 108.4\ \text{J mol}^{-1}\end{aligned}$$

$$E°(\text{thermal, elec}) = E°(\text{thermal, nuc}) = 0$$

Summing these gives $E°(\text{thermal}) = 7540\ \text{J mol}^{-1}$, and then (*6.42*) gives

$$H°(\text{thermal}) = 7540 + (8.314)(298) = 10.018\ \text{kJ mol}^{-1}$$

6.8. Calculate C_V° and C_P° for CH_4(g) at 25 °C.

Using (*6.43*) gives

$$C_V^\circ(\text{trans}) = \frac{3}{2}(8.314) = 12.471\ \text{J mol}^{-1}\ \text{K}^{-1}$$

$$C_V^\circ(\text{rot}) = \frac{3}{2}(8.314) = 12.471\ \text{J mol}^{-1}\ \text{K}^{-1}$$

and, with the values of x_i determined in Problem 6.7,

$$C_V^\circ(\text{vib}) = R\left[\frac{(14.08)^2e^{14.08}}{(e^{14.08}-1)^2} + \frac{(2)(7.404)^2e^{7.404}}{(e^{7.404}-1)^2} + \frac{(3)(14.58)^2e^{14.58}}{(e^{14.58}-1)^2} + \frac{(3)(6.307)^2e^{6.307}}{(e^{6.307}-1)^2}\right]$$

$$= (8.314)(1.5\times10^{-4} + 6.7\times10^{-2} + 3.0\times10^{-4} + 2.19\times10^{-1}) = 2.382 \text{ J mol}^{-1}\text{ K}^{-1}$$

$$C_V^\circ(\text{elec}) = C_V^\circ(\text{nuc}) = 0$$

Summing these contributions gives $C_V^\circ = 27.324 \text{ J mol}^{-1}\text{ K}^{-1}$ and (*2.22*) then gives

$$C_P^\circ = 27.324 + 8.314 = 35.638 \text{ J mol}^{-1}\text{ K}^{-1}$$

6.9. The expressions for the translational and rotational contributions in (*6.44*) can be simplified to

$$S^\circ(\text{trans}) = 36.9588 + 12.471615 \ln(MT) \qquad (6.52a)$$

$$S^\circ(\text{rot}) = \begin{cases} -22.4137 + 8.31441 \ln[(I\times10^{47})T/\sigma] \\ 229.5910 + 12.471615\ln T - 8.31441\ln\sigma + 4.15721\ln(I_xI_yI_z\times10^{114}) \end{cases} \qquad (6.52b)$$

where S° is in EU mol^{-1}, M is in g mol^{-1}, I is in kg m^2, and the first form of (*6.52b*) is valid for a linear molecule and the second form is valid for a nonlinear molecule. Calculate S_{298}° for a mole of O_2 using the data in Problems 6.4 through 6.6.

Substituting $M = 32.0$ g mol^{-1} and $I = 1.937\times10^{-46}$ kg m^2 into (*6.52*) gives

$$S^\circ(\text{trans}) = 36.9588 + 12.471615\ln[(32.0)(298)] = 151.98 \text{ EU mol}^{-1}$$

$$S^\circ(\text{rot}) = -22.4137 + 8.31441\ln[(19.37)(298)/(2)] = 43.81 \text{ EU mol}^{-1}$$

The other contributions to S_{298}° using $x = 7.64$ and $\omega_0 = 3$ are calculated from (*6.44*) as

$$S^\circ(\text{vib}) = (8.314)\left[\frac{7.64}{e^{7.64}-1} - \ln(1-e^{-7.64})\right] = (8.314)\left[\frac{7.64}{2070} - \ln(0.99952)\right]$$

$$= 3\times10^{-2} \text{ EU mol}^{-1}$$

$$S^\circ(\text{elec}) = (8.314)\ln 3 = 9.14 \text{ EU mol}^{-1}$$

$$S^\circ(\text{nuc}) = 0$$

Summing these contributions gives $S_{298}^\circ = 204.96$ EU mol^{-1}.

6.10. Calculate the heat of combustion of CH_4(g) at 500 K, if $\Delta H_{298}^\circ = -191.77$ kcal for the reaction if gaseous water is formed. Spectroscopic data for CH_4(g) are given in Problem 6.7; for O_2(g) in Problem 6.6; for H_2O in Example 6.9; and for CO_2(g), $\bar{\nu} = 1342.86$ cm^{-1}, 667.30 cm^{-1} (doubly degenerate) and 2349.30 cm^{-1}.

For water at 298 K,

$$E^\circ(\text{thermal, trans}) = E^\circ(\text{thermal, rot}) = \frac{3}{2}(8.314)(298) = 3716 \text{ J mol}^{-1}$$

Using $\bar{\nu}_1$, $\bar{\nu}_2$ and $\bar{\nu}_3$ from Example 6.9 in (*2.5*), we find $x_1 = 17.65$, $x_2 = 7.699$ and $x_3 = 18.13$, so that

$$E^\circ(\text{thermal, vib}) = (8.314)(298)\left(\frac{17.65}{e^{17.65}-1} + \frac{7.699}{e^{7.699}-1} + \frac{18.13}{e^{18.13}-1}\right)$$

$$= (8.314)(298)(3.8 \times 10^{-7} + 3.50 \times 10^{-3} + 2.4 \times 10^{-7}) = 8.67 \text{ J mol}^{-1}$$

$$E^\circ(\text{thermal, elec}) = E^\circ(\text{thermal, nuc}) = 0$$

The total of the contributions is $E^\circ(\text{thermal}) = 7.441$ kJ mol^{-1}, and adding RT gives $H^\circ(\text{thermal}) = 9.919$ kJ mol^{-1}. Performing the same operations for O_2(g) gives $E^\circ(\text{thermal}) = 6.203$ kJ mol^{-1} and $H^\circ(\text{thermal}) = 8.681$ kJ mol^{-1}. From Problem 6.7, $H^\circ(\text{thermal}) = 10.018$ kJ mol^{-1} for CH_4(g) and from Problem 6.27, $H^\circ(\text{thermal}) = 9.355$ kJ mol^{-1} for CO_2(g).

Using (*6.45*) for the reaction

$$CH_4(g) + 2O_2(g) = CO_2(g) + 2H_2O(g)$$

gives

$$\Delta H^\circ_{298}(\text{thermal}) = [(1)(9.355) + (2)(9.919)] - [(1)(10.018) + (2)(8.681)] = 1.813 \text{ kJ}$$

Solving for ΔE°_0 in (*6.46*) gives

$$\Delta E^\circ_0 = (-191.77)(4.184) - (1.813) = -804.18 \text{ kJ}$$

Repeating the above calculations for $H^\circ(\text{thermal})$ for the substances at 500 K gives 17.670 kJ mol^{-1} for CO_2(g), 16.827 kJ mol^{-1} for H_2O(g), 18.229 kJ mol^{-1} for CH_4(g) and 14.753 kJ mol^{-1} for O_2(g). Using (*6.45*) gives

$$\Delta H^\circ_{500}(\text{thermal}) = [(1)(17.670) + (2)(16.827)] - [(1)(18.229) + (2)(14.753)] = 3.589 \text{ kJ}$$

and (*6.46*) gives

$$\Delta H_{500}(\text{combustion}) = -804.18 + 3.589 = -800.59 \text{ kJ}$$

6.11. Calculate ΔG° at 298 K and 500 K for the combustion of CH_4(g) forming gaseous water if $(G^\circ - E^\circ_0)/T = -42.06$ and -45.68 cal mol^{-1} K^{-1} for O_2(g), -36.46 and -40.75 cal mol^{-1} K^{-1} for CH_4(g), -43.56 and -47.67 cal mol^{-1} K^{-1} for CO_2(g), and -37.17 and -41.29 cal mol^{-1} K^{-1} for H_2O(g), at 298 K and 500 K, respectively.

Using (*6.48*) with $\Delta E^\circ_0 = -804.18$ kJ (see Problem 6.10),

$$\Delta G^\circ_{298} = -804.18 + (298)[(2)(-37.17) + (1)(-43.56) - (2)(-42.06) - (1)(-36.46)](4.184 \times 10^{-3})$$

$$= -804.18 + (298)(2.68)(4.184 \times 10^{-3}) = -800.84 \text{ kJ}$$

$$\Delta G^\circ_{500} = -804.18 + (500)[(2)(-41.29) + (1)(-47.67) - (2)(-45.68) - (1)(-40.75)](4.184 \times 10^{-3})$$

$$= -804.18 + (500)(1.86)(4.184 \times 10^{-3}) = -800.29 \text{ kJ}$$

6.12. The relation between G and the thermodynamic partition function is

$$G = -NkT(\partial \ln Q/\partial N)_{V,T}$$

(*a*) Derive (*6.47a*). (*b*) Find a general expression for $(G^\circ - E^\circ_0)/T$ for ideal diatomic gases. (*c*) Evaluate $(G^\circ - E^\circ_0)/T$ for 1 mol of O_2 at 298 K given that $\omega_0 = 3$, $x = 7.64$, $\sigma = 2$, $I = 1.937 \times 10^{-46}$ kg m^2 and $M = 32.0$ g mol^{-1}.

(*a*) The logarithm of (*6.21*) is

$$\ln Q = N(\ln q_{\text{trans}} + \ln q_{\text{rot}} + \ln q_{\text{vib}} + \ln q_{\text{elec}} + \ln q_{\text{nuc}}) - \ln N!$$

and taking the derivative gives

$$\left(\frac{\partial \ln Q}{\partial N}\right)_{V,T} = \ln q_{\text{trans}} + \ln q_{\text{rot}} + \ln q_{\text{vib}} + \ln q_{\text{elec}} + \ln q_{\text{nuc}} - \left(\frac{\partial \ln N!}{\partial N}\right)_{V,T}$$

where

$$\left(\frac{\partial \ln N!}{\partial N}\right)_{V,T} = \frac{\partial(N \ln N - N)}{\partial N} = \ln N$$

upon using (*6.11*) for $\ln N!$. Therefore,

$$G = -NkT(\ln q_{\text{trans}} + \ln q_{\text{rot}} + \ln q_{\text{vib}} + \ln q_{\text{elec}} + \ln q_{\text{nuc}} - \ln N)$$

Evaluating G at 0 K gives $G_0^\circ = E_0^\circ = 0$, so

$$G^\circ - E_0^\circ = -NkT[\ln(q_{\text{trans}}^\circ/N) + \ln q_{\text{rot}}^\circ + \ln q_{\text{vib}}^\circ + \ln q_{\text{elec}}^\circ + \ln q_{\text{nuc}}^\circ]$$

which is another form of (*6.47a*).

(*b*) For one mole of an ideal diatomic gas,

$$\frac{G^\circ - E_0^\circ}{T} = \left\{\frac{G^\circ - E_0^\circ}{T}\right\}_{\text{trans}} + \left\{\frac{G^\circ - E_0^\circ}{T}\right\}_{\text{rot}} + \left\{\frac{G^\circ - E_0^\circ}{T}\right\}_{\text{vib}} + \left\{\frac{G^\circ - E_0^\circ}{T}\right\}_{\text{elec}} + \left\{\frac{G^\circ - E_0^\circ}{T}\right\}_{\text{nuc}}$$

where

$$\left\{\frac{G^\circ - E_0^\circ}{T}\right\}_{\text{trans}} = -R\ln\frac{q_{\text{trans}}^\circ}{L} = -R\ln\frac{(2\pi mkT)^{3/2}RT}{h^3L}$$

$$= 30.472 \text{ J mol}^{-1}\text{ K}^{-1} - 1.5\,R\ln M - 2.5\,R\ln T \qquad (6.53a)$$

$$\left\{\frac{G^\circ - E_0^\circ}{T}\right\}_{\text{rot}} = -R\ln q_{\text{rot}} = -R\ln\frac{8\pi^2 IkT}{h^2\sigma}$$

$$= 30.728 \text{ J mol}^{-1}\text{ K}^{-1} + R\ln\frac{\sigma}{T} - R\ln(I\times 10^{47}) \qquad (6.53b)$$

$$\left\{\frac{G^\circ - E_0^\circ}{T}\right\}_{\text{vib}} = R\ln(1-e^{-x}) \qquad (6.53c)$$

$$\left\{\frac{G^\circ - E_0^\circ}{T}\right\}_{\text{elec}} = -R\ln\omega_0 \qquad (6.53d)$$

$$\left\{\frac{G^\circ - E_0^\circ}{T}\right\}_{\text{nuc}} = -R\ln 1 = 0 \qquad (6.53e)$$

upon substitution of (*6.23*), (*6.27*), (*6.30*), (*6.33*) and (*6.34*), respectively.

(*c*) Equations (*6.53*) give

$$\left\{\frac{G^\circ - E_0^\circ}{T}\right\}_{\text{trans}} = 30.472 - (1.5)(8.314)\ln 32.0 - (2.5)(8.314)\ln 298$$

$$= 30.472 - 43.22 - 118.47 = -131.22 \text{ J K}^{-1}\text{ mol}^{-1}$$

$$\left\{\frac{G^\circ - E_0^\circ}{T}\right\}_{\text{rot}} = 30.728 + (8.314)\ln(2/298) - (8.314)\ln(19.37)$$

$$= 30.728 - 41.61 - 24.64 = -35.52 \text{ J K}^{-1}\text{ mol}^{-1}$$

$$\left\{\frac{G^\circ - E_0^\circ}{T}\right\}_{\text{vib}} = (8.314)\ln(1-e^{-7.64}) = -4.0\times 10^{-3} \text{ J K}^{-1}\text{ mol}^{-1}$$

$$\left\{\frac{G^\circ - E_0^\circ}{T}\right\}_{\text{elec}} = -(8.314)\ln 3 = -9.14\ \text{J K}^{-1}\ \text{mol}^{-1}$$

$$\left\{\frac{G^\circ - E_0^\circ}{T}\right\}_{\text{nuc}} = 0$$

Summing these gives for $(G^\circ - E_0^\circ)/T$ at 298 K the value $-175.88\ \text{J K}^{-1}\ \text{mol}^{-1}$.

6.13. Consider the chemical reaction $A = B$, where the molecules of A have three equally-spaced energy states (similar to electronic states) 1×10^{-22} J apart and those of B have a triply-degenerate level which is 2×10^{-22} J above the ground state of A. What is K for this reaction at 25 °C and 1000 K?

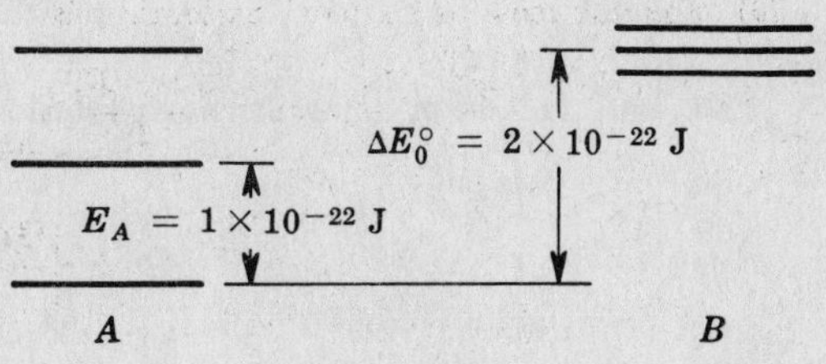

Fig. 6-1

The system is diagramed in Fig. 6-1. Using (*6.47b*) for the reaction gives

$$\Delta\left(\frac{G^\circ - E_0^\circ}{T}\right) = \left\{-k\ln\left[\left(\frac{q_{\text{trans}}^\circ}{N}\right)^N (q_{\text{rot}}^\circ q_{\text{vib}}^\circ q_{\text{elec}}^\circ q_{\text{nuc}}^\circ)^N\right]_B\right\}$$

$$- \left\{-k\ln\left[\left(\frac{q_{\text{trans}}^\circ}{N}\right)^N (q_{\text{rot}}^\circ q_{\text{vib}}^\circ q_{\text{elec}}^\circ q_{\text{nuc}}^\circ)^N\right]_A\right\}$$

$$= -Nk\ln\left(\frac{q_{\text{elec},B}^\circ}{q_{\text{elec},A}^\circ}\right)$$

From (*6.16*),

$$q_{\text{elec},B}^\circ = (3)e^{-0/kT} = 3$$

$$q_{\text{elec},A}^\circ = (1)e^{-0/kT} + (1)e^{-(1\times10^{-22})/(1.3807\times10^{-23})(298)} + (1)e^{-(2\times10^{-22})/(1.3807\times10^{-23})(298)}$$

$$= 2.929$$

at 298 K. Recognizing that $N = L$ and $\Delta E_0^\circ = (2\times10^{-22}\ \text{J})(L)$, we have from (*5.39b*):

$$K = e^{-(2\times10^{-22})(6.022\times10^{23})/(8.314)(298)}(3/2.929) = 0.976$$

Repeating the calculations at 1000 K gives $q_{\text{elec},B}^\circ = 3$, $q_{\text{elec},A}^\circ = 2.978$ and $K = 1.010$. Note that at lower temperatures the equilibrium lies on the side of the reactants and at higher temperatures the situation is reversed.

Monatomic Crystals

6.14. Find $E^\circ - E_0^\circ$, $A^\circ - E_0^\circ$ and S° for Al at 298 K.

For $\Theta_D/T = 1.43$ (see Example 2.8) the right-hand sides of (*6.49*), (*6.50*) and (*6.51*) have the values 0.5637, 0.4619 and 1.0255, respectively. Therefore

$$E^\circ - E_0^\circ = (3)(8.314\times10^{-3})(298)(0.5637) = 4.190\ \text{kJ mol}^{-1}$$

$$A^\circ - E_0^\circ = (3)(8.314\times10^{-3})(298)(0.4619) = 3.433\ \text{kJ mol}^{-1}$$

$$S^\circ = (3)(8.314)(1.0255) = 25.58\ \text{EU mol}^{-1}$$

Supplementary Problems

Ensembles

6.15. What is the number of different "Greek" names for organizations, assuming each chooses some combination of three of the 24 letters in the Greek alphabet?

Ans. $(24)^3 = 13{,}824$

6.16. How many ways can two indistinguishable balls be placed in three boxes if no more than one ball can be in a box? *Ans.* 3

6.17. Evaluate 11! (*a*) by using Stirling's approximation, (*6.11*); (*b*) by using the improved approximation

$$\ln N! = N \ln N - N + \frac{1}{2} \ln 2N$$

and (*c*) by actual calculation. *Ans.* (*a*) 4.77×10^6, (*b*) 2.24×10^7, (*c*) 39,916,800

6.18. Find the overall probability of finding system A in E_1 for the acceptable distributions given in Example 6.1.

Ans. $\Omega(1,1,1,0,0,\ldots) = 6$, $\Omega(2,0,0,1,0,\ldots) = 3$, $\Omega(0,3,0,0,0,\ldots) = 1$; $P_1 = 0.300$

6.19. Consider a system of energy states where $E_n = nE_1$. Find the possible distributions of three particles such that $E_t = 10E_1$. Determine Ω for each distribution. Find the overall probability of finding a chosen system in E_1.

Ans. $(2,0,0,0,0,0,0,1,0,0,\ldots)$, $(1,1,0,0,0,0,1,0,0,0,\ldots)$, $(1,0,1,0,0,1,0,0,0,0,\ldots)$, $(0,2,0,0,0,1,0,0,0,0,\ldots)$, $(1,0,0,1,1,0,0,0,0,0,\ldots)$, $(0,1,1,0,1,0,0,0,0,0,\ldots)$, $(0,1,0,2,0,0,0,0,0,0,\ldots)$, $(0,0,2,1,0,0,0,0,0,0,\ldots)$; $\Omega = 3, 6, 6, 3, 6, 6, 3, 3$; 0.222

Ideal-Gas Partition Functions

6.20. Calculate $\varepsilon_{trans}(1,1,1)$ for an oxygen molecule in a container that has $a = 1.00$ m and determine $N^*_{1,1,2}/N^*_{1,1,1}$ at 25 °C (see Problem 6.4).

Ans. 3.10×10^{-42} J, $e^{-7.53\times10^{-22}} \approx 1$

6.21. Calculate ε_{rot} for $J = 2$ for an oxygen molecule and determine $N^*_{J=2}/N^*_{J=1}$ at 25 °C (see Problem 6.5).

Ans. 17.23×10^{-23} J, $\frac{5}{3}e^{-0.0279} = 1.621$

6.22. Calculate the number of molecules in the first three vibrational states for a mole of O_2 molecules at 25 °C. See Problem 6.6 for pertinent data.

Ans. $x = 7.630$, $N_0 = 0.99951\,L$, $N_1 = 4.9 \times 10^{-4}L$, $N_2 = 2.4 \times 10^{-7}L$

6.23. If the first excited electronic level of O_2 is 15.72×10^{-20} J above the ground level, calculate N^*_1/N^*_0 at 298 K and 1500 K. The degeneracies are $\omega_0 = 3$ and $\omega_1 = 2$.

Ans. $(2/3)e^{-38.2} = 1.6 \times 10^{-17}$; 3.3×10^{-4}

6.24. Derive (*6.31*) through (*6.33*) beginning with (*6.18*).

6.25. Derive (*6.27*) beginning with (*6.19*) and (*6.24*). (*Hint*: Use the technique shown in Example 6.7 for the evaluation of the summation.)

Application to Thermodynamics Involving Ideal Gases

6.26. Show that H°(thermal) for O(g) is equal to that for H(g) at the same temperature.

Ans. $H^\circ(\text{thermal}) = (5/2)RT$ for all monatomic gases

6.27. Calculate E°(thermal) and H°(thermal) for one mole of $CO_2(g)$ at 25 °C if $\nu = 1342.86\ \text{cm}^{-1}$, $667.30\ \text{cm}^{-1}$(doubly-degenerate) and $2349.30\ \text{cm}^{-1}$ for the linear molecule.

Ans. $E^\circ(\text{thermal}) = 6861\ \text{J mol}^{-1}$, $H^\circ(\text{thermal}) = 9339\ \text{J mol}^{-1}$

6.28. Calculate C_V° and C_P° for $CO_2(g)$ at 25 °C using the data in Problem 6.27.

Ans. $C_V^\circ = 28.848\ \text{J mol}^{-1}\ \text{K}^{-1}$, $C_P^\circ = 37.162\ \text{J mol}^{-1}\ \text{K}^{-1}$

6.29. Calculate S_{298}° for a mole of CO(g) using $r = 1.1281$ Å, $\bar{\nu} = 2169.52\ \text{cm}^{-1}$ and $\omega_0 = 1$.

Ans. 197.43 EU mol^{-1}

6.30. Calculate the heat of reaction at 1000 K for the reaction

$$N_2(g) + 2O_2(g) = 2NO_2(g)$$

if $\Delta H_{298}^\circ(\text{reaction}) = 15.86$ kcal. Spectroscopic data are: $\bar{\nu} = 2357.55\ \text{cm}^{-1}$ for $N_2(g)$; 1580.246 cm^{-1} for $O_2(g)$; and 1357.8, 756.8 and 1665.5 cm^{-1} for the nonlinear $NO_2(g)$ molecule.

Ans. $H^\circ(\text{thermal}, N_2) = 8.672$ and $30.079\ \text{kJ mol}^{-1}$, $H^\circ(\text{thermal}, O_2) = 8.673$ and $31.266\ \text{kJ mol}^{-1}$, $H^\circ(\text{thermal}, NO_2) = 10.180$ and $42.527\ \text{kJ mol}^{-1}$, at 298 K and 1000 K respectively; $\Delta E_0^\circ = 72.02$ kJ; $\Delta H_{1000}^\circ(\text{reaction}) = 64.46$ kJ

6.31. Evaluate $(G^\circ - E_0^\circ)/T$ for 1 mol of $N_2(g)$ at 1000 K, given that $\omega_0 = 1$, $\bar{\nu} = 2357.55\ \text{cm}^{-1}$, $\sigma = 2$, $r = 1.08758$ Å and $M = 28.0134\ \text{g mol}^{-1}$.

Ans. $I = 27.5 \times 10^{-47}\ \text{kg m}^2$, $x = 3.392$;
$(G^\circ - E_0^\circ)/T = (-154.72) + (-48.54) + (-0.28) + 0 + 0 = -203.54\ \text{J K}^{-1}\ \text{mol}^{-1}$

6.32. Calculate ΔG_{1000}° for the reaction

$$N_2(g) + 2O_2(g) = 2NO_2(g)$$

if $\Delta G_{298}^\circ(\text{reaction}) = 24.52$ kcal and $(G^\circ - E_0^\circ)/T = -38.82$ and $-47.31\ \text{cal mol}^{-1}\ \text{K}^{-1}$ for $N_2(g)$, -42.06 and $-50.70\ \text{cal mol}^{-1}\ \text{K}^{-1}$ for $O_2(g)$, and -49.19 and $-60.23\ \text{cal mol}^{-1}\ \text{K}^{-1}$ for $NO_2(g)$, at 298 K and 1000 K, respectively.

Ans. $\Delta(G^\circ - E_0^\circ)/T = 24.56\ \text{cal K}^{-1} = 102.76\ \text{J K}^{-1}$ at 298 K and $118.20\ \text{J K}^{-1}$ at 1000 K, $\Delta E_0^\circ = 71.970$ kJ, $\Delta G_{1000}^\circ(\text{reaction}) = 190.170$ kJ

6.33. Consider the equilibrium between system A having three singly-degenerate levels spaced 8×10^{-22} J apart (similar to electronic levels) and system B having a triply-degenerate ground level 3×10^{-22} J above the ground level of A and a doubly-degenerate level 1×10^{-22} J above its own ground level. Calculate K at 10 K and 1000 K.

Ans. $Q_A^\circ = 1.003$, $Q_B^\circ = 3.969$, $K = 0.450$; $Q_A^\circ = 2.834$, $Q_B^\circ = 4.986$, $K = 1.722$

6.34. Predict K for the isotopic exchange reaction

$$^{16}O_2(g) + {}^{18}O(g) = {}^{16}O\,{}^{18}O(g) + {}^{16}O(g)$$

making assumptions similar to those in Example 6.15. What is the driving force of this reaction?

Ans. 2, entropy increase

6.35. (*a*) Calculate $H°$(thermal) for $Cl_2(g)$, $F_2(g)$ and ClF(g) at 298 K and 1000 K given that $\omega_0 = 1$, 1 and 1; $\bar{\nu} = 561.1$, 923.1 and 784.39 cm^{-1}; $r = 1.986$, 1.409 and 1.62813 Å; $\sigma = 2$, 2 and 1; and $M = 70.906$, 38.00 and 54.4514 g mol^{-1}, for $Cl_2(g)$, $F_2(g)$ and ClF(g), respectively. (*b*) Using the values of $H°$(thermal) and the fact that ΔH°_{298}(formation) of ClF(g) is -12.140 kcal mol^{-1}, calculate ΔE°_0 and ΔH°_{1000}(formation). (*c*) Calculate $S°$ for the gases at 298 K and 1000 K and $\Delta S°$(formation) at 298 K and 1000 K. (*d*) Using the values of $\Delta H°$(formation) and $\Delta S°$(formation), calculate $\Delta G°$(formation) at both temperatures. (*e*) If $(G° - E^\circ_0)/T = -45.93$ and -55.43 cal K^{-1} mol^{-1} for $Cl_2(g)$, -41.37 and -50.44 cal K^{-1} mol^{-1} for $F_2(g)$, and -44.92 and -54.11 cal K^{-1} mol^{-1} for ClF(g), at 298 K and 1000 K, respectively, calculate $\Delta G°$(formation) at both temperatures.

Ans. (*a*) 9.151, 8.801 and 8.890 kJ mol^{-1} at 298 K and 34.501, 33.085 and 33.590 kJ mol^{-1} at 1000 K.

(*b*) $\Delta E^\circ_0 = -50.708$ kJ, ΔH°_{1000}(formation) $= -50.911$ kJ mol^{-1}.

(*c*) $S° = 222.84$ and 266.17 EU mol^{-1} for $Cl_2(g)$, 202.53 and 243.77 EU mol^{-1} for $F_2(g)$, and 217.71 and 259.78 EU mol^{-1} for ClF(g), at 298 K and 1000 K, respectively; $\Delta S° = 5.03$ and 4.81 EU mol^{-1} at 298 K and 1000 K, respectively.

(*d*) -52.293 and -55.721 kJ mol^{-1} at 298 K and 1000 K, respectively.

(*e*) -52.292 and -55.624 kJ mol^{-1} at 298 K and 1000 K, respectively.

Monatomic Crystals

6.36. If the value of the right-hand side of (*6.49*) is 0.5806 and 0.8580 for W at 298 K and 1000 K, respectively, calculate $\Delta E°$ for heating one mole from 25 °C to 1000 K.

Ans. E(thermal) $= 4.315$ kJ mol^{-1} at 298 K and 21.400 kJ mol^{-1} at 1000 K,
$\Delta E°$(thermal) $= \Delta E° = 17.085$ kJ mol^{-1}

6.37. Prepare plots of $C^\circ_V/3R$ against $\log T$ for Au using (*a*) the Einstein result

$$\frac{C^\circ_V}{3R} = \left(\frac{\Theta}{T}\right)^2 \frac{e^{\Theta/T}}{(e^{\Theta/T}-1)^2}$$

assuming $\Theta = \Theta_D = 165$ K, and (*b*) the Debye result (*2.20*) omitting electronic terms,

$$\frac{C^\circ_V}{3R} = \frac{3}{(\Theta_D/T)^3}\int_0^{\Theta_D/T} \frac{x^4 e^x}{(e^x-1)^2}\,dx \equiv \mathcal{D}(\Theta_D/T)$$

where the Debye function is tabulated as follows:

Θ_D/T	$\mathcal{D}(\Theta_D/T)$	Θ_D/T	$\mathcal{D}(\Theta_D/T)$	Θ_D/T	$\mathcal{D}(\Theta_D/T)$	Θ_D/T	$\mathcal{D}(\Theta_D/T)$
0.5	0.9876	4.5	0.4320	8.5	0.1182	12.5	0.0397
1.0	0.9517	5.0	0.3686	9.0	0.1015	13.0	0.0354
1.5	0.8960	5.5	0.3133	9.5	0.0875	13.5	0.0316
2.0	0.8254	6.0	0.2656	10.0	0.0758	14.0	0.0284
2.5	0.7459	6.5	0.2251	10.5	0.0660	14.5	0.0255
3.0	0.6628	7.0	0.1909	11.0	0.0577	15.0	0.0231
3.5	0.5807	7.5	0.1622	11.5	0.0507	15.5	0.0209
4.0	0.5031	8.0	0.1382	12.0	0.0448	16.0	0.0190

$\mathcal{D}(\Theta_D/T) = 77.927(T/\Theta_D)^3$ for $\Theta_D/T \geqq 16$.

Compare the curves to a plot of $C_P^\circ/3R$ for Au, where

T, K	$C_P^\circ/3R$	T, K	$C_P^\circ/3R$	T, K	$C_P^\circ/3R$
5	0.002	40	0.449	100	0.859
10	0.017	45	0.515	125	0.913
15	0.059	50	0.573	150	0.945
20	0.128	60	0.664	175	0.965
25	0.210	70	0.733	200	0.978
30	0.295	80	0.787	250	1.001
35	0.376	90	0.828	298	1.018

assuming that $C_P^\circ = C_V^\circ$.

Ans. Same general shape and values, but (*2.20*) fits the experimental data somewhat better.

Chapter 7

Electrochemistry

Oxidation-Reduction

7.1 BALANCING EQUATIONS

Of the several techniques used for balancing redox equations, the ion-electron half-reaction method illustrated in Examples 7.1 and 7.2 is the best because the results are in the proper format for assigning values of voltage and for performing stoichiometric calculations.

EXAMPLE 7.1. The chemical reaction in a "lead storage" cell of a car battery during charging involves the reduction of $PbSO_4(s)$ to Pb(s) and the oxidation of $PbSO_4(s)$ to $PbO_2(s)$, both reactions occurring in the presence of $H_2SO_4(aq)$. Write the balanced reaction.

The species undergoing changes in oxidation numbers are

$$PbSO_4(s) = Pb(s) + PbO_2(s)$$

and writing individual half reactions gives

$$PbSO_4(s) = Pb(s) \qquad PbSO_4(s) = PbO_2(s)$$

The first half reaction can be balanced by adding a $SO_4^{2-}(aq)$ to the right side, giving

$$PbSO_4(s) = Pb(s) + SO_4^{2-}(aq)$$

The second equation also requires a $SO_4^{2-}(aq)$ on the right side, but to balance the oxygen and hydrogen atoms, $xH^+(aq)$ and $yH_2O(liq)$ are added because the reaction is occurring in neutral or acidic media:

$$PbSO_4(s) = PbO_2(s) + SO_4^{2-}(aq) + xH^+(aq) + yH_2O(liq)$$

Counts of the hydrogen atoms and the oxygen atoms give

$$0 = x + 2y \qquad 4 = 2 + 4 + y$$

which yield $x = 4$ and $y = -2$. The overall half reaction becomes

$$PbSO_4(s) + 2H_2O(liq) = PbO_2(s) + SO_4^{2-}(aq) + 4H^+(aq)$$

Balancing the half reactions electrically by adding electrons gives

$$PbSO_4(s) + 2e^- = Pb(s) + SO_4^{2-}(aq)$$

$$PbSO_4(s) + 2H_2O(liq) = PbO_2(s) + SO_4^{2-}(aq) + 4H^+(aq) + 2e^-$$

Because the number of electrons required for the first half reaction is equal to the number released in the second, these half reactions may be added directly giving

$$2PbSO_4(s) + 2H_2O(liq) = Pb(s) + PbO_2(s) + 2SO_4^{2-}(aq) + 4H^+(aq)$$

for the net ionic equation. Upon checking, the equation is balanced with respect to mass and charge.

EXAMPLE 7.2. The "Ni-Cd alkali" cell has an electrode at which Cd is oxidized to $Cd(OH)_2(s)$ and an electrode at which $Ni_2O_3(s)$ is reduced to $Ni(OH)_2(s)$. Write the balanced chemical reaction describing this cell.

The species undergoing changes in oxidation states are

$$Cd(s) + Ni_2O_3(s) = Cd(OH)_2(s) + Ni(OH)_2(s)$$

which gives the following half reactions:

$$Cd(s) = Cd(OH)_2(s) \qquad Ni_2O_3(s) = Ni(OH)_2(s)$$

The first half reaction can be balanced by simply adding $2OH^-(aq)$ to the left side, giving

$$Cd(s) + 2OH^-(aq) = Cd(OH)_2(s)$$

To balance the second reaction, a 2 is placed in front of the $Ni(OH)_2(s)$, and because the reaction is occurring in a basic medium, $xOH^-(aq)$ and $yH_2O(liq)$ are added:

$$Ni_2O_3(s) + xOH^-(aq) + yH_2O(liq) = 2Ni(OH)_2(s)$$

The count of H and O atoms gives the following equations:

$$x + 2y = 4 \qquad 3 + x + y = 4$$

which yield $x = -2$ and $y = 3$. The final half reaction becomes

$$Ni_2O_3(s) + 3H_2O(liq) = 2Ni(OH)_2(s) + 2OH^-(aq)$$

Balancing electrically by adding electrons gives

$$Cd(s) + 2OH^-(aq) = Cd(OH)_2(s) + 2e^-$$

$$Ni_2O_3(s) + 3H_2O(liq) + 2e^- = 2Ni(OH)_2(s) + 2OH^-(aq)$$

Because the number of electrons in each half reaction is the same, adding the reactions directly and canceling $2OH^-(aq)$ common to both sides gives

$$Cd(s) + Ni_2O_3(s) + 3H_2O(liq) = Cd(OH)_2(s) + 2Ni(OH)_2(s)$$

Upon checking, the equation is balanced with respect to mass and charge.

7.2 GALVANIC AND ELECTROLYTIC CELLS

The relationship between the voltage of an electrochemical cell and the spontaneity of the chemical reaction is

$$\Delta G = -n\mathcal{F}\mathcal{E} \tag{5.6}$$

where n is the number of moles of electrons (equivalents) in the balanced reaction. For a negative value of ΔG (a positive value of $\mathcal{E}$), the reaction is spontaneous and the cell will serve as a "seat of emf" or galvanic cell. If ΔG and $\mathcal{E}$ are zero, a state of equilibrium exists. If ΔG is positive ($\mathcal{E}$ is negative), a nonspontaneous reaction has been written, which will occur as written only if the cell is supplied energy from the surroundings, giving an electrolytic cell. The reverse reaction will be spontaneous. If there is a choice of reactions that may occur, the one with the most positive value of $\mathcal{E}$ will occur.

EXAMPLE 7.3. During the charging of the lead storage cell, the following reaction takes place:

$$2PbSO_4(s) + 2H_2O(liq) = Pb(s) + PbO_2(s) + 2H_2SO_4(aq)$$

If ΔG°_{298}(formation) $= -194.36$ kcal mol^{-1} for $PbSO_4(s)$, -56.687 kcal mol^{-1} for $H_2O(liq)$, 0 for Pb(s), -51.95 kcal mol^{-1} for $PbO_2(s)$ and -217.32 kcal mol^{-1} for $H_2SO_4(aq, m = 1)$, calculate ΔG°_{298}(reaction) and $\mathcal{E}^\circ$. Is this reaction spontaneous under standard conditions or is an outside source of energy required for it to proceed?

Using (*5.11*) for the reaction gives

$$\Delta G^\circ(\text{reaction}) = [(1)(0) + (1)(-51.95) + (2)(-217.32)] - [(2)(-194.36) + (2)(-56.687)]$$

$$= 15.50 \text{ kcal} = 64.85 \text{ kJ}$$

and using $n = 2$ (see Example 7.1) in (*5.6*) gives

$$\mathcal{E}^\circ = \frac{-64.85 \text{ kJ}}{(2 \text{ mol})(96.485 \text{ kJ mol}^{-1} \text{ V}^{-1})} = -0.336 \text{ V}$$

The reaction is not spontaneous as written and can occur only if an external power source such as a battery charger is used. The reverse reaction would be spontaneous.

7.3 STOICHIOMETRY

The *equivalent weight* of a material, $W(i)$, is given by

$$W(i) = \frac{M}{n} \tag{7.1}$$

where M is the molecular weight (g mol^{-1}) of material i and n is the number of moles of electrons in the balanced half reaction for one mole of material. In electrochemistry, one equivalent weight of a material always reacts with one equivalent weight of a material. The electric charge carried by one equivalent is equal to 96,484.56 coulombs. The amount of charge transferred in t seconds by a constant current of I amperes is given by

$$q = It \tag{7.2}$$

EXAMPLE 7.4. If 10.0 A were passed through a lead storage cell for 1.50 hr during a charging process, how much $PbSO_4$ would decompose?

The number of coulombs of electricity passed through the cell is given by (*7.2*) as

$$q = (10.0\ \text{A})(1.50\ \text{hr})(3600\ \text{s hr}^{-1}) = 5.40 \times 10^4\ \text{C}$$

This amount of electricity corresponds to

$$\frac{5.40 \times 10^4\ \text{C}}{9.6485 \times 10^4\ \text{C mol}^{-1}} = 0.560\ \text{mol}$$

that is, to 0.560 L electronic charges.

Recalling that $n = 2$ for each of the balanced half reactions in Example 7.1 and that two moles of $PbSO_4$(s) are reacting, (*7.1*) gives

$$W(PbSO_4) = M = 303.25\ \text{g mol}^{-1} = 0.30325\ \text{kg mol}^{-1}$$

The mass of $PbSO_4$(s) reacting is then

$$(0.560\ \text{mol})(0.30325\ \text{kg mol}^{-1}) = 0.170\ \text{kg}$$

half being oxidized and half being reduced.

Conductivity

7.4 EQUIVALENT CONDUCTANCE

The measurement of the resistance to the flow of electricity of a cell is made using a bridge circuit similar to that shown in Fig. 7-1. The resistance of the cell, R, is given in terms of the other resistances which are necessary to balance the circuit by

$$R = R_3 \frac{R_1}{R_2} \tag{7.3}$$

Conductance is the reciprocal of resistance, or

$$L = \frac{1}{R} \tag{7.4}$$

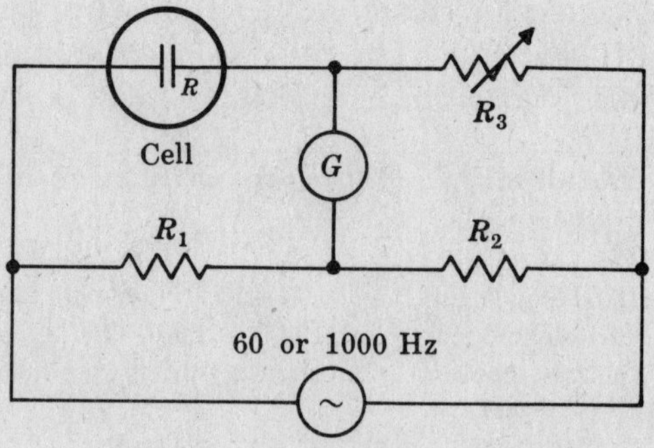

Fig. 7-1

and can be shown to be equal to

$$L = \frac{kA}{l} \tag{7.5}$$

where k is the *specific conductance*, A is the area of an electrode surface (m^2) and l is the distance between the electrodes (m). The cell constant, l/A, is rather difficult to measure directly, so it is usually determined by measuring L for a KCl(aq) solution at a concentration for which k is known and using (*7.5*). A common unit for L is the *mho*: 1 mho = 1 Ω^{-1}.

The *equivalent conductance*, Λ, of an electrolytic solution is defined by

$$\Lambda = \frac{k}{1000c} \tag{7.6}$$

where c is the concentration expressed in terms of equivalents dm^{-3} of solution (normality, N) and k is in $\Omega^{-1}\,m^{-1}$. A plot of Λ against $c^{1/2}$ is nearly linear for a strong electrolyte, i.e. one that is highly ionized or dissociated in solution, and is highly curved for a weak electrolyte, i.e. one that is not highly ionized or dissociated in solution. The value of Λ at infinite dilution, Λ_0, can be considered the sum of the contributions of the conductivities of the individual ions, $\lambda_{0,i}$:

$$\Lambda_0 = \lambda_{0,+} + \lambda_{0,-} \tag{7.7}$$

Because (*7.7*) is valid for all electrolytes, it can be shown that

$$\Lambda_0(WZ) = \Lambda_0(WX) + \Lambda_0(YZ) - \Lambda_0(YX) \tag{7.8}$$

For a weak electrolyte, the fraction of molecules ionized, α, is given by

$$\alpha = \Lambda/\Lambda_0 \tag{7.9}$$

EXAMPLE 7.5. If the equivalent conductances at 25 °C are 422.74, 421.36, 412.00 and 391.32 $cm^2\,mol^{-1}\,\Omega^{-1}$ for HCl; 89.2, 88.5, 83.76 and 72.80 for $NaC_2H_3O_2$; and 124.50, 123.74, 118.51 and 106.74 for NaCl, at 0.0005 N, 0.001 N, 0.01 N and 0.1 N, respectively, find Λ_0 for $HC_2H_3O_2$. If $\Lambda = 14.3\ cm^2\,mol^{-1}\,\Omega^{-1}$ in a 0.01 N solution of $HC_2H_3O_2$, find α.

The values of Λ_0 for HCl, $NaC_2H_3O_2$ and NaCl are found by extrapolation of a plot of Λ against $c^{1/2}$, see Fig. 7-2, giving 426.1, 91.0 and 126.45 $cm^2\,mol^{-1}\,\Omega^{-1}$, respectively. Using (*7.8*) to predict $\Lambda_0(HC_2H_3O_2)$:

$$\Lambda_0(HC_2H_3O_2) = \Lambda_0(HCl) + \Lambda_0(NaC_2H_3O_2) - \Lambda_0(NaCl) = 390.6\ cm^2\,mol^{-1}\,\Omega^{-1}$$

The percent ionization is given by (*7.9*) as $\alpha = 14.3/390.6 = 3.66\%$.

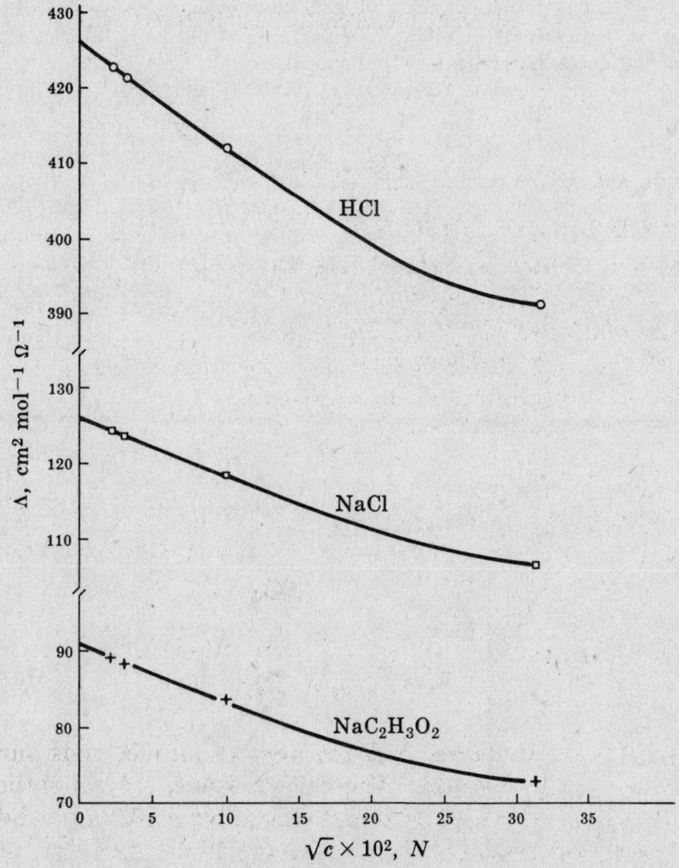

Fig. 7-2

7.5 TRANSFERENCE (TRANSPORT) NUMBERS

The *transference number*, t_i, of an ion is defined as the fraction of the total current carried by that ion. For a single electrolyte in a solution

$$t_+ + t_- = 1 \tag{7.10}$$

There are two common experimental techniques used for determining t_i, the Hittorf method and the moving boundary method. In the former, the cell is divided into three sections and after the passage of current, the cell sections are analyzed for electrolyte content. The transference number is

$$t_i = \frac{|N_0 - N_f \pm N_e'|}{N_e} \tag{7.11}$$

where N_f is the final number of equivalents present, N_0 is the original number, N_e' is the number of equivalents involved in the electrode reaction (the positive sign is used if the equivalents are generated and the negative sign is used if the equivalents are removed), and N_e is the number of equivalents passed through the cell. The value of N_e' will be either 0 or N_e depending on whether inert electrodes are used or not.

For the moving boundary method,

$$t_i = \frac{\mathcal{F}1000c_i}{I}\frac{dV}{dt} \tag{7.12}$$

where c_i is the concentration of the ion in equivalents dm^{-3}, I is the current in amperes, t is the time in seconds and V is the volume through which the moving boundary passes expressed in m^3.

EXAMPLE 7.6. Consider a hypothetical Hittorf cell having inert electrodes, in which each of the compartments contains seven equivalents of electrolyte as represented by + and − signs in Fig. 7-3(*a*). Construct a diagram showing the arrangement of the ions after passing six equivalents of electricity, assuming negligible migration. Construct a diagram showing the arrangement of the equivalents after ionic migration with $t_+ = 2t_-$.

The discharge of 6 eq at the electrodes requires six of the − signs in the left side of the cell to be removed at the electrode, leaving one in that compartment, and six of the + signs in the right side of the cell to be removed at the electrode, leaving one in that compartment, see Fig. 7-3(*b*). For the passing of 6 eq through the solution, four + signs move to the right for every two − signs moving to the left across each boundary, because $t_+ = 2t_-$. This leaves 3 eq in the left side, 7 eq in the middle and 5 eq in the right side, see Fig. 7-3(*c*). As a check, applying (*7.11*) to the left portion of the cell with $N_0 = 7$, $N_f = 3$, $N_e' = 0$ for the cation and 6 for the anion, and $N_e = 6$, gives

$$t_+ = \frac{|7 - 3 \pm 0|}{6} = \frac{2}{3} \qquad t_- = \frac{|7 - 3 - 6|}{6} = \frac{1}{3}$$

so that $t_+ = 2t_-$ and (*7.10*) is satisfied.

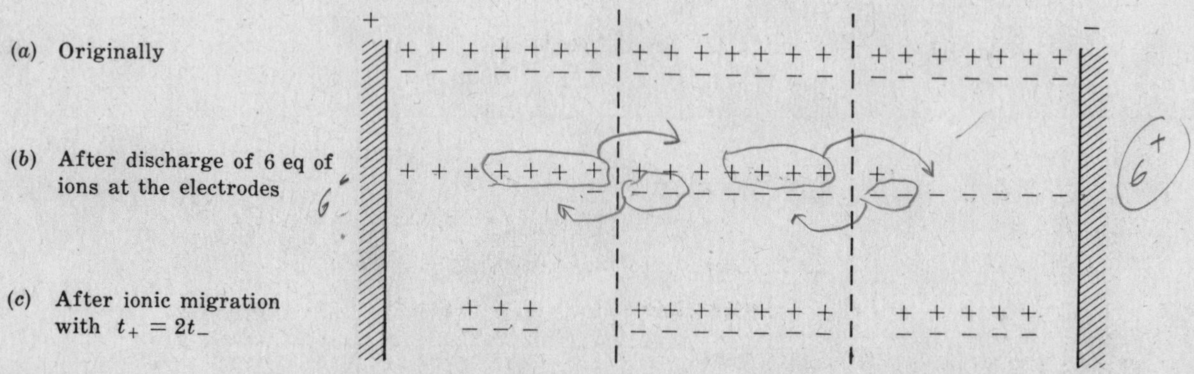

Fig. 7-3

7.6 IONIC MOBILITIES

The *ionic mobility*, u_i, is given by

$$u_i = \frac{l}{t\left(\frac{d\mathcal{E}}{dl}\right)} \tag{7.13}$$

where l is the distance in m that a moving boundary moves, t is the time in seconds and $d\mathcal{E}/dl$ is the electric field strength and can be calculated by

$$\frac{d\mathcal{E}}{dl} = \frac{I}{Ak} \tag{7.14}$$

The relationship between ionic mobility and transference number is

$$t_i = \frac{u_i}{u_+ + u_-} \tag{7.15}$$

EXAMPLE 7.7. The moving boundary technique was used to determine t_+ in 0.0100 N HCl at 25 °C. A current of 3.00 mA was passed through the cell having a cross-sectional area of 3.25 cm² for 45.0 min and the observed boundary moved 2.13 cm. Using these data, find u_+ and u_- given that $\Lambda = 412.00\ \text{cm}^2\ \text{mol}^{-1}\ \Omega^{-1}$.

Using (*7.6*) gives the specific conductance as

$$k = 1000(0.0100)(412.00 \times 10^{-4}) = 0.412\ \Omega^{-1}\ \text{m}^{-1}$$

which upon substitution into (*7.14*) gives

$$\frac{d\mathcal{E}}{dl} = \frac{3.00 \times 10^{-3}\ \text{A}}{(3.25 \times 10^{-4}\ \text{m}^2)(0.412\ \Omega^{-1}\ \text{m}^{-1})} = 22.4\ \text{V m}^{-1}$$

Using (*7.13*) gives

$$u_+ = \frac{2.13 \times 10^{-2}\ \text{m}}{(45 \times 60\ \text{s})(22.4\ \text{V m}^{-1})} = 3.52 \times 10^{-7}\ \text{m}^2\ \text{V}^{-1}\ \text{s}^{-1}$$

Substituting $t_+ = 0.825$, see Problem 7.7, and $u_+ = 3.52 \times 10^{-7}$ into (*7.15*) gives

$$0.825 = \frac{3.52 \times 10^{-7}}{3.52 \times 10^{-7} + u_-}$$

which upon solving gives $u_- = 7.47 \times 10^{-8}\ \text{m}^2\ \text{V}^{-1}\ \text{s}^{-1}$.

7.7 IONIC EQUIVALENT CONDUCTANCE

The *ionic equivalent conductance*, λ_i, is defined as

$$\lambda_i = t_i \Lambda \tag{7.16}$$

where

$$\lambda_+ + \lambda_- = \Lambda \tag{7.17}$$

EXAMPLE 7.8. Find λ_+ and λ_- for the 0.0100 N HCl solution described in Example 7.7.

With $\Lambda = 412.00 \times 10^{-4}\ \text{m}^2\ \Omega^{-1}\ \text{mol}^{-1}$ and $t_+ = 0.825$, (*7.16*) gives

$$\lambda_+ = (0.825)(412.00 \times 10^{-4}) = 0.03399\ \text{m}^2\ \Omega^{-1}\ \text{mol}^{-1}$$

and (*7.17*) gives $\lambda_- = 0.00721\ \text{m}^2\ \Omega^{-1}\ \text{mol}^{-1}$.

Electrochemical Cells

7.8 SIGN CONVENTION AND DIAGRAMS

In a galvanic cell the anode (site of oxidation) is negatively charged as a result of the spontaneous chemical reactions releasing electrons to the electrode. The electrons will move from the anode to the cathode in the external circuit. The cathode (site of reduction) is positively charged with respect to the anode. The positively charged cations move toward the cathode to undergo chemical reactions with the incoming electrons.

In an electrolytic cell an external source of voltage causes the anode (site of oxidation) to be positively charged with respect to the cathode. As a result the negatively charged anions move toward the anode to be oxidized. The cathode (site of reduction) is negatively charged and the positively charged cations move toward the cathode to be reduced. Electrons are forced into the electrolytic cell at the cathode by the outside voltage source and leave the cell from the anode. These conventions are summarized in Fig. 7-4.

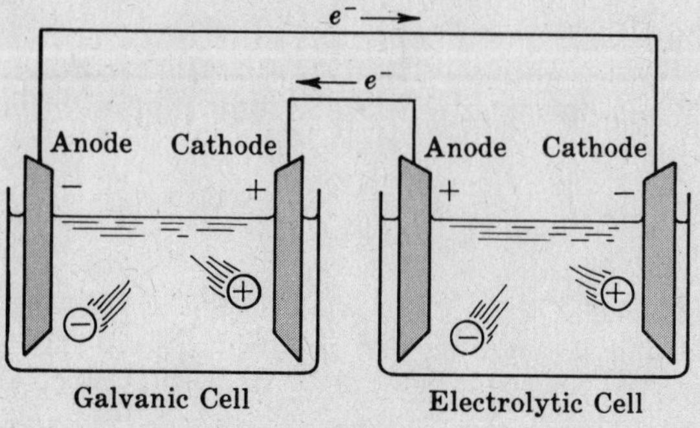

Fig. 7-4

A shorthand notation is used for describing the physical arrangement of electrochemical cells. The first terms in the notation refer to the anode reaction (oxidation) and the latter terms to the cathode reaction (reduction). A slash or semicolon is used to represent phase

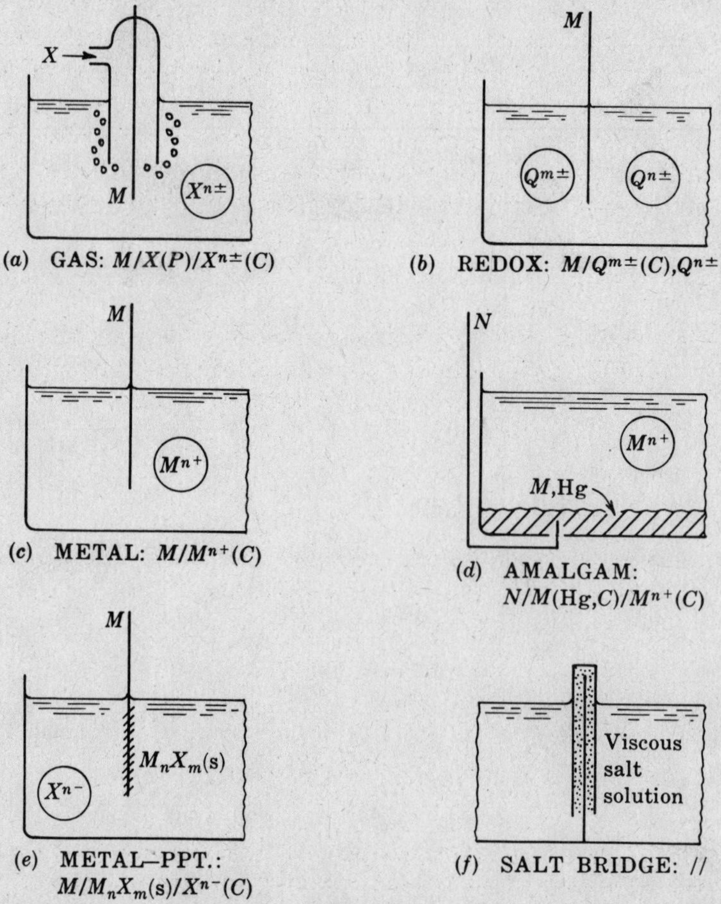

(*a*) GAS: $M/X(P)/X^{n\pm}(C)$

(*b*) REDOX: $M/Q^{m\pm}(C),Q^{n\pm}(C)$

(*c*) METAL: $M/M^{n+}(C)$

(*d*) AMALGAM: $N/M(\text{Hg},C)/M^{n+}(C)$

(*e*) METAL–PPT.: $M/M_nX_m(\text{s})/X^{n-}(C)$

(*f*) SALT BRIDGE: //

Fig. 7-5

boundaries, a comma to separate different species in the same phase and a double slash to represent a salt bridge. Although far from being the most technologically advanced electrode designs, those modules illustrated in Fig. 7-5 will give an idea of what the cell will look like when constructed from the notation.

EXAMPLE 7.9. Construct a diagram using the modules shown in Fig. 7-5 for the electrochemical cell given by Pt/Ag(s)/AgCl(s)/Cl^-(0.1 *M*)//Br^-(0.1 *M*)/Br_2(1 atm)/C(graph)/Pt.

The Ag-AgCl anode will be represented by module (*e*), the salt bridge by module (*f*) and the Br_2 cathode by module (*a*). See Fig. 7-6 for the complete sketch.

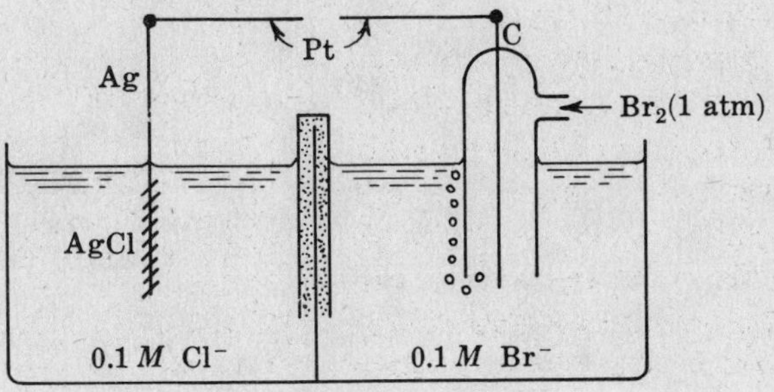

Fig. 7-6

7.9 STANDARD HALF-CELL AND OVERALL CELL POTENTIALS

Each redox half reaction (Section 7.1) has a voltage assigned to it. Many older references give values for oxidation potentials and many newer ones give values for reduction potentials. For the reduction half reaction, the voltage from the reduction potential tables is used directly and the voltage from the oxidation tables is used with its sign changed. For the oxidation half reaction, the voltage from the reduction tables is used with its sign changed and the voltage from the oxidation tables is used directly. Some tables list values of the *electric tension*, $\mathcal{V}°$, which is related to the potential by

$$\mathcal{E}° = -\mathcal{V}° \tag{7.18}$$

To find a value of $\mathcal{E}°$ for a new half reaction from known standard half reactions, the values of $\mathcal{E}°$ for the standard half reactions are converted to $\Delta G°$ using (*5.6*), the values of $\Delta G°$ are added and the $\Delta G°$(reaction) is converted back to $\mathcal{E}°$ using (*5.6*).

7.10 OVERALL CELL POTENTIALS

To determine the overall cell potential, $\mathcal{E}$, for nonstandard state conditions, $\mathcal{E}°$ is first determined as in Example 7.10 and the Nernst equation,

$$\mathcal{E} = \mathcal{E}° - \frac{RT}{n\mathcal{F}} \ln Q \tag{5.40}$$

is applied. At 25 °C, (*5.40*) becomes

$$\mathcal{E} = \mathcal{E}° - \frac{0.059157}{n} \log Q \tag{7.19}$$

EXAMPLE 7.10. To find the overall standard potential (also known as voltage or emf) of a cell the procedure outlined in Section 7.9 is used. Show that for the overall standard emf of a cell, identical results are obtained if the half-cell potentials are simply added.

For the general half reactions

$$\text{reactants}_1 = \text{products}_1 + pe^- \qquad \text{reactants}_2 + me^- = \text{products}_2$$

having standard half-cell potentials $\mathcal{E}_1^\circ$ and $\mathcal{E}_2^\circ$, respectively, the values of ΔG° for the half reactions are

$$\Delta G_1^\circ = -p\mathcal{F}\mathcal{E}_1^\circ \qquad \Delta G_2^\circ = -m\mathcal{F}\mathcal{E}_2^\circ$$

Multiplying the oxidation half reaction by m and the reduction half reaction by p to eliminate electrons and adding gives the overall cell reaction, and

$$\Delta G^\circ(\text{reaction}) = -pm\mathcal{F}\mathcal{E}_1^\circ - pm\mathcal{F}\mathcal{E}_2^\circ = -pm\mathcal{F}(\mathcal{E}_1^\circ + \mathcal{E}_2^\circ)$$

Recognizing that $n = pm$ in *(5.6)*, the overall standard cell potential is

$$\mathcal{E}^\circ = -\frac{-pm\mathcal{F}(\mathcal{E}_1^\circ + \mathcal{E}_2^\circ)}{pm\mathcal{F}} = \mathcal{E}_1^\circ + \mathcal{E}_2^\circ$$

EXAMPLE 7.11. What is $\mathcal{E}$ for the cell $Ag/AgBr(s)/Br^-(a = 0.34),Fe^{3+}(a = 0.1),Fe^{2+}(a = 0.02)/Pt$ if the standard half-cell reduction potentials are 0.0713 V for AgBr/Ag and 0.770 V for Fe^{3+}/Fe^{2+}?

Writing the equations and half-cell voltages gives

$$Ag(s) + Br^-(a = 0.34) = AgBr(s) + 1e^- \qquad \mathcal{E}^\circ = -0.0713\ \text{V}$$

$$Fe^{3+}(a = 0.1) + 1e^- = Fe^{2+}(a = 0.02) \qquad \mathcal{E}^\circ = 0.770\ \text{V}$$

and adding gives

$$Ag(s) + Fe^{3+}(a = 0.1) + Br^-(a = 0.34) = AgBr(s) + Fe^{2+}(a = 0.02) \qquad \mathcal{E}^\circ = 0.669\ \text{V}$$

Observe that the half cell with the larger reduction potential was written as the reduction reaction, making the overall voltage positive (spontaneous reaction) at standard conditions. Using *(5.38)* for the overall reaction gives

$$Q = (a_{AgBr})(a_{Fe^{2+}})/(a_{Ag})(a_{Fe^{3+}})(a_{Br^-})$$

$$= (1)(0.02)/(1)(0.1)(0.34) = 0.588$$

and using *(7.19)* gives

$$\mathcal{E} = 0.699 - \frac{0.059157}{1}\log(0.588) = 0.699 + 0.014 = 0.713\ \text{V}$$

The positive value for $\mathcal{E}$ implies the reaction is spontaneous as written and even more so than at standard conditions.

7.11 CONCENTRATION CELLS AND THERMOCELLS

In either of these galvanic cells, the electrode reactions are identical except for a difference in activities or temperatures of the materials.

Because the reactions in a concentration cell are similar, $\mathcal{E}^\circ = 0$ and the potential arises from the nonstandard conditions of the reactants and products. Thus

$$\mathcal{E} = -\frac{RT}{n\mathcal{F}}\ln Q \tag{7.20}$$

for cells which have no liquid junction or have nearly eliminated the liquid junction by using a salt bridge, and

$$\mathcal{E} = -\frac{RT}{n\mathcal{F}}t_i \ln Q \tag{7.21}$$

for cells with transference, where t_i is the transference number of the ion to which the electrodes are not reversible (the *spectator ion*).

The voltage of a thermocell is approximately given by

$$\mathcal{E} = -\int_{T_1}^{T_2} \frac{\partial \mathcal{E}}{\partial T}\, dT \tag{7.22}$$

where $\partial\mathcal{E}/\partial T$ is the temperature dependence of the cell voltage.

Solved Problems

Oxidation-Reduction

7.1. An electrochemical cell is prepared using a "quinhydrone" electrode at which hydroquinone, HOC_6H_4OH, is oxidized to quinone, OC_6H_4O, and an electrode at which $Cr_2O_7^{2-}$ is reduced to Cr^{3+}. Write the balanced net ionic reaction for this cell.

Summarizing the statement of the problem gives

$$HOC_6H_4OH + Cr_2O_7^{2-} = OC_6H_4O + Cr^{3+}$$

from which the following half reactions are generated:

$$HOC_6H_4OH = OC_6H_4O \qquad Cr_2O_7^{2-} = Cr^{3+}$$

The "quinhydrone" reaction is balanced with respect to C and O atoms and only needs $2H^+$ added to the right side of the reaction to complete the mass balance:

$$HOC_6H_4OH = OC_6H_4O + 2H^+$$

Upon adding $2e^-$, the complete half reaction is

$$HOC_6H_4OH = OC_6H_4O + 2H^+ + 2e^-$$

For the reduction reaction, the Cr atoms are balanced by placing a 2 before the Cr^{3+}, and xH^+ and yH_2O are added giving

$$Cr_2O_7^{2-} = 2Cr^{3+} + xH^+ + yH_2O$$

Counting H and O atoms gives

$$0 = x + 2y \qquad 7 = y$$

respectively, whence $x = -14$ and $y = 7$. The half reaction becomes

$$Cr_2O_7^{2-} + 14H^+ = 2Cr^{3+} + 7H_2O$$

which requires $6e^-$ for the electrical balance:

$$Cr_2O_7^{2-} + 14H^+ + 6e^- = 2Cr^{3+} + 7H_2O$$

Multiplying the oxidation reaction by 3 and the reduction reaction by 1 and adding gives

$$3HOC_6H_4OH + Cr_2O_7^{2-} + 8H^+ = 3OC_6H_4O + 2Cr^{3+} + 7H_2O$$

after canceling common terms.

7.2. The "dry cell" or Leclanché cell involves the reaction at one electrode in which Zn(s) is oxidized to Zn^{2+}(aq); at the other electrode MnO_2(s) is reduced to Mn_2O_3(s) in the presence of NH_4Cl(aq), generating NH_3(aq). Write the balanced net ionic equation for this reaction.

For the reaction $Zn(s) + MnO_2(s) = Mn_2O_3(s) + Zn^{2+}(aq)$, the following half reactions can be written

$$Zn(s) = Zn^{2+}(aq) \qquad MnO_2(s) = Mn_2O_3(s)$$

The oxidation reaction is balanced by adding $2e^-$ to the right side:

$$Zn(s) = Zn^{2+}(aq) + 2e^-$$

The reduction reaction is balanced by placing a 2 before the MnO_2, assuming the excess O atoms to become OH^- by combining with a H^+ from the $NH_4^+(aq)$, and adding $2e^-$, giving

$$2e^- + NH_4^+(aq) + 2MnO_2(s) = Mn_2O_3(s) + OH^-(aq) + NH_3(aq)$$

Adding the half reactions gives

$$Zn(s) + 2MnO_2(s) + NH_4^+(aq) = Mn_2O_3(s) + NH_3(aq) + OH^-(aq) + Zn^{2+}(aq)$$

7.3. **The chemical reaction for the Daniell cell is**

$$Zn(s) + Cu^{2+}(aq) = Zn^{2+}(aq) + Cu(s)$$

If ΔG°_{298}(formation) $= 0$ for Zn(s) and Cu(s), -35.14 kcal mol^{-1} for $Zn^{2+}(aq)$ and 15.66 kcal mol^{-1} for $Cu^{2+}(aq)$, calculate the cell potential and discuss the spontaneity of the reaction under standard conditions.

Applying (*5.11*) to the reaction gives

$$\Delta G^\circ_{298}(\text{reaction}) = [(1)(-35.14) + (1)(0)] - [(1)(0) + (1)(15.66)]$$

$$= -50.80 \text{ kcal} = -212.55 \text{ kJ}$$

and using (*5.6*) gives

$$\mathcal{E}^\circ = \frac{-(-212.55 \text{ kJ})}{(2 \text{ mol})(96.485 \text{ kJ mol}^{-1} \text{ V}^{-1})} = 1.101 \text{ V}$$

which is spontaneous as written.

7.4. **During the electrolysis of a NaCl solution using inert electrodes, the following chemical reactions are possible at the anode:**

$$Cl^-(aq) = \tfrac{1}{2}Cl_2(g) + 1e^-$$

$$2H_2O(liq) = O_2(g) + 4H^+(aq) + 4e^-$$

and at the cathode:

$$Na^+(aq) + 1e^- = Na(s)$$

$$2H^+(aq) + 2e^- = H_2(g)$$

The voltage of a cell described by the first and third equations is -4.0692 V; first and fourth, -1.3583 V; second and third, -3.940 V; and second and fourth, -1.229 V. Which reaction will proceed under standard conditions?

Choosing the combination which has the most positive value of $\mathcal{E}^\circ$ gives

$$2H_2O(liq) = O_2(g) + 2H_2(g)$$

as the reaction most favored.

7.5. **What is the minimum mass of reactants for a dry cell if it is to generate 0.0100 A for 10.0 hr?**

The amount of charge to be generated is given by (*7.2*) as

$$q = (0.0100 \text{ A})(10.0 \text{ hr})(3600 \text{ s hr}^{-1}) = 360 \text{ C}$$

Changing to equivalents gives

$$\frac{360 \text{ C}}{9.6485 \times 10^4 \text{ C mol}^{-1}} = 3.73 \times 10^{-3} \text{ mol}$$

From the half reactions

$$Zn = Zn^{2+} + 2e^- \qquad 2MnO_2 + NH_4^+ + 2e^- = Mn_2O_3 + NH_3 + OH^-$$

the equivalent weights as determined using (*7.1*) are

$$W(\text{Zn}) = \frac{65.37 \text{ g mol}^{-1}}{2 \text{ mol mol}^{-1}} = 32.69 \text{ g mol}^{-1} \qquad W(\text{MnO}_2) = \frac{86.94}{1} = 86.94 \text{ g mol}^{-1}$$

giving $$(32.69 \text{ g mol}^{-1})(3.73 \times 10^{-3} \text{ mol}) = 0.122 \text{ g Zn}$$

and $$(86.94)(3.73 \times 10^{-3}) = 0.324 \text{ g MnO}_2$$

Conductivity

7.6. **(*a*) A conductivity cell was calibrated using 0.01 *N* KCl ($k = 0.14087\ \Omega^{-1}\,\text{m}^{-1}$) in the cell and the measured resistance was 688 Ω. Find the cell constant. (*b*) A 0.0100 *N* $AgNO_3$ solution in the same cell had a resistance of 777 Ω. What is Λ?**

(*a*) From (*7.4*) and (*7.5*),

$$\frac{l}{A} = kR = (0.14087\ \Omega^{-1}\,\text{m}^{-1})(688\ \Omega) = 97.0 \text{ m}^{-1}$$

(*b*) Using the cell constant from (*a*), we have

$$k = \frac{l/A}{R} = \frac{97.0 \text{ m}^{-1}}{777\ \Omega} = 0.1248\ \Omega^{-1}\,\text{m}^{-1}$$

The equivalent conductance is given by (*7.6*) as

$$\Lambda = \frac{0.1248\ \Omega^{-1}\,\text{m}^{-1}}{(1000 \text{ dm}^3\text{ m}^{-3})(0.0100 \text{ mol dm}^{-3})} = 0.01248\ \Omega^{-1}\,\text{m}^2\,\text{mol}^{-1}$$

7.7. **Using the data in Example 7.7, find t_+.**

Assuming dV/dt to be given by V/t, where $V = Al$, (*7.12*) gives

$$t_+ = \left[\frac{(96{,}485)(1000)(0.0100)}{3.00 \times 10^{-3}}\right]\left[\frac{(3.25 \times 10^{-4})(2.13 \times 10^{-2})}{45.0 \times 60}\right] = 0.825$$

7.8. **Current was passed through a 0.100 *N* solution of KCl at 25 °C. A silver coulometer in series with the KCl cell showed that 0.6136 g of Ag had been transferred from one electrode to the other during the electrolysis. The cathode portion weighing 117.51 g was drained and found to contain 0.56662% KCl. The anode portion weighing 121.45 g was drained and found to contain 0.57217% KCl. The middle portion of the Hittorf cell contained 0.74217% KCl. If inert electrodes were used, find t_+.**

The composition of the middle compartment is equal to the original composition of the anode and cathode compartments. In the cathode compartment there are

$$(117.51 \text{ g soln}) - (117.51 \text{ g soln})\left(5.6662 \times 10^{-3}\ \frac{\text{g KCl}}{\text{g soln}}\right)$$

$$= 117.51 \text{ g soln} - 0.6658 \text{ g KCl} = 116.84 \text{ g H}_2\text{O}$$

after the electrolysis, and for the same amount of water there were

$$\frac{116.84}{1 - 7.4217 \times 10^{-3}} = 117.71 \text{ g soln}$$

before the electrolysis containing

$$(117.71)(7.4217 \times 10^{-3}) = 0.8736 \text{ g KCl}$$

Thus

$$N_0 = \frac{0.8736 \text{ g}}{74.56 \text{ g mol}^{-1}} = 1.172 \times 10^{-2} \text{ mol}, \qquad N_f = \frac{0.6658}{74.56} = 0.893 \times 10^{-2} \text{ mol}$$

The number of equivalents of charge passed is

$$N_e = \frac{0.6136 \text{ g Ag}}{107.868 \text{ g mol}^{-1}} = 5.688 \times 10^{-3} \text{ mol}$$

Using *(7.11)* with $N_e' = 0$ gives

$$t_+ = \frac{|(1.172 \times 10^{-2}) - (0.893 \times 10^{-2}) \pm 0|}{5.688 \times 10^{-3}} = 0.491$$

Electrochemical Cells

7.9. Write the notation for the diagram shown in Fig. 7-7.

The anode compartment consists of a Pt electrode in contact with a 5% Na-Hg amalgam, which in turn is in contact with a 0.1 *M* solution of Na^+. The shorthand notation for the anode is

$$\text{Pt/Na(5\% amalgam)/Na}^+(0.1\ M)$$

The cathode compartment consists of a Pt electrode immersed in a 1*M* Cu^{2+} and 0.1 *M* Cu^+ solution, giving the notation $Cu^+(0.1\ M),Cu^{2+}(1M)/Pt$. Recognizing the compartments to be separated by a salt bridge, the complete cell notation becomes

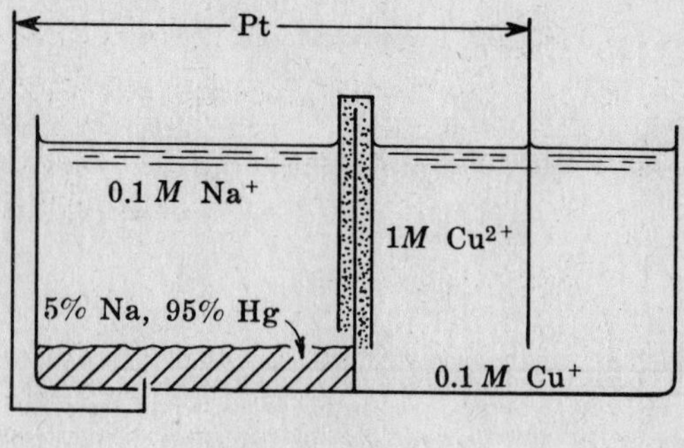

Fig. 7-7

$$\text{Pt/Na(5\% amalgam)/Na}^+(0.1\ M)//\text{Cu}^+(0.1\ M),\text{Cu}^{2+}(1M)/\text{Pt}$$

7.10. What is $\mathcal{E}^\circ$ for the cell Pt/Ag(s)/AgCl(s)/$Cl^-(a=1)$/Cl_2(1 atm)/C(graph)/Pt if the standard half-cell reduction potentials are 0.2223 V for AgCl/Ag and 1.3583 V for Cl_2/Cl^-?

The half reaction with the smaller reduction potential is written as the oxidation, giving

$$\text{Ag(s)} + \text{Cl}^-(a=1) = \text{AgCl(s)} + 1e^- \qquad \mathcal{E}^\circ = -0.2223 \text{ V}$$

and for the reduction reaction

$$\text{Cl}_2(1 \text{ atm}) + 2e^- = 2\text{Cl}^-(a=1) \qquad \mathcal{E}^\circ = 1.3583 \text{ V}$$

We multiply the first reaction by 2 and the second reaction by 1 (leaving the voltages alone) and add to obtain

$$2\text{Ag(s)} + \text{Cl}_2(1 \text{ atm}) = 2\text{AgCl(s)} \qquad \mathcal{E}^\circ = 1.1360 \text{ V}$$

which is spontaneous.

7.11. If the standard half-cell reduction potentials are 0.522 V for Cu^+/Cu and 0.3402 V for Cu^{2+}/Cu, find the standard half-cell reduction potential for Cu^{2+}/Cu^+.

Writing the reaction for the Cu^{2+}/Cu couple and calculating ΔG° gives

$$\text{Cu}^{2+} + 2e^- = \text{Cu} \qquad \Delta G^\circ = -(2)\mathcal{F}(0.3402)$$

and for the reverse of the Cu^+/Cu couple gives

$$\mathrm{Cu} = \mathrm{Cu}^+ + 1e^- \qquad \Delta G^\circ = -(1)\mathcal{F}(-0.522)$$

Adding gives the desired reaction and ΔG° as

$$\mathrm{Cu}^{2+} + 1e^- = \mathrm{Cu}^+ \qquad \Delta G^\circ(\text{reaction}) = -\mathcal{F}(0.158)$$

and applying (*5.6*) with $n = 1$ gives $\mathcal{E}^\circ = 0.158$ V.

7.12. The standard half-cell reduction potential for Ag^+/Ag is 0.7996 V at 25 °C. Given the experimental value $K_{sp} = 1.56 \times 10^{-10}$ for AgCl, calculate the standard half-cell reduction potential for the Ag/AgCl electrode.

For the desired reaction, $\mathrm{AgCl} + 1e^- = \mathrm{Ag} + \mathrm{Cl}^-$, the value of $\mathcal{E}^\circ$ is given by (*5.6*) as

$$\mathcal{E}^\circ = \frac{-\Delta G^\circ(\text{reaction})}{(1)\mathcal{F}}$$

The needed ΔG°(reaction) can be obtained by adding the values of ΔG°(reaction) for the reactions

$$\mathrm{Ag}^+ + 1e^- = \mathrm{Ag} \qquad \Delta G^\circ = -n\mathcal{F}\mathcal{E}^\circ$$

$$\mathrm{AgCl} = \mathrm{Ag}^+ + \mathrm{Cl}^- \qquad \Delta G^\circ = -RT \ln K_{sp}$$

giving

$$\begin{aligned}\Delta G^\circ(\text{reaction}) &= -(1\ \text{mol})(9.6485 \times 10^4\ \text{J mol}^{-1}\ \text{V}^{-1})(0.7996\ \text{V}) \\ &\qquad - (8.314\ \text{J mol}^{-1}\ \text{K}^{-1})(298\ \text{K}) \ln (1.56 \times 10^{-10}) \\ &= -77.15\ \text{kJ} + 55.95\ \text{kJ} = -21.20\ \text{kJ}\end{aligned}$$

The voltage is

$$\mathcal{E}^\circ = \frac{-(-21.20)}{(1)(96.485)} = 0.220\ \text{V}$$

7.13. What is $\mathcal{E}$ for the cell $\mathrm{Mg/Mg^{2+}}(a = 10^{-3})//\mathrm{H^+}(a = 10)/\mathrm{H_2}(0.1\ \text{atm})/\mathrm{Pt}$ if the standard half-cell reduction potentials are -2.375 V for Mg^{2+}/Mg and 0.000 V for H^+/H_2?

For the reaction

$$\mathrm{Mg(s)} + 2\mathrm{H}^+(a = 10) = \mathrm{H_2}(0.1\ \text{atm}) + \mathrm{Mg}^{2+}(a = 10^{-3})$$

$\mathcal{E}^\circ = 2.375$ V and (*5.38*) gives

$$Q = (a_{\mathrm{H_2}})(a_{\mathrm{Mg^{2+}}})/(a_{\mathrm{Mg}})(a_{\mathrm{H^+}})^2 = (0.1)(10^{-3})/(1)(10)^2 = 10^{-6}$$

which upon substitution into (*7.19*) gives

$$\mathcal{E} = 2.375 - \frac{0.059157}{2} \log 10^{-6} = 2.375 + 0.177 = 2.552\ \text{V}$$

The cell is spontaneous as written, with the Mg electrode negative and the H_2 electrode positive.

7.14. What is the voltage of the cell $\mathrm{C/Br_2}(0.1\ \text{atm})/\mathrm{Br^-}(0.5\ M)/\mathrm{Br_2}(1\ \text{atm})/\mathrm{C}$ at 25 °C?

For the half reactions

$$2\mathrm{Br}^-(0.5\ M) = \mathrm{Br_2}(0.1\ \text{atm}) + 2e^- \qquad \mathrm{Br_2}(1\ \text{atm}) + 2e^- = 2\mathrm{Br}^-(0.5\ M)$$

the overall reaction is $\mathrm{Br_2}(1\ \text{atm}) = \mathrm{Br_2}(0.1\ \text{atm})$, and from (*7.20*)

$$\mathcal{E} = -\frac{0.059157}{2} \log\left(\frac{0.1}{1}\right) = 0.029579\ \text{V}$$

7.15. What is the voltage at 25 °C of the cell

$$Pt/H_2(1\ atm)/HCl(0.5\ M)/HCl(1.0\ M)/H_2(1\ atm)/Pt$$

if $t_+ = 0.83$?

For this cell having a liquid junction, (*7.21*) with $t_- = 0.17$ gives for the net reaction $HCl(1.0\ M) = HCl(0.5\ M)$

$$\mathcal{E} = -\frac{0.059157}{1}(0.17)\log\left(\frac{0.5}{1.0}\right) = 0.0030\ V$$

7.16. The voltage of a neutral, saturated Weston cell is given by

$$\mathcal{E}(T') = 1.018410 - 4.93\times10^{-5}(T'-25) - 8.0\times10^{-7}(T'-25)^2 + 1\times10^{-8}(T'-25)^3$$

where T' is the temperature between 5 °C and 50 °C. What is the approximate voltage of the thermocell given below if $T_1' = 5$ °C and $T_2' = 50$ °C?

$$\underset{T_1}{Pt/Cd(amal)/CdSO_4,Hg_2SO_4/Hg/Pt}{-}{-}{-}{-}\underset{T_2}{Pt/Hg/Hg_2SO_4,CdSO_4/Cd(amal)/Pt}$$

The symbol———— represents an external electrical connector between the two halves of the thermocell.

Equation (*7.22*) is equivalent to $\mathcal{E} = -\mathcal{E}(T)\Big|_{T_1}^{T_2} = -\mathcal{E}(T')\Big|_{T_1'}^{T_2'}$. Thus

$$\mathcal{E} = -\{(-4.93\times10^{-5})[(25)-(-20)] - (8.0\times10^{-7})[(25)^2-(-20)^2] + (1\times10^{-8})[(25)^3-(-20)^3]\}$$

$$= -(-2.22\times10^{-3} - 0.18\times10^{-3} + 0.24\times10^{-3}) = 2.16\ mV$$

Supplementary Problems

Oxidation-Reduction

7.17. In the cells of the Edison battery, iron is oxidized to $Fe(OH)_2(s)$ in a 21% KOH solution (containing some LiOH) and $NiO_2(s)$ is reduced to $Ni(OH)_2(s)$. Write the balanced reaction for this cell.

Ans. $Fe(s) + NiO_2(s) + 2H_2O(liq) = Fe(OH)_2(s) + Ni(OH)_2(s)$

7.18. During the electrolysis of a $CuCl_2$ solution using inert electrodes, the following chemical reactions are possible at the anode:

$$Cl^-(aq) = \tfrac{1}{2}Cl_2(g) + 1e^-$$

$$2H_2O(liq) = O_2(g) + 4H^+(aq) + 4e^-$$

and at the cathode:

$$Cu^{2+}(aq) + 2e^- = Cu(s)$$

$$2H^+(aq) + 2e^- = H_2(g)$$

The voltage of a cell described by the first and third equations is −1.0181 V; the first and fourth, −1.3583 V; the second and third, −0.889 V; and the second and fourth, −1.229 V. Which reaction will proceed under standard conditions?

Ans. Reaction with most positive voltage is $2Cu^{2+}(aq) + 2H_2O(liq) = O_2(g) + 4H^+(aq) + 2Cu(s)$.

7.19. During the electrolysis of $CdSO_4$, what volume of O_2 at 25 °C and 1.00 atm will be produced for every gram of Cd?

Ans. $W(Cd) = 56.2$, $W(O_2) = 8.00$, 1.78×10^{-2} eq, 0.142 g O_2; 0.109 dm^3

Conductivity

7.20. The resistance of a conductivity cell was 702 Ω when filled with 0.0100 N KCl (k = 0.14087 $\Omega^{-1}\ m^{-1}$) and 6920 Ω when filled with 0.0100 N $HC_2H_3O_2$. Find the cell constant and Λ for the acid.

Ans. 98.9 m^{-1}, $1.429 \times 10^{-3}\ \Omega^{-1}\ m^2\ mol^{-1}$

7.21. The equivalent conductances at 18 °C are 124.25, 118 and 106.6 $\Omega^{-1}\ cm^2\ mol^{-1}$ for NH_4NO_3; 234, 228 and 213 for KOH; and 123.7, 118.2 and 104.8 for KNO_3, at 0.001 N, 0.01 N and 0.1 N, respectively. (*a*) Find Λ_0 for these substances and calculate Λ_0 for NH_4OH. (*b*) If Λ = 28, 9.6 and 3.3 Ω^{-1} $cm^2\ mol^{-1}$ at 0.001 N, 0.01 N and 0.1 N, respectively, for NH_4OH, find α for these concentrations and comment.

Ans. (*a*) Plot of Λ against $c^{1/2}$ gives Λ_0 = 128 for NH_4NO_3, 237 for KOH, 126 for KNO_3; Λ_0 for NH_4OH = 239.

(*b*) 11.7%, 4.0% and 1.4%; ionization becomes larger as the solution becomes more dilute.

7.22. From the conductivity data given below, find α, K_a and K at each concentration of acetic acid at 25 °C:

$c \times 10^4$, N	0.28014	1.1135	1.5321	2.1844	10.2831	13.6340
Λ, $\Omega^{-1}\ cm^2\ mol^{-1}$	210.38	127.75	112.05	96.493	48.146	42.227

Assume Λ_0 = 390.13 $\Omega^{-1}\ cm^2\ mol^{-1}$.

Ans. α = 0.53925, 0.32745, 0.28721, 0.24733, 0.12341, 0.10824;
$K_a = \alpha^2 c/(1-\alpha)$, giving $K_a \times 10^5$ = 1.768, 1.775, 1.773, 1.775, 1.787, 1.791;
plot of K_a against c or $c^{1/2}$ gives intercept (where $K_\gamma = 1.000$) as $K = 1.764 \times 10^{-5}$

7.23. Repeat Example 7.6 with $t_+ = 5t_-$. *Ans.* See Fig. 7-8.

(*a*) Originally

(*b*) After discharge of 6 eq of ions at the electrodes

(*c*) After ionic migration with $t_+ = 5t_-$

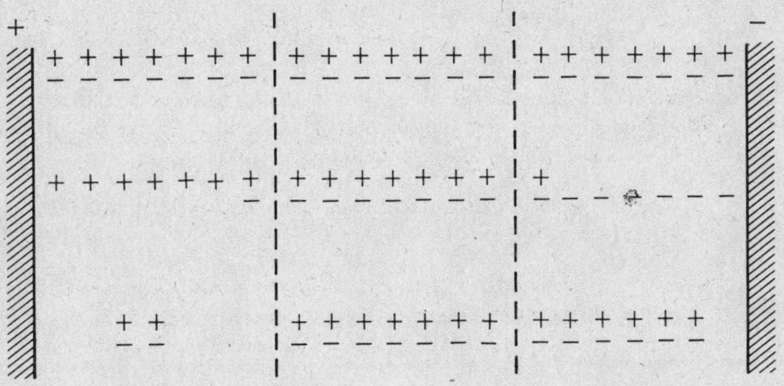

Fig. 7-8

7.24. Calculate t_- for the KCl experiment described in Problem 7.8 by analyzing the anode compartment data.

Ans. 120.76 g H_2O, 121.66 g solution, 0.9029 g KCl,
$N_0 = 0.01211$, $N_f = 0.00932$, $N'_e = 0.005688$; $t_- = 0.509$

7.25. You are to design a moving boundary experiment for students to determine t_+ for 0.0100 N LiCl at 25 °C. The value is 0.3289. Suppose the useful laboratory time is about 1.5 hr and the current source is capable of producing 1.00 mA. To reduce the error in measurement of volume, the desired length change for the boundary should be 2.5 cm. If the cell is to be made from glass tubing, what size tubing should be chosen, to the nearest mm?

Ans. A = 0.736 cm^2, I.D. = 9.68 mm ≈ 10 mm

7.26. If $\Lambda_0 = 91.0\ \text{cm}^2\ \text{mol}^{-1}\ \Omega^{-1}$ for $NaC_2H_3O_2$ and 426.16 for HCl and if $t_+ = 0.556$ for $NaC_2H_3O_2$ and 0.821 for HCl, find Λ_0 for $HC_2H_3O_2$.

Ans. $\lambda_{0,+} = 349.88$, $\lambda_{0,-} = 40.4$, $\Lambda_0 = 390.28\ \text{cm}^2\ \text{mol}^{-1}\ \Omega^{-1}$

7.27. Calculate u_+ and u_- for 0.0100 N LiCl given that $\Lambda = 0.010732\ \Omega^{-1}\ \text{m}^2\ \text{mol}^{-1}$ using the experimental setup described in Problem 7.25.

Ans. $3.657 \times 10^{-8}\ \text{m}^2\ \text{V}^{-1}\ \text{s}^{-1}$, $7.461 \times 10^{-8}\ \text{m}^2\ \text{V}^{-1}\ \text{s}^{-1}$

7.28. Consider a titration between a strong acid and a strong base. Sketch a plot of L against volume of added base. Sketch a similar diagram for the titration of a weak acid and a strong base. Identify the endpoints of the titrations.

Ans. The plot for the strong acid and strong base will be nearly V-shaped (with rather steep slopes because of the high values of λ_i for H^+ and OH^-) with the endpoint at the lowest part of the plot. In the plot for the weak acid and strong base the slope before the neutralization endpoint is not as great as after the endpoint because the concentration of ions present in a weak acid is not large.

7.29. Calculate K_{sp} for AgCl if $k = 2 \times 10^{-4}\ \Omega^{-1}\ \text{m}^{-1}$ at 25 °C and it is assumed that Λ differs very little from Λ_0. Assume $\lambda_{0,i} = 6.192 \times 10^{-3}\ \text{m}^2\ \Omega^{-1}\ \text{mol}^{-1}$ for Ag^+ and $7.634 \times 10^{-3}\ \text{m}^2\ \Omega^{-1}\ \text{mol}^{-1}$ for Cl^-.

Ans. $\Lambda_0 = 0.013826\ \text{m}^2\ \Omega^{-1}\ \text{mol}^{-1}$, $c = 1.5 \times 10^{-5}\ N$, $K_{sp} = 2.3 \times 10^{-10}$

7.30. If $k = 5.7 \times 10^{-6}\ \Omega^{-1}\ \text{m}^{-1}$ for water at 25 °C, find K_w. The values of $\lambda_{0,i}$ are $0.03498\ \text{m}^2\ \Omega^{-1}\ \text{mol}^{-1}$ for H^+ and $0.01967\ \text{m}^2\ \Omega^{-1}\ \text{mol}^{-1}$ for OH^-.

Ans. $\Lambda_0 = 0.05465\ \text{m}^2\ \Omega^{-1}\ \text{mol}^{-1}$, $c = 1.04 \times 10^{-7}\ N$, $K_w = 1.08 \times 10^{-14}$

Electrochemical Cells

7.31. Prepare a sketch for the cell Pt/Na($a = 0.1$, amalgam)/Na^+($a = 0.01$)//Cu^{2+}($a = 0.01$)/Cu(s)/Pt. If the standard half-cell reduction potentials at 25 °C are −2.7109 V for Na^+/Na and 0.3402 V for Cu^{2+}/Cu, calculate $\mathcal{E}^\circ$ and $\mathcal{E}$ for the cell.

Ans. The sketch will consist of modules (*d*), (*f*) and (*c*) from Fig. 7-5; $\mathcal{E}^\circ = \mathcal{E} = 3.0511$ V for the reaction $2Na(a = 0.1) + Cu^{2+}(a = 0.01) = 2Na^+(a = 0.01) + Cu(a = 1)$.

7.32. Calculate the potential of the cell described in Problem 7.31, assuming the Debye-Hückel theory, (*5.36*), to be applicable for the 0.01 M solutions of Na^+ and Cu^{2+}. Compare answers.

Ans. $\gamma_{Na^+} = 0.888$, $\gamma_{Cu^{2+}} = 0.442$; $\mathcal{E} = 3.0436$ V (7.5 mV lower)

7.33. What is $\mathcal{E}^\circ$ for the cell Cu/Ca(s)/Ca^{2+}($a = 1$)//Fe^{3+}($a = 1$)/Fe(s)/Cu if the standard half-cell reduction potentials are −2.76 V for Ca^{2+}/Ca and −0.036 V for Fe^{3+}/Fe?

Ans. 2.72 V for the reaction $3Ca + 2Fe^{3+} = 3Ca^{2+} + 2Fe$

7.34. If the standard half-cell reduction potentials are 1.45 V for ClO_3^-/Cl^- and 1.47 V for ClO_3^-/Cl_2, find $\mathcal{E}^\circ$ for Cl_2/Cl^-. *Ans.* 1.35 V

7.35. The $\mathcal{E}^\circ$ for the cell Pt/H_2(1 atm)/HCl(C)/AgCl(s)/Ag(s)/Pt was to be determined experimentally. Write the Nernst equation for this reaction and show that

$$\mathcal{E} + 0.118314 \log C_{HCl} = \mathcal{E}^\circ - 0.118314 \log \gamma_\pm$$

Because $\log \gamma_{\pm}$ is a function of $C^{1/2}$, see (*5.35*), a plot of $\mathcal{E} + 0.118314 \log C_{HCl}$ against $C^{1/2}$ will have an intercept of $\mathcal{E}°$. Find $\mathcal{E}°$ for the cell from the following data:

$\mathcal{E}$, V	0.3598	0.3892	0.4650	0.5791	0.6961	0.8140	0.9322
C, N	10^{-1}	5×10^{-2}	10^{-2}	10^{-3}	10^{-4}	10^{-5}	10^{-6}

Ans. 0.2223 V

7.36. The value of K_w can be determined from emf data. If the standard half reaction potentials are 0.0000 V for H^+/H_2 and −0.8277 V for the half reaction

$$2H_2O + 2e^- = H_2 + 2OH^-$$

find K_w from these data. Compare your answer to that obtained in Problem 7.30.

Ans. $\mathcal{E}° = -0.8277$ V, $K_w = 1.02 \times 10^{-14}$; essentially the same

7.37. What is the voltage of the cell Pt/Na(10 mole% amalgam)/Na^+(0.1 M)/Na(5 mole% amalgam)/Pt at 25 °C? *Ans.* $\mathcal{E}° = 0$, $\mathcal{E} = 0.0178$ V

7.38. The cell described in Problem 7.15 was changed to

$$Pt/H_2(1\ atm)/HCl(0.5\ M)/AgCl/Ag{-}{-}{-}{-}Ag/AgCl/HCl(1.0\ M)/H_2(1\ atm)/Pt$$

to eliminate the liquid junction. What is the voltage of this cell at 25 °C?

Ans. $\mathcal{E}° = 0$, $\mathcal{E} = 0.0178$ V

7.39. For the thermocell

$$\underset{T_1}{Ag}/AgCl(liq)/\underset{T_2}{Ag}$$

operating between 500 °C and 700 °C, Metz and Seifert reported $d\mathcal{E}/dT = -0.378$ mV K^{-1}. Find $\mathcal{E}$ for this cell operating with $T_1 = 500$ °C and $T_2 = 700$ °C. *Ans.* 75.6 mV

7.40. The potential of the Daniell cell Zn/$ZnSO_4$(1M)//$CuSO_4$(1M)/Cu was reported by Buckbee, Surdzial and Metz as $\mathcal{E}° = 1.1028 - 0.641 \times 10^{-3}T' + 0.72 \times 10^{-5}(T')^2$, where T' is the Celsius temperature. (*a*) Calculate $\Delta G°$, $\Delta S°$ and $\Delta H°$ from this equation at 25 °C. (*b*) Compare the results to the answers found in Problem 7.3. (*c*) The value of $\Delta S° = -15.6$ EU from thermochemical tables is several times less than the cell value. Why?

Ans. (*a*) $\Delta G° = -210.59$ kJ, $\Delta S° = -54.2$ EU, $\Delta H° = -226.74$ kJ.

(*b*) $\Delta G°$ is 0.92% higher.

(*c*) A negligible error in emf from small liquid junction potential gives a significant error in $\Delta S°$ because the liquid junction has a different temperature coefficient than the reaction of interest.

Chapter 8

Heterogeneous Equilibria

Phase Rule

8.1 PHASES

A *phase* can be defined as a portion of the system under consideration that is submacroscopically homogeneous and is separated from other such portions by definite physical boundaries. The symbol for the number of phases present in a system will be p. There can be only one gaseous phase in a system because all gases are completely miscible.

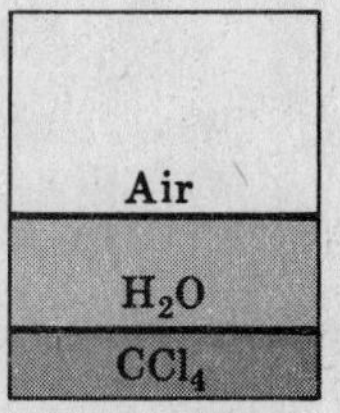

Fig. 8-1

EXAMPLE 8.1. Consider the system shown in Fig. 8-1. Find p and describe the various phases.

The system consists of the CCl_4-rich layer, which contains small amounts of air and H_2O; the H_2O-rich layer, which contains small amounts of air and CCl_4; and the gaseous phase, which contains air, H_2O vapor and CCl_4 vapor. Here $p = 3$.

8.2 COMPONENTS

The number of *components* in a system, c, is the minimum number of independently variable chemical species necessary to describe the composition of each phase. The establishment of chemical equilibrium often reduces c.

EXAMPLE 8.2. Determine the number of components in a mixture of $H_2(g)$, $O_2(g)$ and $H_2O(g)$.

Depending on the method used to prepare the system and the final status of the system, $c = 1$, 2 or 3. If simply a mixture of gases, three components must be specified. If a mixture of three gases that have been allowed to equilibrate, only two components must be specified because the information concerning the third can be calculated from the equilibrium constant for the reaction: $K = a_{H_2O}/a_{H_2}(a_{O_2})^{1/2}$. If a mixture of gases produced by the decomposition of H_2O, then only one component must be specified because the information concerning the other two can be calculated from the equilibrium constant and the known stoichiometry, where $a_{H_2} = 2a_{O_2}$.

8.3 DEGREES OF FREEDOM (VARIANCE)

The number of *degrees of freedom*, f, is the minimum number of intensive variables (mass-independent properties such as T, P and concentration) that must be specified to fix the values of all remaining intensive variables. Systems with $f = 0$ are known as *invariant*, or having no degrees of freedom; with $f = 1$, *univariant* (one degree of freedom); with $f = 2$, *divariant* (two degrees of freedom); etc.

8.4 GIBBS PHASE RULE

The number of degrees of freedom is given by

$$f = c - p + 2 \tag{8.1}$$

EXAMPLE 8.3. Determine f for the system described in Example 8.2.

In all cases $p = 1$, giving $f = c + 1$. For the case where $c = 3$, $f = 4$ implying that T, P and the composition of two of the three components are required to fix the remaining variables. For $c = 2$, $f = 3$ requiring T, P and one composition to be specified. For $c = 1$, $f = 2$ requiring only T and P to be specified. The remaining information can be calculated using the ideal gas law, etc.

Phase Diagrams for One-Component Systems

For a one-component system (*8.1*) becomes

$$f = 3 - p \tag{8.2}$$

Because p is at least 1, a maximum of two variables are needed to fix the remaining properties. Usually T and P are chosen and the system described by a phase diagram expressed in terms of these variables.

EXAMPLE 8.4. Discuss the hypothetical phase diagram shown in Fig. 8-2.

Figure 8-2 consists of a plot of the vapor pressure curve of the liquid between points a and b; the sublimation pressure curves of the α-solid and the β-solid between points b and c and points c and d, respectively; the pressure dependence of the melting point of the α-solid, the β-solid and the γ-solid between points b and e, points e and f, and points f and g, respectively; and the pressure dependence of the phase transition between the β-solid and the α-solid between points c and e, and between the β-solid and the γ-solid between points f and h. The points b, c, e, and f at which three phases are present are known as *triple points*. Point a and the vertical dashed line represent the *critical point* and the *critical isotherm*, respectively.

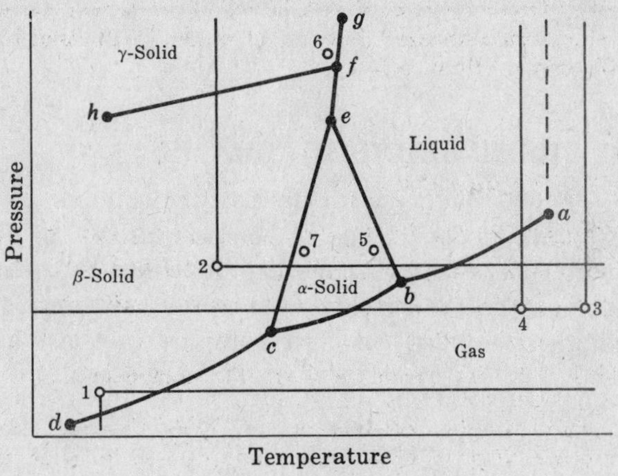

Fig. 8-2

Phase Diagrams for Two-Component Systems

8.5 INTRODUCTION

For two components (*8.1*) becomes

$$f = 4 - p \tag{8.3}$$

Because p can be as low as 1, three variables may be necessary to describe a system. Because three variables are difficult to graph, usually P is held constant on a diagram of T plotted against concentration. Useful measures of concentration are weight percentage of component i in phase j, $(\text{wt}\%\ i)_j$, and mole fraction, x_i.

EXAMPLE 8.5. Consider the hypothetical phase diagram shown in Fig. 8-3. In such a diagram certain areas will be one-phase areas and others will be two-phase areas. The compositions of the phases in equilibrium in the two-phase areas will be determined by horizontal "tie lines." The respective masses of these two phases can be determined by

$$\frac{m_1}{m_2} = \frac{(\text{wt\%}\ B)_2 - (\text{wt\%}\ B)_{AB}}{(\text{wt\%}\ B)_{AB} - (\text{wt\%}\ B)_1} \tag{8.4}$$

where $$m_1 + m_2 = m_{AB} \tag{8.5}$$

What would be the masses of the phases for a system containing 0.050 kg of A and 0.050 kg of B in equilibrium if $(\text{wt\%}\ B)_1 = 30.0\%$ and $(\text{wt\%}\ B)_2 = 85.5\%$?

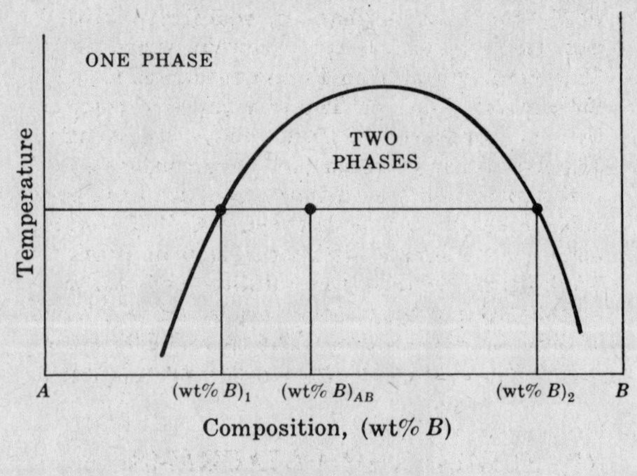

Fig. 8-3

The bulk composition of the system is

$$(\text{wt\%}\ B)_{AB} = \frac{0.050\ \text{kg}}{0.050\ \text{kg} + 0.050\ \text{kg}} = 50.0\%$$

Using (8.4) gives

$$\frac{m_1}{m_2} = \frac{85.5 - 50.0}{50.0 - 30.0} = 1.775$$

Using this result with (8.5), where $m_{AB} = 0.100$ kg, gives $m_1 = 0.064$ kg for phase 1 and $m_2 = 0.036$ kg for phase 2.

8.6 LIQUID-LIQUID DIAGRAMS

Typical diagrams for partially miscible liquids are shown in Fig. 8-4. Figures 8-4(*a*) and 8-4(*b*) can be considered to be special cases of Fig. 8-4(*c*) in which one or both of the components have solidified before reaching the *lower consolute temperature,* point *b*, or have vaporized before reaching the *upper consolute temperature,* point *a*, respectively. There is a single one-phase area and a single two-phase area in these diagrams.

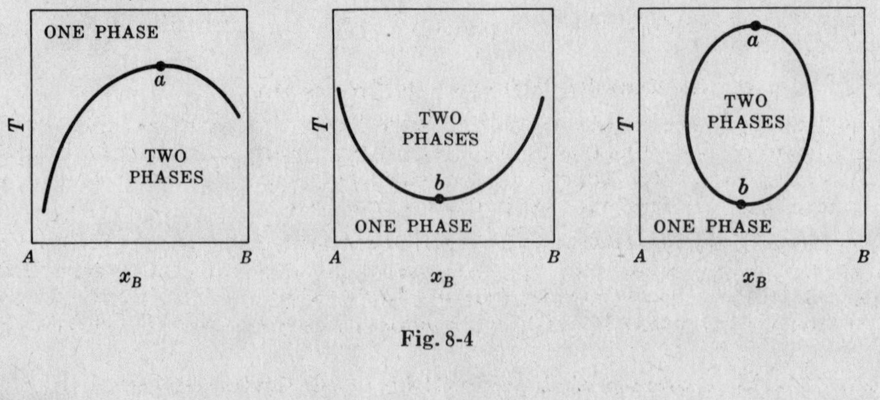

Fig. 8-4

EXAMPLE 8.6. Consider the typical diagram for completely miscible liquids shown in Fig. 8-5. There are two one-phase areas and one two-phase area. Note that pressure is constant for this diagram. Determine the number of *theoretical equivalent plates,* TEP, in a distillation column necessary to separate pure B from a mixture having an original composition x_1.

If a solution having composition x_1 is heated to T_1, the gaseous phase in equilibrium with it has the composition x_2, somewhat richer in B. This vapor is cooled to T_2 and condenses to liquid with composition x_2. The new vapor of composition x_3 is allowed to form above the solution. The new vapor is cooled to T_3 and condensed, yet new vapor is allowed to form, etc., until the more volatile component is isolated. A TEP can be defined as a simple distillation step in which an equilibrium between the solution and vapor is established and the vapor is condensed to a liquid of different composition. The three TEP's shown in the figure will perform the desired separation.

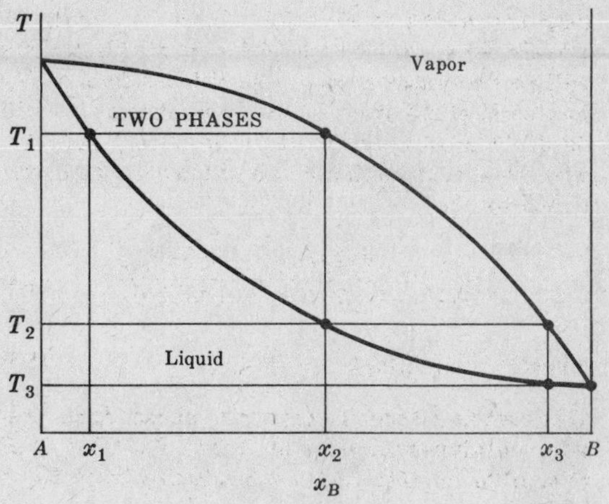

Fig. 8-5

8.7 SOLID-LIQUID DIAGRAMS

There are several features that may appear on these diagrams, such as partial, complete or no mutual solubility of the solids; congruent, incongruent or no compound formation; and solid-solid phase transitions.

Generally these diagrams are determined by cooling-curve measurements at various concentrations. The cooling curves for a pure compound or at the eutectic composition will consist of a plateau or "arrest." At other compositions the cooling curve will consist of (1) a "break" where the solid begins to solidify and the liquid changes composition and (2) an "arrest" at which the remaining liquid solidifies at the eutectic composition.

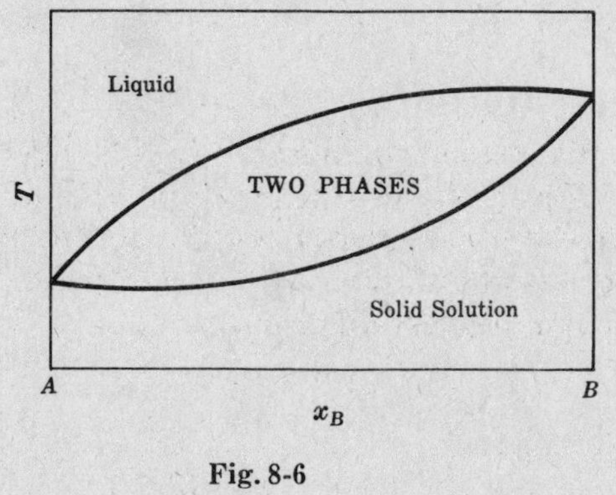

Fig. 8-6

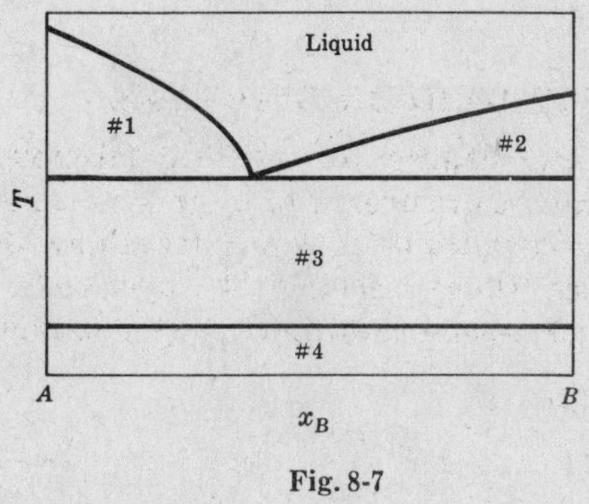

Fig. 8-7

EXAMPLE 8.7. Compare the phase diagrams shown in Figs. 8-6 and 8-7.

Figure 8-6 illustrates complete miscibility of the materials in the solid phase. There are two one-phase areas and one two-phase area. This type of diagram results from the ability of one substance to substitute freely for the other in the crystal lattice because of similarity in size of molecules (atoms or ions), charge (if any), etc. Horizontal "tie lines" are used in the two-phase area.

Figure 8-7 illustrates two substances that are completely immiscible in the solid phase. There are four two-phase areas and one one-phase area. The horizontal "tie lines" indicate that in area #1 the two phases in equilibrium will be solid A and liquid; in area #2, solid B and liquid; and in areas #3 and #4, solid A and solid B, with one of the materials undergoing a phase transition to a second solid state.

EXAMPLE 8.8. The temperature at which pure solid i is in equilibrium with liquid having a concentration x_i is given by

$$\frac{\Delta H(\text{fusion}, i)}{R}\left(\frac{1}{T_{mp,i}} - \frac{1}{T}\right) = \ln x_i \tag{8.6}$$

where $T_{mp,i}$ is the melting point of pure i. If $\Delta H(\text{fusion}, A)$ is 500 cal mol^{-1} and $T_{mp,A} = 400\ ^\circ\text{C}$, find the solubility of B in A at 350 °C.

Using (*8.6*) gives

$$\ln x_A = \frac{(500 \text{ cal mol}^{-1})(4.184 \text{ J cal}^{-1})}{8.314 \text{ J mol}^{-1}\text{ K}^{-1}}\left(\frac{1}{673 \text{ K}} - \frac{1}{623 \text{ K}}\right) = -0.0300$$

or $x_A = 0.9704$. Recognizing that $x_B = 1 - x_A$ gives $x_B = 0.0296$.

EXAMPLE 8.9. Predict the eutectic temperature and composition for a binary solid-liquid system if $\Delta H(\text{fusion}, i) = 500$ and $1000 \text{ cal mol}^{-1}$ and $T_{mp,i} = 400\ °\text{C}$ and $600\ °\text{C}$, respectively, for A and B.

Substituting the data into (*8.6*) gives

$$\ln x_A = \frac{(500)(4.184)}{8.314}\left(\frac{1}{673} - \frac{1}{T}\right)$$

$$\ln x_B = \frac{(1000)(4.184)}{8.314}\left(\frac{1}{873} - \frac{1}{T}\right)$$

which upon solving simultaneously with $x_A + x_B = 1$ gives $x_A = 0.647$ and $T = 38\ °\text{C}$.

Phase Diagrams for Three-Component Systems

For a three-component system (*8.1*) becomes

$$f = 5 - p \tag{8.7}$$

For a system having only one phase, the phase diagram must illustrate four variables, which is difficult. For this reason P and T are fixed for a given diagram and triangular graph paper used to illustrate the system in terms of the remaining variables—two of the three concentrations—as in Fig. 8-8. The "tie lines," which are experimentally determined, must be specified on the phase diagram in the two-phase regions because they are no longer horizontal as in two-component diagrams. "Tie lines" are not used in the three-phase regions.

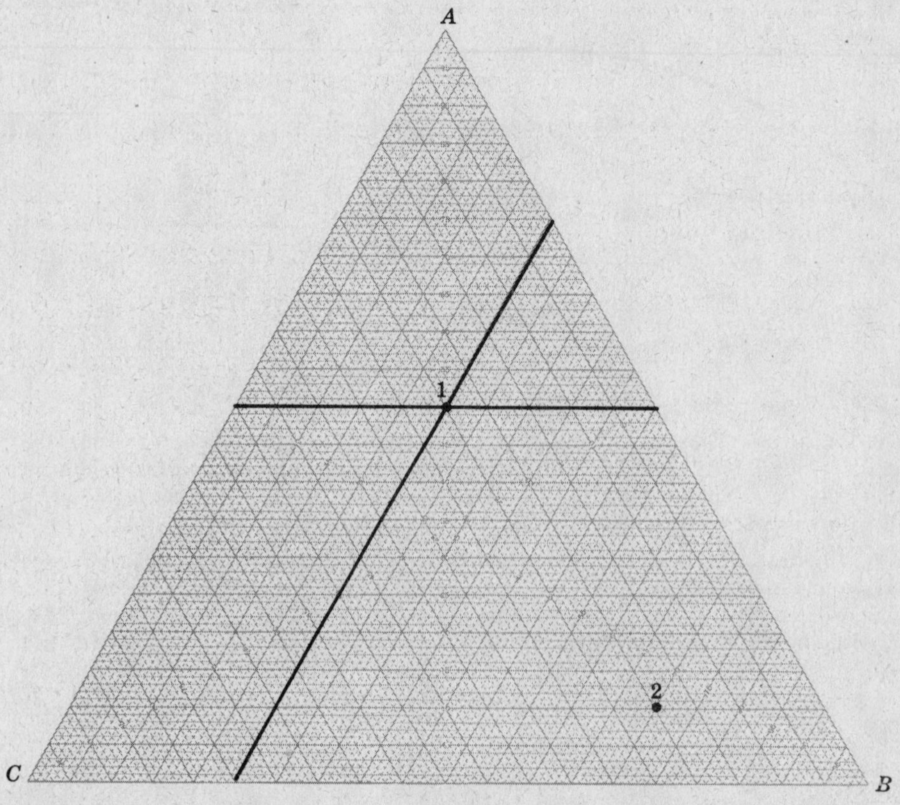

Fig. 8-8

EXAMPLE 8.10. Construct the point $x_A = 0.50$, $x_B = x_C = 0.25$ in Fig. 8-8.

Starting with $x_A = 0.50$, the point will be located one half the distance between side BC and vertex A. This is indicated on the graph by a heavy horizontal line at $x_A = 0.50$. Similarly for x_B, the point will be located on a line one fourth the distance from side AC to vertex B, which line is also drawn heavy. The intersection of these two lines (point 1) is the desired point. As a check, point 1 has $x_C = 0.25$, since the point lies one fourth the distance from side AB to vertex C.

Solved Problems

Phase Rule

8.1. Determine the number of components in the following systems: (*a*) an aqueous solution of sugar; (*b*) an aqueous solution of $HC_2H_3O_2$; (*c*) an aqueous solution of KCl; (*d*) a mixture of $CaCO_3(s)$, $CaO(s)$ and $CO_2(g)$; and (*e*) $Fe(s) + H_2O(g) = FeO(s) + H_2(g)$.

(*a*) Here $c = 2$: the amounts of H_2O and sugar must be known to define the system.

(*b*) Here $c = 2$: the amounts of H_2O and $HC_2H_3O_2$ will define the system even though other species, such as $H^+(aq)$ and $C_2H_3O_2^-(aq)$, are present.

(*c*) Here $c = 2$: the amounts of H_2O and KCl will define the system even though other species, such as $K^+(aq)$, $Cl^-(aq)$, $H^+(aq)$ and $OH^-(aq)$, are present.

(*d*) Here $c = 2$ or 3, depending on the method of preparation and final status of the system. If simply a mixture, all three components must be specified If a mixture produced by the decomposition of $CaCO_3$, only two components need to be specified because the third can be calculated using the stoichiometry of the reaction. The equilibrium expression cannot be used to reduce the number of components needed because it contains only one useful term, $K = a_{CO_2}$.

(*e*) Here $c = 3$: the chemical reaction implies that equilibrium exists, so only one gaseous component must be specified along with the two solid species, because the second may be calculated from $K = a_{H_2}/a_{H_2O}$.

8.2. Determine f for the systems described in Problem 8.1.

For systems (*a*), (*b*) and (*c*), $p = 1$ and $c = 2$ for the aqueous solutions, giving $f = 3$. The usual choice of variables is T, P and one concentration.

For both cases of system (*d*), $p = 3$, giving $f = c - 1$. For the case where $c = 3$, $f = 2$ and knowing T and P is sufficient to fix the system. For $c = 2$, $f = 1$ and only T or P needs to be defined.

For system (*e*), $p = 3$ and $c = 3$, giving $f = 2$. Usually T and P are used to define the system, but other possibilities, such as T and the concentration of one of the gases, would work for a specific application.

Phase Diagrams for One-Component Systems

8.3. Determine f at point c, and along the line between points a and b, and at point 1, for the hypothetical phase diagram shown in Fig. 8-2.

At point c, $p = 3$ which upon substitution into (*8.2*) gives $f = 0$; T and P are fixed. Along a line there are two phases present, in this case liquid and gas, giving $p = 2$ and $f = 1$; either T or P must be specified. At point 1, $p = 1$ and $f = 2$; both T and P must be given.

8.4. Describe the changes in the system shown in Fig. 8-2 for (*a*) isobarically heating from point 1, (*b*) isobarically heating from point 2, (*c*) isothermally compressing from point 3, (*d*) isothermally compressing from point 4, and (*e*) isothermally and isobarically removing heat at point *b*.

For the isobaric heatings, horizontal lines are drawn from the points and for the isothermal compressions, vertical lines are drawn. The changes are:

(*a*) Heating β-solid until reaching the line at which sublimation occurs (isothermally) and then heating the gas.

(*b*) Heating β-solid until reaching the line between points *c* and *e* at which α-solid is isothermally formed, heating α-solid until reaching the line between points *b* and *e* at which isothermal melting occurs, heating the liquid until reaching the line between points *a* and *b* at which isothermal boiling occurs, and heating the gas.

(*c*) Pressure increases for the gas.

(*d*) Pressure increases for the gas until reaching the line between points *a* and *b* at which condensation occurs and the liquid undergoes further compression.

(*e*) The amount of gas phase decreases as more of the condensed phases is formed.

Phase Diagrams for Two-Component Systems

8.5. Consider a liquid-liquid system containing 10.0 kg of *A* and 5.0 kg of *B* at a temperature such that two phases are present, one with $(\text{wt\%}\ B)_1 = 10.0\%$ and the other with $(\text{wt\%}\ B)_2 = 40.0\%$. Calculate the masses of the two phases in equilibrium.

The system has a bulk composition, $(\text{wt\%}\ B)_{AB}$, of

$$(\text{wt\%}\ B)_{AB} = \frac{5.0\ \text{kg}}{5.0\ \text{kg} + 10.0\ \text{kg}} = 33.3\%$$

Using (*8.4*) gives

$$\frac{m_1}{m_2} = \frac{40.0 - 33.3}{33.3 - 10.0} = 0.288$$

which solving simultaneously with (*8.5*), where $m_{AB} = 15.0$ kg, gives $m_1 = 3.4$ kg for the *A*-rich phase and $m_2 = 11.6$ kg for the *B*-rich phase.

8.6. Consider the liquid-vapor phase diagram, Fig. 8-9, for the C_6H_6/C_2H_5OH binary system. If a sample from a packed distillation tower contained $x_{C_6H_6} = 0.10$ and a second sample taken from the tower the proper distance equivalent to one TEP contained $x_{C_6H_6} = 0.25$, what is the operating temperature of this part of the tower? Discuss the separation of C_6H_6 from an alcohol-rich solution using distillation.

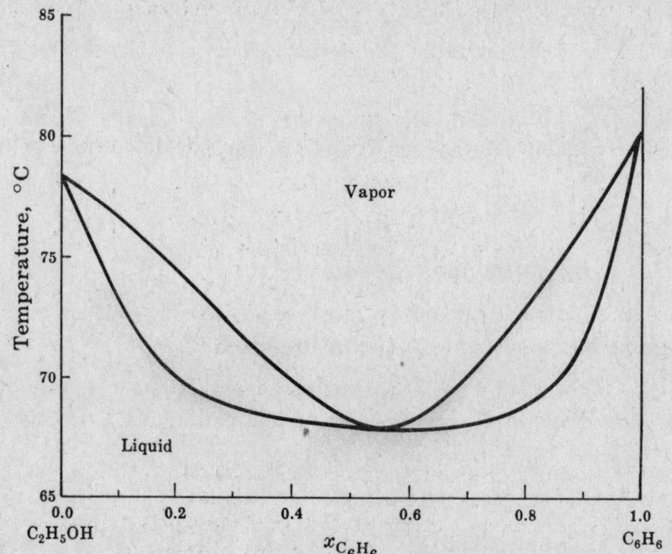

Fig. 8-9

A horizontal line corresponding to $x_{C_6H_6} = 0.10$ on the liquid line and $x_{C_6H_6} = 0.25$ on the vapor line lies at 73 °C.

As the sketches representing the TEP's are drawn in the two-phase area from the alcohol-rich side toward the benzene-rich side, a constant-boiling mixture (*azeotrope*) is reached at 67.8 °C and $x_{C_6H_6} = 0.552$, at which the liquid and vapor above it have identical composition and further separation by distillation is not possible. If the total pressure of the system is changed or a third component is added, the composition and temperature of the azeotrope will change and further separation is possible.

8.7. Identify the phases present in the numbered areas of Fig. 8-10.

A *congruent-melting compound* is formed at $x_B = 0.667$, which means that there are two moles of B for every mole of A; thus the empirical formula of the compound is AB_2. Horizontal "tie lines" indicate that in area #1, solid A and liquid are in equilibrium; in areas #2 and #4, liquid and solid AB_2; in area #3, solid A and solid AB_2; in area #5, solid B and liquid; and in area #6, solid B and solid AB_2.

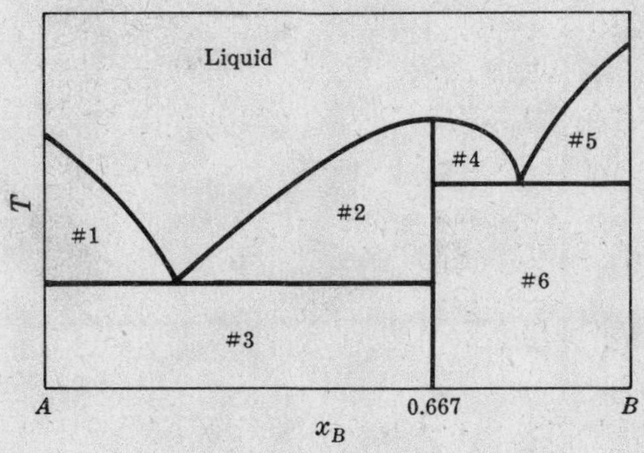

Fig. 8-10

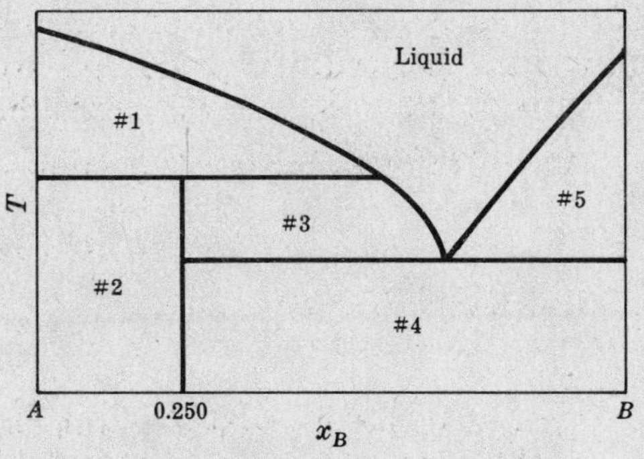

Fig. 8-11

8.8. Identify the phases present in the numbered areas of Fig. 8-11.

An *incongruent-melting compound* is formed at $x_B = 0.250$, which means it has an empirical formula of A_3B. Horizontal "tie lines" indicate that in area #1, solid A and liquid are in equilibrium; in #2, solid A and solid A_3B; in #3, liquid and solid A_3B; in #4, solid B and A_3B; and in #5, solid B and liquid.

8.9. Figure 8-12 is a diagram for two substances that show partial miscibility with each other in the solid state. This type of diagram results from the ability of one substance to penetrate the empty spaces, etc., of the lattice of the other. There are limitations on this type of solubility and the maximum is indicated by the curved lines enclosing areas #1 and #4. Identify the phases present in the numbered areas.

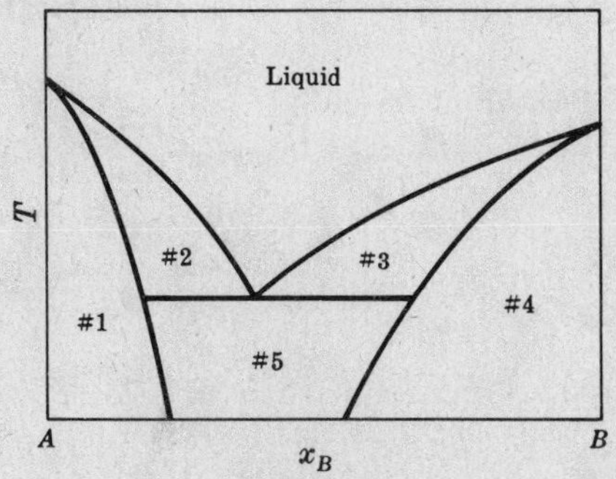

Fig. 8-12

Horizontal "tie lines" indicate that in area #2, liquid and solid solution of B in A (saturated) are in equilibrium; in #3, liquid and solid solution of A in B (saturated); and in #5, solid solution of B in A (saturated) and solid solution of A in B (saturated). Areas #1 and #4 are single phases consisting of an unsaturated solid solution of B in A and of A in B, respectively.

Phase Diagrams for Three-Component Systems

8.10. Describe the changes in the system shown in Fig. 8-13 as salt *B* is added to a solution of composition given by point 1.

As pure *B* is added, the system becomes richer in *B* and less rich in *A* and *C*, as indicated by the line drawn from point 1 to vertex *B*. As *B* is added, it dissolves until sufficient *B* is present so that the bulk concentration reaches point 2, at which solid *B* becomes a second phase in equilibrium with a solution phase of composition given by point 2. Further addition of *B* changes only the relative amounts of each phase, not the composition.

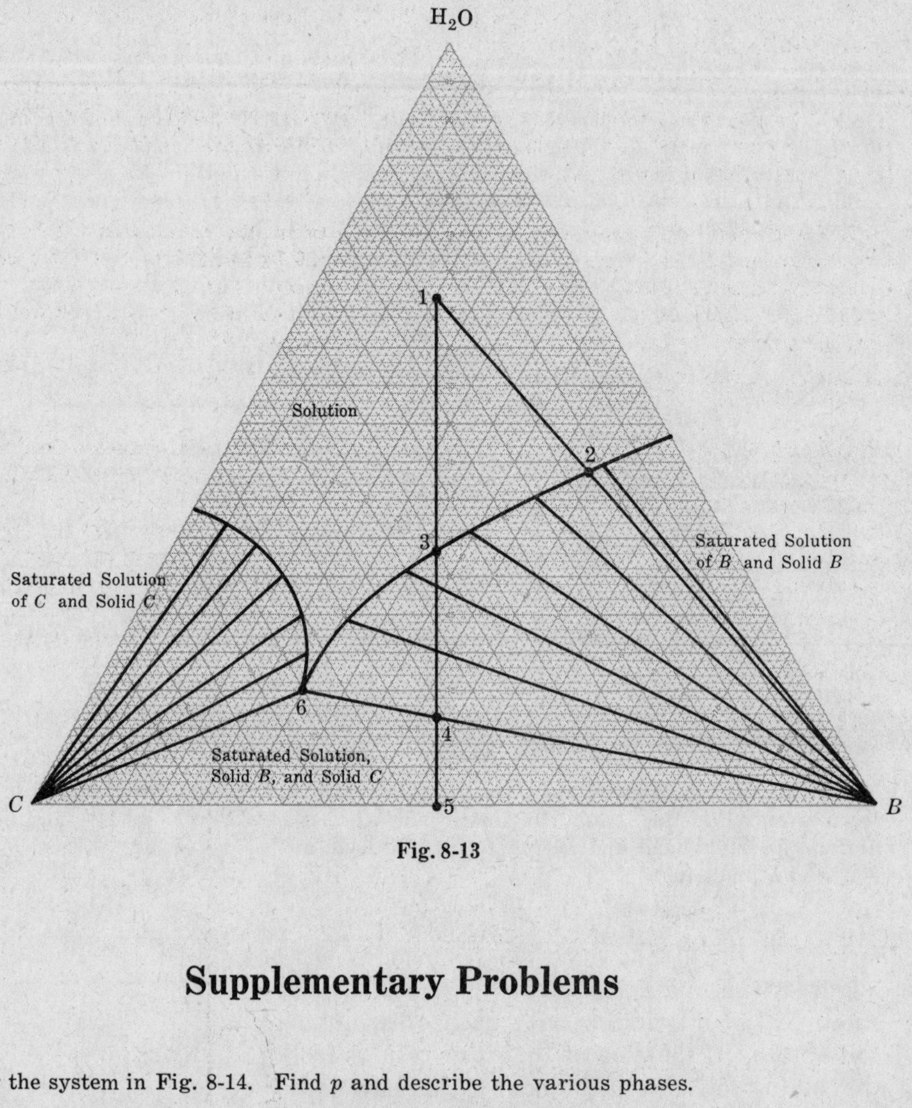

Fig. 8-13

Supplementary Problems

Phase Rule

8.11. Consider the system in Fig. 8-14. Find p and describe the various phases.

Ans. $p = 4$; (1) solid NaCl, (2) aqueous solution of NaCl which contains a small amount of air, (3) ice, and (4) air which contains small amounts of H_2O vapor and NaCl vapor

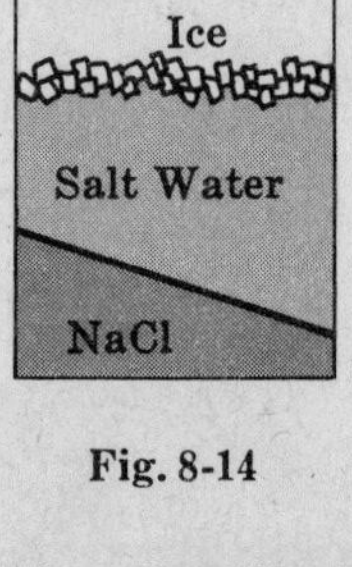

Fig. 8-14

8.12. Determine c for the following systems: (*a*) Br_2 dissolved in CCl_4; (*b*) a mixture of $N_2(g)$, $H_2(g)$ and $NH_3(g)$; (*c*) $2KClO_3(s) = 3O_2(g) + 2KCl(s)$.

Ans. (*a*) 2; (*b*) 1, 2 or 3; (*c*) 2 or 3

8.13. Determine f for the systems described in Problem 8.12.

Ans. (*a*) 3; (*b*) 2, 3 or 4; (*c*) 1 or 2

8.14. Can there be a "quadruple" point on a phase diagram for a one-component system?

Ans. No: $f = 1 - 4 + 2 = -1$.

Phase Diagrams for One-Component Systems

8.15. Determine f at points b and e, along the line between points b and c, and at point 4 for the hypothetical phase diagram shown in Fig. 8-2. *Ans.* 0, 0, 1, 2

8.16. Describe the changes in the system shown in Fig. 8-2 for (*a*) an isothermal expansion from point 1, (*b*) an isothermal compression from point 2, (*c*) an isobaric cooling from point 3, and (*d*) adding heat isothermally and isobarically at point e.

Ans. (*a*) β-solid expanding, subliming, gas expanding; (*b*) β-solid compressing, changing to γ-solid, γ-solid compressing; (*c*) gas cooling, condensing to α-solid, α-solid cooling and changing to β-solid, β-solid cooling; (*d*) increasing the amount of liquid present compared to the amounts of α- and β-solids.

8.17. (*a*) Water has a solid-liquid line similar to that between the points b and e in Fig. 8-2. Describe what happens to ice if pressure is applied at point 5 isothermally. (*b*) What happens to dry ice, which has a solid-liquid line similar to that between points f and g in Fig. 8-2, if pressure is applied at point 6 isothermally? (*c*) What happens to the system in Fig. 8-2 if pressure is applied isothermally at point 7 or the system is cooled isobarically at point 7?

Ans. (*a*) melts; (*b*) nothing; (*c*) α-solid changes to β-solid

8.18. Consider the phase diagram for sulfur shown in Fig. 8-15. The diagram does not show the various transitions that occur in the liquid state as the S_8 molecules become fragmented. (*a*) What is the stable form of S under room conditions? (*b*) Suppose a sample of S were dissolved in CS_2(b.p. = 46.3 °C) and the solvent evaporated. What would be the stable form of the S? (*c*) Suppose a sample of S were heated in boiling water for a short time and removed quickly. What would be observed? (*d*) What would be observed if rhombic S were heated rather quickly? (*e*) What would be observed if molten S at 115 °C were poured into boiling water? (*f*) If molten S at 115 °C were allowed to cool to room temperature and allowed to remain at room temperature for a week, what change would occur?

Ans. (*a*) rhombic; (*b*) rhombic; (*c*) perhaps a little monoclinic would form; (*d*) melt at 114.5 °C; (*e*) monoclinic would form; (*f*) change to rhombic

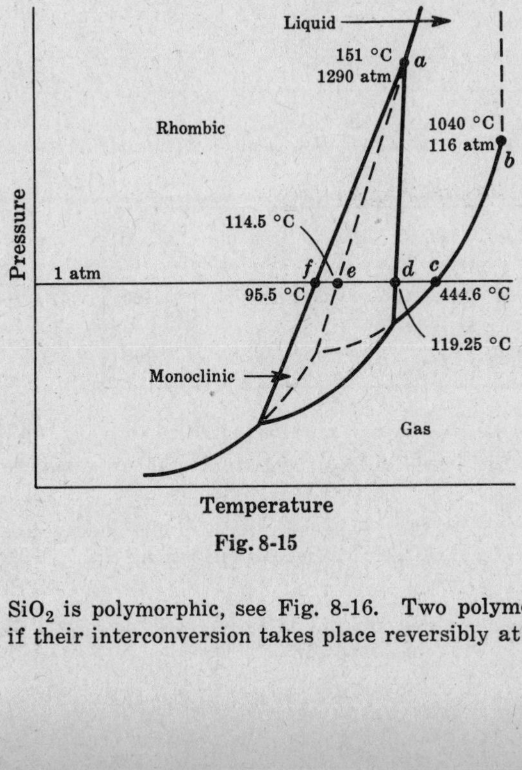

Fig. 8-15

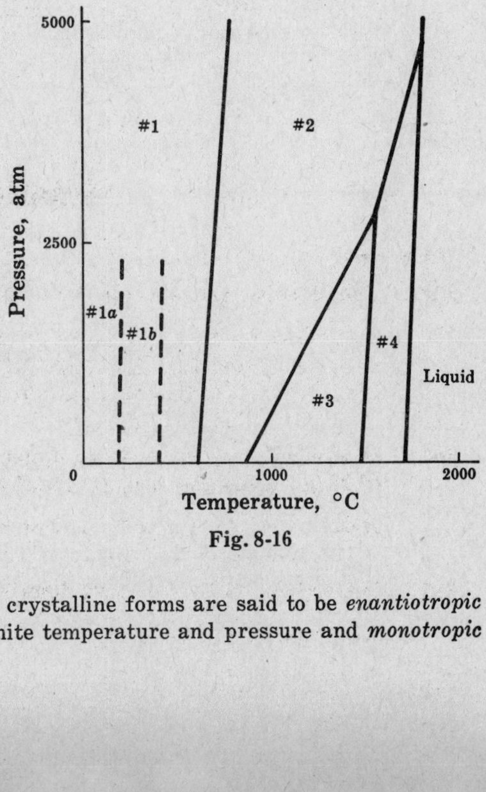

Fig. 8-16

8.19. SiO_2 is polymorphic, see Fig. 8-16. Two polymorphic crystalline forms are said to be *enantiotropic* if their interconversion takes place reversibly at a definite temperature and pressure and *monotropic* if their interconversion occurs irreversibly with the inherently unstable form going into the inherently stable form. Classify the following possible transitions into these two categories: #1/#2, #1*a*/#3, #1*b*/#4, #2/#3, #2/#4, #3/#4, #1*a*/#1, and #1*b*/#1.

Ans. The last two are monotropic, the rest are enantiotropic.

Phase Diagrams for Two-Component Systems

8.20. (*a*) Prepare a liquid-liquid phase diagram for the system of partially miscible liquids *A* and *B*, where the $(\text{wt\%}\ B)_i$ at various temperatures are:

T, °C	0	10	20	30	40
$(\text{wt\%}\ B)_1$	30	37	45	53	64
$(\text{wt\%}\ B)_2$	94	90	87	84	80

(*b*) What is the upper consolute temperature?

(*c*) If a mixture containing 0.0600 kg of *B* and 0.0400 kg of *A* was at 25 °C, what is the composition of the two phases in equilibrium and how much of each phase is present?

Ans. (*a*) diagram will look like Fig. 8-4(*a*); (*b*) 46 °C; (*c*) 0.0702 kg of the phase having composition 49% *B* and 0.0298 kg of the phase having composition 86% *B*

8.21. (*a*) Prepare a liquid-liquid phase diagram for the system of completely miscible liquids *A* and *B* from the following data:

T, °C	0	10	20	30	40	50	60
x_B of liquid	0.00	0.39	0.62	0.77	0.87	0.95	1.00
x_B of vapor	0.00	0.09	0.21	0.35	0.55	0.76	1.00

(*b*) How many TEP's would be required to separate 99% pure *A* from a solution originally containing $x_B = 0.80$?

Ans. (*a*) diagram will look like the reverse of Fig. 8-5; (*b*) 3–4 plates

8.22. (*a*) Construct the liquid-vapor phase diagram for the H_2O/D_2O binary system from the following data at 1 atm:

T, °C	100.00	100.35	100.71	101.06	101.41
x_{D_2O} for liquid	0.000	0.246	0.505	0.752	1.000
x_{D_2O} for vapor	0.000	0.237	0.493	0.743	1.000

(*b*) The natural abundance of D_2O is 1 part in 6900, which may be increased to $x_{D_2O} = 0.15$ by an enrichment technique using H_2S. From the phase diagram determine the approximate change in concentration that one TEP would give.

(*c*) Assuming that a technique which operates in the reverse direction of distillation exists, give an estimate of the number of TEP's necessary to prepare a solution having $x_{D_2O} = 0.95$ from the enrichment product.

Ans. (*a*) diagram has a very narrow two-phase area; (*b*) one TEP averages $\Delta x_{D_2O} = 0.01$; (*c*) 80

8.23. Identify the phases present in the liquid-vapor diagram shown in Fig. 8-17. This type of system is useful for steam distillations.

Ans. #1, vapor; #2, vapor and liquid solution of A saturated with B; #3, liquid solution of B in A; #4, vapor and liquid solution of B saturated with A; #5, liquid solution of A in B; #6, two liquid solutions of B saturated with A and liquid solution of A saturated with B

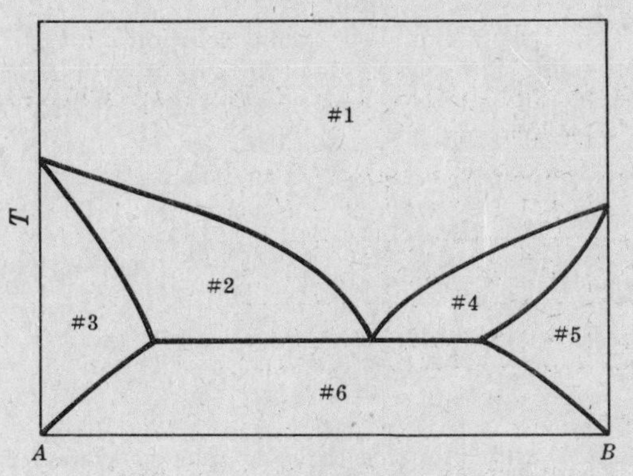

Fig. 8-17

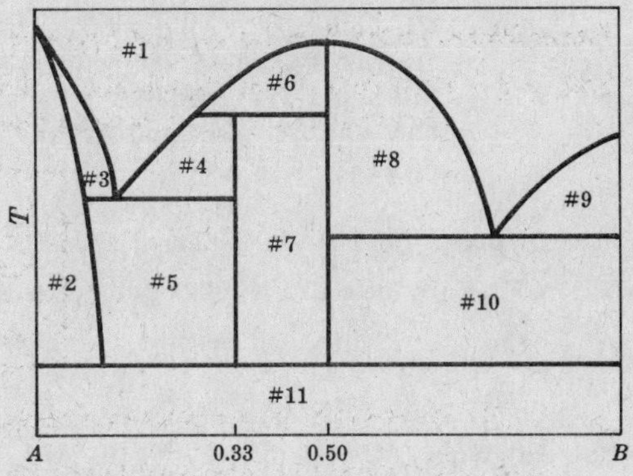

Fig. 8-18

8.24. Construct a liquid-vapor diagram for C_2H_5OH/H_2O from the following data:

T, °C	100	95	90	85	80	79
$x_{C_2H_5OH}$ in liquid	0.00	0.02	0.05	0.13	0.45	1.00
$x_{C_2H_5OH}$ in vapor	0.00	0.18	0.33	0.47	0.68	1.00

and the fact that an azeotrope (constant-boiling mixture) is formed at $x_{C_2H_5OH} = 0.89$ at 79 °C. Find the number of TEP's required to separate 190 proof alcohol (the azeotrope concentration of 95 wt%) from "corn squeezins" with $x_{C_2H_5OH} = 0.10$. *Ans.* 3 plates

8.25. (*a*) Prepare a solid-solid phase diagram for the completely miscible substances A and B from the following data:

T, °C	60	70	80	90	100
x_B for liquid	0.00	0.19	0.42	0.65	1.00
x_B for solid	0.00	0.58	0.78	0.90	1.00

(*b*) If 1.00 kg of a solution having $x_B = 0.50$ were just melted, what would be the composition of the liquid phase in equilibrium with it?

Ans. (*a*) diagram will look like Fig. 8-6; (*b*) $x_B = 0.14$

8.26. (*a*) Construct a solid-liquid phase diagram for substances A and B that are mutually insoluble in the solid state from the following data:

x_B	0.00	0.10	0.20	0.30	0.40	0.50	0.60	0.70	0.80	0.90	1.00
"break", °C		53	46		46		43	42	64	75	
"arrest", °C	60	39	40	40	40	50	31	30	30	30	80

(*b*) What phases will be in equilibrium at $x_B = 0.90$ and 70 °C?

Ans. (*a*) diagram will look like the reverse of Fig. 8-9; (*b*) compound AB formed, eutectics at $x_B = 0.30$ and 0.66 at 40 °C and 30 °C, solid B and liquid having $x_B = 0.85$

8.27. Identify the phases present in the solid-liquid diagram shown in Fig. 8-18.

Ans. #1, liquid; #2, solid solution of A_2B in A; #3, liquid and solid solution of A_2B in A (saturated); #4, liquid and solid A_2B; #5, solid A_2B and solid solution of A_2B in A (saturated); #6, liquid and solid AB; #7, solid A_2B and solid AB; #8, liquid and solid AB; #9, liquid and solid B; #10, solid AB and solid B; #11, solid A and solid B

Phase Diagrams for Three-Component Systems

8.28. What are the coordinates of point 2 in Fig. 8-8?

Ans. $x_A = 0.10$, $x_B = 0.70$, $x_C = 0.20$

8.29. (*a*) What is the composition of the two phases in equilibrium if a three-component system having the bulk composition of (wt% A) = 20.5%, (wt% B) = 49.5% and (wt% C) = 30.0% obeyed the phase diagram shown in Fig. 8-19? (*b*) What is the mass of each phase for 1.000 kg of mixture? (*c*) What mass of A is in each phase?

Hint: Use a ruler to measure $(\text{wt\%})_2 - (\text{wt\%})_{ABC}$ and $(\text{wt\%})_{ABC} - (\text{wt\%})_1$.

Ans. (*a*) $m_2/m_1 = 2.54$.

(*b*) 0.718 kg of (wt% A) = 21.5%, (wt% B) = 63.0% and (wt% C) = 15.5%; 0.282 kg of (wt% A) = 18.0%, (wt% B) = 16.9% and (wt% C) = 66.0%.

(*c*) 0.051 kg of A in the C-rich phase and 0.154 kg of A in the B-rich phase.

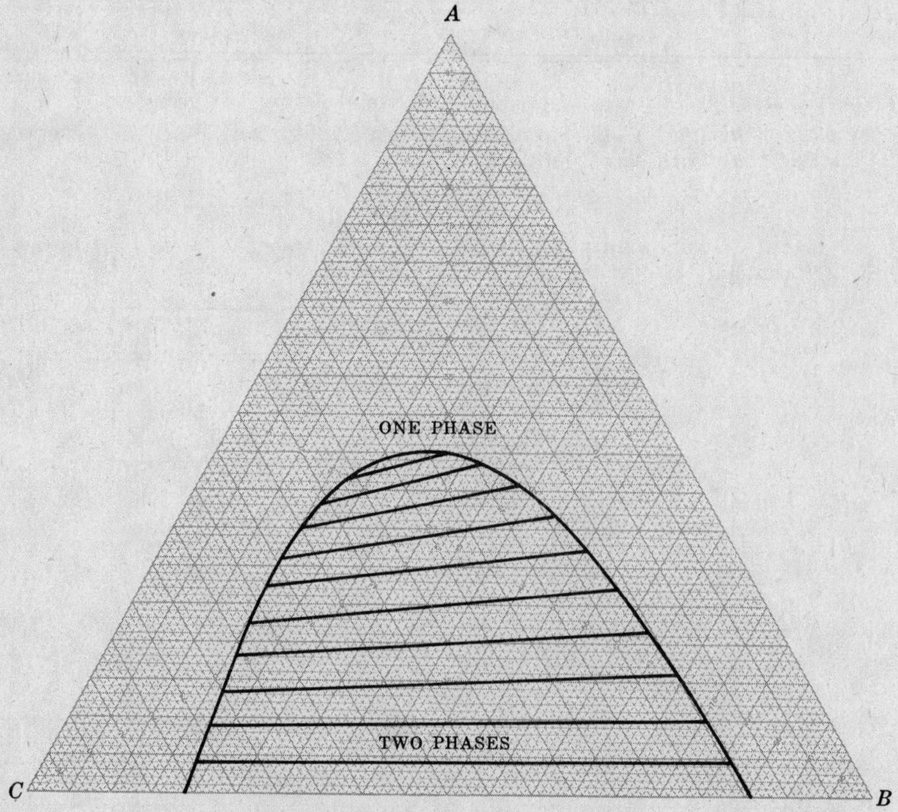

Fig. 8-19

8.30. Describe the changes in the system in Fig. 8-13 as water is evaporated from the composition given by point 1.

Ans. A solution until point 3 is reached, where two phases are in equilibrium: solid B and solution saturated with B. These phases continue until the bulk composition reaches point 4, where three phases are in equilibrium: solid A, solid B and solution saturated with B and C having composition given by point 6. These phases continue until all the water is gone, giving solid A and solid B, a two-component system, with composition given by point 5.

Chapter 9

Solutions

Concentrations

9.1 INTRODUCTION

A *solution* is a homogeneous mixture of two or more substances. The *solvent,* indicated by the subscript 1 or A, is usually the more abundant component, although it may be a minor component chosen for convenience (e.g. if the resulting solution is a liquid the solvent may be chosen as the liquid component). The *solutes,* indicated by the subscripts $2, 3, \ldots$ or $B, C, \ldots$, are the substances dissolved in the solvent. Because the solvent and solute in a binary mixture can be solid, liquid or gas, there are nine possible combinations and all are known to exist.

9.2 CONCENTRATION UNITS

The amount of solute in a solution can be expressed in terms of two systems of units. The "Group A" units specify the amount of solute in a given volume of solution, such as (g solute)(dm^3 soln)$^{-1}$ = (kg solute)(m^3 soln)$^{-1}$; molarity, M or C, (mol solute)(dm^3 soln)$^{-1}$; and normality, N, (eq solute)(dm^3 soln)$^{-1}$. "Group B" units specify the amount of solute for a given mass of solvent or solution, such as (wt% 2); (g solute)(kg solvent)$^{-1}$; molality, m, (mol solute)(kg solvent)$^{-1}$; and mole fraction, x_2. The advantage of "Group A" units is the ease of solution preparation and that of "Group B" units is the temperature independence. To convert from one group to the other requires knowledge of the solution density, d.

EXAMPLE 9.1. A solution containing 13.00 g NaOH (M = 40.01 g mol^{-1}) and 87.00 g H_2O had a density of 1.1421×10^3 kg m^{-3}. Find (*a*) (wt% NaOH), (*b*) (wt% H_2O), (*c*) m, (*d*) x_{NaOH}, (*e*) x_{H_2O}, (*f*) (g solute)(dm^3 soln)$^{-1}$ and (*g*) C.

This type of conversion problem is most easily solved by choosing a "basis" for all calculations, e.g., 13.00 g NaOH and 87.00 g H_2O or 100.00 g solution.

(*a*)
$$(\text{wt\% NaOH}) = \frac{(\text{g NaOH})}{(\text{g NaOH}) + (\text{g H}_2\text{O})} = \frac{13.00}{13.00 + 87.00} = 13.00\%$$

(*b*)
$$(\text{wt\% H}_2\text{O}) = 100.00 - 13.00 = 87.00\%$$

(*c*) The numbers of moles of solute and solvent, respectively, are

$$n_{\text{NaOH}} = \frac{13.00\ \text{g}}{40.01\ \text{g mol}^{-1}} = 0.325\ \text{mol}$$

$$n_{\text{H}_2\text{O}} = \frac{87.00\ \text{g}}{18.015\ \text{g mol}^{-1}} = 4.83\ \text{mol}$$

and the mass of the solvent is 8.700×10^{-2} kg, giving a molality of

$$\frac{0.325 \text{ mol}}{8.700 \times 10^{-2} \text{ kg}} = 3.73\,m$$

(*d*)
$$x_{\text{NaOH}} = \frac{0.325}{0.325 + 4.83} = 0.0631$$

(*e*)
$$x_{\text{H}_2\text{O}} = 1.0000 - 0.0631 = 0.9369$$

(*f*) The volume of solution corresponding to the basis is

$$V = \frac{(100.00 \text{ g})(10^{-3} \text{ kg g}^{-1})}{1.1421 \times 10^3 \text{ kg m}^{-3}} = 87.56 \times 10^{-6} \text{ m}^3 = 87.56 \times 10^{-3} \text{ m}^3$$

and
$$(\text{g solute})(\text{dm}^3 \text{ soln})^{-1} = \frac{13.00 \text{ g}}{87.56 \times 10^{-3} \text{ dm}^3} = 148.5 \text{ g NaOH } (\text{dm}^3 \text{ soln})^{-1}$$

(*g*) The molarity is

$$C = \frac{0.325 \text{ mol NaOH}}{87.56 \times 10^{-3} \text{ dm}^3} = 3.71\,M$$

9.3 DILUTIONS

The required volume of the concentrated solution, V_{conc}, required to prepare a volume of dilute solution, V_{dil}, is given by

$$V_{\text{conc}} = V_{\text{dil}}\left(\frac{C_{\text{dil}}}{C_{\text{conc}}}\right) \tag{9.1}$$

where C_i are the concentrations of the solutions expressed in "Group A" units.

9.4 HENRY'S LAW

At a fixed temperature the amount of a gas dissolved in a given quantity of solvent is proportional to the partial pressure of the gas above the solution, or in equation form,

$$P_2 = x_2 K_2 \tag{9.2}$$

where K_2 is the *Henry's law constant.*

EXAMPLE 9.2. If $K_2 = 3.30 \times 10^7$ torr for a solution of O_2(g) in water at 25 °C, find the solubility of oxygen under room conditions.

Under room conditions, assuming air to be 20% O_2, $P_2 = (0.20)(760 \text{ torr}) = 152$ torr. Using (*9.2*) gives

$$x_2 = \frac{P_2}{K_2} = \frac{152}{3.30 \times 10^7} = 4.6 \times 10^{-6}$$

Assuming that $n_2 + n_1 \approx n_1$ for this very dilute solution,

$$x_2 = \frac{n_2}{n_1 + n_2} \approx \frac{n_2}{n_1} = 4.6 \times 10^{-6}$$

which upon substitution of $n_1 = 5.55$ mol for 100 g of water gives $n_2 = 2.6 \times 10^{-5}$ mol, or 8.3×10^{-4} g O_2 in 100 g H_2O.

9.5 DISTRIBUTION COEFFICIENTS

At a given temperature a substance present in two phases in equilibrium is distributed between them in a definite ratio of concentrations, given by the *Nernst distribution law* as

$$\frac{C_2'}{C_2} = k_d \tag{9.3}$$

where k_d is the *distribution coefficient.* It is assumed that the solute in both phases is chemically the same, i.e. no association taking place, etc.

EXAMPLE 9.3. If the fraction of unextracted solute remaining after n extractions is given by

$$f_n = \left(1 + k_d \frac{V'}{V}\right)^{-n}$$

where V' is the volume of the extracting liquid and V is the volume containing the unextracted solute, find n for a 99.9% extraction of a solute having $k_d = 10$ using equal volumes of solvent.

Taking logarithms and solving for n gives

$$n = \frac{-\log f_n}{\log(1 + k_d V'/V)} = \frac{-\log(0.001)}{\log[1 + (10)(1/1)]} = \frac{3}{1.042} \approx 3$$

Thermodynamic Properties of Solutions

9.6 IDEAL SOLUTIONS

An *ideal solution* is one for which

$$\Delta H(\text{mixing}) = 0, \quad V_{\text{soln}} = \sum_i^{\text{components}} V_i$$

and *Raoult's law,*

$$P_i = P_i^\circ x_i \tag{9.4}$$

are obeyed, where P_i is the partial pressure of component i in the vapor phase above the solution, P_i° is the vapor pressure of the pure component i at that temperature and x_i is the mole fraction of the component in the solution.

9.7 VAPOR PRESSURE

For an ideal solution, the partial pressure of each component is given by (*9.4*) and the total pressure above the solution by

$$P_{\text{soln}} = \sum_i^{\text{components}} P_i \tag{9.5}$$

Those solutions with P_i and P_{soln} less than as predicted by (*9.4*) and (*9.5*) are said to show *negative deviations* and those greater are said to show *positive deviations.*

EXAMPLE 9.4. If $P^\circ_{HNO_3} = 57$ torr and $P^\circ_{H_2O} = 23.756$ torr at 25 °C, prepare plots of P_{HNO_3}, P_{H_2O}, and P_{soln} against x_{HNO_3} assuming the solutions to be ideal. On the same graph, plot the following data for the real solutions:

(wt% HNO_3)	20	25	30	35	40	45	50	55	60	65	70	80	90	100
P_{HNO_3}, torr					0.12	0.23	0.39	0.66	1.21	2.32	4.10	10.5	27.0	57.0
P_{H_2O}, torr	20.6	19.2	17.8	16.2	14.6	12.7	10.7	9.1	7.7	6.6	5.5	3.2	1.0	

Describe the system. Find $x_{HNO_3,\text{vap}}$ at $x_{HNO_3} = 0.500$ if the solution were ideal and for the real solution.

The plots of P_{HNO_3}(ideal) and P_{soln}(ideal) against x_{HNO_3} are linear, see Fig. 9-1, going from 0 to $P^\circ_{HNO_3}$ and from $P^\circ_{H_2O}$ to $P^\circ_{HNO_3}$, respectively. Because the data for the real solutions are given in terms of (wt% HNO_3), they must be converted to x_{HNO_3} before plotting. As a sample calculation, for the 20 wt% solution, on a basis of 100.0 g of solution, there are 20.0 g HNO_3 and 80.0 g H_2O or

$$n_{HNO_3} = \frac{20.0\ \text{g}}{63.01\ \text{g mol}^{-1}} = 0.317\ \text{mol}$$

$$n_{H_2O} = \frac{80.0\ \text{g}}{18.015\ \text{g mol}^{-1}} = 4.44\ \text{mol}$$

giving $$x_{HNO_3} = \frac{0.317}{0.317 + 4.44} = 0.0666$$

The plots of actual data, see Fig. 9-1, show large negative deviations from the plots of (*9.4*) and (*9.5*).

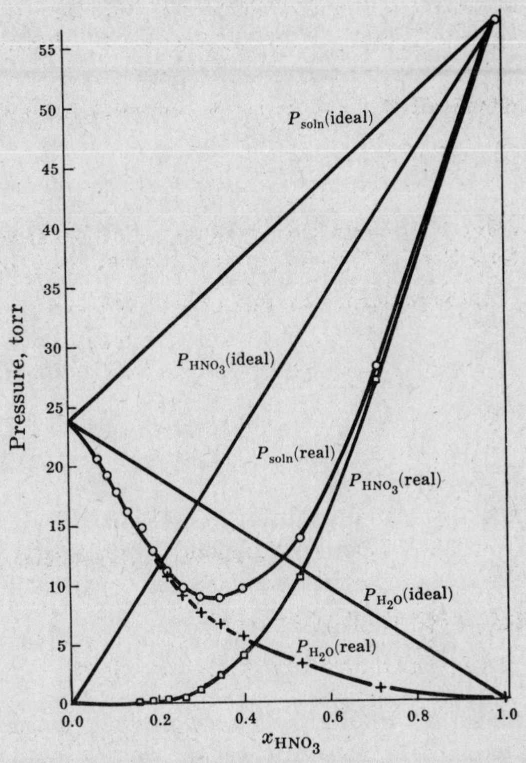

Fig. 9-1

If the solution were ideal, using (*9.4*) and (*9.5*) at $x_{HNO_3} = 0.500$ gives

$$P_{HNO_3} = (57\ \text{torr})(0.500) = 28.5\ \text{torr}$$

$$P_{H_2O} = (23.756)(0.500) = 11.878\ \text{torr}$$

$$P_{\text{soln}} = 28.5 + 11.878 = 40.4\ \text{torr}$$

and the gaseous mole fractions given by (*1.8*) are

$$x_{HNO_3,\text{vap}} = \frac{28.5}{40.4} = 0.705 \qquad x_{H_2O,\text{vap}} = 1.000 - 0.705 = 0.295$$

For the real solution, the values of P_i read from Fig. 9-1 are 8.7 torr for HNO_3 and 3.5 torr for H_2O, giving $P_{\text{soln}} = 12.2$ torr and

$$x_{HNO_3,\text{vap}} = \frac{8.7}{12.2} = 0.71 \qquad x_{H_2O,\text{vap}} = \frac{3.5}{12.2} = 0.29$$

The composition of the vapor for the real solution does not differ greatly from that for the ideal solution in this case, but the total pressure is much lower.

9.8 ΔS, ΔH AND ΔG OF MIXING

For an ideal solution

$$\Delta S(\text{mixing}) = -R \sum_i^{\text{components}} n_i \ln x_i \qquad (4.11a)$$

$$\Delta H(\text{mixing}) = 0 \qquad (9.6)$$

$$\Delta G(\text{mixing}) = RT \sum_i^{\text{components}} n_i \ln x_i \qquad (9.7a)$$

For one mole of solution (*4.11a*) and (*9.7a*) can be written as

$$\Delta S(\text{mixing}) = -R \sum_i^{\text{components}} x_i \ln x_i \qquad (4.11b)$$

$$\Delta G(\text{mixing}) = RT \sum_i^{\text{components}} x_i \ln x_i \qquad (9.7b)$$

EXAMPLE 9.5. Why may real solutions show positive and negative deviations from (*4.11*), (*9.6*) and (*9.7*)?

Usually, negative deviations are caused by association between the solvent and solute molecules, giving a negative ΔH(solution) and a lower value for ΔS(mixing), which results in a more negative value of ΔG(mixing). Positive deviations are usually due to the dissociation of an associated solution component, which results in a positive ΔH(solution) and a higher value for ΔS(mixing), giving a less favorable ΔG(mixing).

9.9 ACTIVITIES AND ACTIVITY COEFFICIENTS

If a solution consists of two volatile liquids, the *activity coefficient*, γ_i, is given by

$$\gamma_i = \frac{P_i}{x_i P_i^\circ} \tag{9.8}$$

and the *activity*, a_i, by

$$a_i = \gamma_i x_i \tag{9.9}$$

For a solution containing two volatile liquids for which it is not possible to vary the mole fractions of both components up to unity, or for a gaseous solute, the activity coefficient for the solvent is given by (*9.8*) and for the solute by

$$\gamma_2 = \frac{P_2}{K_2 x_2} \tag{9.10}$$

where K_2, the Henry's law constant, is the value of the intercept at $x_2 = 0$ of a plot of P_2/x_2 against x_2. Even though the values of γ_2 calculated by (*9.8*) and (*9.10*) differ, as long as the same standard state is used for the substance throughout a calculation, the final result will not be changed.

If the activity of the solvent is known over a range of concentrations and the activity of the solute at one of these concentrations, the Gibbs-Duhem equation (*9.34*), in the form

$$d(\ln a_2) = -\frac{x_1}{x_2}\, d(\ln a_1) \tag{9.11}$$

can be used to determine the value of the solute activity at another concentration by performing a graphical integration of a plot of x_1/x_2 against $\ln a_1$.

EXAMPLE 9.6. The partial pressure of water over an aqueous solution of NH_3 at 70 °F (22.11 °C) is 0.34 psi for $x_{NH_3} = 0.05$. The partial pressure of NH_3 is 0.83 psi over the same solution. Calculate γ_{H_2O}, a_{H_2O}, γ_{NH_3} and a_{NH_3}.

The value of γ_{H_2O} using (*9.8*), where $P^\circ_{H_2O} = 18.77$ torr, is

$$\gamma_{H_2O} = \frac{(0.34 \text{ psi})(760 \text{ torr atm}^{-1}/14.6960 \text{ psi atm}^{-1})}{(0.95)(18.77 \text{ torr})} = 0.986$$

and by (*9.9*), $a_{H_2O} = (0.986)(0.95) = 0.937$.

For NH_3, assuming the value of K_2 as 725 torr, (*9.10*) gives

$$\gamma_{NH_3} = \frac{(0.83)(760/14.6960)}{(0.05)(725)} = 1.18$$

and (*9.9*) gives $a_{NH_3} = (1.18)(0.05) = 0.059$.

Colligative Properties of Solutions Containing Nonelectrolytic Solutes

9.10 VAPOR PRESSURE LOWERING

The vapor pressure of a solution containing a volatile solvent and a nonvolatile solute is given by

$$P_{\text{soln}} = P_1^\circ(1 - x_2) \tag{9.12}$$

EXAMPLE 9.7. The vapor pressure of water is 23.756 torr at 25 °C. What would be the vapor pressure of a solution of sucrose with $x_2 = 0.100$ and of a solution of levulose with $x_2 = 0.100$?

Equation (*9.12*) involves only solvent and concentration terms and so

$$P_{\text{soln}} = (23.756)(1.000 - 0.100) = 21.380 \text{ torr}$$

for both solutions.

9.11 BOILING POINT ELEVATION

The boiling point of a solution containing a nonvolatile solute is given by

$$T_{\text{bp, soln}} = T_{\text{bp},1} + K_{x,\text{bp}}x_2 \tag{9.13}$$

where

$$K_{x,\text{bp}} = \frac{RT^2_{\text{bp},1}}{\Delta H(\text{vaporization, 1})} \tag{9.14}$$

or in terms of molality

$$T_{\text{bp, soln}} = T_{\text{bp},1} + K_{\text{bp}}m \tag{9.15}$$

where the *ebullioscopic constant* is given by

$$K_{\text{bp}} = \frac{RT^2_{\text{bp},1}M_1}{1000\Delta H(\text{vaporization, 1})} \tag{9.16}$$

EXAMPLE 9.8. Calculate $K_{x,\text{bp}}$ for water if $\Delta H(\text{vaporization}) = 9.7171 \text{ kcal mol}^{-1}$ at 373.15 K. What is the boiling point of a solution of urea with $x_2 = 0.100$?

Using (*9.14*) gives

$$K_{x,\text{bp}} = \frac{(8.314 \times 10^{-3} \text{ kJ mol}^{-1}\text{ K}^{-1})(373.15 \text{ K})^2}{(9.7171 \text{ kcal mol}^{-1})(4.184 \text{ kJ kcal}^{-1})} = 28.5 \text{ K}$$

and using (*9.13*) gives $T_{\text{bp}} = 373.15 \text{ K} + (28.5 \text{ K})(0.100) = 376.00 \text{ K}$.

9.12 FREEZING POINT DEPRESSION

The freezing point of a solution containing a nonvolatile solute is given by

$$T_{fp,\text{soln}} = T_{fp,1} - K_{x,fp}x_2 \tag{9.17}$$

where

$$K_{x,fp} = \frac{RT^2_{fp,1}}{\Delta H(\text{fusion, 1})} \tag{9.18}$$

or by

$$T_{fp,\text{soln}} = T_{fp,1} - K_{fp}m \tag{9.19}$$

where the *cryoscopic constant* is given by

$$K_{fp} = \frac{RT^2_{fp,1}M_1}{1000\Delta H(\text{fusion, 1})} \tag{9.20}$$

9.13 OSMOTIC PRESSURE

Osmotic pressure, Π, is the external pressure required to stop the spontaneous flow of solvent from a supply of pure solvent across a semipermeable membrane into a solution. In general,

$$\Pi = -\frac{RT}{v_1}\ln\frac{P_{\text{soln}}}{P_1^\circ}$$

where v_1 is the molar volume of the solvent. If the solution is assumed to be ideal this equation becomes

$$\Pi = -\frac{RT}{v_1}\ln x_1 \tag{9.21a}$$

For ideal dilute solutions, two of the several approximations for (*9.21a*) that are commonly used are

$$\Pi = RT\frac{x_2}{v_1} \tag{9.21b}$$

$$\Pi = CRT \tag{9.21c}$$

In (*9.21c*), C is the molarity of the solution and R is expressed in dm^3 atm K^{-1} mol^{-1}.

EXAMPLE 9.9. For dilute real solutions the semi-empirical formula

$$\frac{\Pi}{C'} = \frac{RT}{M_2} + bC' \tag{9.22}$$

is used to determine the molecular weights of solutes, where C' is the concentration expressed in (g solute)(dm^3 soln)$^{-1}$ and b is known as the *interaction constant.* Determine the molecular weight of sucrose from the following data at 20 °C:

C', (g solute)(dm^3 soln)$^{-1}$	103.8	50.9	40.6	30.3	20.1	10.0
Π, atm	8.14	3.78	2.97	2.21	1.44	0.68

To determine the molecular weight, the values of Π/C' are calculated—e.g. for $C' = 103.8$,

$$\Pi/C' = 8.14/103.8 = 7.84 \times 10^{-2}$$

—and are plotted against C', see Fig. 9-2. The intercept is 7.04×10^{-2} giving

$$M_2 = (0.0821)(293)/7.04 \times 10^{-2} = 342 \text{ g mol}^{-1}$$

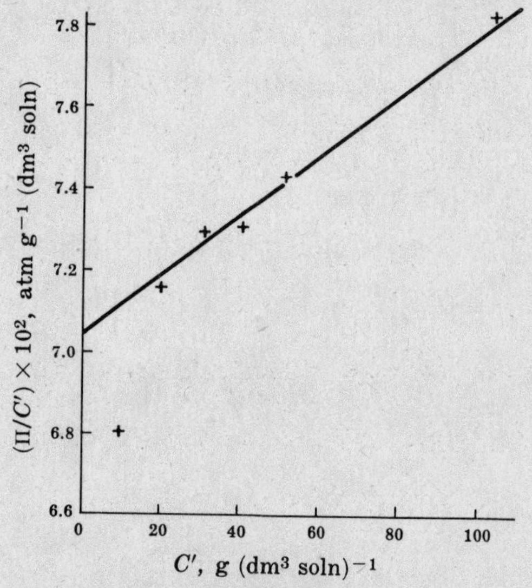

Fig. 9-2

Solutions of Electrolytes

9.14 CONDUCTIVITY (See Sections 7.4–7.7)

9.15 COLLIGATIVE PROPERTIES OF STRONG ELECTROLYTES

For strong electrolytes, (*9.12*), (*9.13*), (*9.15*), (*9.17*), (*9.19*) and (*9.21*) become

$$P_{\text{soln}} = P_1^\circ\left(1 - \frac{n_2 i}{n_2 i + n_1}\right) \tag{9.23}$$

$$T_{\text{bp, soln}} = T_{\text{bp},1} + K_{x,\text{bp}}\frac{n_2 i}{n_2 i + n_1} \tag{9.24}$$

$$T_{\text{bp, soln}} = T_{\text{bp},1} + K_{\text{bp}} m i \tag{9.25}$$

$$T_{fp,\text{soln}} = T_{fp,1} - K_{x,fp}\frac{n_2 i}{n_2 i + n_1} \tag{9.26}$$

$$T_{fp,\text{soln}} = T_{fp,1} - K_{fp} m i \tag{9.27}$$

$$\Pi = -\frac{RT}{v_1}\ln\frac{n_1}{n_1 + n_2 i} \tag{9.28}$$

$$\Pi = \frac{RT}{v_1}\left(\frac{n_2 i}{n_2 i + n_1}\right) \tag{9.29}$$

$$\Pi = iCRT \tag{9.30}$$

where i is the *van't Hoff factor*. The value of i in very dilute solutions approaches the number of ions, ν, that the electrolyte forms in solution. The quantity mi is known as the *apparent molality*.

EXAMPLE 9.10. A 0.001 m solution of $Pt(NH_3)_4Cl_4$ in water had a freezing point depression of 0.0054 °C. Discuss the bonding in the compound.

Substituting the data and $K_{fp,H_2O} = 1.860\ \text{K}\ m^{-1}$ (see Problem 9.10) into (*9.27*) gives $i = 2.9$, which implies that the compound forms 3 ions upon ionization. Recognizing that the NH_3 will take preference over Cl^- in forming ligand bonds, the data imply that the structure is $[Pt(NH_3)_4Cl_2]Cl_2$.

9.16 COLLIGATIVE PROPERTIES OF WEAK ELECTROLYTES

Equations (*9.23*) through (*9.30*) are valid for weak electrolytes as well as strong electrolytes, but the value of i is related to the degree of ionization, α, for the weak electrolyte by

$$\alpha = \frac{i-1}{\nu-1} \tag{9.31}$$

Partial Molar (Molal) Quantities

If X is an extensive (mass-dependent) property of a system such that

$$X = X(P, T, n_1, n_2, \ldots)$$

then

$$dX = \left(\frac{\partial X}{\partial T}\right)_{P,n_1,n_2,\ldots} dT + \left(\frac{\partial X}{\partial P}\right)_{T,n_1,n_2,\ldots} dP + \sum_i^{\text{components}} \left(\frac{\partial X}{\partial n_i}\right)_{T,P,n_j\neq n_i} dn_i$$

If $\bar{X}_i$ is defined as the *partial molar property*, where

$$\bar{X}_i \equiv \left(\frac{\partial X}{\partial n_i}\right)_{T,P,n_j \neq n_i} \tag{9.32}$$

then at constant P and T

$$dX = \sum_i^{\text{components}} \bar{X}_i \, dn_i$$

which integrates to

$$X = \sum_i^{\text{components}} \bar{X}_i n_i \tag{9.33}$$

It follows that for a binary solution

$$n_1 \, d\bar{X}_1 = -n_2 \, d\bar{X}_2 \tag{9.34}$$

which is one form of the *Gibbs-Duhem equation*. If n_j in (*9.32*) is specified as 1 kg of component j, then $\bar{X}_i$ is known as a *partial molal quantity*.

Three important partial molar properties are the *partial molar volumes* of the components in a solution, the *partial molar heat of solution* (which is also known as the *differential heat of solution*), and the *partial molar free energy* (which is also known as the *chemical potential*). These properties can be determined by numerical differentiation of a function relating X to n_i (see Problem 9.40), from the slope of a plot of X against n_i for $n_{j \neq i} = 1$ (see Problems 9.14, 9.16 and Example 9.11), from a numerical calculation involving the *apparent molar quantity*, ϕ_i, where

$$\phi_i \equiv \frac{X - n_1 X_1^\circ}{n_i} \tag{9.35}$$

where X_1° is the molar value for the pure solvent (see Problem 9.42), and from the "method of intercepts" (see Problems 9.17 and 9.39).

EXAMPLE 9.11. Because the total volume of a solution is an extensive property, (*9.32*) through (*9.35*) are valid with $X = V$. Determine $\bar{V}_2$ in a 0.5 m aqueous NaCl solution from the following data:

m	0.349	0.439	0.529	0.621
$d \times 10^{-3}$, kg m^{-3}	1.0125	1.0155	1.0196	1.0233

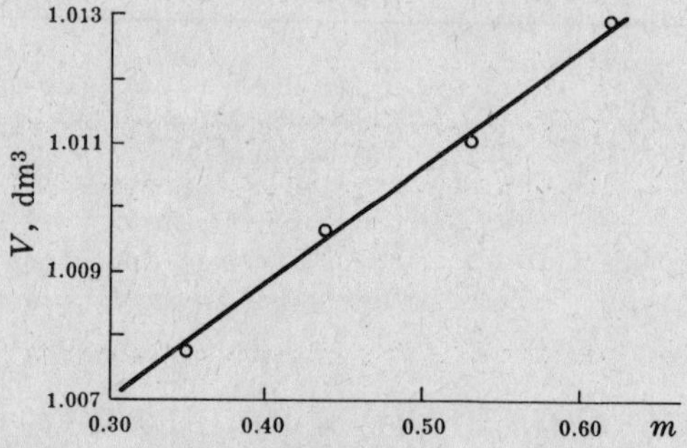

Fig. 9-3

Assume a basis of 1.0000 kg of water, so that $n_2 = (1\text{ kg})m$. The volume of the 0.621 m solution is

$$V_{\text{soln}} = \frac{(0.621\text{ mol})(58.45\text{ g mol}^{-1})(10^{-3}\text{ kg g}^{-1}) + 1.0000\text{ kg}}{1.0233 \times 10^3\text{ kg m}^{-3}} = 1.0127 \times 10^{-3}\text{ m}^3 = 1.0127\text{ dm}^3$$

Volumes for the remaining solutions were calculated as above and appear in Fig. 9-3. By (*9.32*), $\bar{V}_2 = (\partial V/\partial n_2)_{T,P,n_1}$; thus the slope of the line,

$$\frac{dV}{dm} = (1\text{ kg})\frac{dV}{dn_2}$$

gives 0.0181 dm^3 mol^{-1} = $\bar{V}_2$.

Solved Problems

Concentrations

9.1. Specify the solvent and solute(s) in the following solutions: (*a*) 95 wt% ethanol and 5 wt% water; (*b*) 82.3 g HCl in 100 g H_2O; (*c*) 50 g toluene and 50 g benzene; (d) 79 dm³ N_2, 1 dm³ CO_2 and 20 dm³ O_2; (*e*) 5 mole% Ag in Cu.

Choosing as solvent the major component or liquid component gives: (*a*) ethanol as solvent and water as solute; (*b*) water as solvent and HCl as solute; (*c*) an arbitrary choice; (*d*) N_2 as solvent and O_2 and CO_2 as solutes; (*e*) Cu as solvent and Ag as solute.

9.2. How would 1 dm³ of a 2.50 wt% Na_2CO_3 solution be prepared from $Na_2CO_3 \cdot 10H_2O$ and water? The solution density is 1.0178×10^3 kg m^{-3} and the molecular weights are 286.16 g mol^{-1} for the hydrate and 106.00 g mol^{-1} for the anhydrate.

Assuming a basis of 1 dm³ of solution or

$$(1\ \text{dm}^3)(1.0178 \times 10^3\ \text{kg m}^{-3})(10^{-3}\ \text{m}^3\ \text{dm}^{-3}) = 1017.8\ \text{g soln}$$

the weight of anhydrous salt is

$$(1017.8\ \text{g})(2.50\ \text{wt\%}) = 25.4\ \text{g Na}_2\text{CO}_3$$

Converting to moles gives

$$\frac{25.4\ \text{g Na}_2\text{CO}_3}{106.00\ \text{g mol}^{-1}} = 0.240\ \text{mol Na}_2\text{CO}_3$$

To obtain this amount of Na_2CO_3 from the hydrate, the mass of hydrate needed is

$$(286.16\ \text{g mol}^{-1})(0.240\ \text{mol}) = 68.7\ \text{g hydrate}$$

The preparation would consist in weighing 68.7 g of the hydrate, placing it in a 1-dm³ (1-liter) volumetric flask, and adding sufficient water to make 1 dm³ of solution (dilute to "the mark").

9.3. Commercial acetic acid is 17.4 *N*. How would 10 dm³ of 3*M* acid be prepared?

Because acetic acid is monoprotic, 17.4 *N* = 17.4 *M* and (*9.1*) gives

$$V_{\text{conc}} = (10\ \text{dm}^3)\frac{3M}{17.4\,M} = 1.72\ \text{dm}^3$$

which is diluted with sufficient water to produce 10 dm³ of solution.

9.4. If the value of K_2 in (*9.2*) is 5.34×10^7 torr for H_2(g) in water and 2.75×10^6 torr in benzene, how many times more soluble is H_2 in benzene than in water?

Taking a ratio of x_2 as expressed by (*9.2*) in the solvents gives

$$x_{2,\text{C}_6\text{H}_6}/x_{2,\text{H}_2\text{O}} = K_{2,\text{H}_2\text{O}}/K_{2,\text{C}_6\text{H}_6} = (5.34 \times 10^7)/(2.75 \times 10^6) = 19.4$$

9.5. If the value of k_d in (*9.3*) is 410 for the distribution of I_2 between water and CS_2, find the fraction of I_2 remaining in the water phase after an amount of CS_2 equal to the water has been allowed to equilibrate with the aqueous phase.

Letting $C_2' = n_2'/V'$ be the amount of I_2 in the CS_2 layer and $C_2 = n_2/V$ the amount of I_2 in the water layer, we have from (*9.3*)

$$\frac{n_2'/V'}{n_2/V} = 410$$

Letting $V' = V$ gives $n_2' = 410n_2$, which upon substitution into $n_2 + n_2' = 1.00$ gives $n_2 = 2.43 \times 10^{-3}$ of the original amount.

Thermodynamic Properties of Solutions

9.6. At 75 °C, $P_{HNO_3} = 35.0$ torr and $P_{H_2O} = 86$ torr over a 65.0 wt% HNO_3 solution. If $P^\circ_{HNO_3} = 540$ torr and $P^\circ_{H_2O} = 289.1$ torr, calculate P_i for the ideal solution, P_{soln} for the ideal and real solutions, and $x_{i,vap}$ for the ideal and real solutions.

A basis of 100.0 g of solution contains (100.0 g soln)(65.0 wt%) = 65.0 g HNO_3. Then:

$$n_{HNO_3} = \frac{65.0 \text{ g } HNO_3}{63.01 \text{ g mol}^{-1}} = 1.032 \text{ mol } HNO_3$$

$$n_{H_2O} = \frac{35.0 \text{ g } H_2O}{18.015 \text{ g mol}^{-1}} = 1.943 \text{ mol } H_2O$$

so that

$$x_{HNO_3} = \frac{1.032}{1.032 + 1.943} = 0.347 \qquad x_{H_2O} = 1.000 - 0.347 = 0.653$$

For the ideal solution, (*9.4*) and (*9.5*) give

$$P_{HNO_3} = (540 \text{ torr})(0.347) = 187 \text{ torr}$$

$$P_{H_2O} = (289.1 \text{ torr})(0.653) = 189 \text{ torr}$$

$$P_{soln} = 187 + 189 = 376 \text{ torr}$$

The composition of the vapor would be given by (*1.8*) as

$$x_{HNO_3,vap} = \frac{187 \text{ torr}}{376 \text{ torr}} = 0.497 \qquad x_{H_2O,vap} = 1.000 - 0.497 = 0.503$$

For the real solution, (*9.5*) gives $P_{soln} = 35.0 + 86 = 121$ torr, and (*1.8*) gives the composition as

$$x_{HNO_3,vap} = \frac{35.0}{121} = 0.289 \qquad x_{H_2O,vap} = \frac{86}{121} = 0.711$$

a considerable deviation from ideality.

9.7. Prepare plots of (*4.11b*), (*9.6*) and (*9.7b*) against x_i for one mole of an ideal solution at 25 °C. To make the plot of (*4.11b*) more meaningful, it is usually plotted as $T\,\Delta S$(mixing). On the same graph, plot values of ΔH(mixing) against x_{CH_3OH} for one mole of solution, calculated from the following data for solutions of CH_3OH in C_6H_6:

ΔH°_{298}(formation), kcal mol^{-1}	−57.04	−57.004	−56.986	−56.969	−56.952	−56.875
$n_{C_6H_6}$	pure CH_3OH(liq)	0.10	0.15	0.20	0.25	0.50
ΔH°_{298}(formation)	−56.742	−56.634	−56.532	−56.441	−56.359	−56.208
$n_{C_6H_6}$	1.00	1.50	2.00	2.50	3.00	4.00
ΔH°_{298}(formation)	−56.074	−55.950	−55.738	−55.562	−55.212	−54.950
$n_{C_6H_6}$	5.00	6.00	8.00	10.00	15.00	20.00

Qualitatively discuss ΔS(mixing) and ΔG(mixing).

The values of $T\,\Delta S$(mixing) and ΔG(mixing) were calculated at various values of x_i and plotted, see Fig. 9-4. As a sample calculation, at $x_{CH_3OH} = 0.1$,

$$\Delta S(\text{mixing}) = -(8.314\ \text{J mol}^{-1}\ \text{K}^{-1})[(0.1)\ln(0.1) + (0.9)\ln(0.9)]$$
$$= -(8.314)[(-0.230) + (-0.095)] = 2.70\ \text{EU}$$

$$T\,\Delta S(\text{mixing}) = (2.70)(298) = 805\ \text{J}$$

$$\Delta G(\text{mixing}) = (8.314)(298)[(0.1)\ln(0.1) + (0.9)\ln(0.9)] = -805\ \text{J}$$

As a sample calculation of ΔH(mixing) for one mole of solution, consider the data for one mole of CH_3OH in 5 moles of C_6H_6. According to (*3.7*)

$$\Delta H^\circ_{298}(\text{solution}) = [(1)(-56.074)] - [(1)(-57.04)]$$
$$= 970\ \text{cal (mol CH}_3\text{OH)}^{-1} = 4060\ \text{J (mol CH}_3\text{OH)}^{-1}$$

Thus, for one mole of solution, corresponding values are

$$\Delta H(\text{mixing}) = \frac{4060\ \text{J}}{6} = 677\ \text{J} \qquad \text{and} \qquad x_{CH_3OH} = \frac{1}{6} = 0.167$$

Qualitatively, ΔH(mixing) is the endothermic result of breaking the association between the alcohol molecules as the solution is formed. As a result, ΔS(mixing) will be more positive than in the ideal case and ΔG(mixing) will be less favorable than in the ideal case. Thus the solution will show positive deviations from ideality.

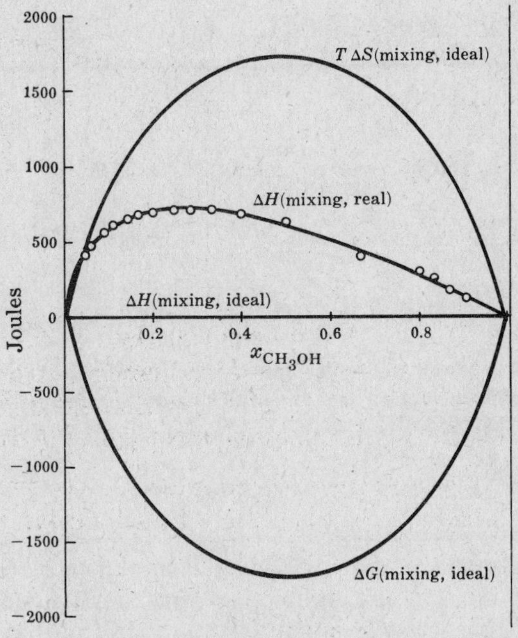

Fig. 9-4

9.8. The partial pressure of ether over a solution of acetone in ether at 30 °C is 535 torr at $x_2 = 0.200$. The partial pressure of acetone at this same concentration is 90 torr. Calculate γ_i given that $P_2^\circ = 283$ torr and $P_1^\circ = 646$ torr. If $P_2 = 148$ torr at $x_2 = 0.400$, use the data from these two solutions to determine K_2 and calculate γ_2.

Using (*9.8*) gives

$$\gamma_{\text{acetone}} = \frac{90}{(0.200)(283)} = 1.59 \qquad \gamma_{\text{ether}} = \frac{535}{(0.800)(646)} = 1.04$$

To estimate K_2, (*9.2*) is applied to each solution giving

$$K_2 = \frac{90}{0.200} = 450 \qquad K_2 = \frac{148}{0.400} = 370$$

and the extrapolated value, see Section 9.9, is 530. Upon substitution into (*9.10*),

$$\gamma_{\text{acetone}} = \frac{90}{(530)(0.200)} = 0.85$$

Colligative Properties of Solutions Containing Nonelectrolytic Solutes

9.9. The vapor pressure above a solution of 5.00 g $HC_2H_3O_2$ in 100.0 g H_2O ($P^\circ_{H_2O} = 23.756$ torr at 25 °C) was 23.40 torr and in 100.0 g C_6H_6 ($P^\circ_{C_6H_6} = 72.5$ torr at 25 °C) was 70.0 torr. Assuming $HC_2H_3O_2$ to be nonvolatile, use these data to discuss the intermolecular bonding in $HC_2H_3O_2$.

For the solutions, (*9.12*) gives

$$x_{2,H_2O} = 1 - \frac{23.40}{23.756} = 0.0150 \qquad x_{2,C_6H_6} = 1 - \frac{70.0}{72.5} = 0.0345$$

In 100.0 g of solvent, there are

$$\frac{100.0\ \text{g}}{18.015\ \text{g mol}^{-1}} = 5.551\ \text{mol } H_2O \qquad \frac{100.0}{78.12} = 1.280\ \text{mol } C_6H_6$$

which upon substituting into (*1.9*) gives

$$0.0150 = \frac{n_{2,H_2O}}{n_{2,H_2O} + 5.551} \qquad 0.0345 = \frac{n_{2,C_6H_6}}{n_{2,C_6H_6} + 1.280}$$

and solving gives $n_{2,H_2O} = 0.0846$ and $n_{2,C_6H_6} = 0.0458$. For 5.00 g, the corresponding values of M are

$$M_{2,H_2O} = \frac{5.00}{0.0846} = 59.1\ \text{g mol}^{-1} \qquad M_{2,C_6H_6} = \frac{5.00}{0.0458} = 109.2\ \text{g mol}^{-1}$$

The factor of 2 between the molecular weights can be attributed to the formation of a dimeric species in the nonpolar solvent as two molecules orient themselves with considerable hydrogen bonding between the mutual —COOH groups.

9.10. If a freezing point change of 1.01 °C was observed in a 15.00 wt% solution of sucrose in water, find the molecular weight of sucrose. ΔH(fusion) = 1.4363 kcal mol^{-1} for water at 273.15 K.

Using (*9.20*) gives for water

$$K_{fp} = \frac{(8.314 \times 10^{-3}\ \text{kJ mol}^{-1}\ \text{K}^{-1})(273.15\ \text{K})^2(18.015\ \text{g mol}^{-1})}{(1000\ \text{g kg}^{-1})(1.4363\ \text{kcal mol}^{-1})(4.184\ \text{kJ kcal}^{-1})} = 1.860\ \text{K kg mol}^{-1}$$

and (*9.19*) gives

$$m = \frac{T_{fp,1} - T_{fp,\text{soln}}}{K_{fp}} = \frac{1.01\ \text{K}}{1.860\ \text{K kg mol}^{-1}} = 0.543\ \text{mol (kg soln)}^{-1}$$

For 1.000 kg of solution there is 0.150 kg solute and 0.850 kg solvent, giving

$$0.543\ \text{mol kg}^{-1} = \frac{0.150\ \text{kg}/(M_2 \times 10^{-3}\ \text{kg mol}^{-1})}{0.850\ \text{kg}}$$

which upon solving yields $M_2 = 325$ g mol^{-1}. The correct answer, 342.30 g mol^{-1}, implies that the solution is not quite ideal.

9.11. Predict the osmotic pressure for a 0.100 m aqueous solution of sucrose at 20 °C using (*9.21*). A 0.100 m solution is equivalent to 0.098 M.

In a 0.100 m solution there is 0.100 mol of solute for 1.000 kg (55.56 mol) of water, giving

$$x_1 = \frac{55.56}{55.56 + 0.10} = 0.9982 \qquad x_2 = \frac{0.100}{55.56 + 0.10} = 0.00180$$

Using $v_1 = 0.0180$ dm^3 mol^{-1}, the most general equation, (*9.21a*), gives

$$\Pi = \frac{-(0.0821 \text{ dm}^3 \text{ atm K}^{-1} \text{ mol}^{-1})(293 \text{ K})}{0.0180 \text{ dm}^3 \text{ mol}^{-1}} \ln(0.9982) = 2.41 \text{ atm}$$

The approximate equations (*9.21b*) and (*9.21c*) give respectively

$$\Pi = (0.0821)(293)\frac{0.00180}{0.0180} = 2.41 \text{ atm}$$

$$\Pi = (0.098)(0.0821)(293) = 2.36 \text{ atm}$$

The observed value is 2.59 atm, indicating that even at this relatively low concentration, the solution is not quite ideal.

Solutions of Electrolytes

9.12. Prepare plots of i against m for the following aqueous solutions.

m, acetone	1.003	0.812	0.625	0.442	0.262	0.087
$T_{fp,1} - T_{fp,\text{soln}}$, °C	1.79	1.46	1.13	0.81	0.48	0.16

m, $NaNO_3$	0.685	0.555	0.427	0.303	0.179	0.059
$T_{fp,1} - T_{fp,\text{soln}}$, °C	2.08	1.70	1.33	0.95	0.58	0.21

m, $(NH_4)_2SO_4$	0.441	0.357	0.275	0.195	0.115	0.038
$T_{fp,1} - T_{fp,\text{soln}}$, °C	1.63	1.35	1.07	0.78	0.48	0.17

Why is i nonintegral?

Using the value of $K_{fp} = 1.860$ K kg mol^{-1}, see Problem 9.10, (*9.27*) gives for the 1.003 m acetone solution

$$i = \frac{1.79}{(1.860)(1.003)} = 0.96$$

Performing the same calculations for the rest of the solutions generates the points shown in Fig. 9-5. As can be seen in the figure, the van't Hoff factors approach 1, 2 and 3, respectively, as molality approaches zero. The value of i represents the actual number of moles of particles present for each mole of solute added, which includes ion pairs, etc., at finite concentrations. Consequently, i will be smaller than the integer ν.

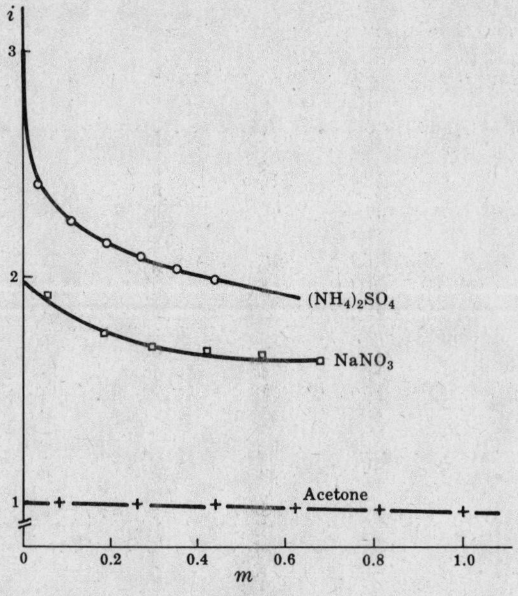

Fig. 9-5

9.13. The observed freezing point depression for a 0.100 m aqueous solution of acetic acid is 0.190 °C. Find K_a at this concentration.

Using (*9.27*) gives $i = (0.190)/(1.860)(0.100) = 1.02$, and (*9.31*) gives

$$\alpha = \frac{1.02 - 1}{2 - 1} = 0.02$$

For the equilibrium

$$HC_2H_3O_2(aq) = H^+(aq) + C_2H_3O_2^-(aq)$$

the equilibrium constant expressed in terms of α becomes

$$K_a = (C_{H^+})(C_{C_2H_3O_2^-})/(C_{HC_2H_3O_2}) = \alpha^2 C/(1-\alpha)$$
$$= (0.02)^2(0.100)/(0.98) = 4 \times 10^{-5}$$

assuming that $0.100\,m = 0.100\,M$. Because the values of α and K_a determined from freezing point depression measurements are precise only to one or two significant figures, values determined from conductivity measurements are usually preferred (see Example 7.5).

Partial Molar (Molal) Quantities

9.14. Graphically determine $\overline{\Delta H(\text{solution})_i}$ for water and H_2SO_4 in a $1m$ solution, using the following data:

ΔH°_{298}(formation), kcal mol^{-1}	−194.548	−211.755	−211.869	−211.944
n_{H_2O}	pure H_2SO_4(liq)	30	40	50
ΔH°_{298}(formation)	−212.068	−212.150	−212.192	−212.282
n_{H_2O}	75	100	115	150

From (*9.33*) calculate ΔH(solution) for preparing 1 mol of the $1m$ solution.

The integral heat of solution for $n_{H_2O} = 30$ is

$$\Delta H(\text{solution}) = -211.755 - (-194.548) = -17.207 \text{ kcal} = -71.994 \text{ kJ}$$

The heat of solution for preparing the amount of solution containing 1 mol of water is

$$\frac{-71.994 \text{ kJ}}{30 \text{ mol } H_2O} = -2.400 \text{ kJ (mol } H_2O)^{-1}$$

and the number of moles of H_2SO_4 for each mole of water is

$$n_2 = \frac{1 \text{ mol } H_2SO_4}{30 \text{ mol } H_2O} = 0.0333 \text{ (mol } H_2SO_4)(\text{mol } H_2O)^{-1}$$

The results of similar calculations for the remainder of the solutions are shown in Fig. 9-6. The slope of the plot at $1m$ ($n_2 = 0.0180$) is

$$\overline{\Delta H(\text{solution})}_{H_2SO_4} = -71.46 \text{ kJ (mol } H_2SO_4)^{-1}$$

The integral heat of solution, e.g. -71.994 kJ (mol H_2SO_4)$^{-1}$ for 30 mol of H_2O, is the heat of solution for preparing the amount of solution containing 1 mol of H_2SO_4. Figure 9-7 is a plot of these values, and the slope at $1m$, where $n_1 = 55.56$, is

$$\overline{\Delta H(\text{solution})}_{H_2O} = -25.0 \text{ J (mol } H_2O)^{-1}$$

For 1 mol of a $1m$ solution, the data needed for (*9.33*) are

$$n_2 = \frac{1.000}{1.000 + 55.56} = 0.0177 \qquad n_1 = \frac{55.56}{1.000 + 55.56} = 0.9823$$

giving

$$\Delta H(\text{solution}) = n_1 \overline{\Delta H(\text{solution})}_1 + n_2 \overline{\Delta H(\text{solution})}_2$$
$$= (0.9823)(-0.025) + (0.0177)(-71.46) = -1.29 \text{ kJ}$$

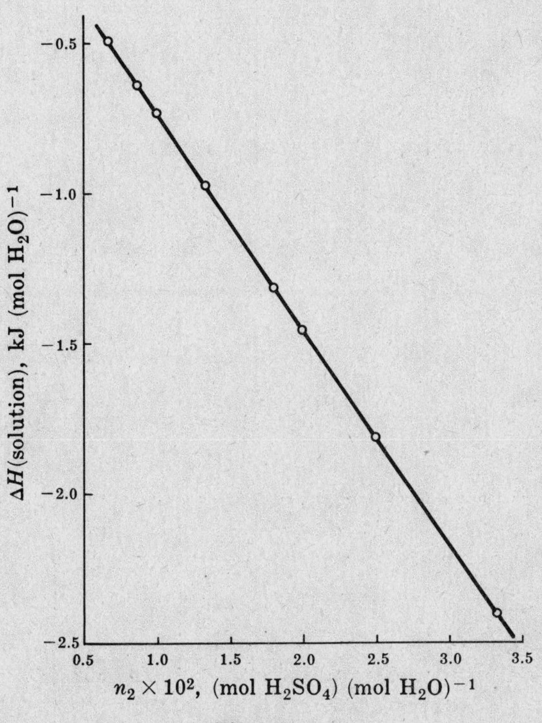

Fig. 9-6

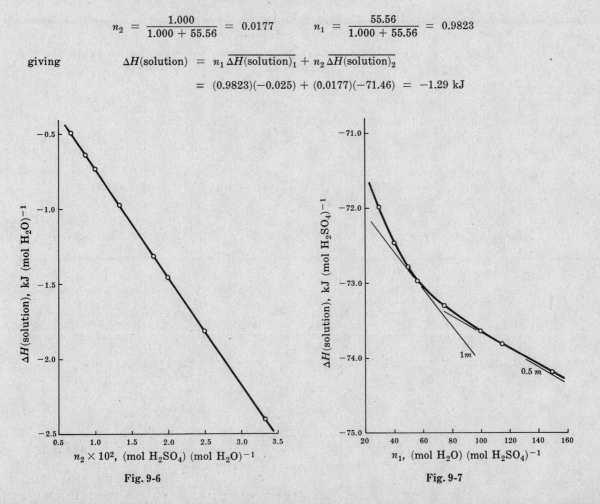

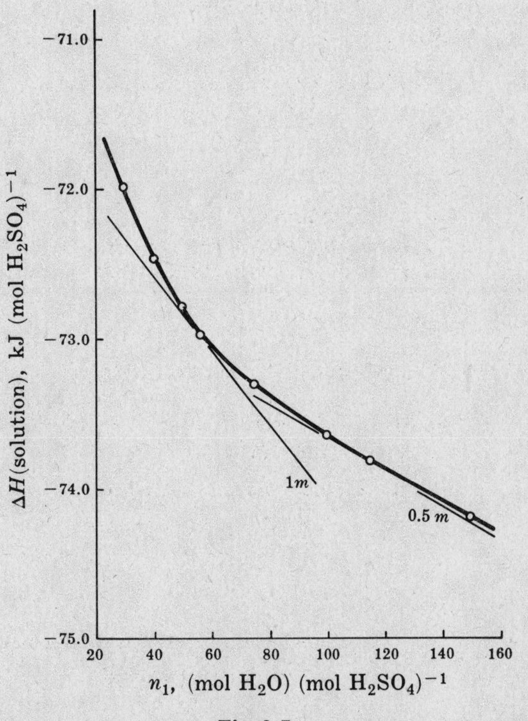

Fig. 9-7

9.15. Although $\overline{\Delta H(\text{solution})_1}$ as shown in Fig. 9-7 changes from -25.0 to -11.4 J (mol H_2O)$^{-1}$ as the concentration changes from $1m$ to $0.5\,m$, $\overline{\Delta H(\text{solution})_2}$ essentially remains constant. Show this to be true from (*9.34*).

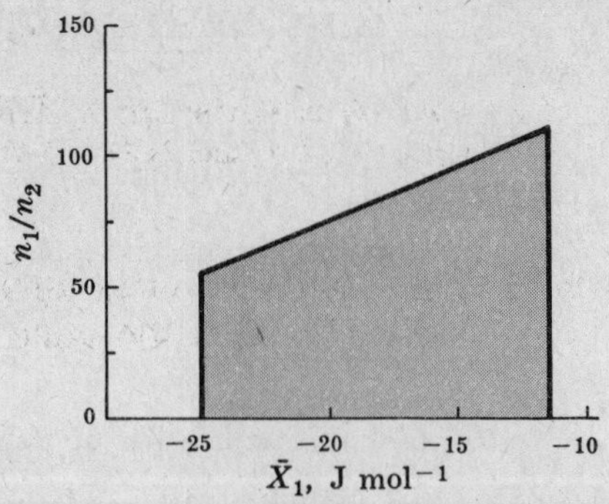

Fig. 9-8

Rearranging (*9.34*) gives

$$d\bar{X}_2 = -\frac{n_1}{n_2}\,d\bar{X}_1$$

where, in this case, $\bar{X} = \Delta H$. Integration gives

$$\Delta\bar{X}_2 = -\int_{-25.0}^{-11.4} \frac{n_1}{n_2}\,d\bar{X}_1$$

The integration is performed graphically, see Fig. 9-8, giving $\Delta\bar{X}_2 = -1.13$ kJ (mol H_2SO_4)$^{-1}$. This change would not be significant on Fig. 9-6.

9.16. Using the data in Problem 9.14 for the H_2SO_4/H_2O solutions, prepare a plot of the heat of solution for preparing one mole of the above solutions and check the answer of -1.29 kJ for a $1m$ solution. Using the value of $\overline{\Delta H(\text{solution})_2} = -71.46$ kJ (mol H_2SO_4)$^{-1}$ at $0.5\,m$ from Fig. 9-6 and the value of ΔH(solution) read from the new plot, determine $\overline{\Delta H(\text{solution})_1}$ at $0.5\,m$.

For $n_{H_2O} = 30$, ΔH(solution) for one mole of solution is

$$\frac{-71.994\ \text{kJ}}{30+1} = -2.322\ \text{kJ}$$

Figure 9-9 contains a plot of the data as calculated above. From the plot, ΔH(solution) $= -1.296$ kJ, a difference of 0.5% for the $1m$ solution. For the $0.5\,m$ solution, ΔH(solution) $= -0.663$ kJ. By (*9.33*)

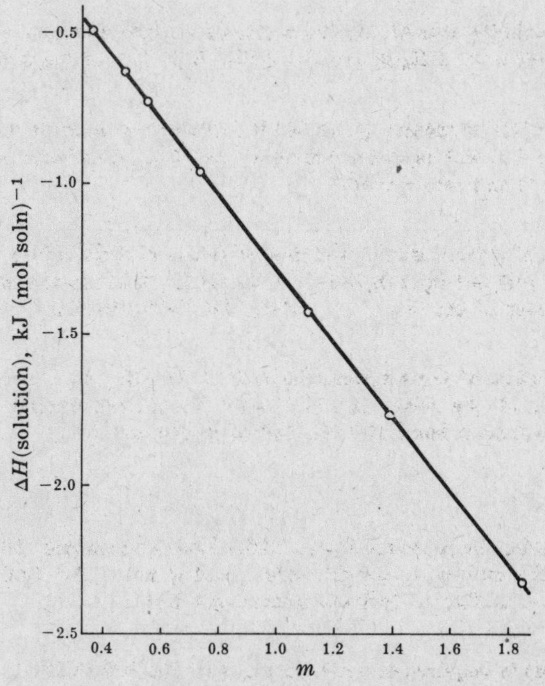

Fig. 9-9

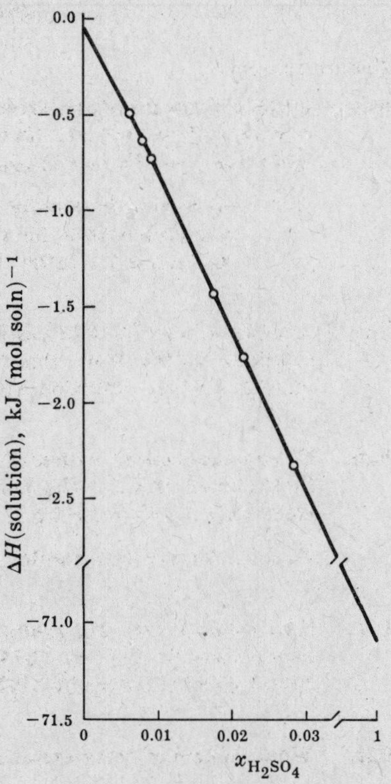

Fig. 9-10

$$-0.663 = \frac{55.56}{56.06}\overline{\Delta H(\text{solution})}_1 + \frac{0.50}{56.06}(-71.46)$$

which upon solving gives $\overline{\Delta H(\text{solution})}_1 = -26$ J (mol $H_2O)^{-1}$. The slope of the curve in Fig. 9-7 gives -11.4 J (mol $H_2O)^{-1}$, which is more precise.

9.17. The "method of intercepts" is a convenient method for determining both partial molar quantities from the same graph. A plot of X', where

$$X' \equiv \frac{X}{n_1 + n_2}$$

against x_2 is prepared and a tangent is drawn to the curve at the desired concentration. The intercept of the tangent on the x_1-axis is $\bar{X}_1$ and on the x_2-axis is $\bar{X}_2$. Using the data in Problem 9.14 for the H_2SO_4/H_2O solutions, prepare a plot of ΔH(solution) for one mole of solution against $x_{H_2SO_4}$ and determine $\overline{\Delta H(\text{solution})}_i$ for a 1m solution.

For $n_{H_2O} = 30$ mol H_2O,

$$x_2 = \frac{1}{31} = 0.0323 \qquad X' = \frac{-71.994\ \text{kJ}}{31\ \text{mol}} = -2.322\ \text{kJ (mol soln)}^{-1}$$

The results of similar calculations are plotted in Fig. 9-10. The intercepts of the tangent (superimposed on the plot of the data) give

$$\overline{\Delta H(\text{solution})}_{H_2SO_4} = -71.1\ \text{kJ (mol } H_2SO_4)^{-1} \quad \text{and} \quad \overline{\Delta H(\text{solution})}_{H_2O} = 25\ \text{J (mol } H_2O)^{-1}$$

for the 1m solution. These values agree well with those obtained in Problem 9.14.

Supplementary Problems

Concentrations

9.18. Specify the solvent and solute in the following solutions: (*a*) 60 g ethanol and 40 g water, (*b*) 50 g ethanol and 50 g water, (*c*) 89.9 g (about 100 dm³) NH_3(g) and 100 g H_2O(liq), (*d*) 116.8 g NaBr and 100 g H_2O, (*e*) Pt and H_2(g).

Ans. (*a*) solvent is usually ethanol and solute is water; (*b*) choice is arbitrary, but water might be more convenient for the solvent; (*c*) solvent is water and solute is NH_3; (*d*) solvent is water and solute is NaBr; (*e*) solvent is Pt and solute is H_2

9.19. The *formality* of a solution is the number of gram-formula weights of solute contained in 1 dm³ of solution. In this book, this concentration unit has been included as *molarity*. What is the molarity of a 1F $Pb(NO_3)_2$ solution with respect to each of the ions? *Ans.* 1M Pb^{2+}, 2M NO_3^-

9.20. What is the concentration of a 0.509 M solution of D-mannitol, $CH_2OH(CHOH)_4CH_2OH$, expressed in (wt% D-mannitol)? The molecular weight of the solute is 182.17 g mol^{-1} and the density of the solution is 1.0302×10^3 kg m^{-3}. (*Hint:* Assume a basis of 1.000 dm³ of solution.)

Ans. 9.00 wt% D-mannitol

9.21. How would 1 dm³ of a 1.00 wt% $CaCl_2$ solution be prepared from $CaCl_2 \cdot 2H_2O$ and water? The solution density is 1.0065×10^3 kg m^{-3} and the molecular weights are 110.99 g mol^{-1} for $CaCl_2$ and 147.03 g mol^{-1} for $CaCl_2 \cdot 2H_2O$. *Ans.* 13.33 g of hydrate diluted to 1 dm³

9.22. What volume of commercial NH_4OH (7.4 M) is required to produce 1 dm³ of 3M NH_4OH?

Ans. 0.405 dm³ diluted to 1 dm³

9.23. The value of K_2 in (*9.2*) is 3.30×10^7 torr for $O_2(g)$ in water at 25 °C and 3.52×10^7 torr at 30 °C. What change in the solubility of O_2 at 0.20 atm in water will occur if thermal pollution of water changes the temperature by 5 °C?

Ans. $x_2 = 4.61 \times 10^{-6}$ at 25 °C and 4.32×10^{-6} at 30 °C, a 6.3% decrease

9.24. Repeat Problem 9.5, now using two extraction samples of CS_2, each with $V_2' = 0.5\,V$.

Ans. $n_2 = 4.85 \times 10^{-3}$ of the original after the first extraction and $n_2 = 2.35 \times 10^{-5}$ of the original after the second equilibrium

9.25. Repeat Problem 5.54 if K_2 in (*9.2*) is 1.18×10^6 torr and $P_2 = 3.3 \times 10^{-4}$ atm.

Ans. $x_2 = 2.1 \times 10^{-7}$, $C_{CO_2} = 1.17 \times 10^{-5} M$, $C_{H^+} = 2.03 \times 10^{-6}$, pH = 5.7

Thermodynamic Properties of Solutions

9.26. Using the data in Example 3.10 for ΔH°_{298}(formation) for various solutions of HNO_3, prepare a plot of ΔH(mixing) for one mole of solution against x_{HNO_3}. Include plots for (*4.11b*) as $T\,\Delta S$(mixing), (*9.6*) and (*9.7b*) on the same graph. Discuss qualitatively the results for ΔH(mixing) for the real solution and what the plots for ΔS(mixing) and ΔG(mixing) would look like.

Ans. The plots for the ideal solutions would look like those in Fig. 9-4. The ΔH(mixing) curve shows very negative deviations from ideality as it goes to −1670 cal = −6987 J at x_{HNO_3} = 0.500. The very large exothermic ΔH(mixing) is the result of forming H^+(aq) and NO_3^-(aq) in the solution. Qualitatively, ΔS(mixing) will be less positive and ΔG(mixing) more negative than in the ideal case; thus the solution will show negative deviations from ideality.

9.27. Using the following data, prepare a plot of P_i and P_{soln} against x_B:

P_A, torr	600	540	475	411	347	269	160	81	50	25	0
P_B, torr	0	13	25	42	88	179	350	467	543	622	700
x_B	0.0	0.1	0.2	0.3	0.4	0.5	0.6	0.7	0.8	0.9	1.0

Include plots of (*9.4*) and (*9.5*) on the graph. Describe the system. Calculate γ_i at $x_B = 0.2$ using the convention given by (*9.8*). Calculate γ_B using the convention given by (*9.10*) at the same concentration.

Ans. both substances show negative deviations from ideality; $\gamma_A = 0.990$, $\gamma_B = 0.179$; plot of P_2/x_2 against x_2 has intercept $= K_B = 135$, $\gamma_B = 0.926$

9.28. At $x_B = 0.3$, the partial pressure of component B in Problem 9.27 no longer agrees with the value predicted by Henry's law, but the value for component A agrees fairly well with the value predicted by Raoult's law. From points on the graph prepared for Problem 9.27, find γ_A from $x_B = 0.2$ to 0.3 at 0.01 intervals. Using (*9.9*), calculate a_A for these concentrations. Prepare a plot of x_A/x_B against $\ln a_A$ and graphically integrate (*9.11*) to determine $\ln a_{B,0.3} - \ln a_{B,0.2}$. Using the value of $a_{B,0.2} = 0.185$, find $a_{B,0.3}$.

Ans. P_A = 475, 469, 463, 456, 450, 444, 438, 432, 425, 417 and 411 torr;
γ_A = 0.990, 0.989, 0.989, 0.987, 0.987, 0.987, 0.986, 0.986, 0.984, 0.979, and 0.979;
a_A = 0.792, 0.781, 0.771, 0.760, 0.750, 0.740, 0.730, 0.720, 0.708, 0.695, and 0.685;
coordinates of plot are (4.00, −0.233), (3.76, −0.247), (3.55, −0.260), (3.35, −0.275), (3.17, −0.288), (3.00, −0.301), (2.85, −0.315), (2.70, −0.329), (2.57, −0.345), (2.45, −0.364), (2.33, −0.379); area corresponds to 0.442; $a_{B,0.3} = 0.288$

Colligative Properties of Solutions Containing Nonelectrolytic Solutes

9.29. The vapor pressure of water is 23.756 torr at 25 °C. If the vapor pressure over a 4.50 wt% solution of urea is 23.426 torr, find the molecular weight of urea.

Ans. $x_2 = 1.39 \times 10^{-2}$, $M = 60.2$ g mol^{-1}

9.30. Calculate K_{bp} for water and the boiling point of a 0.100 m solution of urea. ΔH(vaporization) = 9.7171 kcal mol^{-1} for water at 373.15 K. *Ans.* 0.513 K m^{-1}, 373.20 K

9.31. What freezing point depression would be predicted for a 0.1 m solution of benzoic acid in benzene if ΔH(fusion) = 30.45 cal g^{-1} at 278.69 K for benzene?

Ans. ΔH(fusion) = 9.951 kJ mol^{-1}, K_{fp} = 5.07 K m^{-1}; -0.507 °C

9.32. The melting points and heats of fusion for Bi and Cd are 544.2 K and 2.63 kcal mol^{-1} and 594.1 K and 1.46 kcal mol^{-1}, respectively. Using (*9.17*) and (*9.18*) predict the temperature and composition of the simple eutectic formed by these metals, by plotting the freezing points of solutions with various compositions for each substance against mole fraction and observing where the curves meet. The observed values are 144 °C and 40 wt% Cd.

Ans. $K_{x,fp}$ = 224 °C for Bi and 480 °C for Cd; 134 °C at x_{Cd} = 0.612 (46 wt%)

9.33. Using (*9.21*), predict the osmotic pressure for a 1.000 m (0.825 M) aqueous solution of sucrose at 20 °C. Assume x_1 = 0.0180 dm^3 mol^{-1}. The observed value is 26.64 atm.

Ans. x_1 = 0.9823, x_2 = 0.0177; Π = 23.9, 23.7 and 19.8 atm

9.34. Determine the molecular weight of inulin, $(C_6H_{10}O_5)_x$, from the following data at 20 °C:

C', (g solute)(dm^3 soln)$^{-1}$	103.8	77.1	50.9	25.2
Π, atm	0.86	0.58	0.31	0.14

Ans. The intercept of a plot of Π/C' against C' is 4.65×10^{-3}, giving 5200 g mol^{-1}.

Solutions of Electrolytes

9.35. Assuming 100% dissociation of the solutes, what would be the freezing point depression for an aqueous solution that is 0.1 m in NaCl and 0.1 m in $CaCl_2$? K_{fp} = 1.860 K m^{-1} for water.

Ans. m = 0.5, 0.93 °C

9.36. Prepare a plot of i against m for the KH_2PO_4 solutions given below:

m	0.037	0.074	0.112	0.227	0.306	0.427	0.552	0.683	0.771
$T_{fp,1} - T_{fp,\text{soln}}$, °C	0.13	0.25	0.37	0.74	0.97	1.31	1.64	1.94	2.14

What conclusions from the graph can be made concerning the species present at these concentrations?

Ans. Values of i lie between 1.49 and 1.89 for the concentrations given. Intercept at $m = 0$ will be above 2, implying that $H_2PO_4^-$ is mainly associated.

9.37. The major solutes in surface seawater expressed in ppm by weight are: Cl^-, 18,980; Na^+, 10,560; SO_4^{2-}, 2700; Mg^{2+}, 1270; Ca^{2+}, 400; K^+, 380; HCO_3^-, 140; and Br^-, 65. Express these concentrations as m and predict the boiling and freezing points of a sample of seawater if K_{bp} = 0.513 K m^{-1} and K_{fp} = 1.860 K m^{-1}.

Ans. 965,505 ppm H_2O; 0.554 m Cl^-, 0.475 m Na^+, 0.029 m SO_4^{2-}, 0.054 m Mg^{2+}, 0.010 m Ca^{2+}, 0.010 m K^+, 0.002 m HCO_3^-, 0.001 m Br^-; m = 1.135; 100.58 °C; -2.11 °C

9.38. Find K_a for tartaric acid if a $0.100\,m$ solution freezes at $-0.205\,^\circ\text{C}$. Assume that only the first ionization is of importance and that $0.100\,m = 0.100\,M$. $K_{fp} = 1.860\text{ K }m^{-1}$.

Ans. $i = 1.10$, $\alpha = 0.10$, $K_a = 1.1 \times 10^{-3}$

Partial Molar (Molal) Quantities

9.39. Determine $\overline{\Delta H(\text{solution})}_i$ for CCl_4 and C_6H_6 at $x_i = 0.500$, using the following data:

ΔH°_{298}(formation), kcal mol^{-1}	-32.370	-32.348	-32.333	-32.315	-32.303	-32.295
$n_{C_6H_6}$	pure CCl_4(liq)	0.25	0.50	1.0	1.5	2.0

by preparing plots of ΔH(solution) against n_{CCl_4} and $n_{C_6H_6}$ and determining the slopes. Using *(9.33)* calculate ΔH(solution) for preparing 1 mol of this solution. Prepare a plot of the heat of solution for preparing 1 mol of the above solutions against $x_{C_6H_6}$ and find ΔH(solution). From this same plot, determine $\overline{\Delta H(\text{solution})}_i$ using the method of intercepts.

Ans. $\overline{\Delta H(\text{solution})}_i = 122\text{ J (mol }C_6H_6)^{-1}$ and $111\text{ J (mol }CCl_4)^{-1}$; $\Delta H(\text{solution}) = 117\text{ J}$; $\Delta H(\text{solution}) = 115\text{ J}$, $\overline{\Delta H(\text{solution})}_i = 121\text{ J (mol }C_6H_6)^{-1}$ and $109\text{ J (mol }CCl_4)^{-1}$

9.40. Determine $\bar{V}_2$ in a $0.5\,m$ aqueous HCl solution from the following data:

m	0.418	0.560
$d \times 10^{-3}$, kg m^{-3}	1.0057	1.0081

by finding V as a function of m and using *(9.32)*.

Ans. For 1 kg of water, $V = 1.0016 + (0.0190)m$; $\bar{V}_2 = 0.0190\text{ dm}^3\text{ mol}^{-1}$

9.41. The *chemical potential*, μ, is defined as the partial molar free energy, i.e.

$$\mu_i \equiv \left(\frac{\partial G}{\partial n_i}\right)_{T,P,n_j \neq n_i} \tag{9.36}$$

Beginning with *(5.7)*, show that

$$\left(\frac{\partial\,\Delta\mu_2}{\partial P}\right)_T = \Delta\bar{V}_2$$

Will the solubility of the solute increase or decrease for an increase in P if $\Delta\bar{V}_2 = \bar{V}_2 - V_2^\circ > 0$ where V_2° is the molar volume of the pure state?

Ans. As P increases, $\Delta\mu_2$ increases, giving a larger μ_2 for the solution. There is a net driving force for solute to leave solution, so that solubility decreases.

9.42. Beginning with *(9.35)*, show that

$$\bar{X}_2 = \phi_2 + n_2\frac{\partial\phi_2}{\partial n_2} = \phi_2 + \frac{\partial\phi_2}{\partial(\ln n_2)}$$

Using the data in Example 9.11 for the $NaCl/H_2O$ solutions, prepare a plot of ϕ_2 against $\ln n_2$ and find $\bar{V}_2$ for a $0.5\,m$ solution. Assume that $V_1^\circ = 0.01809\text{ dm}^3\text{ mol}^{-1}$

Ans. At $0.5\,m$, $\phi = 11.05$, $d\phi/d(\ln n_2) = 7.84$, $\bar{V} = 0.01889\text{ dm}^3\text{ mol}^{-1}$

Chapter 10

Kinetics

Rate Equations for Simple Reactions

10.1 CONCENTRATION DEPENDENCE

The rate of the chemical reaction

$$aA + bB + \cdots \longrightarrow cC + dD + \cdots$$

can be expressed as $-dC_A/dt, -dC_B/dt, \ldots, +dC_C/dt, +dC_D/dt, \ldots$, where the negative sign signifies the decrease in the concentration of one of the reactants and the positive sign signifies the increase in the concentration of one of the products.

The rate equation for a single chemical reaction contains a proportionality constant, k, known as the *rate constant* (or *specific rate*), and concentrations of each reactant entering into the actual reaction equation raised to a power equal to the number of molecules involved in the actual reaction equation. The actual reaction equation may or may not be the same as the overall stoichiometric equation for the reaction. The value of the exponent for each reactant is known as the *order of reaction* for that component and the overall order of the reaction is the sum of the exponents. The dimensions of k are $[(\text{concentration})^{1-\text{overall order}}(\text{time})^{-1}]$.

EXAMPLE 10.1. For the chemical reaction

$$H_2O + Cr_2O_7^{2-}(aq) \longrightarrow 2CrO_4^{2-}(aq) + 2H^+(aq)$$

evaluate the various expressions for the rate in terms of $-dC_{Cr_2O_7^{2-}}/dt$. If the actual reaction equation for the chromate-dichromate system is identical to the stoichiometric equation, write the rate equation. If C_{H_2O} is large enough to remain essentially constant, write the revised rate equation. What is the overall order of both of these rate equations?

Both of the product ions are being formed twice as fast as the dichromate ion is reacting, which gives

$$\frac{d}{dt}(C_{CrO_4^{2-}}) = \frac{d}{dt}(C_{H^+}) = -2\frac{d}{dt}(C_{Cr_2O_7^{2-}})$$

The water is reacting in a 1 : 1 ratio to $Cr_2O_7^{2-}$, giving

$$-\frac{d}{dt}(C_{H_2O}) = -\frac{d}{dt}(C_{Cr_2O_7^{2-}})$$

The complete rate equation is the second-order equation

$$\text{rate} = kC_{H_2O}\,C_{Cr_2O_7^{2-}}$$

For C_{H_2O} a constant, the revised rate equation will be the pseudo-first-order equation

$$\text{rate} = k'C_{Cr_2O_7^{2-}} \quad \text{where} \quad k' = kC_{H_2O}$$

10.2 ZERO-ORDER REACTIONS

Zero-order reactions are those having the differential rate equation

$$-\frac{dC}{dt} = k \qquad (10.1)$$

which upon integration ($C = C_0$ at $t = 0$) gives

$$C = C_0 - kt \qquad (10.2)$$

For a reaction that is zero-order, a plot of C against t will give a straight line having a slope of k and an intercept of C_0.

EXAMPLE 10.2. The *half-life* of a chemical reaction, $t_{1/2}$, is defined by the condition $C = \frac{1}{2}C_0$ at $t = t_{1/2}$. For a zero-order reaction, (*10.2*) gives

$$t_{1/2} = \frac{C_0}{2k}$$

10.3 FIRST-ORDER REACTIONS

First-order reactions are those having the differential rate equation

$$-\frac{dC}{dt} = kC \qquad (10.3)$$

which upon integration gives

$$\ln C = \ln C_0 - kt \qquad (10.4)$$

For a first-order reaction, a plot of $\ln C$ against t will be linear with a slope of k and an intercept of $\ln C_0$.

EXAMPLE 10.3. The liquid-phase dissociation of dicyclopentadiene has been studied by Langer and Patton using gas chromatographic techniques. The technique involved measured a quantity proportional to dC/dt rather than $-dC/dt$, so (*10.4*) becomes

$$\ln C' = \ln C'_0 + kt$$

where C' and C'_0 are the quantities that are proportional to the concentration. Note that k has not changed. Determine k from the following data at 190 °C:

C'	1.85	2.04	2.34	2.70	3.83	5.28
t, s	524	620	752	876	1188	1452

For the first-order reaction, the plot of $\ln C'$ against t is linear, see Fig. 10-1, with slope $k = 1.12 \times 10^{-3}\ \text{s}^{-1}$.

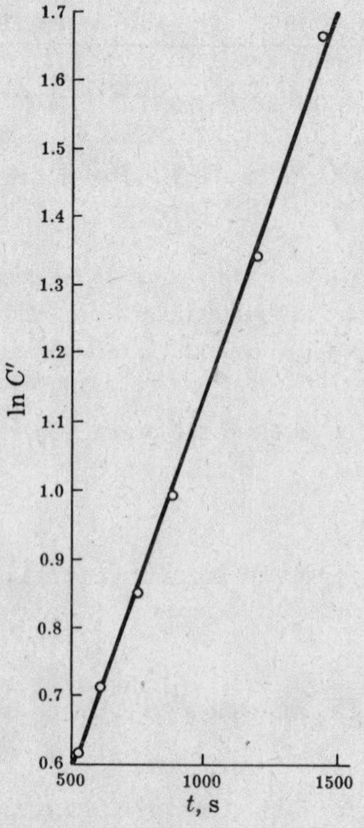

Fig. 10-1

10.4 SECOND-ORDER REACTIONS

The most general second-order reaction is one in which the stoichiometry is given by

$$aA + bB \longrightarrow \text{products}$$

where $a \neq b$ and $C_{A,0} \neq C_{B,0}$. For this reaction the integrated rate equation is

$$\frac{1}{bC_{A,0} - aC_{B,0}} \ln\left(\frac{C_{B,0}}{C_{A,0}}\frac{C_A}{C_B}\right) = kt \qquad (10.5)$$

If $a = b$ with $C_{A,0} \neq C_{B,0}$, the differential rate equation is

$$-\frac{dC_A}{dt} = -\frac{dC_B}{dt} = kC_AC_B \tag{10.6}$$

which integrates to

$$\frac{1}{C_{A,0} - C_{B,0}} \ln\left(\frac{C_{B,0}}{C_{A,0}} \frac{C_B}{C_A}\right) = kt \tag{10.7}$$

For (*10.6*) with $a = b = 1$ and $C_{A,0} = C_{B,0}$ or for the reaction $2A \longrightarrow$ products, the differential rate equation is

$$-\frac{dC}{dt} = kC^2 \tag{10.8}$$

which integrates to

$$\frac{1}{C} = \frac{1}{C_0} + kt \tag{10.9}$$

Plots of the left-hand sides of (*10.5*), (*10.7*) and (*10.9*) against t will be linear, with a slope in each case equal to k.

EXAMPLE 10.4. What are the dimensions of k for a second-order reaction?

Upon inspection of (*10.5*), (*10.7*) and (*10.9*), it can be seen that the dimensions of the left-hand sides are $[C^{-1}]$. (The coefficients a and b in (*10.5*) represent numbers of reacting molecules of A and B, and so these coefficients are pure numbers.) Hence the dimensions of k are $[C^{-1}t^{-1}]$, in agreement with the general rule presented in Section 10.1.

10.5 THIRD-ORDER REACTIONS

For the reaction $A + B + C \longrightarrow$ products, with $C_{A,0} \neq C_{B,0} \neq C_{C,0}$, the differential rate equation is

$$-\frac{dC_A}{dt} = kC_AC_BC_C \tag{10.10}$$

and the integrated equation is

$$\frac{\ln(C_A/C_{A,0})}{(C_{A,0} - C_{B,0})(C_{C,0} - C_{A,0})} + \frac{\ln(C_B/C_{B,0})}{(C_{A,0} - C_{B,0})(C_{B,0} - C_{C,0})} + \frac{\ln(C_C/C_{C,0})}{(C_{B,0} - C_{C,0})(C_{C,0} - C_{A,0})} = kt \tag{10.11}$$

For the case where $C_{B,0} \neq C_{A,0} = C_{C,0}$ in (*10.10*) or for the reaction

$$2A + B \longrightarrow \text{products}$$

with $C_{A,0} \neq C_{B,0}$ or $C_{A,0} \neq 2C_{B,0}$, the differential rate equation is

$$-\frac{dC_A}{dt} = kC_A^2C_B \tag{10.12}$$

and the integrated form is

$$\frac{2}{(2C_{B,0} - C_{A,0})^2}\left[\frac{2(2C_{B,0} - C_{A,0})(C_{A,0} - C_A)}{C_{A,0}C_A} + \ln\frac{C_{B,0}C_A}{C_{A,0}C_B}\right] = kt \tag{10.13}$$

For the reaction $A + B \longrightarrow$ products, with $C_{A,0} \neq C_{B,0}$ where (*10.12*) is valid, the integrated form is

$$\frac{1}{(C_{B,0}-C_{A,0})^2}\left[\frac{(C_{B,0}-C_{A,0})(C_{A,0}-C_A)}{C_{A,0}C_A}+\ln\frac{C_{B,0}C_A}{C_{A,0}C_B}\right] = kt \tag{10.14}$$

For the case where $C_{A,0}=C_{B,0}=C_{C,0}$ for (*10.10*), or $C_{A,0}=C_{B,0}$ or $C_{A,0}=2C_{B,0}$ for (*10.12*), or for the reaction $3A \longrightarrow$ products, the differential rate equation is

$$-\frac{dC}{dt} = kC^3 \tag{10.15}$$

which integrates to

$$\frac{1}{2}\left(\frac{1}{C^2}-\frac{1}{C_0^2}\right) = kt \tag{10.16}$$

Plots of the left-hand sides of (*10.11*), (*10.13*), (*10.14*) and (*10.16*) against t will be linear, having a slope in each case equal to k.

10.6 PSEUDO-ORDER REACTIONS

If one of the reactants is in great excess or is regenerated (catalyst) so that its concentration is essentially constant, the concentration term in the rate equation for that component will appear as part of k unless special effort is taken to separate its contribution.

EXAMPLE 10.5. Consider the reaction $A + H_2O + H^+(aq) \longrightarrow$ products. Write the complete rate equation and the pseudo-order rate equation if $C_{H_2O} \gg C_A$ and if H^+ is regenerated. If $k' = 1.00 \times 10^{-5}\ s^{-1}$ for the pseudo-first-order reaction, find k for the complete rate equation, given that $C_{H_2O} = 55.5\ M$ and $C_{H^+} = 0.10\ M$.

The complete rate equation is

$$-\frac{dC_A}{dt} = kC_AC_{H_2O}C_{H^+}$$

If C_{H_2O} and C_{H^+} are constant, the pseudo-order equation is

$$-\frac{dC_A}{dt} = k'C_A \qquad \text{where} \qquad k' = kC_{H_2O}C_{H^+}$$

Substituting the values of concentrations gives

$$k = \frac{k'}{C_{H_2O}C_{H^+}} = \frac{1.00\times10^{-5}\ s^{-1}}{(55.5\ M)(0.10\ M)} = 1.8\times10^{-6}\ M^{-2}\ s^{-1}$$

Rate Equations for Complex Reactions

10.7 DIFFERENTIAL RATE EQUATIONS

The rate equation for a series of reactions in a complex mechanism is written as a sum of the rate equations for the simple reactions making up the complex mechanism. In the expression for dC_i/dt, a term appears for each reaction in which substance i appears or disappears.

EXAMPLE 10.6. For the set of reactions

$$A + B \underset{k_{-1}}{\overset{k_1}{\rightleftharpoons}} C \qquad\qquad C + B \xrightarrow{k_2} D$$

find $-dC_A/dt$, $-dC_B/dt$, dC_C/dt and dC_D/dt.

The substance A appears only in the first equation, but because it both reacts in and is formed by this reaction, the rate equation contains two terms:

$$-\frac{dC_A}{dt} = k_1 C_A C_B - k_{-1} C_C$$

The substance B appears in both equations, reacting and being formed in the first and reacting in the second, giving three terms for the rate expression:

$$-\frac{dC_B}{dt} = k_1 C_A C_B - k_{-1} C_C + k_2 C_C C_B$$

In the same manner,

$$\frac{dC_C}{dt} = k_1 C_A C_B - k_{-1} C_C - k_2 C_C C_B \qquad \frac{dC_D}{dt} = k_2 C_C C_B$$

10.8 STEADY-STATE APPROXIMATION

The *steady-state approximation* assumes that the concentrations of certain intermediate substances reach constant values (i.e. $dC_i/dt = 0$ for these substances).

EXAMPLE 10.7. Assuming that $dC_C/dt = 0$ for the set of reactions given in Example 10.6, find $-dC_A/dt$, $-dC_B/dt$ and dC_D/dt in terms of C_A, C_B and C_D.

Assuming that $dC_C/dt = k_1 C_A C_B - k_{-1} C_C - k_2 C_C C_B = 0$ gives

$$C_C = \frac{k_1 C_A C_B}{k_{-1} + k_2 C_B}$$

which upon substitution into the rate expressions for the other substances gives

$$-\frac{dC_A}{dt} = k_1 C_A C_B - \frac{k_{-1} k_1 C_A C_B}{k_{-1} + k_2 C_B} = \frac{k_1 k_2 C_A C_B^2}{k_{-1} + k_2 C_B}$$

$$-\frac{dC_B}{dt} = k_1 C_A C_B - \frac{k_{-1} k_1 C_A C_B}{k_{-1} + k_2 C_B} + \frac{k_2 C_B k_1 C_A C_B}{k_{-1} + k_2 C_B} = \frac{2 k_1 k_2 C_A C_B^2}{k_{-1} + k_2 C_B}$$

$$\frac{dC_D}{dt} = \frac{k_1 k_2 C_A C_B^2}{k_{-1} + k_2 C_B}$$

EXAMPLE 10.8. If $k_2 C_B \gg k_{-1}$, what is the pseudo-order of the formation of D in Example 10.7? If $k_2 C_B \ll k_{-1}$, what is the pseudo-order?

If $k_2 C_B \gg k_{-1}$, $k_{-1} + k_2 C_B$ can be replaced by $k_2 C_B$, giving $dC_D/dt = k_1 C_A C_B$, which is pseudo-second-order. For $k_2 C_B \ll k_{-1}$, $k_{-1} + k_2 C_B$ can be replaced by k_{-1}, giving $dC_D/dt = k_3 C_A C_B^2$, a pseudo-third-order reaction, where $k_3 = k_1 k_2 / k_{-1}$.

10.9 OPPOSING REACTIONS AND EQUILIBRIUM

At equilibrium opposing reactions proceed at equal rates, yielding a net rate of change of zero for each component. It is possible to collect all concentration terms on one side, and all rate constants on the other side, of an equation and equate the latter side to the thermodynamic equilibrium constant, K.

EXAMPLE 10.9. Consider the opposing second-order reactions

$$A_2 + B_2 \underset{k_{-2}}{\overset{k_2}{\rightleftharpoons}} 2AB$$

Derive an expression for K in terms of k_2 and k_{-2}.

For component A at equilibrium

$$-\frac{d}{dt}(C_{A_2}) = k_2 C_{A_2} C_{B_2} - k_{-2} C_{AB}^2 = 0$$

To find K we solve the above equation for the ratio of product concentrations to reactant concentrations (see Section 5.9), obtaining

$$\frac{C_{AB}^2}{C_{A_2} C_{B_2}} = \frac{k_2}{k_{-2}} = K$$

10.10 CONSECUTIVE FIRST-ORDER REACTIONS

Consider the consecutive first-order reactions

$$A \xrightarrow{k_1} B \qquad B \xrightarrow{k_2} C$$

The concentrations at time t will be

$$C_A = C_{A,0} e^{-k_1 t} \tag{10.17a}$$

$$C_B = \frac{k_1 C_{A,0}}{k_2 - k_1}(e^{-k_1 t} - e^{-k_2 t}) \tag{10.17b}$$

$$C_C = C_{A,0}\left(1 - \frac{k_2 e^{-k_1 t} - k_1 e^{-k_2 t}}{k_2 - k_1}\right) \tag{10.17c}$$

assuming that $C_{B,0} = C_{C,0} = 0$. As a check, note that $C_A + C_B + C_C = C_{A,0}$.

10.11 COMPETING (PARALLEL) REACTIONS

Quite often the reactants can form several different sets of products. The proper choice of a catalyst or temperature conditions can often alter the values of the parallel rate constants so as to favor one reaction.

EXAMPLE 10.10. For the series of competing reactions

$$H + HO_2 \xrightarrow{k_1} H_2 + O_2 \qquad H + HO_2 \xrightarrow{k_2} 2OH \qquad H + HO_2 \xrightarrow{k_3} H_2O + O$$

Westenberg and deHass report $k_1 / k_2 / k_3 = 0.62 / 0.27 / 0.11$. Find the ratio of the products at time t.

The rate equation for the reactions is

$$\text{rate} = k_1 C_H C_{HO_2} + k_2 C_H C_{HO_2} + k_3 C_H C_{HO_2} = k C_H C_{HO_2}$$

where $k = k_1 + k_2 + k_3$. The given ratio of rate constants implies that 62% of the reactants will form the products of the first reaction, 27% will form the products of the second reaction, etc. Thus the ratio of the products will be

$$(C_{H_2} = C_{O_2}) / C_{OH} / (C_{H_2O} = C_O) = 0.62 / 0.54 / 0.11$$

Determination of Reaction Order and Rate Constants

10.12 DIFFERENTIAL METHOD

The *differential method* determines $\pm dC_i/dt$ for substance i as a function of concentration for that substance when an excess or fixed amount of the remaining materials is used. The rate equation for the pseudo-order reaction in that component only is

$$\pm\frac{dC_i}{dt} = kC_i^n$$

which upon taking logarithms gives

$$\log\left(\pm\frac{dC_i}{dt}\right) = \log k + n \log C_i \tag{10.18}$$

A plot of $\log(\pm dC_i/dt)$ against $\log C_i$ will give a straight line with a slope of n for that component and an intercept of $\log k$, where k is the rate constant for the pseudo-order reaction.

10.13 INTEGRAL METHODS

The *graphical integral method* for determining n and k in (*10.18*) is a trial-and-error procedure. It begins by plotting $\log C_i$ against t, giving a linear plot only if $n = 1$ and a curved plot if $n \neq 1$; it continues by plotting C_i^{1-n} against t for various values of $n \neq 1$. The plot that turns out to be linear specifies n and has a slope given by $(n-1)k$. The *mathematical integral method* is another trial-and-error procedure, which solves for the value of k in the integrated form of the rate equation for various values of n until one value of n is found that gives the same rate constant for all the data.

10.14 HALF-LIFE METHOD

The *half-life method* is based on measurements of the time required for one-half of the substance to disappear, as a function of $C_{i,0}$. For a first-order reaction, $t_{1/2}$ is independent of $C_{i,0}$, and for order $n \neq 1$,

$$\log t_{1/2} = \log\frac{2^{n-1}-1}{(n-1)k} - (n-1)\log C_{i,0} \tag{10.19}$$

Thus a plot of $\log t_{1/2}$ against $\log C_{i,0}$ will give a straight line having slope $n-1$ and intercept $\log[(2^{n-1}-1)/(n-1)k]$.

10.15 RELAXATION METHODS

Relaxation methods allow the study of fast reactions. A reaction mixture at equilibrium is disturbed by a pressure, thermal, or electrical shock and allowed to return to equilibrium. The restoration is always first-order for small displacements from equilibrium, giving

$$\Delta C_i = \Delta C_{i,0} e^{-t/\tau} \tag{10.20}$$

where ΔC_i is the displacement from equilibrium at time t, $\Delta C_{i,0}$ is the initial displacement from equilibrium and τ is the *relaxation time*. Upon differentiation, (*10.20*) gives

$$\frac{d(\Delta C_i)}{dt} = -\Delta C_i\left(\frac{1}{\tau}\right) \tag{10.21}$$

EXAMPLE 10.11. Derive the relationship between the relaxation time and k_1 and k_2, for the reaction

$$A + B \underset{k_2}{\overset{k_1}{\rightleftharpoons}} C$$

Assuming $\tau = 2.0\ \mu s$ for $C_{A,e} = C_{B,e} = 1.0\ M$ and $3.3\ \mu s$ for $C_{A,e} = C_{B,e} = 0.5\ M$, find k_1, k_2 and K.

The rate equation for the system is

$$\frac{dC_C}{dt} = k_1 C_A C_B - k_2 C_C$$

and at equilibrium $k_1 C_{A,e} C_{B,e} - k_2 C_{C,e} = 0$. For a small increase in C_C, ΔC_C,

$$C_C = C_{C,e} + \Delta C_C \qquad C_B = C_{B,e} - \Delta C_C \qquad C_A = C_{A,e} - \Delta C_C$$

The rate equation for the decay of ΔC_C is

$$\begin{aligned}\frac{d(\Delta C_C)}{dt} &= k_1(C_{A,e} - \Delta C_C)(C_{B,e} - \Delta C_C) - k_2(C_{C,e} + \Delta C_C)\\ &= k_1(C_{A,e}C_{B,e} - C_{B,e}\Delta C_C - C_{A,e}\Delta C_C + \Delta C_C^2) - k_2(C_{C,e} + \Delta C_C)\\ &= (k_1C_{A,e}C_{B,e} - k_2C_{C,e}) - (k_1C_{A,e} + k_1C_{B,e} + k_2)\Delta C_C\\ &= -(k_1C_{A,e} + k_1C_{B,e} + k_2)\Delta C_C\end{aligned}$$

where the results at equilibrium were substituted and the term ΔC_C^2 was neglected. Upon comparison to (*10.21*)

$$\frac{1}{\tau} = k_1C_{A,e} + k_1C_{B,e} + k_2 = k_2 + k_1(C_{A,e} + C_{B,e})$$

which implies that a plot of $1/\tau$ against $C_{A,e} + C_{B,e}$ will be linear with a slope of k_1 and an intercept of k_2. Rather than making a plot for two sets of data, the simultaneous equations

$$\frac{1}{2.0 \times 10^{-6}} = k_2 + k_1(1+1) \qquad \frac{1}{3.3 \times 10^{-6}} = k_2 + k_1(0.5+0.5)$$

can be solved, giving $k_1 = 2 \times 10^5$ and $k_2 = 1 \times 10^5$. Then

$$K = \frac{k_1}{k_2} = 2$$

10.16 EXPERIMENTAL PARAMETERS

In many experiments C_i is not measured, but some related property (P, pH, absorbancy, etc.) may be the basis for writing the rate equation. For a first-order reaction there is no change in the value of k, but for other orders the value and units of k must be changed.

EXAMPLE 10.12. Consider the chromate-dichromate reaction

$$H_2O + Cr_2O_7^{2-}(aq) \longrightarrow 2CrO_4^{2-}(aq) + 2H^+(aq)$$

How is pH related to $C_{Cr_2O_7^{2-}}$?

From Example 10.1,

$$\frac{d}{dt}(C_{H^+}) = -2\frac{d}{dt}(C_{Cr_2O_7^{2-}})$$

which integrates into

$$C_{H^+} = C_{H^+,0} - 2(C_{Cr_2O_7^{2-}} - C_{Cr_2O_7^{2-},0})$$

By definition, $pH = -\log C_{H^+}$. Hence the desired relation is

$$pH = -\log[10^{-(pH)_0} - 2(C_{Cr_2O_7^{2-}} - C_{Cr_2O_7^{2-},0})]$$

Influence of Temperature

Over moderate temperature intervals, a plot of $\log k$ against $1/T$ is linear, giving

$$\ln k = \ln \mathcal{A} - \left(\frac{\Delta E^*}{R}\right)\frac{1}{T} \qquad (10.22a)$$

where $\mathcal{A}$ is known as the *pre-exponential factor* and ΔE^* is known as the *activation energy*. Values of the rate constant at different temperatures are related by

$$\ln\frac{k_2}{k_1} = -\left(\frac{\Delta E^*}{R}\right)\left(\frac{1}{T_2} - \frac{1}{T_1}\right) \qquad (10.22b)$$

Equations (*10.22*) require that the units on ΔE^* be those of (energy)(mol^{-1}) so that the right-hand side of each equation is dimensionless. The (mol^{-1}) term is simply a reminder that molar quantities of reagents are involved in a chemical reaction, although the equation which describes the reaction on a molecular scale does not refer to numbers of moles. Some authors ignore the (mol^{-1}) term completely, while others retain it throughout all calculations even though it may not be dimensionally correct in some of its applications. In keeping with the convention adopted earlier in this book for ΔE, ΔG, etc., the (mol^{-1}) term will not appear in values of ΔE^* for a specific equation unless the term is needed to give the correct units in a calculation.

If a plot of E against the progress of the reaction is prepared (*reaction coordinate diagram*), ΔE^* represents the energy hump that must be surmounted before the products are formed. If the reverse reaction occurs as written in the equation, the energy of activation for the reverse reaction, ΔE^*_-, is related to ΔE^* by

$$\Delta E^\circ = \Delta E^* - \Delta E^*_- \qquad (10.23)$$

where ΔE° is the change in internal energy for the reaction, see Section 3.1.

EXAMPLE 10.13. The average rate constants for dicyclopentadiene dissociation in *n*-hexatriacontane on Gas Chrom Q are $1.92 \times 10^{-4}\ \mathrm{s}^{-1}$ at 170.0 °C, $4.61 \times 10^{-4}\ \mathrm{s}^{-1}$ at 180.1 °C, $7.10 \times 10^{-4}\ \mathrm{s}^{-1}$ at 185.2 °C and $10.52 \times 10^{-4}\ \mathrm{s}^{-1}$ at 189.9 °C, as reported by Langer and Patton. Prepare an *Arrhenius plot* ($\log k$ against $1/T$) and determine ΔE^* for the decomposition. If ΔE° is about -545 kJ for the reaction

$$(C_5H_6)_2 \longrightarrow 2C_5H_6$$

prepare a reaction coordinate diagram and find ΔE^*_-, assuming the reverse reaction to be a simple bimolecular collision as shown in the equation.

The slope of a plot of $\log k$ against $1/T$ is equal to -7610 K, see Fig. 10-2. Then (*10.22a*) gives

$$\begin{aligned}\Delta E^* &= -(2.303)R(\text{slope})\\ &= -(2.303)(8.314\ \mathrm{J\ mol^{-1}\ K^{-1}})(-7610\ \mathrm{K})\\ &= 145.7\ \mathrm{kJ\ mol^{-1}}\end{aligned}$$

for the decomposition. The reaction coordinate diagram inserted in Fig. 10-2 shows this potential-energy barrier above the reactant, with the product 545 kJ below the reactant. The value of ΔE^*_- is given by (*10.23*) as

$$\Delta E^*_- = 145.7\ \mathrm{kJ} - (-545\ \mathrm{kJ}) = 691\ \mathrm{kJ}$$

for the reverse reaction.

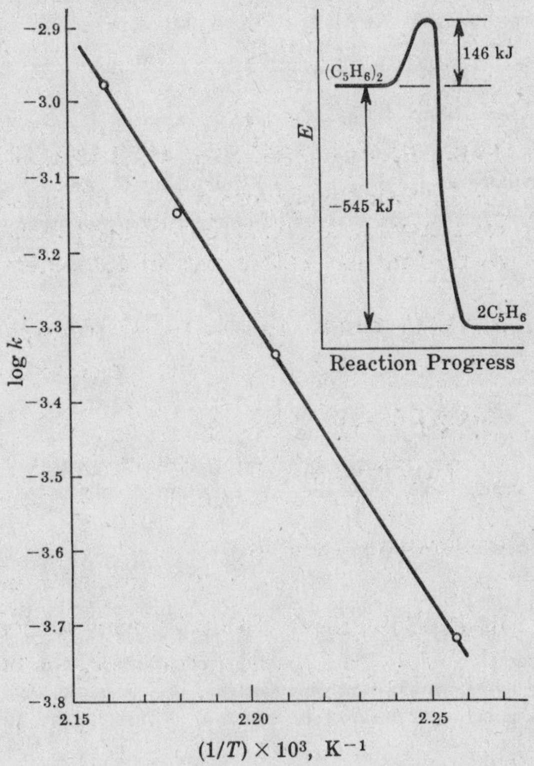

Fig. 10-2

Catalysis

10.17 HOMOGENEOUS CATALYSIS

A *catalyst* is a substance that alters the rate of a chemical reaction without undergoing any permanent chemical change. The presence of a catalyst will not influence equilibrium conditions once these are attained. Because the catalyst may enter into the reaction, the complete rate equation should include catalytic terms. In *homogeneous catalysis*, the catalyst is found in the same physical state as the reactants.

EXAMPLE 10.14. One of the proposed mechanisms for the recombination of bromine atoms in the presence of a third body or *chaperon*, M, is

$$Br + Br \underset{k_2}{\overset{k_1}{\rightleftharpoons}} Br_2^* \qquad Br_2^* + M \xrightarrow{k_3} Br_2 + M$$

where * indicates a highly excited molecule having an energy content of the order of the Br—Br bond dissociation energy. Why are CCl_4 and SF_6 better catalysts than Ne or other monatomic and diatomic species?

The more simple molecules have only translational—and perhaps two rotational and one vibrational—degrees of freedom available to absorb the energy from the Br_2^*, whereas the more complicated molecules have three rotational and many more vibrational degrees of freedom. Thus the energy transfer in a collision with the more complicated molecule will be more effective in increasing the rate of formation of Br_2.

EXAMPLE 10.15. Consider the following mechanism describing enzyme catalysis:

$$E + S \underset{k_{-1}}{\overset{k_1}{\rightleftharpoons}} X \underset{k_{-2}}{\overset{k_2}{\rightleftharpoons}} E + P$$

where E is the enzymatic site, S is the substrate, X is the enzyme substrate complex and P is the product of the reaction. Derive the rate equation for this process assuming $dC_X/dt = 0$ and discuss the results for the reaction during the initial stages.

The rate equations for this mechanism are

$$\frac{dC_X}{dt} = 0 = k_1 C_E C_S - k_{-1} C_X - k_2 C_X + k_2 C_E C_P \qquad \frac{dC_P}{dt} = k_2 C_X - k_{-2} C_E C_P$$

where $C_{E,0} = C_E + C_X$. Eliminating C_X and C_E gives

$$\frac{dC_P}{dt} = \frac{(V_S/K_S)C_S - (V_P/K_P)C_P}{1 + (C_S/K_S) + (C_P/K_P)}$$

where

$$V_S = k_2 C_{E,0} \qquad V_P = k_{-1} C_{E,0}$$

$$K_S = \frac{k_{-1} + k_2}{k_1} \qquad K_P = \frac{k_{-1} + k_2}{k_{-2}}$$

If the measurements of the reaction rate are made during the early stages of the reaction, C_P will be nearly zero and the rate equation simplifies to give the *Michaelis-Menten equation:*

$$\frac{dC_P}{dt} = \frac{(V_S/K_S)C_S}{1 + (C_S/K_S)} = \frac{V_S}{1 + (K_S/C_S)}$$

If $C_S \ll K_S$, the reaction rate is first-order with respect to C_S and if $C_S \gg K_S$, the reaction rate is zero-order with respect to C_S. In both cases the reaction is dependent on V_S, which is first-order with respect to $C_{E,0} \approx C_E$. The Michaelis constant for the substrate, K_S, represents the value of C_S necessary to reduce the maximum reaction rate, V_S, by a factor of two. The rate constant for the product reaction, k_2, is known as the *turnover constant.* Casting the rate equation into the *Lineweaver-Burk linear form* gives

$$\left(\frac{dC_P}{dt}\right)^{-1} = \left(\frac{K_S}{V_S}\right) C_S^{-1} + V_S^{-1}$$

Thus a plot of $(dC_P/dt)^{-1}$ against C_S^{-1} will be linear, having an intercept of V_S^{-1} and a slope of K_S/V_S.

10.18 ADSORPTION AND HETEROGENEOUS CATALYSIS

Heterogeneous catalysis occurs as the reactant collects or adsorbs on the surface of the catalyst. The amount of reactant adsorbed at a given temperature is described by various equations called *adsorption isotherms.* For example, at rather low pressures, P, the volume, V, of adsorbed gas on a solid is given by the *Freundlich isotherm* as

$$V = kP^n \tag{10.24}$$

where k and n are constants with $n < 1$. More complete equations are the *Langmuir isotherm,*

$$V = V_m\theta \tag{10.25}$$

where V_m represents the volume of gas to form a monolayer over the entire surface of the solid, where

$$\theta = \frac{bP}{1+bP} \tag{10.26}$$

and where b is the ratio of the rate constant for adsorption to that for desorption; and the *Brunauer-Emmett-Teller (BET) isotherm,*

$$V = \frac{V_m c(P/P^\circ)}{1-(P/P^\circ)}\,\frac{1-(n+1)(P/P^\circ)^n + n(P/P^\circ)^{n+1}}{1+(c-1)(P/P^\circ) - c(P/P^\circ)^{n+1}} \tag{10.27}$$

Here n is the number of layers of adsorbed molecules, P° is the vapor pressure of the pure liquid, and

$$c = e^{[\Delta H(\text{mono}) - \Delta H(\text{vaporization})]/RT} \tag{10.28}$$

where ΔH(mono) is the heat of vaporization for the first layer, assumed to be different from the heat of vaporization of the liquid, ΔH(vaporization). For $n = \infty$, (*10.27*) becomes

$$V = \frac{V_m cP}{(P^\circ - P)[1+(c-1)(P/P^\circ)]} \tag{10.29}$$

If more than one gas is adsorbed by the catalyst during a gaseous decomposition reaction, (*10.26*) becomes

$$\theta_i = \frac{b_i P_i}{(1 + b_A P_A + b_B P_B + \cdots)} \tag{10.30}$$

for each gas, assuming simple adsorption. The adsorption of additional gases reduces the surface area available for the reaction under consideration and thus causes the inhibition (*poison* or retardation) of the reaction.

The general expression describing the rate of decomposition for the reaction

$$A \longrightarrow \text{products}$$

is given by

$$\text{rate} = k'\theta \tag{10.31}$$

where k' is a proportionality constant and θ is the fraction of the surface covered.

EXAMPLE 10.16. The Langmuir isotherm is useful in describing monolayer adsorption (*chemisorption*), but fails at higher pressures where a second layer begins to form (*physisorption*). Show that (*10.25*) qualitatively predicts the Freundlich isotherm at relatively low pressures and that V is pressure-independent at high pressures.

At low pressures the denominator of (*10.26*) approaches unity, giving $\theta = bP$, and (*10.25*) becomes

$$V = V_m bP$$

which agrees with (*10.24*) for $n = 1$ and $k = V_m b$. At high pressures the denominator of (*10.26*) approaches bP, giving $\theta = 1$, and (*10.25*) becomes

$$V = \frac{V_m bP}{bP} = V_m$$

which is pressure-independent.

EXAMPLE 10.17. The mass, y, of adsorbed solute on a solid is given by a form of the Freundlich isotherm as

$$y = kC_2^n \tag{10.32}$$

where C_2 is the concentration. If C_2 is expressed in (mol dm^{-3}), the values of k and n in (*10.32*) which give y in units of (g acetic acid)(g blood charcoal)$^{-1}$ are $k = 0.160$ and $n = 0.431$. Find the number of moles of acetic acid that 1 kg of charcoal would adsorb from a 5.00-wt% (0.837 M) vinegar solution.

The mass of solute is calculated using (*10.32*) as

$$y = (0.160)(0.837)^{0.431} = 0.148 \text{ (g HAc)(g charcoal)}^{-1} = 148 \text{ (g HAc)(kg charcoal)}^{-1}$$

which upon converting to moles becomes

$$\frac{148 \text{ (g HAc)(kg charcoal)}^{-1}}{60.05 \text{ g mol}^{-1}} = 2.47 \text{ (mol HAc)(kg charcoal)}^{-1}$$

EXAMPLE 10.18. Derive the integrated rate equation for the general case in which A is moderately adsorbed. Show that the following data of Stock and Bodenstein for the decomposition of SbH_3 on Sb at 25 °C satisfy this rate equation:

t, min	0	5	10	15	20	25
P_{SbH_3}, atm	1.000	0.731	0.509	0.327	0.189	0.093

Substituting (*10.26*) into (*10.31*) gives

$$-\frac{d}{dt}(P_{SbH_3}) = \frac{k'bP_{SbH_3}}{1 + bP_{SbH_3}} = \frac{kP_{SbH_3}}{1 + bP_{SbH_3}}$$

which upon rearrangement becomes

$$-k\,dt = [(P_{SbH_3})^{-1} + b]\,dP_{SbH_3}$$

Integration and substitution of proper limits yield

$$\ln(P_{SbH_3,0}/P_{SbH_3}) + b(P_{SbH_3,0} - P_{SbH_3}) = kt$$

Unless b is known, k cannot be determined graphically. However, both b and k can be determined numerically by substitution of data and solving the five equations to give an average of $b = 1.848$ atm^{-1} and $k = 0.160$ min^{-1}. Because of the difficulty in working with this equation, the Freundlich equation is sometimes used for these systems, see Problem 10.63.

EXAMPLE 10.19. Derive the expression for θ describing the reaction

$$A_2 \longrightarrow 2A$$

where A is strongly adsorbed.

For simple adsorption, the rate of condensation is given by $k_1P(1-\theta)$ and the rate of desorption by $k_2\theta$. Setting these rates equal at equilibrium and solving for θ gives (*10.26*). When dissociation accompanies adsorption, the law of mass action gives the rate of condensation as $k_1P(1-\theta)^2$ and the rate of desorption as $k_2\theta^2$. Setting these equal for equilibrium and solving for θ gives

$$\theta = \frac{bP^{1/2}}{1 + bP^{1/2}}$$

where $b = (k_1/k_2)^{1/2}$.

Photochemistry

Only those light quanta which are absorbed by a substance will be effective in producing a photochemical change. The energy of a quantum is given by

$$E = h\nu = \frac{hc}{\lambda} \tag{10.33}$$

where h is Planck's constant, ν is the frequency of the incident light, c is the velocity of light and λ is the wavelength of the incident light. Many authors express the number of quanta in *einsteins*, where

$$1 \text{ einstein} = \text{one mole of quanta} = L \text{ quanta}$$

The primary step in a photochemical reaction involves one molecule being activated by one absorbed quantum of radiation. The *quantum yield*, ϕ, is defined as the number of molecules of reactant consumed or product generated per quantum absorbed.

EXAMPLE 10.20. Bridges and White propose the following mechanism for the photolysis of methanethiol:

$$(1)\quad CH_3SH + h\nu = CH_3S + H^*$$

$$(2)\quad CH_3SH + h\nu = CH_3(\text{or } CH_3^*) + SH(\text{or } SH^*)$$

$$(3)\quad H^* + CH_3SH = CH_3S + H_2$$

$$(4a)\quad H^* + CH_3SH = CH_3 + H_2S$$

$$(4b)\quad H^* + CH_3SH = CH_4 + SH$$

$$(5)\quad CH_3(\text{or } CH_3^*) + CH_3SH = CH_3S + CH_4$$

$$(6)\quad SH(\text{or } SH^*) + CH_3SH = CH_3S + H_2S$$

$$(7)\quad H^* + M = H + M$$

$$(8)\quad H + CH_3SH = CH_3S + H_2$$

$$(9)\quad CH_3S + CH_3S = CH_3SSCH_3$$

Assuming one quantum of light to be absorbed according to reaction (*1*), find the relationships between $\phi(H_2)$, $\phi(CH_4)$, $\phi(H_2S)$ and $\phi(CH_3SSCH_3)$.

The products of (*1*) are CH_3 and H^*. Assuming the H^* to react in (*3*), a second CH_3S is generated, as well as an H_2. The two CH_3S can react according to (*9*), giving one CH_3SSCH_3. For this path for the dissipation of H^*, $\phi(H_2) = 1$, $\phi(CH_3SSCH_3) = 1$ and $\phi(H_2S) = \phi(CH_4) = 0$.

If the H^* reacts according to (*4a*), a CH_3 and H_2S are formed. Letting the CH_3 react with a second CH_3SH according to (*5*) gives CH_4 and a second CH_3S. Again, the two CH_3S fragments react according to (*9*). For this path, $\phi(CH_3SSCH_3) = 1$, $\phi(H_2S) = \phi(CH_4) = 1$ and $\phi(H_2) = 0$.

Assuming the H^* to react according to (*4b*), a CH_4 and SH are formed. Assuming the latter to react according to (*6*) gives H_2S and a second CH_3S. Again, both of the CH_3S react according to (*9*). For this path, $\phi(CH_3SSCH_3) = 1$, $\phi(CH_4) = \phi(H_2S) = 1$ and $\phi(H_2) = 0$.

Finally, letting the H^* dissipate its extra energy by colliding with the inert material M according to (*7*) gives H, which in turn reacts according to (*8*), giving the second CH_3S needed for (*9*) and an H_2. For this path, $\phi(H_2) = 1$, $\phi(CH_3SSCH_3) = 1$ and $\phi(CH_4) = \phi(H_2S) = 0$.

In summary, regardless of which path was chosen for the dissipation of the H^*, $\phi(CH_3SSCH_3) = 1$. Because the paths are competing reactions (Section 10.11), the exact values for the other quantum yields cannot be determined from the information given above, but the relationships $\phi(H_2S) = \phi(CH_4)$ and $\phi(CH_4) + \phi(H_2) = 1$ are valid.

EXAMPLE 10.21. For the reactions described in Example 10.20, Bridges and White reported that $\phi(CH_4) =$ 0.16 at 254 nm and 0.35 at 214 nm. Discuss these results.

The energy of the 214-nm light is given by (*10.24*) as

$$E = \frac{(6.626 \times 10^{-34}\ \text{J s})(2.9979 \times 10^{8}\ \text{m s}^{-1})}{(214\ \text{nm})(10^{-9}\ \text{m nm}^{-1})} = 9.28 \times 10^{-19}\ \text{J}$$

or 559 kJ einstein^{-1}, and the energy of the 254-nm radiation is 471 kJ einstein^{-1}. The energy required to break the S—H bond in reaction (*1*) is roughly 353 kJ mol^{-1} and for the C—S bond in (*2*) it is roughly 305 kJ mol^{-1} (see Section 3.11). Because both wavelengths have sufficient energy to cleave both bond types, both reactions (*1*) and (*2*) are favored and a mixture of CH_4, H_2S and H_2 will result. As the energy is increased by changing to 214-nm light, reaction (*2*) becomes more favored than before and a larger yield of CH_4 and H_2S (see Problem 10.67) will result.

Reaction Rate Theory

10.19 COLLISION THEORY OF BIMOLECULAR REACTIONS

According to the collision theory, the reaction rate is a function of the collision number (z_{12} for unlike molecules and $2z_{11}$ for like molecules) and the fraction of molecules having sufficient energy to react ($e^{-\Delta E^*/RT}$). Using (*1.36*) or (*1.35*), (*1.27*) and (*1.31*), and changing concentrations from molecules m^{-3} to mol dm^{-3}, it can be shown that

$$\text{rate} = p\left[\frac{8\pi RT(M_1+M_2)}{M_1M_2}\right]^{1/2}\sigma_{12}^2(10^3L)e^{-\Delta E^*/RT}C_1C_2$$

$$= (2.753\times10^{29})p\sigma_{12}^2\left[\frac{T(M_1+M_2)}{M_1M_2}\right]^{1/2}e^{-\Delta E^*/RT}C_1C_2 \qquad (10.34a)$$

for unlike molecules colliding, and

$$\text{rate} = 4p\left(\frac{\pi RT}{M}\right)^{1/2}\sigma^2(10^3L)e^{-\Delta E^*/RT}C^2$$

$$= (3.893\times10^{29})p\sigma^2\left(\frac{T}{M}\right)^{1/2}e^{-\Delta E^*/RT}C^2 \qquad (10.34b)$$

for like molecules colliding, where σ_{12} and σ are expressed in m and the *steric factor*, *p*, is dependent on the relative positions of the colliding molecules.

EXAMPLE 10.22. Upon comparison of (*10.22a*) with (*10.34*), the Arrhenius pre-exponential factor is given by the collision theory as

$$\mathcal{A} = (2.753\times10^{29})p\sigma_{12}^2\left[\frac{T(M_1+M_2)}{M_1M_2}\right]^{1/2}$$

for unlike molecules and

$$\mathcal{A} = (3.893\times10^{29})p\sigma^2\left(\frac{T}{M}\right)^{1/2}$$

for like molecules. Although the Arrhenius theory describes $\mathcal{A}$ as a constant and the collision theory predicts a temperature dependence for $\mathcal{A}$, show that these theories are not in conflict for typical reactions over reasonable temperature intervals.

Assuming $\sigma = 2$ Å, $M = 100$ g mol^{-1} and $p = 1.00$, the pre-exponential factor at 100 °C for like molecules would be

$$\mathcal{A} = (3.893\times10^{29})(1.00)(2\times10^{-10})^2\left(\frac{373}{100}\right)^{1/2} = 3.01\times10^{10}\ \text{dm}^3\ \text{mol}^{-1}\ \text{s}^{-1}$$

and at 200 °C would be

$$\mathcal{A} = (3.893\times10^{29})(1.00)(2\times10^{-10})^2\left(\frac{473}{100}\right)^{1/2} = 3.39\times10^{10}\ \text{dm}^3\ \text{mol}^{-1}\ \text{s}^{-1}$$

a 12% change. Over this same temperature interval, the exponential factor increases from 9.92×10^{-22} to 2.73×10^{-17}, a factor of 2.75×10^4, assuming a typical value of $\Delta E^* = 150$ kJ mol^{-1}. Thus the temperature dependence for the exponential factor is many orders of magnitude larger than that for the pre-exponential factor.

10.20 TRANSITION-STATE THEORY

According to the *transition-state*, or *absolute rate, theory* the reactants form an activated complex under equilibrium conditions, which undergoes decomposition to the products according to the mechanism

$$\underset{\text{reactants}}{A + B} \overset{K_c}{\rightleftharpoons} \underset{\substack{\text{activated}\\\text{complex}}}{(AB)^{\#}} \overset{k_1}{\longrightarrow} \text{products}$$

For this process, the rate equation can be shown to be

$$\text{rate} = w\left(\frac{kT}{h}\right)\left(\frac{Q_{\#}}{Q_A Q_B}\right)e^{-E_0^{\circ}/RT}C_A C_B \tag{10.35}$$

where w is the *transmission coefficient* (usually neglected) and the partition functions are given by

$$Q_i = q_{\text{trans}}\,q_{\text{rot}}\,q_{\text{vib}} \tag{10.36}$$

where q_{trans} is given by (*6.23*), q_{rot} is given by (*6.27*) or (*6.28*), and q_{vib} is given by (*6.30*) using $3\Lambda_A + 3\Lambda_B - 7$ degrees of freedom for a nonlinear activated complex and $3\Lambda_A + 3\Lambda_B - 6$ degrees of freedom for a linear activated complex and the usual values of $3\Lambda - 5$ and $3\Lambda - 6$ for linear and nonlinear reactants respectively.

The approximate values of $\mathcal{A}$ at 25 °C, p (assuming $w = 1$), and the exponent of T in $\mathcal{A}$, given in Table 10-1, can often suggest the structure of the activated complex.

Table 10-1

Reactant A	+	Reactant B	=	Activated Complex $(AB)^{\#}$	Exponent of T in $\mathcal{A}$	$\mathcal{A}$ at 25 °C, $\text{dm}^3\ \text{mol}^{-1}\ \text{s}^{-1}$	Approximate p
atom		atom		linear	$\frac{1}{2}$	10^{12}	1
atom		linear molecule		linear	$-\frac{1}{2}$ to $\frac{1}{2}$	10^{10}	10^{-2}
atom		linear molecule		nonlinear	0 to $\frac{1}{2}$	10^{11}	10^{-1}
atom		nonlinear molecule		nonlinear	$-\frac{1}{2}$ to $\frac{1}{2}$	10^{10}	10^{-2}
linear molecule		linear molecule		linear	$-\frac{3}{2}$ to $\frac{1}{2}$	10^{7}	10^{-4}
linear molecule		linear molecule		nonlinear	-1 to $\frac{1}{2}$	10^{8}	10^{-3}
linear molecule		nonlinear molecule		nonlinear	$-\frac{3}{2}$ to $\frac{1}{2}$	10^{7}	10^{-4}
nonlinear molecule		nonlinear molecule		nonlinear	-2 to $\frac{1}{2}$	10^{7}	10^{-5}

EXAMPLE 10.23. Assuming A and B are atomic species which form a diatomic activated complex having $I = m_A m_B \sigma_{AB}^2/m_{\#}$, where $m_{\#} = m_A + m_B$, show that the pre-exponential factor predicted by (*10.35*) is similar to that predicted by (*10.34a*).

For this reaction, (*10.36*) gives the partition functions as

$$Q_{\#} = q_{\text{trans}}\,q_{\text{rot}} \qquad Q_A = Q_B = q_{\text{trans}}$$

which upon substitution of (*6.23*), with $V = 1\ \text{m}^3$, and (*6.27*), with $\sigma = 1$, become

$$Q_{\#} = (2\pi m_{\#} kT)^{5/2}\frac{4\pi m_A m_B \sigma_{AB}^2}{m_{\#}^2 h^5}, \qquad Q_A = \frac{(2\pi m_A kT)^{3/2}}{h^3}, \qquad Q_B = \frac{(2\pi m_B kT)^{3/2}}{h^3}$$

Inserting these expressions into (*10.35*), simplifying, and changing the units from $\text{m}^3\ \text{molecule}^{-1}\ \text{s}^{-1}$ to $\text{dm}^3\ \text{mol}^{-1}\ \text{s}^{-1}$, we find

$$\mathcal{A} = w\left[\frac{8\pi RTM_{\#}}{M_A M_B}\right]^{1/2}\sigma_{AB}^2(10^3 L)$$

This result is identical with (*10.34a*) if we set $p = w$.

10.21 THERMODYNAMIC CONSIDERATIONS

The equilibrium constant (denoted K_c in Section 10.20) for the formation of the transition-state complex from the reactants is given by

$$K_c = \frac{C_{(AB)^\#}}{C_A C_B} = \left(\frac{kT}{h\nu}\right)\left(\frac{Q_\#}{Q_A Q_B}\right)e^{-E_0^\circ/RT} = \left(\frac{kT}{h\nu}\right)K_\# \tag{10.37}$$

where ν is the intramolecular vibrational frequency associated with the decomposition of the complex into the products and $K_\#$ differs from K_c by the same factor, $kT/h\nu$, that relates $Q_\#$ and the entire Q for the activated complex. Although $K_\#$ is rather difficult to calculate, it can be considered using classical thermodynamics; thus (*5.9*) and (*5.39a*) give

$$\Delta G_\#^\circ = \Delta H_\#^\circ + T\,\Delta S_\#^\circ = -RT \ln K_\#$$

Solving for $K_\#$ and substituting into (*10.37*) gives

$$\text{rate} = \frac{kT}{h} e^{\Delta S_\#^\circ/R} e^{-\Delta H_\#^\circ/RT} C_A C_B \tag{10.38}$$

which upon comparison with (*10.22a*) gives

$$\mathcal{A} = e^n \left(\frac{kT}{h}\right) e^{\Delta S_\#^\circ/R} \tag{10.39}$$

if

$$\Delta H_\#^\circ = \Delta E^* - nRT \tag{10.40}$$

where n is 1 for condensed-phase reactions and is the molecularity for gas-phase reactions.

EXAMPLE 10.24. The influence of ionic strength on the rate constant as predicted by the transition-state theory is known as the *primary salt effect.* Discuss the influence on k if ions A and B have like charges.

The thermodynamic equilibrium constant for the formation of the complex is given by

$$K = \frac{a_{(AB)^\#}}{a_A a_B} = \frac{C_{(AB)^\#}}{C_A C_B}\,\frac{\gamma_{(AB)^\#}}{\gamma_A \gamma_B}$$

which upon solving for $C_{(AB)^\#}$ and substituting into the first-order reaction describing the decomposition of the complex into the products gives

$$\text{rate} = k_1 C_{(AB)^\#} = k_1 K\left(\frac{\gamma_A \gamma_B}{\gamma_{(AB)^\#}}\right) C_A C_B = k C_A C_B$$

For charged species in rather dilute solutions, (*5.36*) gives

$$\log \gamma_A = -z_A^2(0.5116)I^{1/2}$$

$$\log \gamma_B = -z_B^2(0.5116)I^{1/2}$$

$$\log \gamma_{(AB)^\#} = -(z_A + z_B)^2(0.5116)I^{1/2}$$

which upon substitution into the logarithm of the last two terms of the rate equation gives

$$\log k = \log(k_1 K) + \log\frac{\gamma_A \gamma_B}{\gamma_{(AB)^\#}} = \log(k_1 K) + (1.0232)z_A z_B I^{1/2} \tag{10.41}$$

For z_A and z_B both positive or both negative, (*10.41*) predicts that $\log k$ will increase for an increase in I.

Solved Problems

Rate Equations for Simple Reactions

10.1. Consider a photochemical reaction in which one molecule of A will react for every photon of light energy absorbed: $A + h\nu = \text{products}$. Assume that five photons are being absorbed each second. If $C_A = 1M$, what will be the rate of the reaction? If $C_A = 2M$, what will be the rate of the reaction?

If five photons are being absorbed each second, only five molecules of A can react each second, no matter what the concentration of A is (so long as it can supply the molecules as needed). The rate of reaction in both cases, pseudo-zero-order in concentration, is the same and independent of C_A.

10.2. The concentrations of bromine at various times after flash photolysis of a bromine-SF_6 mixture with $C_{Br_2}/C_{SF_6} = 3.2 \times 10^{-2}$ were reported by DeGraff and Lang as:

$C_{Br} \times 10^5$, M	2.58	1.51	1.04	0.80	0.67	0.56
t, μs	120	220	320	420	520	620

If these data are for the reaction

$$2\text{Br} \xrightarrow{k} \text{Br}_2$$

show that the reaction is pseudo-second-order and calculate k.

This second-order reaction is described by (*10.8*) and (*10.9*). A plot of $1/C_{Br}$ against t is linear, see Fig. 10-3, having a slope of $2.75 \times 10^8\ M^{-1}\ \text{s}^{-1} = k$.

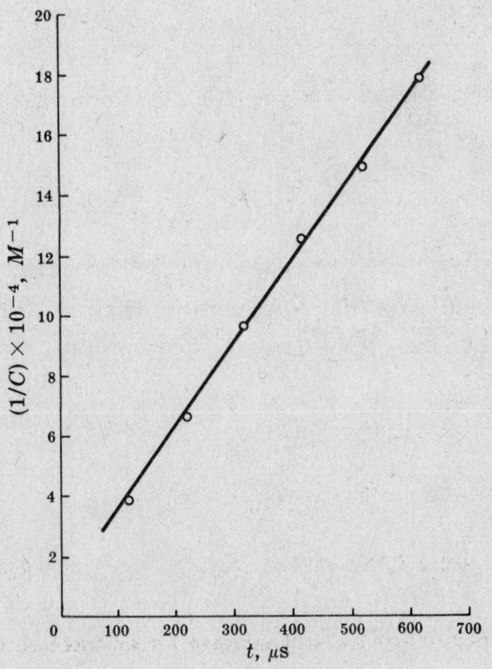

Fig. 10-3

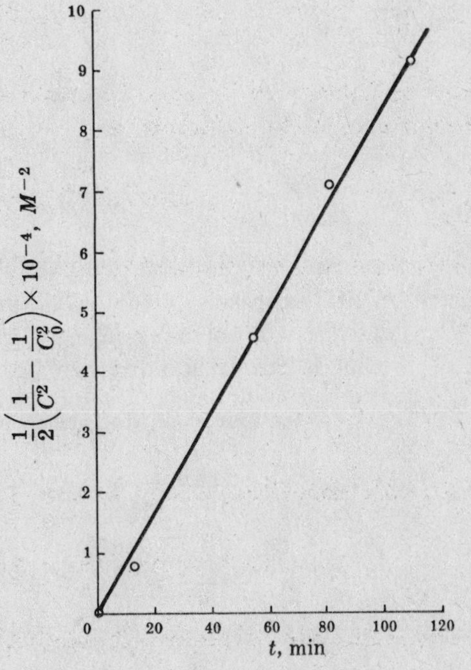

Fig. 10-4

10.3. In the presence of an acidic solution of phenol, the iodate ion is reduced to the iodite ion by Br^-, according to the reaction

$$IO_3^- + 2Br^- + 2H^+ \longrightarrow IO_2^- + Br_2 + H_2O$$

With $C_{IO_3^-,0} = 5.00 \times 10^{-3} M$ and $C_{Br^-,0} = 1.00 \times 10^{-2} M$, the following data are reported by Sharma and Gupta for a solution at 35 °C having $C_{C_6H_5OH} = 2 \times 10^{-2} M$:

$C_{IO_3^-} \times 10^3$, M	5.00	4.23	2.76	2.35	2.12
t, min	0.0	12.8	54.8	82.1	110.1

Show that these data correspond to a pseudo-third-order reaction and find k.

Because $C_{Br^-,0} = 2C_{IO_3^-,0}$, the integrated rate equation (*10.16*) must be used. As a sample calculation, for $t = 12.8$ min,

$$\frac{1}{2}\left(\frac{1}{C^2} - \frac{1}{C_0^2}\right) = \frac{1}{2}\left[\frac{1}{(4.23 \times 10^{-3})^2} - \frac{1}{(5.00 \times 10^{-3})^2}\right]$$

$$= \frac{1}{2}[(2.36 \times 10^2)^2 - (2.00 \times 10^2)^2] = 0.78 \times 10^4 \, M^{-2}$$

A plot of the values of the left-hand side of (*10.16*) against t is linear, see Fig. 10-4, with a slope of $k = 8.29 \times 10^2 \, M^{-2} \, \text{min}^{-1} = 13.8 \, M^{-2} \, \text{s}^{-1}$.

Rate Equations for Complex Reactions

10.4. A proposed mechanism for the reaction between $H_2(g)$ and $Br_2(g)$ is

$$Br_2 \underset{k_5}{\overset{k_1}{\rightleftharpoons}} 2Br$$

$$Br + H_2 \xrightarrow{k_2} HBr + H$$

$$H + Br_2 \xrightarrow{k_3} HBr + Br$$

$$H + HBr \xrightarrow{k_4} H_2 + Br$$

Write expressions for dC_{HBr}/dt, dC_H/dt and dC_{Br}/dt. Assuming that $dC_H/dt = dC_{Br}/dt = 0$, solve for dC_{HBr}/dt in terms of C_{H_2}, C_{Br_2} and C_{HBr}. If $1 \gg (k_4/k_3)(C_{HBr}/C_{Br_2})$, what is the pseudo-order of the reaction?

For the four steps, the rate expressions are

$$\frac{dC_{HBr}}{dt} = k_2 C_{Br} C_{H_2} + k_3 C_H C_{Br_2} - k_4 C_H C_{HBr}$$

$$\frac{dC_H}{dt} = k_2 C_{Br} C_{H_2} - k_3 C_H C_{Br_2} - k_4 C_H C_{HBr} = 0$$

$$\frac{dC_{Br}}{dt} = 2k_1 C_{Br_2} - k_2 C_{Br} C_{H_2} + k_3 C_H C_{Br_2} + k_4 C_H C_{HBr} - 2k_5 C_{Br}^2 = 0$$

Solving the last two equations simultaneously gives

$$C_{\mathrm{Br}} = \left(\frac{k_1}{k_5}\right)^{1/2} (C_{\mathrm{Br}_2})^{1/2}$$

$$C_{\mathrm{H}} = k_2\left(\frac{k_1}{k_5}\right)^{1/2} \frac{(C_{\mathrm{Br}_2})^{1/2} C_{\mathrm{H}_2}}{k_3 C_{\mathrm{Br}_2} + k_4 C_{\mathrm{HBr}}}$$

which upon substitution into the expression for dC_{HBr}/dt gives

$$\frac{dC_{\mathrm{HBr}}}{dt} = 2k_2\left(\frac{k_1}{k_5}\right)^{1/2} \frac{C_{\mathrm{H}_2}(C_{\mathrm{Br}_2})^{1/2}}{1 + (k_4/k_3)(C_{\mathrm{HBr}}/C_{\mathrm{Br}_2})}$$

Upon approximating the denominator, the rate equation can be written as the following pseudo-$1\frac{1}{2}$-order reaction:

$$\frac{dC_{\mathrm{HBr}}}{dt} = k' C_{\mathrm{H}_2}(C_{\mathrm{Br}_2})^{1/2}$$

10.5. $^{214}_{82}\mathrm{Pb}$ undergoes β^--emission forming $^{214}_{83}\mathrm{Bi}$, which undergoes further decomposition by β^--emission to become $^{214}_{84}\mathrm{Po}$. The half-lives of $^{214}_{82}\mathrm{Pb}$ and $^{214}_{83}\mathrm{Bi}$ are 26.8 min and 19.7 min, respectively. Assuming $C_0 = 100$ atoms for $^{214}_{82}\mathrm{Pb}$, prepare a diagram showing the concentrations of $^{214}_{82}\mathrm{Pb}$, $^{214}_{83}\mathrm{Bi}$ and $^{214}_{84}\mathrm{Po}$ as functions of time up to 100 min.

Substituting $t = t_{1/2}$ and $C = \frac{1}{2}C_0$ into (*10.4*) and solving gives

$$k = \frac{\ln 2}{t_{1/2}}$$

whence

$$k_1 = \frac{\ln 2}{26.8\ \mathrm{min}} = 2.59 \times 10^{-2}\ \mathrm{min}^{-1}$$

$$k_2 = \frac{\ln 2}{19.7\ \mathrm{min}} = 3.52 \times 10^{-2}\ \mathrm{min}^{-1}$$

As a sample calculation, (*10.17*) give for t = 10 min:

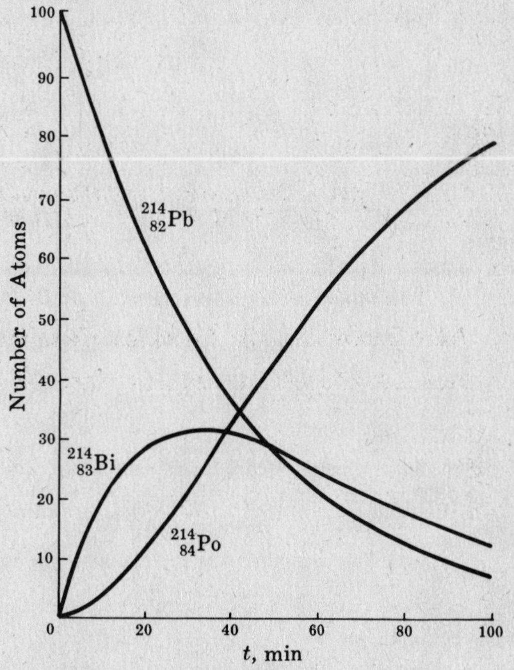

Fig. 10-5

$$C_A = 100e^{-2.59\times10^{-2}(10)} = 100e^{-0.259} = 77.2 \approx 77 \text{ atoms}$$

$$C_B = \frac{(2.59\times10^{-2})(100)}{3.52\times10^{-2} - 2.59\times10^{-2}}[e^{-2.59\times10^{-2}(10)} - e^{-3.52\times10^{-2}(10)}]$$

$$= \frac{2.59}{0.92\times10^{-2}}(0.772 - 0.703) = 19.1$$

$$C_C = 100 - 77.2 - 19.1 = 3.7$$

10.6. How will the plot of the concentrations given by (*10.17*) look for $k_1 > 100k_2$ and for $100k_1 < k_2$?

In both cases C_A will decrease exponentially with a rate constant of k_1; C_B will essentially be given by $C_{A,0}e^{-k_2t}$ and $(k_1C_{A,0}/k_2)e^{-k_1t}$, respectively; and C_C will essentially be given by $C_{A,0}(1 - e^{-k_2t})$ and $C_{A,0}(1 - e^{-k_1t})$, respectively.

Determination of Reaction Order and Rate Constants

10.7. Determine a and b in the rate equation

$$\text{rate} = kC_A^a C_B^b$$

given the following:

rate, $M\ s^{-1}$	0.05	0.10	0.20	0.40
$C_{A,0}$, M	1	1	2	2
$C_{B,0}$, M	1	2	1	2

Calculate k for this reaction.

To determine the order for substance B, substitute the first two entries ($C_{A,0}$ fixed) of the data into (*10.18*), obtaining

$$\log(0.05) = \log k_B + b \log 1 \qquad \log(0.10) = \log k_B + b \log 2$$

which upon solving gives $b = 1$. Likewise using the first and third entries ($C_{B,0}$ fixed) gives

$$\log(0.05) = \log k_A + a \log 1 \qquad \log(0.20) = \log k_A + a \log 2$$

whence $a = 2$. Thus the rate equation is

$$\text{rate} = kC_A^2 C_B$$

The same rate equation could be derived by direct inspection of the data.

To determine k, the rate equation is solved for k and a set of data substituted, giving

$$k = \frac{(\text{rate})}{C_A^2 C_B} = \frac{0.20\ M\ s^{-1}}{(2M)^2(1M)} = 0.05\ M^{-2}\ s^{-1}$$

As a check, the predicted rate for $C_A = C_B = 2M$ is

$$\text{rate} = (0.05)(2)^2(2) = 0.40$$

which agrees with the fourth entry in the data.

10.8. The half-life for a given reaction was halved as the initial concentration of a reactant was doubled. What is n for this component?

Substituting the data into (*10.19*) gives

$$\log t_{1/2} = \log \frac{2^{n-1}-1}{(n-1)k} - (n-1)\log C_{i,0}$$

$$\log \frac{t_{1/2}}{2} = \log \frac{2^{n-1}-1}{(n-1)k} - (n-1)\log 2C_{i,0}$$

and solving by subtraction gives $n = 2$.

10.9. Williams and Petrucci studied the system

$$\text{Ni(NCS)}^+ + \text{NCS}^- \underset{k_r}{\overset{k_f}{\rightleftharpoons}} \text{Ni(NCS)}_2$$

at 25 °C in methanol using a pressure-jump technique and obtained the following data:

$C_{\mathrm{Ni(NCS)_2}}$, M	0.001	0.002	0.005	0.010	0.025	0.05	0.10
τ, ms	4.08	3.74	2.63	1.84	1.31	0.88	0.67

Determine k_f, k_r and K.

In Example 10.11 it was shown that

$$\frac{1}{\tau} = k_r + k_f(C_{\mathrm{Ni(NCS)^+},e} + C_{\mathrm{NCS^-},e})$$

with $C_{\mathrm{Ni(NCS)^+},e} = C_{\mathrm{NCS^-},e}$. As for the third component,

$$C_{\mathrm{Ni(NCS)_2},e} = C_{\mathrm{Ni(NCS)_2}}\left(1 - \frac{\alpha}{100}\right)$$

where $C_{\mathrm{Ni(NCS)_2}}$ is the total (associated plus dissociated) concentration and α is the percent dissociation. Assuming that K will be large, and therefore that α will be small, we have

$$K = \frac{k_f}{k_r} = \frac{C_{\mathrm{Ni(NCS)_2},e}}{[C_{\mathrm{Ni(NCS)^+},e}]^2}$$

$$\approx \frac{C_{\mathrm{Ni(NCS)_2}}}{[C_{\mathrm{Ni(NCS)^+},e}]^2}$$

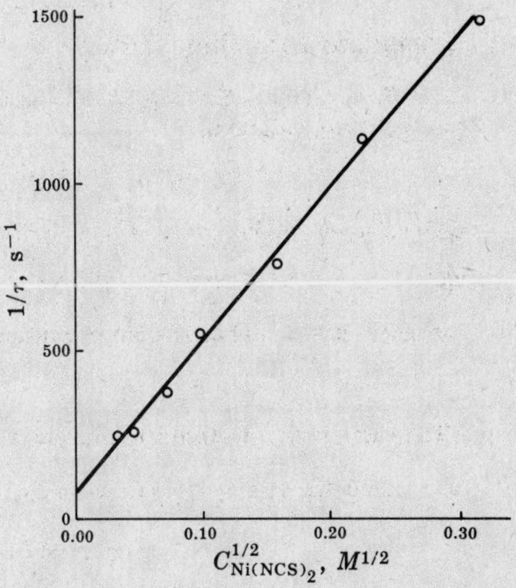

Fig. 10-6

and the formula for the relaxation time becomes

$$\frac{1}{\tau} = k_r + 2(k_f k_r)^{1/2} C^{1/2}_{\mathrm{Ni(NCS)_2}}$$

A plot of $1/\tau$ against $C^{1/2}_{\mathrm{Ni(NCS)_2}}$, see Fig. 10-6, is linear with a slope of 4600 $M^{-1/2}\ \mathrm{s}^{-1}$ and an intercept of $k_r = 78\ \mathrm{s}^{-1}$. The value of k_f is

$$k_f = \left[\frac{\text{(slope)}}{2k_r^{1/2}}\right]^2 = \left[\frac{4600}{(2)(78)^{1/2}}\right]^2 = 6.8 \times 10^4\ M^{-1}\ \mathrm{s}^{-1}$$

and the value of K is

$$K = \frac{6.8 \times 10^4}{78} = 870$$

10.10. Consider the gaseous decomposition reaction of cyclopentene to H_2 and cyclopentadiene:

$$\text{c-}C_5H_8 = H_2 + \text{c-}C_5H_6$$

(*a*) How is dP/dt related to $-dC_{\mathrm{C_5H_8}}/dt$? (*b*) If the reaction is first-order, what are the units on k? (*c*) Derive the first-order integrated rate equation in terms of $P_{\mathrm{C_5H_8},0}$ and P.

(*a*) The total pressure is given by (*1.7*) as

$$P = P_{\mathrm{C_5H_8}} + P_{\mathrm{H_2}} + P_{\mathrm{C_5H_6}}$$

The stoichiometry of the reaction is such that

$$P_{\mathrm{H_2}} = P_{\mathrm{C_5H_6}} = P_{\mathrm{C_5H_8},0} - P_{\mathrm{C_5H_8}}$$

Hence $$P = P_{C_5H_8} + 2(P_{C_5H_8,0} - P_{C_5H_8}) = 2P_{C_5H_8,0} - P_{C_5H_8}$$

Taking derivatives gives $$\frac{dP}{dt} = -\frac{dP_{C_5H_8}}{dt}$$

(*b*) The units of k are s^{-1}, independent of whether concentration or pressure is used.

(*c*) For a first-order reaction
$$-\frac{d}{dt}(P_{C_5H_8}) = kP_{C_5H_8}$$

Then, by (*a*), $$\frac{dP}{dt} = kP_{C_5H_8} = k(2P_{C_5H_8,0} - P)$$

which integrates to $$\ln [P_{C_5H_8,0}/(2P_{C_5H_8,0} - P)] = kt$$

Influence of Temperature

10.11. For the reaction described in Problem 10.9 a more careful analysis of the data gave:

T, °C	19.7	25	30	33.5
$k_f \times 10^{-5}$, $M^{-1}\ s^{-1}$	0.66	1.40	2.21	3.32
k_r, s^{-1}	27	73	72	91

Find ΔE_f^* and ΔE_r^* and prepare a reaction coordinate diagram.

Plots of $\log k$ against $1/T$ are shown in Fig. 10-7. From the slopes of the lines, (*10.22a*) gives

$$\Delta E_f^* = -(2.303)R(\text{slope}) = -(2.303)(8.314\ \text{J mol}^{-1}\ \text{K}^{-1})(-4200\ \text{K}) = 80.4\ \text{kJ mol}^{-1}$$

$$\Delta E_r^* = -(2.303)(8.314)(-7000) = 134.0\ \text{kJ mol}^{-1}$$

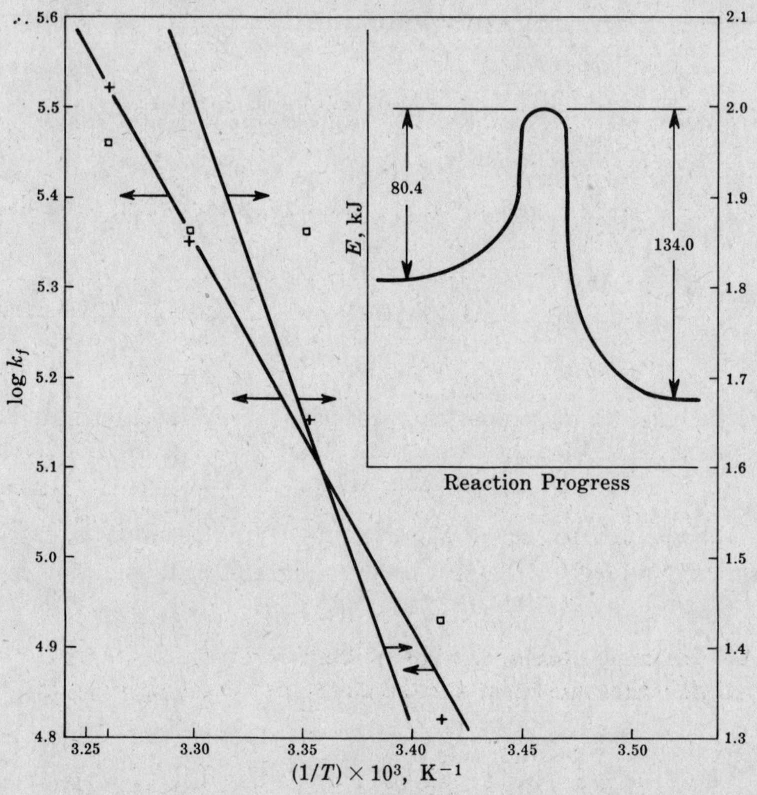

Fig. 10-7

Equation (*10.23*) gives for the reaction

$$\Delta E^\circ = 80.4 - 134.0 = -53.6 \text{ kJ}$$

The reaction coordinate diagram is shown as an insert in Fig. 10-7.

Catalysis

10.12. The pseudo-first-order rate constant for the cobalt-catalyzed autooxidation of toluene in acetic acid at 87 °C was determined for several concentrations of the catalyst, Co(III), by Scott and Chester. The data are

$k \times 10^5$, s^{-1}	1.47	2.93	5.68
$C_{Co(III)}$, M	0.053	0.084	0.1185

for $C_{C_6H_5CH_3,0} = 0.5\,M$. Find the order with respect to $C_{Co(III)}$ and the rate constant.

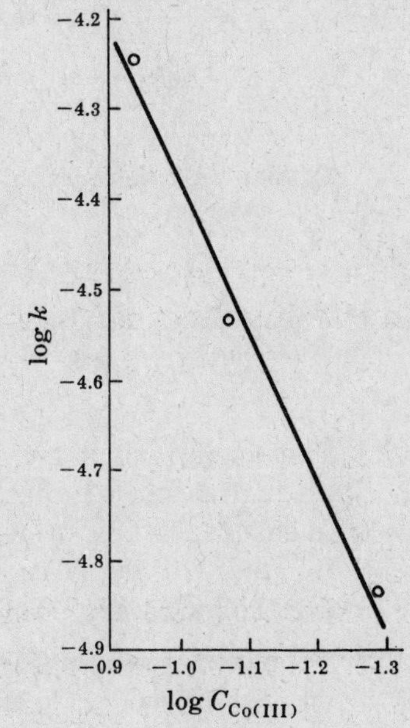

Fig. 10-8

Assuming k to be defined in terms of the rate constant k' as

$$k = k'[C_{Co(III)}]^n$$

this definition can be put into linear form by taking logarithms, giving

$$\log k = \log k' + n \log C_{Co(III)}$$

Thus a plot of $\log k$ against $\log C_{Co(III)}$ will give a straight line with slope n and intercept $\log k'$. From Fig. 10-8, $n = 1.71$ (nearly 2) and then, from the data,

$$k' \approx \frac{2.93 \times 10^{-5}}{(0.084)^2} = 4.15 \times 10^{-3}\ M^{-2}\ s^{-1}$$

10.13. The thermal decomposition of 3-chloro-3-phenyldiazirine in various solvents has been studied by Liu and Toriyama. Show from the data below that the catalytic solvent effect is negligible for the solvents dimethyl sulfoxide (DMSO) and diethylene glycol monoethyl ether (DEGME).

T, °C	60.0	65.0	70.0	75.0	80.0	85.0	90.0
$k \times 10^4$ in DMSO, s^{-1}	0.47		1.60	3.04	5.00		15.8
$k \times 10^4$ in DEGME, s^{-1}		0.70	1.32	2.30	4.00	6.90	

The ΔE^* values for the reaction in the two solvents, as determined from an Arrhenius plot similar to Fig. 10-2, are 117.6 kJ mol^{-1} and 114.7 kJ mol^{-1} for DMSO and DEGME, respectively. Because these values are within 3% of each other, there is very little difference between the solvents in their catalytic effect.

10.14. Consider the following mechanism describing competitive inhibition of an enzyme catalyst in which the substrate and inhibitor are competing in the binding to the enzyme:

$$E + S \underset{k_{-1}}{\overset{k_1}{\rightleftharpoons}} X \underset{k_{-2}}{\overset{k_2}{\rightleftharpoons}} E + P \qquad E + I \underset{k_{-3}}{\overset{k_3}{\rightleftharpoons}} EI$$

where I is the inhibitor and the inhibition can be described by $K_I = C_E C_I / C_{EI}$. Derive the rate equation for this process during the initial stages of the reaction where the formation of X from E reacting with P is negligible. Assume $dC_X/dt = 0$.

The rate equations for this mechanism are

$$\frac{dC_X}{dt} = 0 = k_1 C_E C_S - k_{-1} C_X - k_2 C_X \qquad \frac{dC_P}{dt} = k_2 C_X$$

where $C_{E,0} = C_E + C_X + C_{EI}$. Eliminating C_X, C_E and C_{EI} gives

$$\frac{dC_P}{dt} = \frac{k_1 k_2 C_{E,0} C_S}{k_1 C_S + k_{-1} + k_{-1}(C_I/K_I) + k_2 + k_2(C_I/K_I)} = \frac{V_S C_S}{C_S + K_S[1 + (C_I/K_I)]}$$

Casting the rate equation into the Lineweaver-Burk form (Example 10.15) gives

$$\left(\frac{dC_P}{dt}\right)^{-1} = \frac{K_S}{V_S}\left(1 + \frac{C_I}{K_I}\right) C_S^{-1} + V_S^{-1}$$

A plot of $(dC_P/dt)^{-1}$ against C_S^{-1} will be linear, having an intercept of V_S^{-1}, as in the case of no inhibition, and a slope of $(K_S/V_S)(1 + C_I/K_I)$, greater than in the case of no inhibition.

10.15. The amount of a gas adsorbed on a solid has a rather definite correlation with the critical point of the gas. If 1 kg of charcoal at 15 °C will adsorb 8.0×10^{-3} m³ (measured at STP) of N_2 and 380×10^{-3} m³ of SO_2, approximately what volumes of CO_2 and Cl_2 would be adsorbed under similar conditions? The critical temperatures for the gases are −146.9 °C for N_2, 31 °C for CO_2, 144 °C for Cl_2 and 157.4 °C for SO_2.

Based on the order of the critical temperatures, the volumes of CO_2 and Cl_2 should be greater than the volume of N_2 and less than the volume of SO_2. Less CO_2 should be adsorbed than Cl_2. The observed values are 48×10^{-3} m³ for CO_2 and 235×10^{-3} m³ for Cl_2, which agree with this prediction.

10.16. For an adsorbate on the surface of an adsorbent, the *Gibbs adsorption coefficient* Γ is related to the surface tension, γ, and the activity of the adsorbate, a_2, by

$$\Gamma = -\frac{a_2}{RT}\frac{d\gamma}{da_2} = -\frac{1}{RT}\frac{d\gamma}{d(\ln a_2)} \qquad (10.42)$$

If glycerol raises the surface tension of water as it is added, will adsorption occur at the water-air interface?

For dilute solutions where the activity coefficient is essentially unity, (*9.9*) gives $a_2 = x_2$ and the Gibbs adsorption equation becomes

$$\Gamma = -\frac{x_2}{RT}\frac{d\gamma}{dx_2}$$

Because $d\gamma/dx_2$ is positive, Γ will be negative and glycerol will be negatively adsorbed.

10.17. An equation similar to (*3.15b*) describes the temperature dependence of the amount of gas adsorbed on the surface of a solid. Find ΔH(adsorption) for N_2 at 1 atm if 155 cm³ (measured at STP) is adsorbed by 1 g of charcoal at 88 K, and 15 cm³ at 273 K.

Solving
$$\ln\frac{V_2}{V_1} = -\frac{\Delta H}{R}\left(\frac{1}{T_2} - \frac{1}{T_1}\right) \qquad (10.43)$$

for ΔH and substituting the data gives

$$\Delta H = \frac{-R\ln(V_2/V_1)}{\dfrac{1}{T_2} - \dfrac{1}{T_1}} = \frac{-(8.314\ \text{J mol}^{-1}\ \text{K}^{-1})\ln(155/15)}{\dfrac{1}{88\ \text{K}} - \dfrac{1}{273\ \text{K}}} = -2.52\ \text{kJ mol}^{-1}$$

10.18. Show that for $n = 1$ the BET isotherm gives the Langmuir isotherm.

For $n = 1$, (*10.27*) becomes

$$V = \frac{V_m c(P/P^\circ)}{1-(P/P^\circ)} \frac{1-2(P/P^\circ)+(P/P^\circ)^2}{1+(c-1)(P/P^\circ)-c(P/P^\circ)^2}$$

$$= \frac{V_m c(P/P^\circ)}{1-(P/P^\circ)} \frac{[1-(P/P^\circ)]^2}{[1+c(P/P^\circ)][1-(P/P^\circ)]} = \frac{V_m c(P/P^\circ)}{1+c(P/P^\circ)} = \frac{V_m bP}{1+bP}$$

if $b = c/P^\circ$.

10.19. Langmuir reported the following results for the adsorption of N_2 on mica at 90 K:

P, N m^{-2}	0.28	0.34	0.40	0.49	0.60	0.73	0.94	1.28	1.71	2.35	3.35
V, mm^3(20 °C, 1 atm) g^{-1}	12.0	13.4	15.1	17.0	19.0	21.6	23.9	25.5	28.2	30.8	33.0

(*a*) Show that these data obey the Freundlich isotherm at low pressures. (*b*) Find the number of moles of N_2 equivalent to V_m if $b = 1.56 \text{ m}^2 \text{ N}^{-1}$. (*c*) What is the surface area of the mica phase?

(*a*) Equation (*10.24*) can be transformed into a linear equation by taking logarithms of both sides, giving

$$\log V = \log k + n \log P$$

From a plot of $\log V$ against $\log P$, see Fig. 10-9, the intercept is 1.423, giving

$$k = \text{antilog}(1.423) = 26.5$$

and the slope of the straight line through the low-pressure data is $0.617 = n$.

(*b*) Eliminating θ in (*10.25*) and (*10.26*), solving the resulting equation for V_m, and substituting the value of b and the data for 0.40 N m^{-2} gives

$$V_m = \frac{V(1+bP)}{bP} = \frac{(15.1 \text{ mm}^3 \text{ g}^{-1})[1+(1.56 \text{ m}^2 \text{ N}^{-1})(0.40 \text{ N m}^{-2})]}{(1.56)(0.40)} = 39.3 \text{ mm}^3 \text{ g}^{-1}$$

which upon converting to moles becomes

$$n = \frac{(1 \text{ atm})(39.3\times10^{-9} \text{ m}^3 \text{ g}^{-1})}{(8.21\times10^{-5} \text{ m}^3 \text{ mol}^{-1} \text{ K}^{-1})(293 \text{ K})} = 1.63\times10^{-6} \text{ (mol N}_2\text{)(g mica)}^{-1}$$

(*c*) The number of molecules covering the surface of the mica is

$$[1.63\times10^{-6} \text{ (mol N}_2\text{)(g mica)}^{-1}](6.022\times10^{23} \text{ mol}^{-1}) = 9.82\times10^{17} \text{ g}^{-1}$$

Assuming a density of 0.8081×10^3 kg m^{-3} for liquid N_2, the area covered by a single molecule is approximately

$$\left[\frac{28.0\times10^{-3} \text{ kg mol}^{-1}}{(0.8081\times10^3 \text{ kg m}^{-3})(6.022\times10^{23} \text{ mol}^{-1})}\right]^{2/3} = 14.9\times10^{-20} \text{ m}^2$$

The area of adsorption is the product of these results, i.e.

$$(9.82\times10^{17} \text{ g}^{-1})(14.9\times10^{-20} \text{ m}^2) = 0.146 \text{ m}^2 \text{ g}^{-1}$$

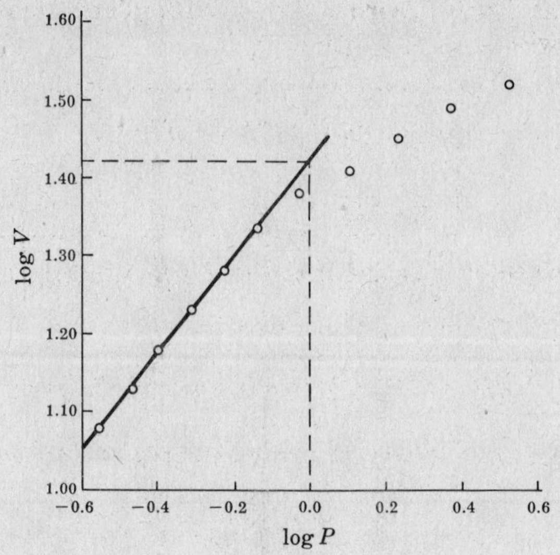

Fig. 10-9

10.20. Derive the integrated rate equation for the special case in which substance A is only slightly adsorbed. Show that the following data describing the decomposition of N_2O on Au at 900 °C satisfy this rate equation:

t, s	0	1800	4800	7200
P_{N_2O}, torr	200	136	70	44

Substituting (*10.26*) into (*10.31*) gives

$$-\frac{d}{dt}(P_{N_2O}) = \frac{k'bP_{N_2O}}{1 + bP_{N_2O}}$$

which upon making the approximation $1 \gg bP_{N_2O}$ becomes

$$-\frac{d}{dt}(P_{N_2O}) = k'bP_{N_2O} = kP_{N_2O}$$

a first-order reaction. Integration and substitution of proper limits give

$$\ln(P_{N_2O}/P_{N_2O,0}) = -kt$$

Although the value of k could be determined from the slope of a plot of the logarithm against t, it is easier to calculate k for the three sets of data and find an average of these values. For $t = 1800$ s,

$$k = -\frac{\ln(136/200)}{1800 \text{ s}} = 2.14 \times 10^{-4} \text{ s}^{-1}$$

and for the other data, $k = 2.19 \times 10^{-4} \text{ s}^{-1}$ and $2.10 \times 10^{-4} \text{ s}^{-1}$, giving an average of $2.14 \times 10^{-4} \text{ s}^{-1}$.

10.21. Derive (*10.30*) for the case of two gases, A and B, being adsorbed.

Recognizing that the fraction of surface uncovered is $1 - \theta_A - \theta_B$, the rates of adsorption are

$$k_{1,A}P_A(1 - \theta_A - \theta_B) \qquad \text{and} \qquad k_{1,B}P_B(1 - \theta_A - \theta_B)$$

and the rates of desorption are $k_{2,A}\theta_A$ and $k_{2,B}\theta_B$. Equating these rates for equilibrium gives

$$\theta_A = \frac{b_AP_A}{1 + b_AP_A + b_BP_B} \qquad \theta_B = \frac{b_BP_B}{1 + b_AP_A + b_BP_B}$$

10.22. Hinshelwood and Burk reported the following data for the decomposition of NH_3 on Pt at 1138 °C with $P_{NH_3,0} = 100$ torr:

$-\Delta P_{NH_3}/\Delta t$, torr s^{-1}	0.275	0.133	0.083
P_{H_2}, torr	50	100	150

Show that these data indicate that the H_2 is strongly adsorbed after it is formed.

The rate of decomposition of NH_3 is given by

$$-\frac{d}{dt}(P_{NH_3}) = k'(1-\theta_{NH_3}-\theta_{H_2}-\theta_{N_2})P_{NH_3} \approx k'(1-\theta_{H_2})P_{NH_3}$$

assuming $\theta_{H_2} \gg \theta_{NH_3}, \theta_{N_2}$. Making the same assumption for the denominator of (*10.30*) gives

$$\theta_{H_2} = \frac{b_{H_2}P_{H_2}}{1+b_{H_2}P_{H_2}}$$

The expression for $1-\theta_{H_2}$ is

$$1-\theta_{H_2} = \frac{1}{1+b_{H_2}P_{H_2}} = \frac{1}{b_{H_2}P_{H_2}}$$

where $b_{H_2}P_{H_2} \gg 1$. Substitution into the rate equation gives

$$-\frac{d}{dt}(P_{NH_3}) = (k'/b_{H_2})(P_{NH_3}/P_{H_2}) = kP_{NH_3}/P_{H_2}$$

The values of $k = (-\Delta P_{NH_3}/\Delta t)(P_{H_2}/P_{NH_3})$ using the above data are 0.138, 0.133 and 0.125 torr s^{-1}, which are reasonably constant and imply that the rate equation is valid.

Photochemistry

10.23. Shapiro and Treinin recommend the following reaction for use as an *actinometer*—a device for counting quanta:

$$HN_3 + H_2O + h\nu \longrightarrow N_2 + NH_2OH$$

Find ϕ for the reaction if $I = 1.00 \times 10^{-7}$ einstein dm^{-3} s^{-1} at 214 nm and $C_{N_2} = C_{NH_2OH} = 24.1 \times 10^{-5}M$ after a period of radiation of 39.38 min.

On a 1-dm^3 basis, the number of moles formed each second is

$$n = \frac{24.1\times10^{-5}\text{ mol}}{(39.38\text{ min})(60\text{ s min}^{-1})} = 1.02\times10^{-7}\text{ mol s}^{-1}$$

and

$$\phi = \frac{1.02\times10^{-7}\text{ mol s}^{-1}}{1.00\times10^{-7}\text{ einstein s}^{-1}} = 1.02$$

10.24. Consider the proposed mechanism for the photodimerization of A:

$$A + h\nu \xrightarrow{k_1} A^* \qquad A^* + A \xrightarrow{k_2} A_2 \qquad A^* \xrightarrow{k_3} A + h\nu'$$

Derive the expression for $\phi(A_2)$.

Under steady-state conditions

$$\frac{dC_{A^*}}{dt} = 0 = k_1I - k_2C_{A^*}C_A - k_3C_{A^*}$$

where I is the intensity of the light absorbed. Upon rearrangement,

$$C_{A*} = \frac{k_1 I}{k_2 C_A + k_3}$$

The formation of A_2 is given by

$$\frac{d}{dt}(C_{A_2}) = k_2 C_{A*} C_A = \frac{k_1 k_2 I C_A}{k_2 C_A + k_3}$$

and

$$\phi(A_2) = \frac{dC_{A_2}/dt}{I} = \frac{k_1 k_2 C_A}{k_2 C_A + k_3}$$

Reaction Rate Theory

10.25. Predict $\mathcal{A}$ for the reaction

$$Cl(g) + H_2(g) \longrightarrow HCl(g) + H(g)$$

if $M = 35.453\ \text{g mol}^{-1}$ for Cl and $2.01594\ \text{g mol}^{-1}$ for H_2 and $\sigma = 2.00$ Å for Cl and 1.50 Å for H_2. If the value of $\log \mathcal{A}$ is 10.08 between 250 K and 450 K, find p and interpret the result.

The pre-exponential factor at 350 K is given by *(10.34a)* as

$$\mathcal{A} = (2.753 \times 10^{29})p\left[\frac{1}{2}(2.00 + 1.50)10^{-10}\right]^2\left[\frac{350(35.453 + 2.01594)}{(35.453)(2.01594)}\right]^{1/2}$$

$$= 1.142 \times 10^{11} p$$

Comparing the predicted value of $\mathcal{A}$ to the observed value, antilog (10.08), gives

$$p = \frac{\text{antilog}\ (10.08)}{1.142 \times 10^{11}} = \frac{1.2 \times 10^{10}}{1.142 \times 10^{11}} = 0.11$$

A reasonably high value for p would be expected for this reaction because the Cl can combine with either end of the H_2 molecule to eventually form the products.

10.26. (*a*) Deduce the structure of the activated complex formed between Cl and H_2 in the reaction described in Problem 10.25 and confirm the entries in Table 10-1 for this configuration by calculating the approximate values of $\mathcal{A}$ and p, assuming $q_{\text{trans}} = 10^{10}$, $q_{\text{rot}} = 10$ and $q_{\text{vib}} = 1$ *for each degree of freedom.* (*b*) If the temperature exponent is 1/2 for each translational and rotational degree of freedom, and 0 to 1 for each vibrational degree of freedom, predict the temperature exponent in $\mathcal{A}$ (maximum value is 1/2).

(*a*) Problem 10.25 gave $\mathcal{A} = 1.2 \times 10^{10}$ and $p = 0.11$. For the reaction between an atom and a linear molecule, the entries in Table 10-1 are $\mathcal{A} = 10^{10}$ and $p = 10^{-2}$ for a linear complex, and $\mathcal{A} = 10^{11}$ and $p = 10^{-1}$ for a nonlinear complex. Giving more weight to the value of p because the errors in its estimation tend to cancel, the predicted activated complex is nonlinear.

To confirm the table value of $\mathcal{A}$, *(10.35)* is applied to the reaction of an atom A with a linear molecule B to form a nonlinear activated complex $(AB)^{\#}$. For each component, every degree of freedom gives rise to a factor in the partition function; hence *(10.36)* gives

$$Q_A = q_{\text{trans}}\, q_{\text{rot}}\, q_{\text{vib}} = (10^{10})^3(10)^0(1)^0 = 10^{30}$$

$$Q_B = q_{\text{trans}}\, q_{\text{rot}}\, q_{\text{vib}} = (10^{10})^3(10)^2(1)^1 = 10^{32}$$

$$Q_{\#} = q_{\text{trans}}\, q_{\text{rot}}\, q_{\text{vib}} = (10^{10})^3(10)^3(1)^2 = 10^{33}$$

Substituting into (*10.35*) and converting to $dm^3\ mol^{-1}\ s^{-1}$ gives

$$\mathcal{A} = \frac{kT}{h}(10^3L)\frac{Q_\#}{Q_AQ_B} = (4\times10^{39})\frac{10^{33}}{10^{30}10^{32}} = 4\times10^{10}$$

which is in good agreement with the table entry of 10^{11}.

The value of p for this reaction is found by comparing the estimated value of $\mathcal{A}$ to that for the reaction of rigid spheres interacting to form a diatomic activated complex. For the latter reaction,

$$Q_A = Q_B = (10^{10})^3(10)^0(1)^0 = 10^{30}$$

As for $Q_\#$, the activated complex has, according to Section 10.20, $3(1)+3(1)-6=0$ degrees of vibrational freedom attributed to it, so that

$$Q_\# = (10^{10})^3(10)^2(1)^0 = 10^{32}$$

Then

$$\mathcal{A} = p(4\times10^{39})\frac{10^{32}}{10^{30}10^{30}} = p(4\times10^{11})$$

from which $p = 10^{-1}$.

(*b*) Multiplying partition functions means adding temperature exponents. Hence, as above

$$Q_A \propto (T^{1/2})^3(T^{1/2})^0(T^\theta)^0 = T^{3/2}$$

$$Q_B \propto (T^{1/2})^3(T^{1/2})^2(T^\theta)^1 = T^{5/2+\theta}$$

$$Q_\# \propto (T^{1/2})^3(T^{1/2})^3(T^\theta)^2 = T^{3+2\theta}$$

where θ stands for a number between 0 and 1. Then,

$$\mathcal{A} \propto T\frac{Q_\#}{Q_AQ_B} \propto T\frac{T^{3+2\theta}}{T^{3/2}T^{5/2+\theta}} = T^\theta$$

Because the exponent cannot exceed 1/2, see Table 10-1, it must be between 0 and 1/2.

10.27. Estimate $\Delta S^\circ_\#$ for the reaction

$$A + B \overset{K}{\rightleftharpoons} (AB)^\#$$

where A is an atom, B is a diatomic molecule and $(AB)^\#$ is a nonlinear triatomic molecule.

Before the formation of the complex, the system had 3 degrees of translational freedom for A and 3 degrees of translational freedom, 2 degrees of rotational freedom and 1 degree of vibrational freedom for B, giving a total of 6 translational, 2 rotational and 1 vibrational degrees of freedom. After the formation of the complex, the system has 3 translational, 3 rotational and 2 vibrational degrees of freedom. Assuming numerical values similar to those calculated in Example 6.14 for the various modes, $\Delta S^\circ_\#$ will be quite negative for this process:

$$\Delta S^\circ_\# = [3S^\circ(\text{trans})+3S^\circ(\text{rot})+2S^\circ(\text{vib})] - [6S^\circ(\text{trans})+2S^\circ(\text{rot})+S^\circ(\text{vib})]$$

$$= S^\circ(\text{rot})+S^\circ(\text{vib})-3S^\circ(\text{trans}) \approx 30+1-3(50) \approx -120\ \text{EU}$$

10.28. Calculate $\Delta S^\circ_\#$ at 350 K for the reaction described in Problem 10.25. Does this value agree with the results of Problems 10.26 and 10.27, which predicted a nonlinear complex being formed with $\Delta S^\circ_\#$ estimated as -120 EU?

Solving (*10.39*) for $\Delta S^\circ_\#$ and substituting $\mathcal{A} = 1.2\times10^{10}$ gives

$$\Delta S^\circ_\# = R\left[\ln\left(\frac{\mathcal{A}h}{kt}\right)-n\right] = (8.314)\left\{\ln\left[\frac{(1.2\times10^{10})(6.626\times10^{-34})}{(1.3807\times10^{-23})(350)}\right]-2\right\}$$

$$= (8.314)[\ln(1.6\times10^{-3})-2] = -70\ \text{EU}$$

This value is about half of the estimate made in Problem 10.27, which is fair agreement.

Supplementary Problems

Rate Equations for Simple Reactions

10.29. For the reaction $I_2(g) + H_2(g) \longrightarrow 2HI(g)$, evaluate the expressions for the rate in terms of $-dC_{I_2}/dt$. *Ans.* $dC_{HI}/dt = 2(-dC_{I_2}/dt)$, $-dC_{H_2}/dt = -dC_{I_2}/dt$

10.30. If the actual reaction equation for the H_2-I_2 system described in Problem 10.29 is identical to the stoichiometric equation, write the simple rate equation. What is the overall order of this reaction and the order with respect to each reactant?

Ans. rate $= kC_{H_2}C_{I_2}$, second, first for each

10.31. Discuss the following overall reactions with respect to order, catalysts, etc.

(*a*) $2A \longrightarrow 4B + C,\quad -\dfrac{dC_A}{dt} = kC_A$

(*b*) $2A + B \longrightarrow 2C + D + B,\quad -\dfrac{dC_A}{dt} = kC_AC_B$

(*c*) $2A + B \longrightarrow 2C,\quad \dfrac{dC_C}{dt} = kC_A^2C_B$

(*d*) $A + B \longrightarrow C,\quad \dfrac{dC_C}{dt} = kC_AC_B^{-1}$

(*e*) $2A + B \longrightarrow 2C,\quad \dfrac{dC_C}{dt} = kC_AC_C^{-1/2}$

(*f*) $A + 2B \longrightarrow C + D,\quad \dfrac{dC_C}{dt} = kC_AC_B^2C_C$

Ans. (*a*) first-order in A, first-order overall

(*b*) first-order in A, first-order in B (catalyst), second-order overall

(*c*) second-order in A, first-order in B, third-order overall

(*d*) first-order in A, negative first-order in B (reactant is inhibitor), zero-order overall

(*e*) first-order in A, negative $\frac{1}{2}$-order in C (product is negative catalyst), $\frac{1}{2}$-order overall

(*f*) first-order in A, second-order in B, first-order in C (product is catalyst), fourth-order overall

10.32. Find the overall order of a reaction for which the half-life and the units of k do not involve molarity.

Ans. For a first-order reaction, $t_{1/2} = (\ln 2)/k$ and units of k are s^{-1}.

10.33. (*a*) Integrate the rate equation

$$-\frac{dC}{dt} = kC^{1/2}$$

(*b*) How could a group of data be checked graphically to see if they describe a half-order reaction?

(*c*) Derive an expression for $t_{1/2}$ in terms of k and C_0. (*d*) What are the units of k?

Ans. (*a*) $2(C_0^{1/2} - C^{1/2}) = kt$

(*b*) plot of $C^{1/2}$ against t would be linear

(*c*) $t^{1/2} = 0.586\, C_0^{1/2}/k$

(*d*) $\text{mol}^{1/2}\ \text{dm}^{-3/2}\ \text{s}^{-1}$

10.34. Consider a decomposition reaction, A = products, which is catalyzed by a finely divided solid. If there are only enough "active sites" on the catalyst so that five molecules of A can react each second, what is the rate of reaction for a $1M$ solution of A? Does this change for a $2M$ solution?

Ans. 5 molecules s^{-1}; no

10.35. In the region of constant Co(III) concentration, the following data were obtained by Scott and Chester for the autooxidation of toluene in acetic acid at 88 °C:

$C_{C_6H_5CH_3}$, M	0.282	0.229	0.200	0.168	0.130
t, min	104	143	192	252	321

Determine k for this first-order reaction. *Ans.* $5.68 \times 10^{-5}\ \mathrm{s}^{-1}$

10.36. The reaction between ozone and CS_2 was studied at 29.3 °C with excess CS_2 to find the order of reaction with respect to O_3. From the following data by Olszyna and Heicklen prove that the reaction is second-order and determine the pseudo-second-order rate constant.

t, min	0.0	0.5	1.0	2.0	3.0	4.0
P_{O_3}, torr	1.76	1.04	0.79	0.52	0.37	0.29

Ans. plot of $1/P_{O_3}$ against t is linear, slope gives $k = 1.20 \times 10^{-2}\ \mathrm{torr}^{-1}\ \mathrm{s}^{-1}$

10.37. The kinetics for the reaction

$$A + B \xrightarrow{k} \text{products}$$

are known to be third-order. From the following data, determine m and n in the rate equation

$$-\frac{dC_A}{dt} = kC_A^m C_B^n$$

by calculating values of k using variations of *(10.14)* until a constant value is reached.

t, s	0	5	10
C_A, M	0.750	0.700	0.665
C_B, M	0.500	0.450	0.415

Ans. $k = 0.0400$ and $0.0352\ M^{-2}\ \mathrm{s}^{-1}$ using *(10.14)* for $m=2$ and $n=1$, not very constant;
$k = 0.0605$ and $0.0579\ M^{-2}\ \mathrm{s}^{-1}$ using *(10.14)* rewritten for $m=1$ and $n=2$, rather constant;
$k = 0.0592\ M^{-2}\ \mathrm{s}^{-1}$

10.38. The second-order reaction

$$OH^- + C_2H_5OH \longrightarrow C_2H_5O^- + H_2O$$

when studied in 0.1 M NaOH gave the pseudo-first-order rate equation

$$-\frac{d}{dt}(C_{C_2H_5OH}) = kC_{C_2H_5OH}$$

with $k = 3 \times 10^5\ \mathrm{s}^{-1}$. Find the rate constant for the second-order reaction.

Ans. $k_2 = k/C_{OH^-} = 3 \times 10^6\ M^{-1}\ \mathrm{s}^{-1}$

Rate Equations for Complex Reactions

10.39. Consider the following mechanism

$$A + A \underset{k_{-2}}{\overset{k_2}{\rightleftharpoons}} A^* + A \qquad\qquad A^* \xrightarrow{k_1} \text{products}$$

used to describe the decomposition of a gaseous molecule. (a) Write the differential rate equations for $-dC_A/dt$ and dC_{A*}/dt and assuming a steady-state approximation for C_{A*}, write $-dC_A/dt$ in terms of C_A and rate constants. (b) Under what conditions is this a pseudo-first-order reaction? (c) A pseudo-second-order reaction?

Ans. (a) $-\dfrac{dC_A}{dt} = k_2 C_A^2 - k_{-2} C_{A*} C_A,$ (b) $k_{-2} C_A \gg 1$

$\dfrac{dC_{A*}}{dt} = k_2 C_A^2 - k_{-2} C_{A*} C_A - k_1 C_{A*},$ (c) $\dfrac{k_{-2} C_A}{k_1} \ll 1$

$-\dfrac{dC_A}{dt} = \dfrac{k_2 C_A^2}{1 + (k_{-2}/k_1) C_A}$

10.40. Consider the opposing first- and second-order reactions

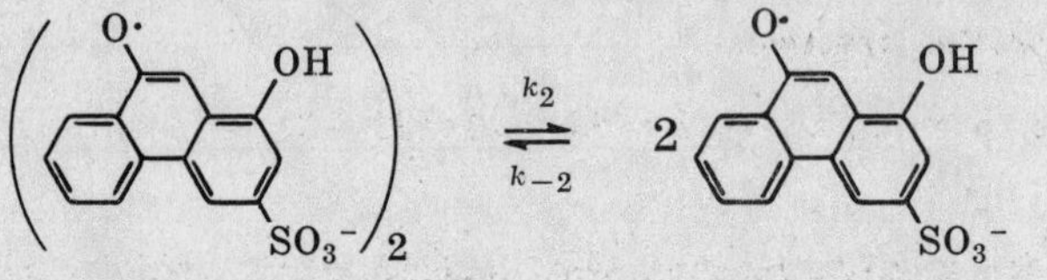

If $k_2 = 1.35 \times 10^3$ s^{-1} and $k_{-2} = 2.41 \times 10^6$ M^{-1} s^{-1}, as reported by Cheung and Swinehart, determine K.   Ans. $K = k_2/k_{-2} = 5.60 \times 10^{-4}$

10.41. The proposed mechanism for the saponification of dimethyl glutarate (DMGL) by NaOH is

$$\text{NaOH} + \text{H}_3\text{COOC(CH}_2)_3\text{COOCH}_3 \xrightarrow{k_1} \text{NaOOC(CH}_2)_3\text{COOCH}_3 + \text{CH}_3\text{OH}$$

$$\text{NaOH} + \text{NaOOC(CH}_2)_3\text{COOCH}_3 \xrightarrow{k_2} \text{NaOOC(CH}_2)_3\text{COONa} + \text{CH}_3\text{OH}$$

If k_1 and k_2 are related to the probability of a Na$^+$ colliding with the CH$_3$-end of the molecule, would k_1 be greater or less than k_2?

Ans. Greater, because Na$^+$ can react with either end of DMGL, but with only one end of the monosubstituted salt.

10.42. $^{214}_{83}$Bi undergoes β^- emission (99.96%) or α emission (0.04%). If the half-life is 19.7 min, find k_α and k_β.   Ans. $k = k_\alpha + k_\beta = 5.86 \times 10^{-4}$ s^{-1}, $k_\alpha = 2.3 \times 10^{-7}$ s^{-1}, $k_\beta = 5.86 \times 10^{-4}$ s^{-1}

10.43. A mixture of products is obtained during the thermal decomposition of cyclobutanone, as shown by the competing reactions

$$\begin{matrix}\text{H}_2\text{C}-\text{C}=\text{O}\\|\qquad|\\\text{H}_2\text{C}-\text{CH}_2\end{matrix} \xrightarrow{k_1} \text{C}_2\text{H}_4 + \text{H}_2\text{C}=\text{C}=\text{O} \qquad \begin{matrix}\text{H}_2\text{C}-\text{C}=\text{O}\\|\qquad|\\\text{H}_2\text{C}-\text{CH}_2\end{matrix} \xrightarrow{k_2} \begin{matrix}\text{H}_2\text{C}\\\quad\diagdown\\\quad\text{H}_2\text{C}\end{matrix}\text{CH}_2 + \text{CO}$$

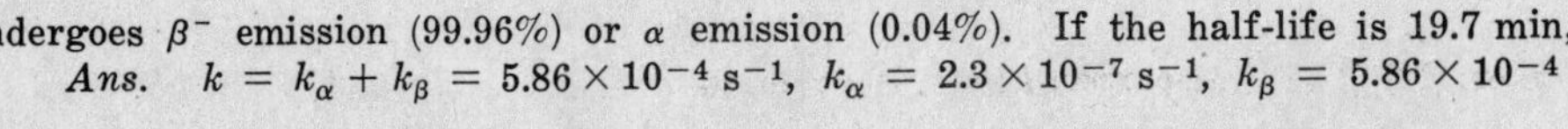

Write the rate equation for $-dC_{\text{C}_4\text{H}_6\text{O}}/dt$ and show that it is first-order. From the following data by McGee and Schleifer at 383 °C for $C_{\text{C}_4\text{H}_6\text{O},0} = 6.50 \times 10^{-5} M$, determine k_1, k_2 and the first-order rate constant for $-dC_{\text{C}_4\text{H}_6\text{O}}/dt$.

t, min	0.5	1.0	3.0	6.0
$C_{\text{C}_2\text{H}_4} \times 10^5$, M	0.31	0.68	1.53	2.63
$C_{\text{c-C}_3\text{H}_6} \times 10^7$, M	0.21	0.47	1.24	2.20

Ans. $-dC_{\text{C}_4\text{H}_6\text{O}}/dt = k_1 C_{\text{C}_4\text{H}_6\text{O}} + k_2 C_{\text{C}_4\text{H}_6\text{O}} = k C_{\text{C}_4\text{H}_6\text{O}}$ where $k = k_1 + k_2$;
plot of $\ln(C_{\text{C}_4\text{H}_6\text{O},0} - C_{\text{C}_2\text{H}_4} - C_{\text{c-C}_3\text{H}_6})$ against t is linear, slope gives $k = 1.39 \times 10^{-3}$ s^{-1};
ratios of $C_{\text{C}_2\text{H}_4}/C_{\text{c-C}_3\text{H}_6}$ give $k_1/k_2 = 120$, $k_1 = 1.38 \times 10^{-3}$ s^{-1}, $k_2 = 1.15 \times 10^{-5}$ s^{-1}

Determination of Reaction Order and Rate Constants

10.44. Determine a, b, and c for the rate equation

$$\text{rate} = kC_A^a C_B^b C_C^c$$

from the following data:

rate $\times 10^5$, $M\ s^{-1}$	5.0	5.0	2.5	14.1
$C_{A,0}$, M	0.010	0.010	0.010	0.020
$C_{B,0}$, M	0.005	0.005	0.010	0.005
$C_{C,0}$, M	0.010	0.015	0.010	0.010

Calculate k for this reaction.

Ans. $a = 3/2$, $b = -1$, $c = 0$, $k = 2.5 \times 10^{-4}\ M^{-1/2}\ s^{-1}$

10.45. The half-life for a given reaction was doubled as the initial concentration of a reactant was doubled. What is n for this component? *Ans.* 0

10.46. Express the relaxation time as a function of k_1 and k_2 for the reaction

$$A \underset{k_2}{\overset{k_1}{\rightleftharpoons}} B$$

Assuming $K = 1.0 \times 10^3$ and $\tau = 10\ \mu s$, find k_1 and k_2.

Ans. $\tau^{-1} = k_1 + k_2$; $K = k_1/k_2$, $k_1 = 1 \times 10^5\ s^{-1}$, $k_2 = 1 \times 10^2\ s^{-1}$

10.47. Show that the relaxation time for the reaction

$$HIn^- \underset{k_2}{\overset{k_1}{\rightleftharpoons}} H^+ + In^{2-}$$

where HIn^- is bromocresol green, is given by

$$\frac{1}{\tau} = k_2(C_{H^+} + C_{In^{2-}}) + k_1$$

From the following data reported by Warrick, Auborn and Eyring, prepare a plot of $1/\tau$ against $C_{H^+} + C_{In^{2-}}$ and determine k_1, k_2 and the equilibrium constant, K.

$(1/\tau) \times 10^6$, s^{-1}	1.01	1.16	3.13	5.56	6.62	7.87	11.24	17.2
$C_{H^+} + C_{In^{2-}}$, μM	4.30	6.91	50.94	85.70	100.5	129.1	176.0	286.5

(Concentrations have been corrected for ionic strength changes.)

Ans. intercept gives $k_1 = 6.75 \times 10^5\ s^{-1}$, slope gives $k_2 = 5.76 \times 10^{10}\ s^{-1}$, $K = 1.17 \times 10^{-5}$

10.48. Consider the gaseous reaction between H_2 and F_2 to give HF:

$$H_2(g) + F_2(g) \longrightarrow 2HF(g)$$

How is dP/dt related to dP_{HF}/dt?

Ans. At any time, $P = P_{H_2,0} + P_{F_2,0}$, giving $dP/dt = 0$; not related.

10.49. (*a*) The thermal decomposition of 3-chloro-3-phenyldiazirine in cyclohexane at 90 °C was observed spectrophotometrically by Liu and Toriyama:

t, min	0	3	6	9	12	15	18	21	24
A	1.924	1.649	1.377	1.165	0.964	0.813	0.683	0.559	0.472

where the absorbancy, A, is directly proportional to C. The reaction was also studied using vapor-phase chromotography, generating the following data:

t, min	0.00	3.00	6.00	9.00	10.00	15.00	25.00	30.00
peak area ratio	2.520	2.098	1.716	1.461	1.245	1.014	0.559	0.421

where the peak area ratio is also directly proportional to the concentration. Show that these two data sets indicate the same reaction order and give the same value for k. If the proposed mechanism for the reaction is

$$\phi\!-\!\!\overset{N}{\underset{Cl}{\overset{\|}{C}}}\!\!\overset{\|}{N} \quad \xrightarrow{k_1} \quad N_2 + \phi ClC\!:$$

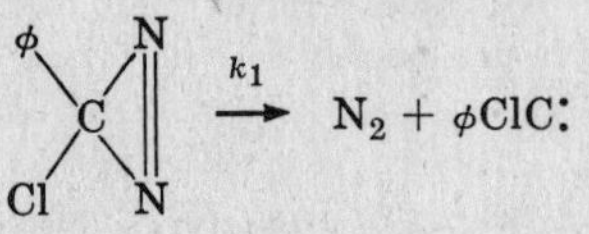

where the carbene can undergo further reaction, e.g.

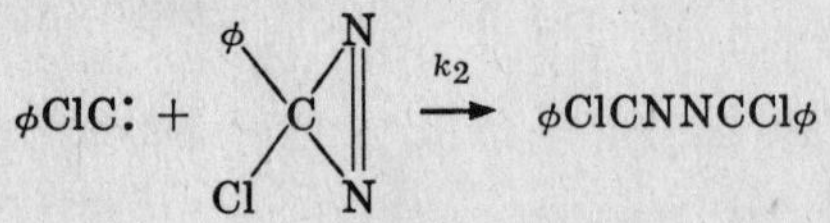

$$\phi ClC\!: + \;\phi\!-\!\!\overset{N}{\underset{Cl}{\overset{\|}{C}}}\!\!\overset{\|}{N} \quad \xrightarrow{k_2} \quad \phi ClCNNCCl\phi$$

$$\phi ClC\!: + S(\text{solvent}) \xrightarrow{k_3} \text{addition and insertion products}$$

derive the overall expression for $-dC_{\phi ClCNN}/dt$ and show that in high concentration of solvent, the reaction is pseudo-first order.

Ans.   (*a*) Plots of $\ln A$ and $\ln$ p.a.r. against t are linear (first-order reaction), slopes give

$$k = 9.8 \times 10^{-4}\ \text{s}^{-1},\ 10.0 \times 10^{-4}\ \text{s}^{-1}$$

(*b*) Using steady state,

$$C_{\phi ClC:} = \frac{k_1 C_{\phi ClCNN}}{k_2 C_{\phi ClCNN} + k_3 C_S}$$

and

$$-\frac{d}{dt}(C_{\phi ClCNN}) = k_1 C_{\phi ClCNN}\left(1 + \frac{k_2 C_{\phi ClCNN}}{k_2 C_{\phi ClCNN} + k_3 C_S}\right) \approx k_1 C_{\phi ClCNN}$$

Influence of Temperature

10.50. Using the reaction coordinate diagrams shown in Fig. 10-10, describe the relation of k_1 to k_2 for the consecutive reactions

$$A \xrightarrow{k_1} B \qquad B \xrightarrow{k_2} C$$

where in each case the overall reaction $A \longrightarrow C$ is exothermic. Describe the possibility of isolation of B in each case.

Ans.   (*a*) k_1 about equal to k_2, fair   (*c*) $k_1 \ll k_2$, little   (*e*) $k_1 > k_2$, good

    (*b*) $k_1 \ll k_2$, little   (*d*) $k_1 > k_2$, excellent

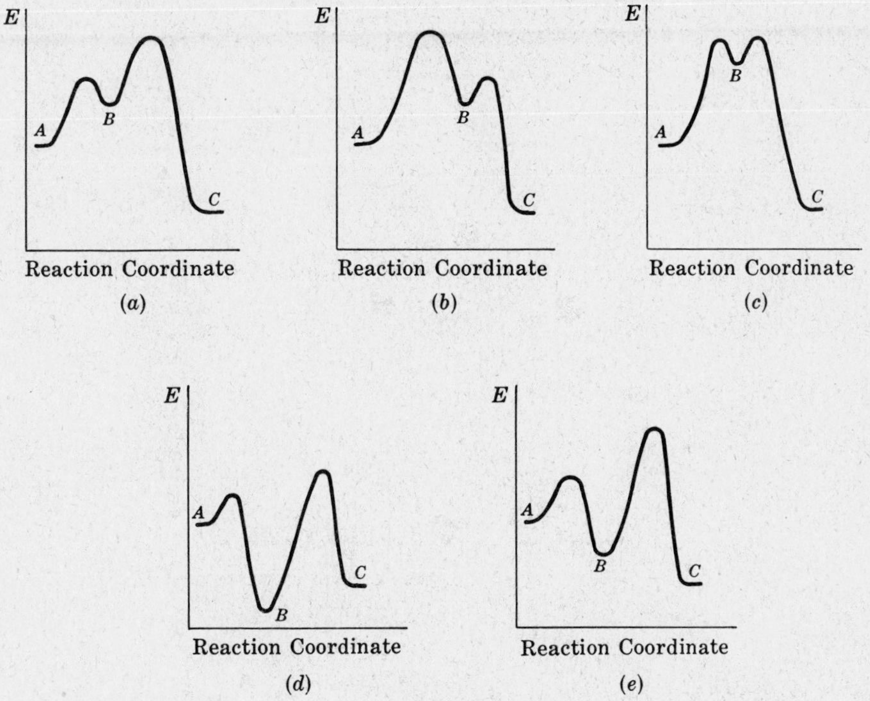

Fig. 10-10

10.51. A rule often quoted in the laboratory is "heat the sample by 10 °C and the reaction will proceed twice as fast." This is true at any given temperature only for reactions having one value of ΔE^*. Find the value of ΔE^* if $t_1 = 25$ °C and $t_2 = 35$ °C. *Ans.* 52.9 kJ mol^{-1}

10.52. The rate constants at several different temperatures for the reaction

$$CH_3CHF_2 \xrightarrow{k} CH_2CHF + HF$$

have been reported by Noble, Carmichael and Bumgardner as

$k \times 10^7$, s^{-1}	7.9	26	52	58	69	230	250	620	1400	1700
T, °C	429	447	460	462	463	483	487	507	521	522

Prepare an Arrhenius plot and determine ΔE^*. If $\Delta E°$ for this reaction is −389 kJ, prepare a reaction coordinate diagram.

Ans. $\Delta E^* = 260$ kJ mol^{-1}; plot similar to Fig. 10-2 with insert having barrier about 70% as high as decrease in E from reactants to products

10.53. Calculate ΔE_1^* and ΔE_2^* for the cyclobutanone decomposition described in Problem 10.43 from the following values of k_1 and k_2:

$k_1 \times 10^4$, s^{-1}	4.6	7.2	14.5	39.8	67.5
T, °C	361	371	383	396	406

$k_2 \times 10^6$, s^{-1}	2.6	6.0	11.5	30.2	53.7
T, °C	360	372	383	396	406

Ans. $\Delta E_1^* = 215\ \text{kJ mol}^{-1}$, $\Delta E_2^* = 235\ \text{kJ mol}^{-1}$

Catalysis

10.54. In Problem 10.12 the second-order behavior with respect to $C_{\text{Co(III)}}$ fails at low concentrations of Co(III). The following alternative expression for k was suggested by Scott and Chester:

$$k = k_a[C_{\text{Co(III)}}]^{1/2}[C_{\text{Co(II)}}]^{-1} + k_b[C_{\text{Co(III)}}]^2$$

which includes the positive catalytic effect of Co(III) in both terms, giving an order between 1 and 2 ($n = 1.71$ in Problem 10.12), and a negative catalytic effect of Co(II) in one term. Upon rearrangement

$$kC_{\text{Co(II)}}[C_{\text{Co(III)}}]^{-1/2} = k_a + k_bC_{\text{Co(II)}}[C_{\text{Co(III)}}]^{3/2}$$

which means that a plot of $kC_{\text{Co(II)}}[C_{\text{Co(III)}}]^{-1/2}$ against $C_{\text{Co(II)}}[C_{\text{Co(III)}}]^{3/2}$ will be linear with a slope of k_b and an intercept of k_a. Prepare such a plot from the following data for $C_{C_6H_5CH_3,0} = 0.5\,M$ at 87 °C and determine k_a and k_b:

$k \times 10^5$, s^{-1}	0.455	1.47	2.93	5.68
$C_{\text{Co(III)}}$, M	0.0179	0.053	0.084	0.1185
$C_{\text{Co(II)}}$, M	0.0446	0.0720	0.1035	0.1315

Ans. $k_a = 1.2 \times 10^{-6}\ M^{1/2}\ s^{-1}$, $k_b = 3.74 \times 10^{-3}\ M^{-2}\ s^{-1}$

10.55. The catalytic effect of various gases on the observed rate constants for the recombination of bromine atoms has been studied by DeGraff and Lang. From the following data determine which chaperon gas is most effective as a positive catalyst.

T, °C	94	76	46	24	96	63	39	26	96	75	54	26
$k \times 10^{-9}$, $M^{-2}\ s^{-1}$	1.07	1.13	1.36	1.48	4.39	6.19	6.87	8.56	9.95	12.01	14.92	22.13
gas	Ne....................				SF_6....................				CCl_4....................			

Ans. $\Delta E^* = -4.2$, -7.7 and $-10.3\ \text{kJ mol}^{-1}$ for Ne, SF_6 and CCl_4, respectively; CCl_4 most effective in absorbing the ΔE^* from the excited molecule

10.56. Consider the following mechanism describing noncompetitive inhibition of an enzyme catalyst in which the substrate and inhibitor bind simultaneously to the enzyme forming an inactive complex, XI:

$$E + S \underset{k_{-1}}{\overset{k_1}{\rightleftharpoons}} X \underset{k_{-2}}{\overset{k_2}{\rightleftharpoons}} E + P$$

$$E + I \underset{k_{-3}}{\overset{k_3}{\rightleftharpoons}} EI$$

$$X + I \underset{k_{-4}}{\overset{k_4}{\rightleftharpoons}} XI$$

$$EI + S \underset{k_{-5}}{\overset{k_5}{\rightleftharpoons}} XI$$

where the inhibitions can be described by K_I, $K_I' = C_X C_I / C_{XI}$ and $K_S' = C_S C_{EI}/C_{XI}$. Derive the rate equation for this process during the initial stages of the reaction where the formation of X from E reacting with P is negligible. Assume $dC_X/dt = 0$.

Ans. $$\left(\frac{dC_P}{dt}\right)^{-1} = \frac{K_S}{V_S}\left(1+\frac{C_I}{K_I}\right)C_S^{-1} + \left(1+\frac{C_I}{K_I'}\right)V_S^{-1};$$

slope same as for competitive inhibition, intercept greater than in competitive and no-inhibition cases

10.57. Substances such as fatty acids, soaps and alcohols lower the surface tension of water as they are added. Will adsorption occur at the water-air interface?

Ans. Yes: $d\gamma/dx_2$ is negative giving a positive Γ.

10.58. Using *(10.43)* and the data in Problem 10.17, predict the amount of N_2 that could be adsorbed under similar conditions at 15 °C. *Ans.* $V_2 = 14\ \text{cm}^3(\text{at STP})\ \text{g}^{-1}$ or $14 \times 10^{-3}\ \text{m}^3\ \text{kg}^{-1}$

10.59. If 1 kg of charcoal at 25 °C will adsorb 0.62 mol of acetic acid from a 0.031 M aqueous solution and 2.48 mol from a 0.882 M solution, verify the constants given in Example 10.17.

Ans. $y = 3.72 \times 10^{-2}$ (g HAc) (g charcoal)$^{-1}$ at 0.031 M and 1.49×10^{-1} at 0.882 M; *(10.32)* then gives $n = 0.412$ and $k = 0.156$.

10.60. Show that *(10.25)* can be put into the linear form

$$\frac{P}{V} = \frac{1}{V_m b} + \frac{P}{V_m}$$

Prepare a plot of P/V against P for the data in Problem 10.19 and confirm the given values of b and V_m.

Ans. slope $= 2.59 \times 10^{-2}\ \text{mm}^{-3}$ g whence $V_m = 38.6\ \text{mm}^3\ \text{g}^{-1} = 1.60 \times 10^{-6}$ (mol N_2) (g charcoal)$^{-1}$; intercept $= 0.0163\ \text{N m}^{-2}\ \text{mm}^{-3}$ g whence $b = 1.59\ \text{m}^2\ \text{N}^{-1}$

10.61. The following data were obtained for the adsorption of N_2 on Al_2O_3 at 77.3 K:

P, torr	31.7	64.5	96.7	128.8	169.3
$n \times 10^4$, (mol N_2) (g Al_2O_3)$^{-1}$	8.31	9.03	9.85	10.45	11.18

(*a*) Prepare a plot of $P/[V(P°-P)]$ against $P/P°$, assuming $P° = 759$ torr. If the intercept and slope give $1/V_m c$ and $(c-1)/V_m c$, respectively, find V_m (expressed in mol N_2 g^{-1}) and c. (*b*) If ΔH(vaporization) $= 5.6$ kJ mol^{-1}, find ΔH(mono). (*c*) If the area covered by one nitrogen molecule is 16.2×10^{-20} m^2, find the surface area of the alumina.

Ans. (*a*) intercept = 7 g mol^{-1}, slope = 1120 g mol^{-1}; $c = 161$; $V_m = 8.87 \times 10^{-4}$ mol g^{-1}
(*b*) 8.9 kJ mol^{-1} (*c*) 86.5 m^2(g alumina)$^{-1}$

10.62. The constant b, in units of atm^{-1}, in *(10.26)* can be estimated from statistical mechanics by

$$b = (7.33 \times 10^{27})q_{AS}\frac{e^{-\Delta E(\text{adsorption})/RT}}{Tq_A q_S}$$

where $q_S = 1$ because the solid adsorbent is rigid; q_A is given by

$$q_A = (2\pi mkT/h^2)^{3/2}q_{A,\text{int}}$$

where $q_{A,\text{int}}$ would contain the internal contributions given by *(6.28)*, *(6.30)*, *(6.33)*, and *(6.34)*; q_{AS} is given by

$$q_{AS} = (1-e^{-h\nu_z/kT})^{-1}(1-e^{-h\nu_x/kT})^{-1}(1-e^{-h\nu_y/kT})^{-1}$$

where the adsorbed molecule might have three different vibrational motions; and ΔE(adsorption) is the internal energy change for the adsorption process. If $\Delta E(\text{adsorption}) = 3.0\ \text{kJ mol}^{-1}$ for Ar at 200 K and $\nu_x = \nu_y = \nu_z = 5 \times 10^{12}\ \text{s}^{-1}$, find b and estimate θ at 1 atm.

Ans. $b = 1.32 \times 10^{-7}\ \text{atm}^{-1}$, $\theta = 1.32 \times 10^{-7}$

10.63. The rate equation for the decomposition described in Example 10.18 is provided by the Freundlich isotherm

$$-\frac{d}{dt}(P_{\text{SbH}_3}) = k(P_{\text{SbH}_3})^n$$

Evaluate k and n from two points on a plot of P_{SbH_3} against t.

Ans. rate = 0.0475 at 0.70 atm and 0.0247 at 0.20 atm; $n = 0.522$; $k = 0.0572$

10.64. Substitute (*10.26*) into (*10.31*) and derive the integrated rate equation for the special case in which A is strongly adsorbed. Show that the following data of Hinshelwood and Burk for the decomposition of NH_3 on W at 856 °C satisfy this rate equation:

t, s	0	100	200	300
P_{NH_3}, torr	200	186	173	162

Note that at longer times the hydrogen that is formed reduces the available area on the surface of the catalyst and this rate equation fails, see Problem 10.22.

Ans. $b_{\text{NH}_3}P_{\text{NH}_3} \gg 1$, $P_{\text{NH}_3} = P_{\text{NH}_3,0} - k't$;
slope of plot of P_{NH_3} against t gives $k' = 0.135\ \text{torr s}^{-1}$.

10.65. Find the expressions for θ_A and θ_B for the case of two gases being adsorbed on a surface such that one of them is diatomic and decomposes upon adsorption.

Ans. $k_{1,A}P_A(1-\theta_A-\theta_B) = k_{2,A}\theta_A$, $k_{1,B}P_B(1-\theta_A-\theta_B)^2 = k_{2,B}\theta_B^2$;
$\theta_A = b_AP_A/[1+b_AP_A+(b_BP_B)^{1/2}]$; $\theta_B = b_BP_B/[1+b_AP_A+(b_BP_B)^{1/2}]$

10.66. Hinshelwood and Prichard reported the following data at 741 °C for the decomposition of N_2O on Pt:

t, s	315	750	1400	2250	3450	5150
P_{O_2}, torr	10	20	30	40	50	60

where $P_{\text{N}_2\text{O},0} = 95$ torr and $P_{\text{N}_2\text{O}} = 95 - P_{\text{O}_2}$. Assuming retardation by O_2 which is moderately adsorbed on Pt, show that

$$(1 + b_{\text{O}_2}P_{\text{N}_2\text{O},0}) \ln \frac{P_{\text{N}_2\text{O},0}}{P_{\text{N}_2\text{O},0} - P_{\text{O}_2}} = k't + b_{\text{O}_2}P_{\text{O}_2}$$

and find b and k'.

Ans. rate $= k'(1-\theta_{\text{O}_2})P_{\text{N}_2\text{O}}$, $\theta_{\text{O}_2} = b_{\text{O}_2}P_{\text{O}_2}/(1+b_{\text{O}_2}P_{\text{O}_2})$;
plot of P_{O_2}/t against $(1/t)\ln\{P_{\text{N}_2\text{O},0}/(P_{\text{N}_2\text{O},0} - P_{\text{O}_2})\}$
is linear with intercept $-0.0128\ \text{torr s}^{-1}$ and slope 1.255×10^2 torr;
$b_{\text{O}_2} = 3.28 \times 10^{-2}$ torr; $k' = 4.21 \times 10^{-4}\ \text{s}^{-1}$

Photochemistry

10.67. Assuming one quantum of light to be absorbed according to reaction (*2*) of Example 10.20, find the relationships between $\phi(H_2)$, $\phi(CH_4)$, $\phi(H_2S)$ and $\phi(CH_3SSCH_3)$.

Ans. Products of (*2*) enter into reactions (*5*) and (*6*) producing CH_4, H_2S and $2CH_3S$, giving $\phi(CH_4) = \phi(H_2S) = 1$; the $2CH_3S$ enter into reaction (*9*) producing CH_3SSCH_3, giving $\phi(CH_3SSCH_3) = 1$; because no H_2 is formed in this path, $\phi(H_2) = 0$.

10.68. Consider the proposed mechanism for the photodimerization of A:

$$A + h\nu \xrightarrow{k_1} A^* \qquad A^* + A \underset{k_{-2}}{\overset{k_2}{\rightleftharpoons}} A_2 \qquad A^* \xrightarrow{k_3} A + h\nu'$$

Is $\phi(A_2)$ dependent on I?

Ans. Using a steady-state approximation, $\phi(A_2) = \dfrac{k_1k_2C_A - k_{-2}k_3C_{A_2}I^{-1}}{k_2C_A + k_3}$; yes.

10.69. Discuss the reaction of acetone with light having $\lambda = 3000$ Å. The average bond energies are 414 kJ mol^{-1} for C—H, 347 kJ mol^{-1} for C—C and 732 kJ mol^{-1} for C=O.

Ans. $E = 399$ kJ mol^{-1}, C—C bond will break giving $CH_3\cdot + CH_3\dot{C}{=}O$

10.70. Find the wavelength of light necessary to photochemically break a H—H bond if the average bond energy is 431 kJ mol^{-1}. Molecular hydrogen does not absorb in this wavelength region, so the energy must be absorbed by another material and transferred to the hydrogen (*photosensitization*). Which substance, Hg(g) or Na(g), would serve as a good photosensitizing agent, if the primary absorption wavelengths are 2536.519 Å and 3302.988 Å, respectively? *Ans.* 2770 Å, Hg

10.71. The actinometer described in Problem 10.23 was used to find the number of quanta absorbed by a sample of HX(g). The concentrations in the actinometer after 30.0 min of light absorption were $C_{N_2} = 43.1 \times 10^{-5}M$ and $51.2 \times 10^{-5}M$, respectively, for the transmitted beam and the incident beam. (*a*) Find the quanta absorbed by the HX(g) sample if the actinometer had a volume of 1 dm^3. (*b*) If 0.158×10^{-3} mol of HX decomposed upon absorption of these quanta, find ϕ. Does this value agree with that predicted by the mechanism

$$HX + h\nu \longrightarrow H + X \qquad H + HX \longrightarrow H_2 + X \qquad X + X \longrightarrow X_2\,?$$

Ans. (*a*) 0.45×10^{-7} einstein s^{-1}; (*b*) $\phi = 1.95$, ϕ(predicted) = 2

Reaction Rate Theory

10.72. Predict k and $\mathcal{A}$ for the reaction

$$Cl(g) + ICl(g) \longrightarrow Cl_2(g) + I(g)$$

if $M = 35.453$ g mol^{-1} for Cl and 162.357 g mol^{-1} for ICl, $\sigma = 2.00$ Å for Cl and 4.65 Å for ICl, and $\Delta E^* = 4.5$ kcal. If $\log \mathcal{A} = 8.7$ for this reaction between 303 K and 333 K, find p and compare the value to that obtained for the reaction described in Problem 10.25.

Ans. $\mathcal{A} = 1.005 \times 10^{11}p$ dm^3 mol^{-1} s^{-1} at 318 K, $k = 7.24 \times 10^7 p$ dm^3 mol^{-1} s^{-1}; $p = 0.005$ (reaction occurs only at one end, therefore less)

10.73. Deduce the structure for the transition-state complex formed between Cl and ICl in the reaction described in Problem 10.72. Confirm the entries in Table 10-1 for this mechanism by calculating the approximate values of $\mathcal{A}$ and p, assuming $q_{trans} = 10^{10}$, $q_{rot} = 10$ and $q_{vib} = 1$ for each degree of freedom. If the temperature exponent is 1/2 for each translational and rotational degree of freedom, predict the temperature exponent in $\mathcal{A}$.

Ans. linear complex; $Q_{\#} = 10^{32}$, $Q_A = 10^{30}$, $Q_B = 10^{32}$, $\mathcal{A} = 4 \times 10^9 \approx 10^{10}$, $p = 10^{-2}$; estimated T-exponent is $-1/2$ to $3/2$, so $-1/2$ to $1/2$

10.74. Qualitatively discuss $\Delta S^\circ_{\#}$ for the reaction

$$M(H_2O)_6^{2+} + Y^{2-} \overset{K}{\rightleftharpoons} (MY)^{\#} + 6H_2O$$

Ans. Negative ΔS in forming $(MY)^{\#}$, large positive ΔS in releasing 6 mol H_2O, positive $\Delta S^\circ_{\#}$.

10.75. Estimate $\Delta S^\circ_\#$ for the reaction

$$A + B \overset{K}{\rightleftharpoons} (AB)^\#$$

where A is an atom, B is a diatomic molecule and $(AB)^\#$ is a linear triatomic molecule.

Ans. $\Delta S^\circ_\# = 2S^\circ(\text{vib}) - 3S^\circ(\text{trans}) = -150$ EU, using values from Problem 10.27.

10.76. Calculate $\Delta S^\circ_\#$ at 318 K for the reaction described in Problem 10.72. Does this value agree with that predicted by Problem 10.75?

Ans. -96 EU, same order of magnitude

10.77. Equation (*10.41*) describes correctly the primary salt effect for all cases except that of $z_A = +n$ and $z_B = -n$, where the resulting charge on $(AB)^\#$ is zero. Show that (*10.41*) gives the correct dependence on I even in this case.

Ans. $\log \gamma_A = -z_A^2(0.5116)I^{1/2}$, $\log \gamma_B = -z_B^2(0.5116)I^{1/2}$, $\gamma_{(AB)^\#} \approx 1$ (by other methods),

$$\log \frac{\gamma_A \gamma_B}{\gamma_{(AB)^\#}} = -(z_A^2 + z_B^2)(0.5116)I^{1/2} = -1.0232\, I^{1/2} n^2$$

10.78. Predict the primary salt effect using (*10.41*) if $z_A = +n$ and $z_B = -m$.

Ans. $z_A z_B < 0$ so $\log k$ will decrease with increasing I.

Chapter 11

Introduction to Quantum Mechanics

Preliminaries

11.1 ELECTROMAGNETIC RADIATION

The properties of electromagnetic radiation are currently explained in terms of a dualistic theory. One part of the theory considers the radiation to obey wave theory, with the frequency ν, wavelength λ, and velocity c of the light related by

$$\nu\lambda = c \tag{11.1}$$

If ν is a large number, a more convenient representation of the wavelength is the *wave number*, $\bar{\nu}$, where

$$\bar{\nu} = \frac{1}{\lambda} \tag{11.2}$$

The second part of the dualistic theory assumes the radiation to act as discrete packets of energy, called quanta. The wave and the corpuscular aspects are related by

$$E = h\nu \tag{11.3}$$

where E is the energy of the quantum and h is Planck's constant.

11.2 DE BROGLIE WAVELENGTH

Any particle with mass m that is moving with a velocity v has associated with it a wavelength given by

$$\lambda = \frac{h}{mv} \tag{11.4}$$

EXAMPLE 11.1. Calculate λ for an electron moving with $v = 0.1\,c$, using the rest mass,

$$m_e = 9.109534 \times 10^{-31}\ \text{kg}$$

as the mass. In what part of the electromagnetic spectrum would this value of λ fall?

Using *(11.4)* gives

$$\lambda = \frac{6.626 \times 10^{-34}\ \text{J s}}{(9.11 \times 10^{-31}\ \text{kg})(0.1)(3.00 \times 10^{8}\ \text{m s}^{-1})} = 2.42 \times 10^{-11}\ \text{m}$$

or 0.242 Å, which falls into the long γ-ray region of the spectrum, assuming it to be divided into the following bands: 0.01 Å, γ-rays; 10 Å, X-rays; 100–2000 Å, vacuum ultraviolet; 2000–4000 Å, ultraviolet; 4000–7000 Å, visible; 0.7–20 μm, near infrared; 20–1000 μm, far infrared; 0.1–100 cm, microwave; and 1 m, radio.

11.3 HEISENBERG UNCERTAINTY (INDETERMINACY) PRINCIPLE

There are no restrictions on the precision of measurement of position, x, alone or on the measurement of momentum in the x-direction, p_x, alone. But the product of the measurement uncertainties, Δx and Δp_x, during a simultaneous measurement must be greater than $\hbar/2$ or, in the limiting case, equal to $\hbar/2$:

$$(\Delta p_x)(\Delta x) \geqq \frac{\hbar}{2} \tag{11.5}$$

where $\hbar = h/2\pi = 1.0545887 \times 10^{-34}$ J s. Likewise for simultaneous measurements of energy and time:

$$(\Delta E)(\Delta t) \geqq \frac{\hbar}{2} \tag{11.6}$$

11.4 RYDBERG EQUATION

Under low resolution, the emission spectra of hydrogenlike elements appear as series of lines fitting the empirical *Rydberg equation*:

$$\bar{\nu} = Z^2 \mathcal{R}\left(\frac{1}{n_2^2} - \frac{1}{n_1^2}\right) \tag{11.7}$$

where Z is the atomic number of the element, $\mathcal{R}$ is the *Rydberg constant*,

$$\mathcal{R} = (109{,}737.3177 \text{ cm}^{-1})\left(\frac{m_{\text{nucleus}}}{m_{\text{nucleus}} + m_e}\right) \tag{11.8}$$

and n_i are integers, with $n_2 < n_1$.

EXAMPLE 11.2. Find the ionization potential for atomic hydrogen.

The ionization potential is the energy required to remove the electron from the lowest energy level ($n_2 = 1$) to ∞ ($n_1 = \infty$). Using $\mathcal{R} = 109{,}677.59$ cm^{-1} for H, see Problem 11.3, (*11.7*) and (*11.3*) give

$$\bar{\nu} = (1)^2(109{,}677.59 \text{ cm}^{-1})\left(\frac{1}{1^2} - \frac{1}{\infty^2}\right) = 109{,}677.59 \text{ cm}^{-1}$$

$$\begin{aligned} E &= (6.626176 \times 10^{-34} \text{ J s})(109{,}677.59 \text{ cm}^{-1})(10^2 \text{ cm m}^{-1})(2.99792458 \times 10^8 \text{ m s}^{-1}) \\ &= 2.178721 \times 10^{-18} \text{ J} \end{aligned}$$

A frequently used unit in quantum mechanics is the *electron volt*, eV. Converting the above answer gives

$$E = \frac{2.178721 \times 10^{-18} \text{ J}}{1.6021892 \times 10^{-19} \text{ J eV}^{-1}} = 13.5984 \text{ eV}$$

11.5 BOHR THEORY FOR HYDROGENLIKE ATOMS

The Bohr theory consists of three main postulates: (1) the electron moves around the nucleus of charge $+Ze$ in a circular orbit of constant energy; (2) the only orbits that are allowed are those in which the electron has an angular momentum equal to $n\hbar$, where n is an integer (quantum number); (3) transitions between orbits generate spectral lines, with the frequency of a line being given by $(\Delta E)/h$, where ΔE is the energy difference between the initial and final orbits.

By applying these postulates to the system shown in Fig. 11-1, it is possible to show that the radii of the orbits, r_n, are given by

$$r_n = n^2 \frac{(4\pi\epsilon_0)\hbar^2}{\mu e^2 Z} \tag{11.9}$$

where $e = 1.6021892 \times 10^{-19}$ C is the electronic charge, $4\pi\epsilon_0 = 1.112650056 \times 10^{-10}\ \text{C}^2\ \text{N}^{-1}\ \text{m}^{-2}$ is the permittivity constant and

$$\mu = \frac{m_e m_{\text{nucleus}}}{m_e + m_{\text{nucleus}}} \tag{11.10}$$

is the reduced mass of the system. The energy of the orbit having quantum number n is

$$E_n = -\frac{\mu Z^2 e^4}{2n^2\hbar^2(4\pi\epsilon_0)^2} \tag{11.11}$$

The Bohr theory explained the Rydberg equation but failed to predict the fine structure of spectra and to describe polyelectronic systems.

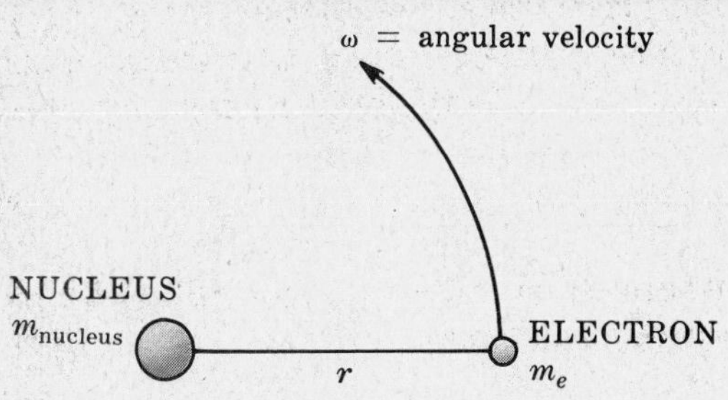

Fig. 11-1

EXAMPLE 11.3. Calculate the radii and energies of the first four orbits of atomic hydrogen. Prepare a sketch of these orbits to scale. Prepare an energy diagram to scale and determine the number of transitions that can occur. Find the values of ν for these transitions.

Using $m_{\text{nucleus}} = 1.6726485 \times 10^{-27}$ kg, $m_e = 9.109534 \times 10^{-31}$ kg and $Z = 1$, (*11.10*) gives $\mu = 9.104575 \times 10^{-31}$ kg. Then, from (*11.9*) and (*11.11*),

$$r_n = n^2 \frac{(1.112650 \times 10^{-10}\ \text{C}^2\ \text{N}^{-1}\ \text{m}^{-2})(1.0545887 \times 10^{-34}\ \text{J s})^2}{(9.104575 \times 10^{-31}\ \text{kg})(1.6021892 \times 10^{-19}\ \text{C})^2(1)}$$

$$= n^2(5.294653 \times 10^{-11})\ \text{m} = n^2(0.5294653)\ \text{Å}$$

$$E_n = -\frac{(9.104575 \times 10^{-31}\ \text{kg})(1)^2(1.6021892 \times 10^{-19}\ \text{C})^4}{2n^2(1.0545887 \times 10^{-34}\ \text{J s})^2(1.112650 \times 10^{-10}\ \text{C}^2\ \text{N}^{-1}\ \text{m}^{-2})^2}$$

$$= -\frac{2.178720 \times 10^{-18}}{n^2}\ \text{J} = -\frac{109{,}677.6}{n^2}\ \text{cm}^{-1}$$

The energy was changed from J to cm^{-1} using the conversion factor $1.986477 \times 10^{-23}\ \text{J}\ (\text{cm}^{-1})^{-1}$. Values corresponding to $n = 1, 2, 3$ and 4 are indicated in Fig. 11-2. The six vertical lines shown in Fig. 11-2(*b*) represent possible transitions, with energies

$$\Delta E_{2\to1} = (-27{,}400\ \text{cm}^{-1}) - (-109{,}700\ \text{cm}^{-1}) = 82{,}300\ \text{cm}^{-1}$$

$\Delta E_{3\to1} = 97{,}500\ \text{cm}^{-1}$; $\Delta E_{3\to2} = 15{,}200\ \text{cm}^{-1}$; $\Delta E_{4\to1} = 102{,}800\ \text{cm}^{-1}$; $\Delta E_{4\to2} = 20{,}500\ \text{cm}^{-1}$; and $\Delta E_{4\to3} = 5300\ \text{cm}^{-1}$.

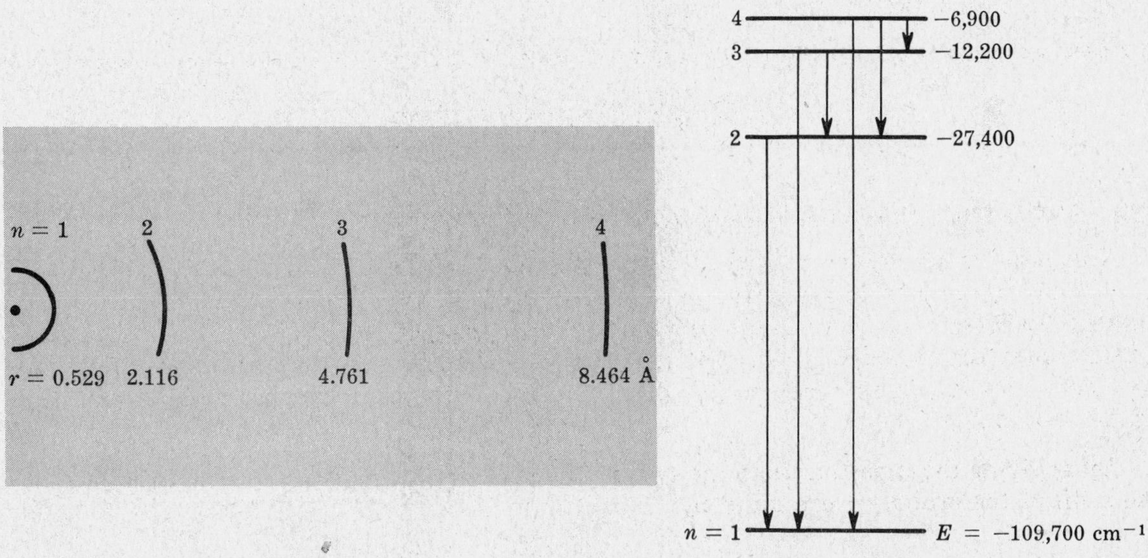

(*a*) (*b*)

Fig. 11-2

Postulates of Quantum Mechanics

11.6 WAVE FUNCTIONS

Any state of a dynamic system containing N particles can be described by a wave function $\psi(q_1, q_2, \ldots, q_{3N}, t)$, where the q_i are coordinates and t is time, such that $\psi^*\psi$ is proportional to the probability of finding the coordinates between q_i and $q_i + dq_i$ at t. The wave function should be continuous, single-valued and square-integrable so that it may be in agreement with physical reality. In addition, the first and second derivatives should be continuous. The symbol ψ^* represents the complex conjugate of ψ, which is formed by changing the sign of the imaginary unit i in the expression for ψ.

If

$$\int_{\text{all space}} \psi^* \psi \, dV \equiv \langle \psi | \psi \rangle = 1 \tag{11.12}$$

where dV is the volume element of the coordinate system, the wave function is said to be *normalized*. If

$$\int_{\text{all space}} \psi_i^* \psi_j \, dV \equiv \langle \psi_i | \psi_j \rangle = 0 \tag{11.13}$$

for two wave functions, the functions are said to be *orthogonal* The notation in (*11.12*) and (*11.13*) is the *Dirac notation,* where the first bracket essentially represents the integral sign, everything to the left of the first slash is the complex conjugate, everything to the right of the last slash is the function itself, and the last bracket represents the volume element. If ψ_i and ψ_j are normalized wave functions that satisfy (*11.13*), they are known as *orthonormal* wave functions.

EXAMPLE 11.4. Consider a particle having mass m located in a one-dimensional potential-energy well (box) with infinitely high walls, as shown in Fig. 11-3(*a*). The wave function describing this system is

$$\psi_n(x) = \begin{cases} K \sin \dfrac{n\pi x}{a} & \text{for } 0 \leqq x \leqq a \\ 0 & \text{otherwise} \end{cases} \tag{11.14}$$

where K is a constant and $n = 1, 2, 3, \ldots$. (Because the potential energy is infinite—an artificial condition—outside the well, it is not possible to make the derivative of ψ continuous at the walls.) Determine $K^*K = |K|^2$.

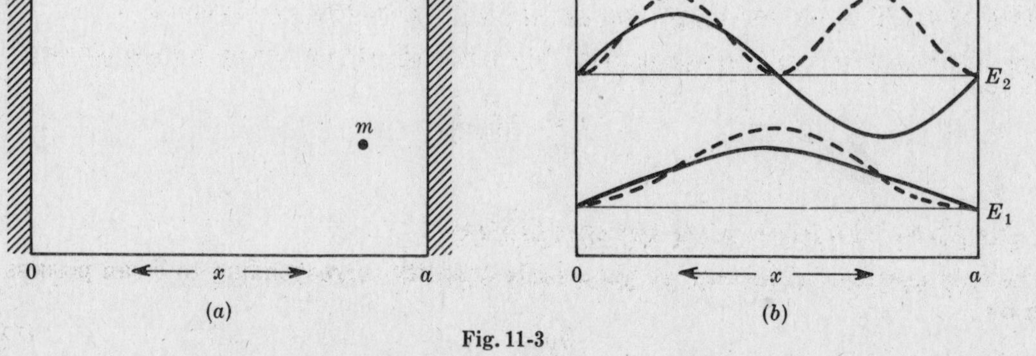

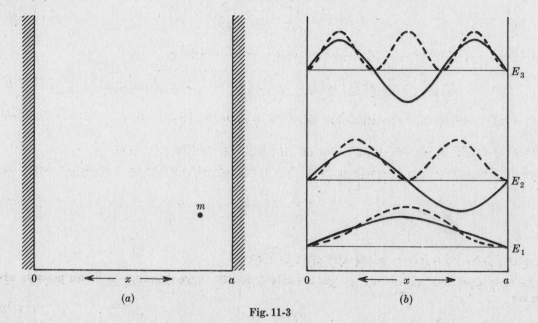

Fig. 11-3

Substituting *(11.14)* and $\psi_n(x)^* = K^* \sin(n\pi x/a)$ into *(11.12)* gives

$$1 = \int_0^a \left(K^* \sin\frac{n\pi x}{a}\right)\left(K \sin\frac{n\pi x}{a}\right) dx = K^* K \int_0^a \sin^2\frac{n\pi x}{a}\, dx$$

The integral can be transformed into one found in most integral tables by letting $z = n\pi x/a$ and $dz = (n\pi/a)\,dx$ giving

$$1 = K^* K\left(\frac{a}{n\pi}\right)\int_0^{n\pi} \sin^2 z\, dz = K^* K \frac{a}{2}$$

Thus $K^* K = 2/a$.

EXAMPLE 11.5. Show that $\psi_n'(x) = W \cos(n\pi x/a)$ and the functions *(11.14)* are orthogonal.

Evaluating $\langle\psi_n(x) \mid \psi_n'(x)\rangle$ gives

$$\langle\psi_n(x) \mid \psi_n'(x)\rangle = \int_0^a \left(K^* \sin\frac{n\pi x}{a}\right)\left(W \cos\frac{n\pi x}{a}\right) dx = K^* W \int_0^a \sin\left(\frac{n\pi x}{a}\right) \cos\left(\frac{n\pi x}{a}\right) dx$$

The integral can be evaluated as described in Example 11.4 giving

$$\langle\psi_n(x) \mid \psi_n'(x)\rangle = K^* W\left(\frac{a}{n\pi}\right)\int_0^{n\pi} \sin z \cos z\, dz = 0$$

which according to *(11.13)* proves orthogonality.

11.7 OPERATORS

For every physically observable property of a system there exists a linear, Hermitian operator, $\hat{o}$, which can operate on ψ. Examples of $\hat{o}$ are: position, $\hat{x} = x$; x-component of linear momentum, $\hat{p}_x = (\hbar/i)(\partial/\partial x)$; x-component of angular momentum, $\hat{l}_x = (\hbar/i)[y(\partial/\partial z) - z(\partial/\partial y)]$; kinetic energy along the x-axis, $\hat{T}_x = -(\hbar^2/2m)(\partial^2/\partial x^2)$; and the total energy (the *Hamiltonian*) for N particles,

$$\hat{H} = \mathcal{H} = -\frac{\hbar^2}{2}\sum_{i=1}^{N}\frac{1}{m_i}\nabla_i^2 + U(x,y,z) \qquad (11.15)$$

in which U is the total potential-energy function. The Laplacian operator is given by

$$\nabla^2 \equiv \frac{\partial^2}{\partial x^2} + \frac{\partial^2}{\partial y^2} + \frac{\partial^2}{\partial z^2} \qquad (11.16a)$$

in Cartesian coordinates and in spherical polar coordinates by

$$\nabla^2 \equiv \frac{1}{r^2}\frac{\partial}{\partial r}\left(r^2\frac{\partial}{\partial r}\right) + \frac{1}{r^2 \sin\theta}\frac{\partial}{\partial\theta}\left(\sin\theta\frac{\partial}{\partial\theta}\right) + \frac{1}{r^2\sin^2\theta}\left(\frac{\partial^2}{\partial\phi^2}\right) \qquad (11.16b)$$

In *(11.15)* ∇_i^2 stands for the Laplacian with respect to the coordinates of the ith particle.

EXAMPLE 11.6. Write the total energy operator for the system described in Example 11.4.

The Hamiltonian is found by substituting $U(x) = 0$ and *(11.16a)* written for one dimension into *(11.15)*, giving

$$\mathcal{H} = -\frac{\hbar^2}{2m}\frac{\partial^2}{\partial x^2} \qquad (11.17)$$

11.8 EIGENFUNCTIONS AND EIGENVALUES

The only possible values that an observable quantity corresponding to $\hat{o}$ can possess are given by

$$\hat{o}\psi = o\psi \qquad (11.18)$$

where an allowed value o is known as an *eigenvalue* and ψ is the corresponding *eigenfunction*. In some cases o can be continuously variable and in others o can have only discrete values.

EXAMPLE 11.7. The eigenvalues for position for the system described in Example 11.4 are continuously variable, but those for energy are discrete and are given by

$$E_n = \frac{n^2h^2}{8ma^2} \tag{11.19}$$

Prepare a sketch of the energy levels E_n and superimpose plots of $\psi_n(x)$ and $\psi_n(x)^*\psi_n(x)$ on the respective levels.

In units of $h^2/8ma^2$ the energies are given by (*11.19*) as $E_1 = 1$, $E_2 = 4$, $E_3 = 9$, etc. These energies are shown in Fig. 11-3(*b*). The plots of $\psi_n(x)$ are shown as solid curves and those of $\psi_n(x)^*\psi_n(x)$ as dashed curves.

11.9 EXPECTATION VALUES

The average of a series of measurements will be given by

$$\langle o \rangle = \frac{\int_{\text{all space}} \psi^* \hat{o} \psi \, dV}{\int_{\text{all space}} \psi^* \psi \, dV} \equiv \frac{\langle \psi | \hat{o} | \psi \rangle}{\langle \psi | \psi \rangle} \tag{11.20}$$

The denominator in (*11.20*) does not appear if normalized wave functions are used. Because of the Hermitian character of the operators,

$$\langle \psi_i | \hat{o} | \psi_j \rangle \equiv \langle \psi_j | \hat{o}^* | \psi_i \rangle \tag{11.21}$$

EXAMPLE 11.8. Find the average position of the particle described in Example 11.4. Would this location be a good place to seek the particle if it is in energy state E_2?

Substituting $\hat{x} = x$ and (*11.14*) with $K^*K = 2/a$ into (*11.20*) gives

$$\langle x \rangle = \int_0^a \left(K^* \sin\frac{n\pi x}{a}\right) x \left(K \sin\frac{n\pi x}{a}\right) dx = \frac{2}{a}\int_0^a x \sin^2\frac{n\pi x}{a}\, dx$$

Evaluating the integral as described in Example 11.4 gives

$$\langle x \rangle = \left(\frac{2}{a}\right)\left(\frac{a}{n\pi}\right)^2 \int_0^{n\pi} z \sin^2 z \, dz = \left(\frac{2}{a}\right)\left(\frac{a}{n\pi}\right)^2\left(\frac{n^2\pi^2}{4}\right) = \frac{a}{2}$$

the center of the potential-energy well. The particle will spend equal amounts of time on either side of the center because $\psi_n(x)^*\psi_n(x)$ is symmetrical about the center. However, for $n = 2$, the probability of finding the particle near the center, where $\psi_2(x)^*\psi_2(x) = 0$, is very low, see Fig. 11-3(*b*).

EXAMPLE 11.9. Show that (*11.19*) is the solution of (*11.20*) for the particle described in Example 11.4.

Substituting $\mathcal{H} = (-\hbar^2/2m)(\partial^2/\partial x^2)$ for $\hat{o}$ and E for o into (*11.20*) gives

$$E_n \equiv \langle E \rangle = \int_0^a \left(K^* \sin\frac{n\pi x}{a}\right)\left(-\frac{\hbar^2}{2m}\frac{\partial^2}{\partial x^2}\right)\left(K \sin\frac{n\pi x}{a}\right) dx = K^*K\left(-\frac{\hbar^2}{2m}\right)\int_0^a \left(\sin\frac{n\pi x}{a}\right)\frac{\partial^2}{\partial x^2}\left(\sin\frac{n\pi x}{a}\right) dx$$

$$= \left(\frac{2}{a}\right)\left(-\frac{\hbar^2}{2m}\right)\left(\frac{n\pi}{a}\right)^2(-1)\int_0^a \sin^2\frac{n\pi x}{a}\, dx = \left(\frac{2}{a}\right)\left(-\frac{\hbar^2}{2m}\right)\left(\frac{n\pi}{a}\right)^2(-1)\left(\frac{a}{2}\right)$$

$$= \frac{n^2\hbar^2\pi^2}{2ma^2} = \frac{n^2h^2}{8ma^2}$$

11.10 TIME DEPENDENCE

The evolution of $\psi(q_i, t)$ is given by $i\hbar(\partial\psi/\partial t) = \mathcal{H}\psi$. Because $\mathcal{H}$ is not a function of time, $\psi(q_i, t)$ can be written as $\psi(q_i)e^{-(i/\hbar)Et}$, giving the *time-independent Schrödinger equation*

$$\mathcal{H}\psi(q_i) = E\psi(q_i) \tag{11.22}$$

for $\psi(q_i)$.

EXAMPLE 11.10. Show that (*11.14*) is a solution to (*11.22*) for the particle described in Example 11.4.

Performing the operation $\mathcal{H}\psi_n(x)$ gives

$$\mathcal{H}\psi_n(x) = \left(-\frac{\hbar^2}{2m}\frac{\partial^2}{\partial x^2}\right)\left(K \sin\frac{n\pi x}{a}\right)$$

$$= \left(-\frac{\hbar^2}{2m}\right)K\left(\frac{n\pi}{a}\right)^2(-1)\sin\frac{n\pi x}{a} = \left(\frac{\hbar^2}{2m}\right)\left(\frac{n\pi}{a}\right)^2\psi_n(x) = E_n\psi_n(x)$$

11.11 THE CORRESPONDENCE PRINCIPLE

Quantum mechanics may be successfully extrapolated to macroscopic systems, generating the classical Newtonian results.

EXAMPLE 11.11. The classical model for an ideal-gas molecule restricted to one dimension predicts that position is continuous. Show that (*11.14*) qualitatively predicts this result.

At room temperature a molecule with one degree of freedom has a kinetic energy given by $E = (1/2)kT = 2.06 \times 10^{-21}$ J. Assuming a molecular weight of 28.0 g mol^{-1}, and $a = 1$ m, (*11.19*) gives

$$n^2 = \frac{E(8ma^2)}{h^2} = \frac{(2.06 \times 10^{-21})(8)(28.0 \times 10^{-3}/6.022 \times 10^{23})(1)^2}{(6.626 \times 10^{-34})^2} = 1.75 \times 10^{21}$$

or $n = 4.18 \times 10^{10}$. Recognizing that the plots of $\psi_n(x)^*\psi_n(x)$ as shown in Fig. 11-3(*b*) contain n maxima, the separation between the most probable locations would be $(1 \text{ m})/(4.18 \times 10^{10}) = 0.239$ Å. Because the molecular size is larger than this value, position is for all purposes continuous.

Approximation Methods

11.12 THE VARIATION METHOD

For most problems of chemical interest, the exact solution of (*11.22*) is not possible. However, an approximate solution corresponding to the quantum state of lowest energy, the *ground state*, can be obtained by choosing a trial wave function, ϕ, and adjusting the parameters in ϕ to give a minimum energy. Then

$$E_{\text{ground}} \leqq E = \frac{\langle\phi|\mathcal{H}|\phi\rangle}{\langle\phi|\phi\rangle} \tag{11.23}$$

that is, the best choice of ϕ provides an upper bound for the true energy of the ground state.

If ϕ is constructed by taking a linear combination of m "basis functions," μ_i, i.e.

$$\phi = \sum_{i=1}^{m} c_i\mu_i \tag{11.24}$$

where c_i are variable parameters, the values of c_i that give the minimum energy satisfy the following set of equations:

$$\begin{array}{l} c_1(H_{11} - ES_{11}) + c_2(H_{12} - ES_{12}) + \cdots + c_m(H_{1m} - ES_{1m}) = 0 \\ c_1(H_{21} - ES_{21}) + c_2(H_{22} - ES_{22}) + \cdots + c_m(H_{2m} - ES_{2m}) = 0 \\ \cdots\cdots\cdots\cdots\cdots\cdots\cdots\cdots\cdots\cdots\cdots\cdots \\ c_1(H_{m1} - ES_{m1}) + c_2(H_{m2} - ES_{m2}) + \cdots + c_m(H_{mm} - ES_{mm}) = 0 \end{array} \tag{11.25}$$

where
$$H_{ij} = \langle \mu_i | \mathcal{H} | \mu_j \rangle \tag{11.26}$$
$$S_{ij} = \langle \mu_i | \mu_j \rangle \tag{11.27}$$

The system (*11.25*) will have a nonzero solution only for those values of E which make the determinant of the coefficients vanish, i.e.

$$\begin{vmatrix} H_{11}-ES_{11} & H_{12}-ES_{12} & \cdots & H_{1m}-ES_{1m} \\ H_{21}-ES_{21} & H_{22}-ES_{22} & \cdots & H_{2m}-ES_{2m} \\ \vdots & \vdots & & \vdots \\ H_{m1}-ES_{m1} & H_{m2}-ES_{m2} & \cdots & H_{mm}-ES_{mm} \end{vmatrix} = 0 \tag{11.28}$$

With E determined as a root of the *secular equation* (*11.28*), the c_i can be found by solving $m-1$ of the equations (*11.25*) and imposing the condition that the wave function be normalized.

EXAMPLE 11.12. The boundary conditions in Example 11.4 are $\psi_n(0) = \psi_n(a) = 0$. Choosing $\mu_1 = x(x-a)$, which also satisfies the boundary conditions, as a simple basis function, find the estimate for E_{ground}.

For the trial function $\phi = c_1 x(x-a)$, (*11.28*) is

$$H_{11} - ES_{11} = 0$$

Substituting the values of H_{11} and S_{11} given by

$$H_{11} = \langle \mu_1 | \mathcal{H} | \mu_1 \rangle = \int_0^a [x(x-a)]\left(-\frac{\hbar^2}{2m}\frac{d^2}{dx^2}\right)[x(x-a)]\,dx$$
$$= \left(-\frac{\hbar^2}{2m}\right)\int_0^a x(x-a)\,dx = \frac{\hbar^2 a^3}{6m}$$
$$S_{11} = \langle \mu_1 | \mu_1 \rangle = \int_0^a x^2(x-a)^2\,dx = \frac{a^5}{30}$$

yields
$$E = \frac{H_{11}}{S_{11}} = \frac{\hbar^2 a^3/6m}{a^5/30} = \frac{5\hbar^2}{ma^2} = \frac{5h^2}{4\pi^2 ma^2}$$

A comparison with the true value, $E_{\text{ground}} = E_1 = h^2/8ma^2$, gives the percent error as

$$\frac{E-E_1}{E_1} = \frac{(5h^2/4\pi^2ma^2) - (h^2/8ma^2)}{(h^2/8ma^2)} = \frac{10}{\pi^2} - 1 = 1.3\%$$

which is rather good considering the crudeness of the trial function (a ramp function instead of a sine wave).

11.13 NONDEGENERATE PERTURBATION THEORY

If the problem for which an approximate solution is desired does not differ greatly from one for which normalized $\psi_n^{(0)}$ and $E_n^{(0)}$ are known for the corresponding $\mathcal{H}^{(0)}$, then the Hamiltonian is written as

$$\mathcal{H} = \mathcal{H}^{(0)} + \lambda \mathcal{H}^{(1)} \tag{11.29}$$

and (*11.22*) has the solutions

$$\psi_n = \psi_n^{(0)} + \lambda\psi_n^{(1)} + \lambda^2\psi_n^{(2)} + \cdots \tag{11.30}$$
$$E_n = E_n^{(0)} + \lambda E_n^{(1)} + \lambda^2 E_n^{(2)} + \cdots \tag{11.31}$$

where the parameter λ is a measure of the deviation of the problem of interest from the unperturbed problem. Normally λ is set equal to 1, signifying that the perturbation is being fully applied. For first-order theory, i.e. retaining terms in λ^1, (*11.30*) and (*11.31*) become

$$\psi_n = \psi_n^{(0)} + \lambda \sum_m{}' \frac{H_{mn}^{(1)}\psi_m^{(0)}}{E_n^{(0)} - E_m^{(0)}} \tag{11.32}$$

$$E_n = E_n^{(0)} + \lambda H_{nn}^{(1)} \tag{11.33}$$

where

$$H_{mn}^{(1)} = \langle \psi_m^{(0)} | \mathcal{H}^{(1)} | \psi_n^{(0)} \rangle \tag{11.34}$$

$$E_m^{(0)} = \langle \psi_m^{(0)} | \mathcal{H}^{(0)} | \psi_m^{(0)} \rangle \tag{11.35}$$

and $\sum_m{}'$ means to sum over all values of $m \neq n$ until an insignificant addition results. The second-order estimate for the energy is

$$E_n = E_n^{(0)} + \lambda H_{nn}^{(1)} + \lambda^2 \sum_m{}' \frac{H_{nm}^{(1)} H_{mn}^{(1)}}{E_n^{(0)} - E_m^{(0)}} \tag{11.36}$$

EXAMPLE 11.13. Consider the particle in the one-dimensional well shown in Fig. 11-4, inside which the potential energy is given by $U(x) = C(x/a)$. What is the first-order estimate of the energy of this system using perturbation theory?

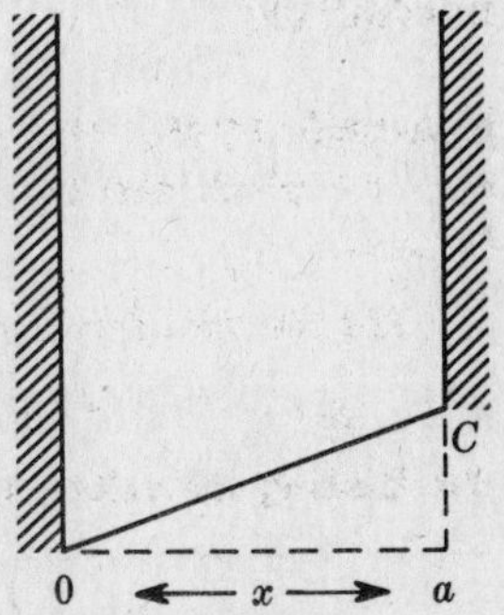

Fig. 11-4

The unperturbed problem, of which the Hamiltonian is

$$\mathcal{H}^{(0)} = \frac{-\hbar^2}{2m}\frac{d^2}{dx^2}$$

has the solution (see Examples 11.4 and 11.7)

$$\psi_n^{(0)} = K \sin \frac{n\pi x}{a}$$

with $K^*K = 2/a$, and

$$E_n^{(0)} = \frac{n^2h^2}{8ma^2}$$

For $0 \leqq x \leqq a$ the Hamiltonian for the perturbed system is

$$\mathcal{H} = -\frac{\hbar^2}{2m}\frac{d^2}{dx^2} + C\frac{x}{a} = \mathcal{H}^{(0)} + \mathcal{H}^{(1)}$$

where $\mathcal{H}^{(1)} = C(x/a)$. Then (*11.34*) gives

$$H_{nn}^{(1)} = \int_0^a \left(K^* \sin\frac{n\pi x}{a}\right)\left(C\frac{x}{a}\right)\left(K \sin\frac{n\pi x}{a}\right) dx = \frac{K^*KC}{a}\int_0^a x \sin^2\frac{n\pi x}{a}\,dx$$

This integral was evaluated in Example 11.8 as $a^2/4$, giving

$$H_{nn}^{(1)} = \frac{K^*KC}{a}\left(\frac{a^2}{4}\right) = \frac{C}{2}$$

Hence (*11.33*) gives

$$E_n = \frac{n^2h^2}{8ma^2} + \frac{C}{2}$$

Solved Problems

Preliminaries

11.1. Commercial FM radio stations operate between 88 and 108 MHz. Calculate λ, $\bar{\nu}$ and E for a radio wave having $\nu = 95.5$ MHz.

Using (*11.1*) through (*11.3*) gives

$$\lambda = \frac{2.9979 \times 10^8 \text{ m s}^{-1}}{95.5 \times 10^6 \text{ s}^{-1}} = 3.14 \text{ m} \qquad \bar{\nu} = \frac{1}{3.14 \text{ m}} = 0.319 \text{ m}^{-1}$$

$$E = (6.626 \times 10^{-34} \text{ J s})(95.5 \times 10^6 \text{ s}^{-1}) = 6.33 \times 10^{-26} \text{ J}$$

Note that the wavelength is about 10 feet, a multiple of the size for various quarter- and half-wave "rabbit-ear" and TV antennas.

11.2. What is the maximum precision with which the momentum may be known if the position of an electron is determined to within ±0.001 Å? Will there be any problems in describing the momentum if it has a value of $\hbar/0.529$ Å?

Using the limiting case of *(11.5)* gives

$$\Delta p_x = \frac{\hbar/2}{\Delta x} = \frac{1.055 \times 10^{-34}\ \text{J s}}{(2)(0.001\ \text{Å})(10^{-10}\ \text{m Å}^{-1})} = 5.28 \times 10^{-22}\ \text{N s}$$

If the momentum is $\hbar/0.529$ Å $= 1.99 \times 10^{-24}$ N s, the uncertainty in the measurement of momentum will be about 265 times as large as the momentum itself. For that reason, the concept of definite electron orbits has been replaced by "probabilities" of locating electrons.

11.3. The "Balmer series" of lines in the spectrum of atomic hydrogen has $n_2 = 2$ in *(11.7)*. Calculate λ for the first six lines of this series.

Substituting $m_{\text{nucleus}} = 1.6726485 \times 10^{-27}$ kg and $m_e = 9.109534 \times 10^{-31}$ kg into *(11.8)* gives the value of the Rydberg constant for hydrogen as $\mathcal{R} = 109{,}677.59\ \text{cm}^{-1}$. Substituting this value of $\mathcal{R}$ with $n_1 = 3$ and $n_2 = 2$ into *(11.7)* gives

$$\bar{\nu} = (1)^2(109{,}677.59\ \text{cm}^{-1})\left(\frac{1}{2^2} - \frac{1}{3^2}\right) = 15{,}233.00\ \text{cm}^{-1}$$

and *(11.2)* gives

$$\lambda = \frac{1}{\bar{\nu}} = \frac{1}{15{,}233.00\ \text{cm}^{-1}} = 6.564696 \times 10^{-5}\ \text{cm} = 6564.696\ \text{Å}$$

Repeating the calculations for $n_1 = 4, 5, 6, 7$ and 8 gives 4862.738, 4341.730, 4102.935, 3971.236 and 3890.190 Å, respectively. Note that the difference between successive lines becomes smaller as n_1 increases.

Postulates of Quantum Mechanics

11.4. If the walls of a potential-energy well have a finite height, V_0, then the wave function describing a particle within the box does not go to zero at the walls but continues into the energy barrier.

(*a*) Find an equation for the allowed energies of the system if the wave functions describing the particle in the three regions shown in Fig. 11.5(*a*) are

$$\psi_{\text{I}}(x) = Ae^{[2m(V_0-E)]^{1/2}(x/\hbar)}$$

$$\psi_{\text{II}}(x) = B \sin[(2mE)^{1/2}(x/\hbar)] + C \cos[(2mE)^{1/2}(x/\hbar)]$$

$$\psi_{\text{III}}(x) = De^{-[2m(V_0-E)]^{1/2}(x/\hbar)}$$

(*b*) Discuss the sketches for the first three energy levels, as shown in Fig. 11-5(*b*).

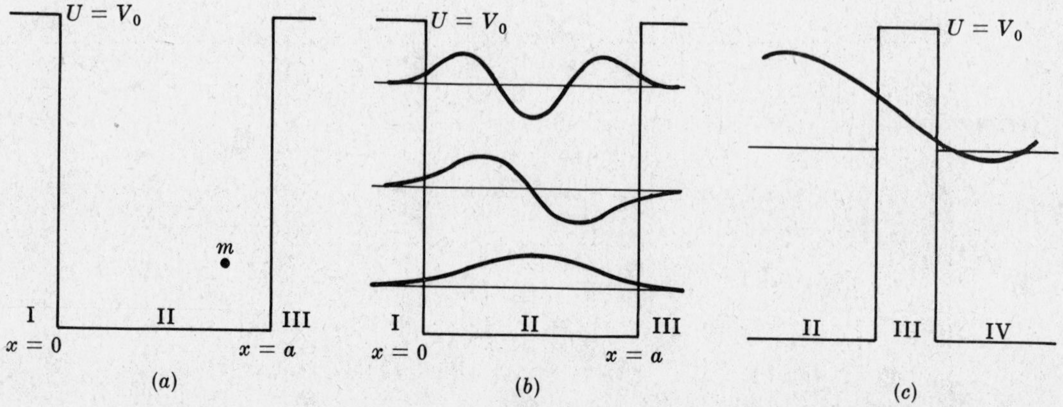

Fig. 11-5

(a) Because $\psi(x)$ must be continuous at $x = 0$, $\psi_{\rm I}(0) = \psi_{\rm II}(0)$, which implies $A = C$. Furthermore, the derivatives

$$\left.\frac{d\psi_{\rm I}}{dx}\right|_{x=0} = A\,\frac{[2m(V_0 - E)]^{1/2}}{\hbar} \qquad \text{and} \qquad \left.\frac{d\psi_{\rm II}}{dx}\right|_{x=0} = B\,\frac{(2mE)^{1/2}}{\hbar}$$

must be equal, giving

$$A = B\left(\frac{E}{V_0 - E}\right)^{1/2}$$

Similarly, the continuity of ψ and its first derivative at $x = a$ require that

$$B \sin\frac{(2mE)^{1/2}a}{\hbar} + C\cos\frac{(2mE)^{1/2}a}{\hbar} = De^{-[2m(V_0-E)]^{1/2}(a/\hbar)}$$

and

$$B\frac{(2mE)^{1/2}}{\hbar}\cos\frac{(2mE)^{1/2}a}{\hbar} - C\frac{(2mE)^{1/2}}{\hbar}\sin\frac{(2mE)^{1/2}a}{\hbar} = -D\,\frac{[2m(V_0 - E)]^{1/2}}{\hbar}\,e^{-[2m(V_0-E)]^{1/2}(a/\hbar)}$$

In view of the relation between A and C and between A and B found above, the last two equations can be rewritten as

$$\sin\frac{(2mE)^{1/2}a}{\hbar} + \left(\frac{E}{V_0 - E}\right)^{1/2}\cos\frac{(2mE)^{1/2}a}{\hbar} = \frac{D}{B}e^{-[2m(V_0-E)]^{1/2}(a/\hbar)}$$

and

$$\cos\frac{(2mE)^{1/2}a}{\hbar} - \left(\frac{E}{V_0 - E}\right)^{1/2}\sin\frac{(2mE)^{1/2}a}{\hbar} = -\frac{D}{B}\left(\frac{V_0 - E}{E}\right)^{1/2}e^{-[2m(V_0-E)]^{1/2}(a/\hbar)}$$

Dividing these two equations yields the desired equation for E, which, after some manipulation, can be put in the form

$$\left(\frac{E}{V_0 - E}\right)^{1/2} = \cot\frac{(2mE)^{1/2}a}{2\hbar} \qquad \text{or} \qquad -\left(\frac{E}{V_0 - E}\right)^{1/2} = \tan\frac{(2mE)^{1/2}a}{2\hbar}$$

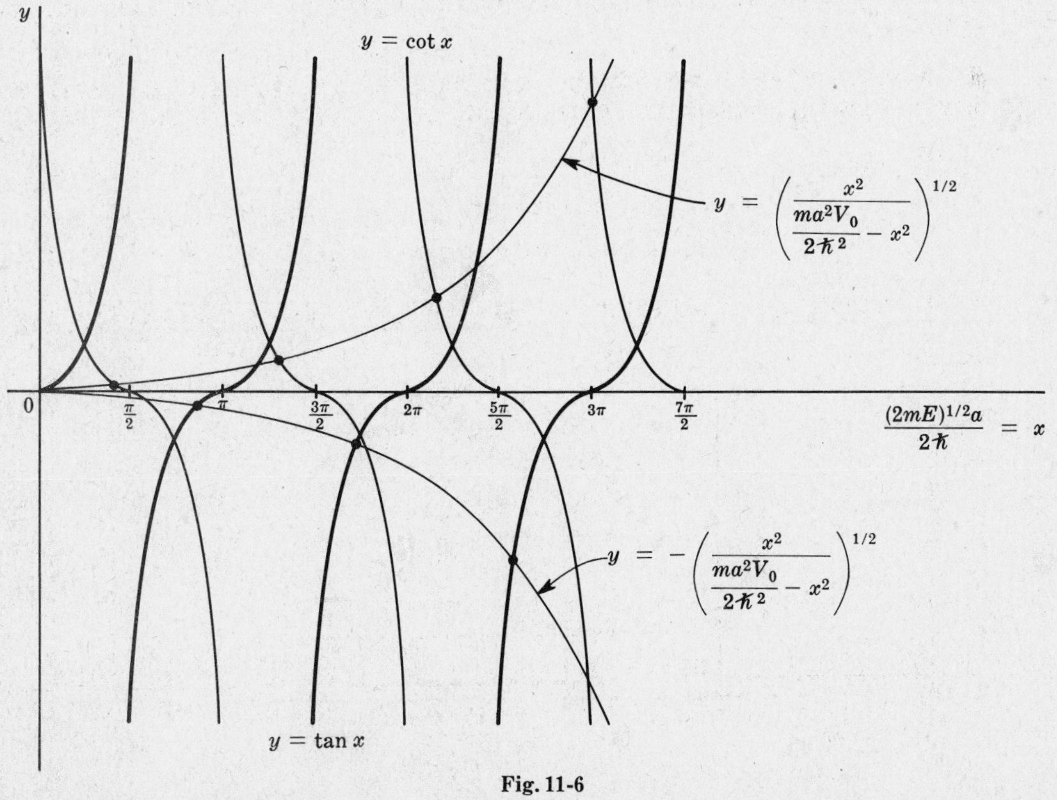

Fig. 11-6

A graphical solution is indicated in Fig. 11-6. The intersections above the x-axis give the energies corresponding to wave functions that are symmetrical about the center of the well; those below the axis correspond to antisymmetric wave functions.

(*b*) As E approaches V_0 from below, the relative amount of "tailing off" in regions I and III increases, see Fig. 11-5(*b*). If the width of the potential barrier for region III is small enough that $\psi_{III}(x)$ has not reached zero before entering the region IV shown in Fig. 11-5(*c*), there is a finite probability for the particle to "tunnel" from II to IV.

11.5. A simple harmonic oscillator (SHO) is characterized by two bodies of mass m_1 and m_2 separated by a distance which can change by an amount x, see Fig. 11-7. For a displacement x, it is assumed that a restoring force equal to $-kx$ is present. Write the Hamiltonian for this system.

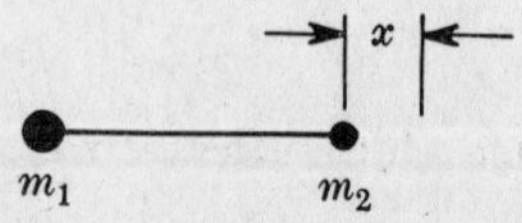

Fig. 11-7

The potential energy for the system may be determined by integrating the negative of the restoring force giving

$$U(x) = -\int_0^x f(y)\,dy = -\int_0^x (-ky)\,dy = \frac{kx^2}{2} \qquad (11.37)$$

Substituting this expression into (*11.15*) gives

$$\mathcal{H} = -\frac{\hbar^2}{2\mu}\frac{d^2}{dx^2} + \frac{kx^2}{2} \qquad (11.38)$$

where μ is the reduced mass expressed in terms of m_1 and m_2, see (*11.10*).

11.6. The eigenvalues describing the energy states for the SHO described in Problem 11.5 are given by

$$E_v = \left(v + \frac{1}{2}\right)h\nu_0 \qquad (11.39)$$

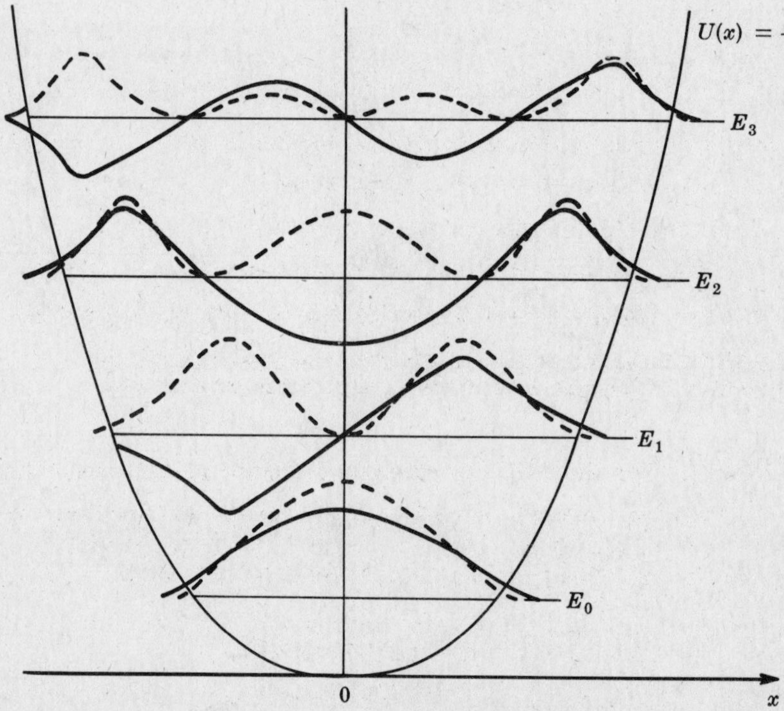

Fig. 11-8

where $v = 0, 1, 2, 3, \ldots$ and

$$\nu_0 = \frac{(k/\mu)^{1/2}}{2\pi} \tag{11.40}$$

Prepare a plot of (*11.37*) and sketch the energy levels given by (*11.39*).

A plot of (*11.37*) gives a parabola, see Fig. 11-8, centered about $x = 0$. The energy levels given by (*11.39*) are equally spaced:

$$\Delta E_v = \left(v + 1 + \frac{1}{2}\right)h\nu_0 - \left(v + \frac{1}{2}\right)h\nu_0 = h\nu_0$$

11.7. The normalized eigenfunctions for the SHO described in Problem 11.5 are

$$\psi_v(x) = (2^v v!)^{-1/2}(a/\pi)^{1/4}e^{-ax^2/2}H_v(a^{1/2}x) \tag{11.41}$$

where
$$a = \frac{2\pi\nu_0\mu}{\hbar} \tag{11.42}$$

and the *Hermite polynomials* are defined as

$$H_n(z) = (-1)^n e^{z^2}\left(\frac{d^n e^{-z^2}}{dz^n}\right) \tag{11.43}$$

Find the first four eigenfunctions and sketch $\psi_v(x)$ and $\psi_v(x)^*\psi_v(x)$ on the corresponding energy levels shown in Fig. 11-8.

The first four Hermite polynomials are given by (*11.43*) as

$$H_0(z) = (-1)^0 e^{z^2}\left(\frac{d^0 e^{-z^2}}{dz^0}\right) = 1$$

$$H_1(z) = (-1)^1 e^{z^2}\left(\frac{de^{-z^2}}{dz}\right) = 2z$$

$$H_2(z) = (-1)^2 e^{z^2}\left(\frac{d^2 e^{-z^2}}{dz^2}\right) = 4z^2 - 2$$

$$H_3(z) = (-1)^3 e^{z^2}\left(\frac{d^3 e^{-z^2}}{dz^3}\right) = 8z^3 - 12z$$

which expressed in terms of $a^{1/2}x$ and substituted into (*11.41*) give

$$\psi_0(x) = (2^0 0!)^{-1/2}(a/\pi)^{1/4}e^{-ax^2/2}(1) = (a/\pi)^{1/4}e^{-ax^2/2}$$

$$\psi_1(x) = (2^1 1!)^{-1/2}(a/\pi)^{1/4}e^{-ax^2/2}(2a^{1/2}x) = (2a)^{1/2}(a/\pi)^{1/4}xe^{-ax^2/2}$$

$$\psi_2(x) = (2^2 2!)^{-1/2}(a/\pi)^{1/4}e^{-ax^2/2}(4ax^2 - 2) = (1/2)^{1/2}(a/\pi)^{1/4}(2ax^2 - 1)e^{-ax^2/2}$$

$$\psi_3(x) = (2^3 3!)^{-1/2}(a/\pi)^{1/4}e^{-ax^2/2}(8a^{3/2}x^3 - 12a^{1/2}x) = (1/3)^{1/2}(a/\pi)^{1/4}(2a^{3/2}x^3 - 3a^{1/2}x)e^{-ax^2/2}$$

Figure 11-8 shows these functions as solid curves and $\psi^*\psi$ as dashed curves. Note that there is a finite probability that the system lies outside the parabolic potential well.

11.8. Verify that $\psi_3(x)$ for the SHO, as given in Problem 11.7, is normalized.

To see if the wave function is normalized, the integral $\langle\psi \mid \psi\rangle$ is evaluated, giving

$$\langle\psi_3(x) \mid \psi_3(x)\rangle = \int_{-\infty}^{\infty}\left[\left(\frac{1}{3}\right)^{1/2}\left(\frac{a}{\pi}\right)^{1/4}(2a^{3/2}x^3 - 3a^{1/2}x)e^{-ax^2/2}\right]^2 dx$$

$$= \left(\frac{1}{3}\right)\left(\frac{a}{\pi}\right)^{1/2}\int_{-\infty}^{\infty} e^{-ax^2}(2a^{3/2}x^3 - 3a^{1/2})^2\,dx$$

$$= \left(\frac{1}{3}\right)\left(\frac{a}{\pi}\right)^{1/2}\left[4a^3\int_{-\infty}^{\infty} x^6 e^{-ax^2}\,dx - 12a^2\int_{-\infty}^{\infty} x^4 e^{-ax^2}\,dx + 9a\int_{-\infty}^{\infty} x^2 e^{-ax^2}\,dx\right]$$

The three integrals can be evaluated using

$$\int_0^\infty x^{2n}e^{-ax^2}\,dx = \frac{(1)(3)(5)\cdots(2n-1)(\pi/a)^{1/2}}{2^{n+1}a^n}$$

and the fact that the three integrands are even functions. Thus

$$\langle\psi_3(x)\mid\psi_3(x)\rangle = 2\left(\frac{1}{3}\right)\left(\frac{a}{\pi}\right)^{1/2}\left[4a^3\frac{(1)(3)(5)(\pi/a)^{1/2}}{2^4a^3} - 12a^2\frac{(1)(3)(\pi/a)^{1/2}}{2^3a^2} + 9a\frac{(1)(\pi/a)^{1/2}}{2^2a}\right]$$

$$= 2\left(\frac{1}{3}\right)\left(\frac{a}{\pi}\right)^{1/2}\left[(1.5)\left(\frac{\pi}{a}\right)^{1/2}\right] = 1$$

The wave function is normalized, see (*11.12*).

11.9. For Hermitian operators, eigenfunctions corresponding to distinct eigenvalues are orthogonal, i.e. they obey (*11.13*). Verify the orthogonality of the first two eigenfunctions of the SHO, $\psi_0(x)$ and $\psi_1(x)$.

$$\langle\psi_0(x)\mid\psi_1(x)\rangle = \int_{-\infty}^{\infty}\left[\left(\frac{a}{\pi}\right)^{1/4}e^{-ax^2/2}\right]\left[(2a)^{1/2}\left(\frac{a}{\pi}\right)^{1/4}xe^{-ax^2/2}\right]dx = a\left(\frac{2}{\pi}\right)^{1/2}\int_{-\infty}^{\infty}xe^{-ax^2}\,dx$$

But the integrand is an odd function, so that the value of the integral is zero.

11.10. Evaluate $\langle x\rangle$ for the SHO system in the lowest energy state.

Substituting the expression derived in Problem 11.7 for $\psi_0(x)$ into (*11.20*) gives

$$\langle x\rangle = \int_{-\infty}^{\infty}\left[\left(\frac{a}{\pi}\right)^{1/4}e^{-ax^2/2}\right]x\left[\left(\frac{a}{\pi}\right)^{1/4}e^{-ax^2/2}\right]dx = \left(\frac{a}{\pi}\right)^{1/2}\int_{-\infty}^{\infty}xe^{-ax^2}\,dx = 0$$

which is the center of the parabola. Thus the $v = 0$ state can be interpreted as a symmetrical oscillation around the equilibrium position.

11.11. Show that the wave function given by (*11.41*) for the lowest energy state of the SHO system is indeed a solution to (*11.22*).

Using the Hamiltonian from (*11.38*), E_0 from (*11.39*) and the expression for $\psi_0(x)$ from Problem 11.7 in (*11.22*) gives

$$-\frac{\hbar^2}{2\mu}\frac{d^2}{dx^2}\left[\left(\frac{a}{\pi}\right)^{1/4}e^{-ax^2/2}\right] + \frac{hx^2}{2}\left[\left(\frac{a}{\pi}\right)^{1/4}e^{-ax^2/2}\right] = \frac{1}{2}h\nu_0\left[\left(\frac{a}{\pi}\right)^{1/4}e^{-ax^2/2}\right]$$

Taking the derivatives and simplifying gives

$$\left(-\frac{\hbar^2}{2\mu}\right)(a^2x^2-a)e^{-ax^2/2} + \left(\frac{hx^2}{2}\right)e^{-ax^2/2} = \frac{h\nu_0}{2}e^{-ax^2/2}$$

which upon canceling the exponentials, substitution of (*11.42*) and (*11.40*), and simplification gives identical terms on both sides of the equation.

11.12. Figure 11-9 is a plot of $\psi^*\psi$ for the $v = 10$ state of the SHO. How does it illustrate the correspondence principle?

According to the correspondence principle, at high quantum numbers the oscillator should approach a macroscopic classical oscillator in behavior, e.g. a pendulum. The figure shows that the probability distribution is concentrated near the "turning points," where the system's energy is purely potential. This indeed describes a pendulum, which spends more time slowing down, reversing direction and accelerating near the extremes of displacement than in the center of the movement where it has its maximum speed.

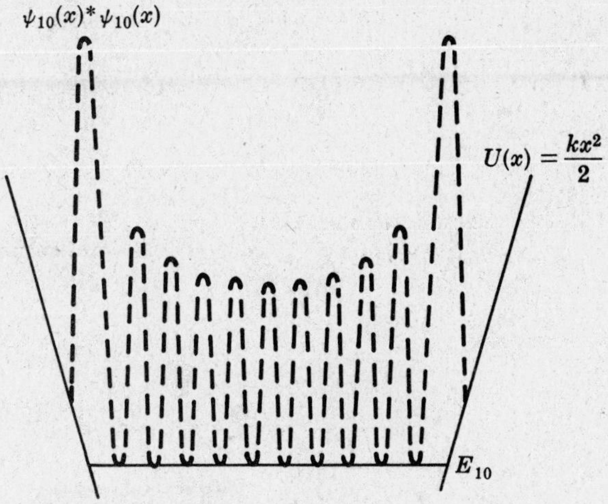

Fig. 11-9

Approximation Methods

11.13. A particle is confined in a one-dimensional potential-energy well where the potential energy is given by $U(x) = U_0 \sin(p\pi x/a)$. Here p is a fixed positive integer. Use perturbation theory to obtain a first-order estimate of the energies of the system.

The given problem is not too different from that of a particle in a box with infinite walls and zero potential energy inside. Choosing this as the unperturbed problem, (*11.17*), (*11.14*) and (*11.19*) give

$$\mathcal{H}^{(0)} = -\frac{\hbar^2}{2m}\frac{d^2}{dx^2} \qquad \psi_n^{(0)} = K\sin\frac{n\pi x}{a} \qquad E_n^{(0)} = \frac{n^2h^2}{8ma^2}$$

With $\lambda = 1$, (*11.29*) gives the perturbation term as $\mathcal{H}^{(1)} = U_0 \sin(p\pi x/a)$. Then, from (*11.34*),

$$H_{nn}^{(1)} = \int_0^a \left(K^*\sin\frac{n\pi x}{a}\right)\left(U_0\sin\frac{p\pi x}{a}\right)\left(K\sin\frac{n\pi x}{a}\right)dx = \frac{2U_0}{a}\int_0^a \sin\frac{p\pi x}{a}\sin^2\frac{n\pi x}{a}\,dx$$

Employing the half-angle formula $\sin^2\alpha = \frac{1}{2} - \frac{1}{2}\cos 2\alpha$, $H_{nn}^{(1)}$ becomes

$$\begin{aligned} H_{nn}^{(1)} &= \frac{U_0}{a}\int_0^a \sin\frac{p\pi x}{a}\,dx - \frac{U_0}{a}\int_0^a \sin\frac{p\pi x}{a}\cos\frac{2n\pi x}{a}\,dx \\ &= -\frac{U_0}{p\pi}\left[\cos\frac{p\pi x}{a}\right]_0^a - \frac{U_0}{a}\int_0^a \sin\frac{p\pi x}{a}\cos\frac{2n\pi x}{a}\,dx \end{aligned}$$

The first term is equal to zero if p is even and $2U_0/p\pi$ if p is odd. The last integral can be evaluated from tables, but three cases must be considered.

Case 1: p is odd. Then $2n \neq p$ and the tabulated integral

$$\int \sin\alpha x\cos\beta x\,dx = -\frac{1}{2}\left[\frac{\cos(\alpha-\beta)x}{\alpha-\beta} + \frac{\cos(\alpha+\beta)x}{\alpha+\beta}\right]$$

can be used to give

$$H_{nn}^{(1)} = \frac{2U_0}{p\pi} - \frac{U_0}{\pi}\left(\frac{1}{p-2n} + \frac{1}{p+2n}\right) = -\frac{8n^2U_0}{p(p^2-4n^2)\pi}$$

Case 2: p is even and $n \neq p/2$. Then the integral in Case 1 still applies, giving

$$H_{nn}^{(1)} = 0 + 0 = 0$$

Case 3: p is even and $n = p/2$. Then

$$H_{p/2,p/2}^{(1)} = 0 - \frac{U_0}{a}\int_0^a \sin\frac{p\pi x}{a}\cos\frac{p\pi x}{a}\,dx = -\frac{U_0}{2a}\int_0^a \sin\frac{2p\pi x}{a}\,dx = 0$$

The perturbed energies are therefore

$$E_n = E_n^{(0)} + H_{nn}^{(1)} = \begin{cases} \dfrac{n^2h^2}{8ma^2} - \dfrac{8n^2U_0}{p(p^2-4n^2)\pi} & \text{if } p \text{ is odd} \\ \dfrac{n^2h^2}{8ma^2} & \text{if } p \text{ is even} \end{cases}$$

The result for even values of p might have been anticipated. When p is even, a whole number of wavelengths of the perturbing function fits into the box. The function thus has average value zero over the box and does not show up in a first-order perturbation.

Supplementary Problems

Preliminaries

11.14. The visible spectrum corresponds to values of λ between 4000 and 7000 Å. Calculate ν, $\bar{\nu}$ and E for yellow light having $\lambda = 5800$ Å.

Ans. 5.169×10^{14} Hz, 17,240 cm^{-1}, 3.425×10^{-19} J

11.15. The speeds of the "Indy-500" racing cars are recorded to ± 0.001 mph. Assuming the track distance to be known to within ± 0.01 mile, is the uncertainty principle violated for a 3.5-ton car?

Ans. $m = 3.2 \times 10^3$ kg, $\Delta v = 4.5 \times 10^{-4}$ m s^{-1}, $\Delta p_x = m\,\Delta v = 1.4$ kg m s^{-1}, $\Delta x = 16$ m, $(\Delta p_x)(\Delta x) = 22$ J s; no

11.16. Compare the emission spectra of atomic hydrogen and deuterium. Assume $m_e = 9.109534 \times 10^{-31}$ kg and $m_{\text{nucleus}} = 1.6726485 \times 10^{-27}$ kg for H and 3.343398×10^{-27} kg for D.

Ans. $\mathcal{R} = 109{,}677.59$ cm^{-1} for H and 109,707.43 cm^{-1} for D, giving slightly higher values of $\bar{\nu}$ and slightly lower values of λ for D.

11.17. Repeat Example 11.3 for He^+, assuming $\mu = m_e$.

Ans. r = 0.265, 1.058, 2.381, 4.233 Å;
E = −438,710, −109,678, −48,746, −27,419 cm^{-1};
ΔE = 329,332, 389,964, 60,932, 411,291, 82,259, 21,327 cm^{-1}

11.18. The element "positronium" consists of an electron moving in space around a nucleus consisting of a positron (see Table 21.1). Using the Bohr theory, calculate the radii of the first four orbits of the electron, the corresponding energies and the predicted electronic spectrum, assuming the positron to be motionless.

Ans. $\mu = m_e/2$; $r = n^2(1.05835)$ Å giving 1.058, 4.233, 9.525, 16.934 Å;
$E = (-54{,}869/n^2)$ cm^{-1} giving −54,869, −13,717, −6097, −3429 cm^{-1};
ΔE = 41,152, 48,772, 7620, 51,440, 10,288, 2668 cm^{-1}

Postulates of Quantum Mechanics

11.19. The general form of the wave function for a free particle moving along the x-axis is

$$\psi = K \cos \frac{[2m(E-U)]^{1/2}x}{\hbar}$$

where $U = \text{constant}$ and $E > U$. Write the wave function describing a particle moving over the potential-energy well shown in Fig. 11-10.

Ans. $\psi_{\text{I}} = \psi_{\text{III}} = A \cos \dfrac{[2m(E - V_0)]^{1/2}x}{\hbar}, \quad \psi_{\text{II}} = B \cos \dfrac{(2mE)^{1/2}x}{\hbar}$

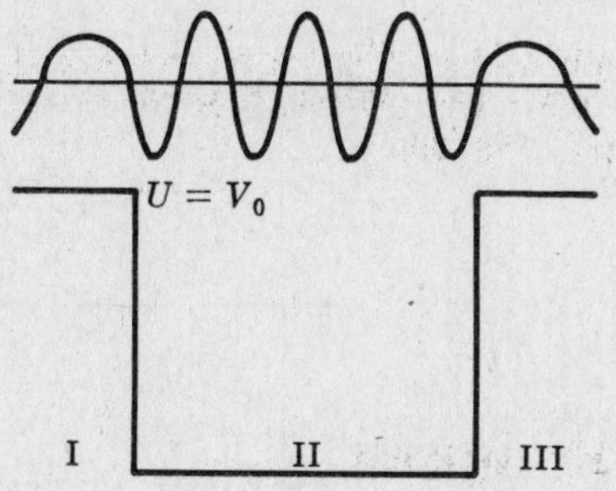

Fig. 11-10

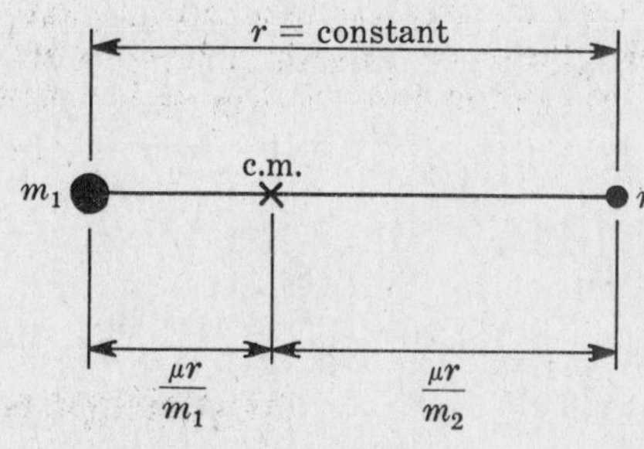

Fig. 11-11

11.20. The normalized wave functions and energies for a particle moving in a three-dimensional potential-energy well which is infinitely deep and has sides of lengths a, b and c are given by

$$\psi(x, y, z) = A \sin \frac{n_x \pi x}{a} \sin \frac{n_y \pi y}{b} \sin \frac{n_z \pi z}{c} \tag{11.44}$$

$$E = \frac{h^2}{8m}\left(\frac{n_x^2}{a^2} + \frac{n_y^2}{b^2} + \frac{n_z^2}{c^2}\right) \tag{11.45}$$

where $A^*A = 8/abc$ and n_x, n_y and n_z are positive integers. What is the degeneracy (the number of different quantum states having the same energy) of the energy level $E = 6h^2/8ma^2$, if the particle is in a cube?

Ans. Triply degenerate: $n_x^2 + n_y^2 + n_z^2 = 6$ if $n_x = 2$, $n_y = 1$, $n_z = 1$ or $n_x = 1$, $n_y = 2$, $n_z = 1$ or $n_x = 1$, $n_y = 1$, $n_z = 2$.

11.21. Find $\langle z \rangle$, $\langle z^2 \rangle$, $\langle p_z \rangle$ and $\langle p_z^2 \rangle$ for a particle in a three-dimensional box using the wave function given by (*11.44*). The operator $\widehat{p_z^2}$ is $(\hbar^2/i^2)(\partial^2/\partial z^2)$. *Ans.* $c/2$, $c^2(2\pi^2 n_z^2 - 3)/6\pi^2 n_z^2$, 0, $\hbar^2\pi^2 n_z^2/c^2$

11.22. The *two-particle rigid rotator* undergoes rotation about its center of mass (see Fig. 11-11). Write the Hamiltonian for this system, using spherical cordinates.

Ans.
$$\mathcal{H} = \left(-\frac{\hbar^2}{2\mu}\right)\left[\frac{1}{r^2 \sin \theta} \frac{\partial}{\partial \theta}\left(\sin \theta \frac{\partial}{\partial \theta}\right) + \frac{1}{r^2 \sin^2 \theta} \frac{\partial^2}{\partial \phi^2}\right] \tag{11.46}$$

11.23. The normalized eigenfunctions for the rigid rotator described in Problem 11.22 are given by

$$\psi_{J,m}(\theta, \phi) = (2\pi)^{-1/2}\Theta_{J,m}(\theta)\, e^{\pm im\phi} \tag{11.47}$$

where
$$\Theta_{J,m}(\theta) = \left[\frac{(2J+1)(J-|m|)!}{2(J+|m|)!}\right]^{1/2} P_J^{|m|}(\cos \theta) \tag{11.48}$$

for $J = 0, 1, 2, \ldots$ and $m = -J, -J+1, \ldots, J-1, J$. Here, the *associated Legendre functions*, $P_\ell^{|m|}(x)$, are defined as

$$P_\ell^{|m|}(x) = \frac{1}{2^\ell \ell!}(1 - x^2)^{|m|/2} \frac{d^{\ell+|m|}}{dx^{\ell+|m|}}(x^2 - 1)^\ell \tag{11.49}$$

Determine $\psi_{J,m}(\theta,\phi)$ for $J = 2$ and $m = \pm 1$ and verify that it is normalized.

Ans. $\psi_{2,\pm 1}(\theta,\phi) = \left(\frac{15}{8\pi}\right)^{1/2} \sin\theta\cos\theta\; e^{\pm i\phi}$;

$\langle\psi\,|\,\psi\rangle = 1$

11.24. The eigenvalues for the rigid rotator described in Problem 11.22 are

$$E_J = \frac{J(J+1)\hbar^2}{2I} \qquad (11.50)$$

where the moment of inertia is given by

$$I = \mu r^2 \qquad (11.51)$$

(*a*) What is the degeneracy of each level? (*b*) Prepare a plot of the energy levels expressed in units of $\hbar^2/2I$.

Ans. (*a*) $2J+1$; (*b*) see Fig. 11-12.

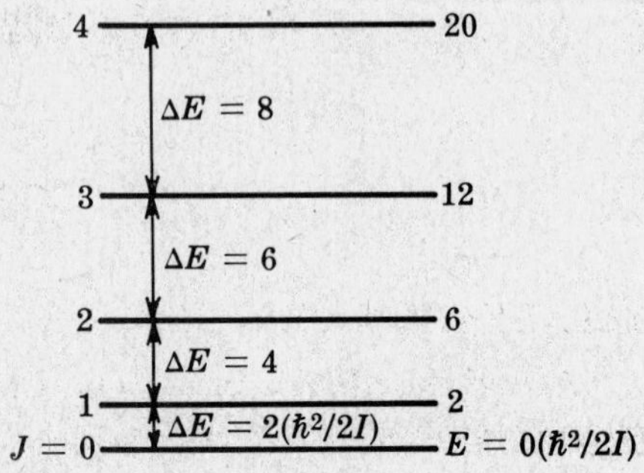

Fig. 11-12

11.25. Determine $\psi(\theta,\phi)$ for a rigid rotator using (*11.47*) if $J = 2$ and $m = 0$ and show that it is a solution to (*11.22*).

Ans. $\left(\frac{5}{16\pi}\right)^{1/2} (3\cos^2\theta - 1)$

Approximation Methods

11.26. Consider a particle in a one-dimensional box $(0 \leqq x \leqq a)$ where $U(x) = U_0 \cos(n\pi x/a)$. Use first-order perturbation theory to determine E.

Ans. $\mathcal{H}^{(1)} = U_0\cos(n\pi x/a)$, $H_{nn}^{(1)} = 0$, $E = n^2h^2/8ma^2$

11.27. Solve the secular equation

$$\begin{vmatrix} H_{aa} - E & H_{ba} - ES \\ H_{ba} - ES & H_{aa} - E \end{vmatrix} = 0$$

Ans. $E = (H_{aa} + H_{ba})/(1+S)$ or $(H_{aa} - H_{ba})/(1-S)$

Chapter 12

Atomic Structure and Spectroscopy

Hydrogenlike Atoms

12.1 SYSTEM DESCRIPTION

A *hydrogenlike* atom is one in which an electron having a charge of $-e$ and mass m_e is moving around a nucleus having a charge of $+Ze$ and a mass of m_{nucleus}. Usually such a system is described using spherical coordinates (r, θ, ϕ), see Fig. 12-1. After separating the kinetic energy terms describing the translational motion of the entire atom (a particle in a three-dimensional box), (*11.22*) becomes

$$\left(-\frac{\hbar^2}{2\mu}\right)\left[\frac{1}{r^2}\frac{\partial}{\partial r}\left(r^2\frac{\partial}{\partial r}\psi(r,\theta,\phi)\right) + \frac{1}{r^2\sin\theta}\frac{\partial}{\partial\theta}\left(\sin\theta\frac{\partial}{\partial\theta}\psi(r,\theta,\phi)\right) + \frac{1}{r^2\sin^2\theta}\frac{\partial^2}{\partial\phi^2}\psi(r,\theta,\phi)\right] + \left(-\frac{Ze^2}{4\pi\epsilon_0 r}\right)\psi(r,\theta,\phi) = E\psi(r,\theta,\phi) \qquad (12.1)$$

where μ is the reduced mass of the system and $-Ze^2/4\pi\epsilon_0 r$ represents the potential energy of the system as a result of the coulombic attraction between the nucleus and the electron.

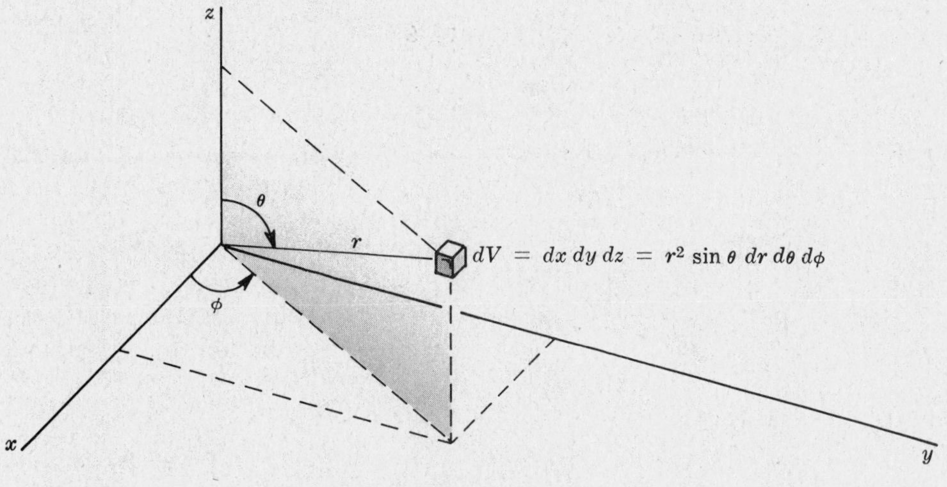

Fig. 12-1

A wave function that satisfies (*12.1*) is

$$\psi(r, \theta, \phi) = R(r)\,\Theta(\theta)\,\Phi(\phi) \tag{12.2}$$

where the new wave functions, $R(r)$, $\Theta(\theta)$ and $\Phi(\phi)$ are functions of only r, θ and ϕ, respectively. Substituting (*12.2*) into (*12.1*) generates the following set of three equations:

$$\frac{1}{r^2}\frac{d}{dr}\left(r^2\frac{d}{dr}R(r)\right) - \frac{\beta}{r^2}R(r) + \left(\frac{2\mu}{\hbar^2}\right)\left(E + \frac{Ze^2}{4\pi\epsilon_0 r}\right)R(r) = 0 \tag{12.3a}$$

$$\left(\frac{m^2}{\sin^2\theta}\right)\Theta(\theta) - \frac{1}{\sin\theta}\frac{d}{d\theta}\left(\sin\theta\frac{d}{d\theta}\Theta(\theta)\right) - \beta\Theta(\theta) = 0 \tag{12.3b}$$

$$\left(-\frac{1}{\Phi(\phi)}\right)\frac{d^2}{d\phi^2}\Phi(\phi) = m^2 \tag{12.3c}$$

where m and β are constants.

12.2 THE ANGULAR FUNCTION

The normalized solution of (*12.3c*) is

$$\Phi(\phi) = (2\pi)^{-1/2}e^{im\phi} \tag{12.4}$$

where $m = 0, \pm1, \pm2, \ldots$. The integer m is known as the *magnetic quantum number* because in the presence of a magnetic field, states with different values of m will have different energies (*Zeeman effect*).

The normalized solution of (*12.3b*) with $\beta = \ell(\ell+1)$ is given by

$$\Theta(\theta) = \left[\frac{(2\ell+1)(\ell-|m|)!}{2(\ell+|m|)!}\right]^{1/2} P_\ell^{|m|}(\cos\theta) \tag{12.5}$$

where $P_\ell^{|m|}(\cos\theta)$ has been defined by (*11.49*) and $\ell = 0, 1, 2, \ldots$. The integer ℓ is known as the *azimuthal quantum number* and describes the general shape of the wave function for an *atomic subshell.* A common notation is to substitute the letter s for $\ell = 0$, p for $\ell = 1$, d for $\ell = 2$, f for $\ell = 3$, g for $\ell = 4$, etc. The magnetic quantum number must be restricted to

$$m = 0, \pm1, \pm2, \ldots, \pm\ell \tag{12.6}$$

if $\Theta(\theta)$ is to be defined by (*12.5*). The combination of the azimuthal and magnetic quantum numbers generates an *atomic orbital.*

The product $\Theta(\theta)\,\Phi(\phi)$ is known as the *angular eigenfunction* and is given the symbol $Y(\theta, \phi)$. Note that the solution for the rigid-rotator problem given by (*11.47*) is identical with $Y(\theta, \phi)$. Unless $m = 0$, the angular wave functions determined by (*12.4*) and (*12.5*) contain imaginary terms, which presents difficulty in visualization of the wave function. For this reason linear combinations of the $Y(\theta, \phi)$ which generate real wave functions are usually chosen to describe the atomic orbitals (without changing the eigenvalues of energy). It is not possible to assign one of these newly created wave functions to a given value of m.

EXAMPLE 12.1. The angular wave functions for $\ell = 2$ and $m = \pm1$ are

$$Y(\theta, \phi) = \left(\frac{15}{8\pi}\right)^{1/2} \sin\theta\cos\theta\; e^{\pm i\phi}$$

Construct two real wave functions, $Y'(\theta, \phi)$ and $Y''(\theta, \phi)$, from these and prepare two-dimensional plots of the new wave functions and of

$$Y'(\theta, \phi)^* Y'(\theta, \phi) = [Y'(\theta, \phi)]^2 \qquad \text{and} \qquad Y''(\theta, \phi)^* Y''(\theta, \phi) = [Y''(\theta, \phi)]^2$$

In view of Euler's formula, $e^{\pm i\phi} = \cos\phi \pm i\sin\phi$, the linear combinations

$$Y'(\theta,\phi) \equiv \sqrt{2}\left[\frac{Y_+(\theta,\phi) + Y_-(\theta,\phi)}{2}\right]$$

$$Y''(\theta,\phi) \equiv \sqrt{2}\left[\frac{Y_+(\theta,\phi) - Y_-(\theta,\phi)}{2i}\right]$$

will be real, where the subscripts on $Y(\theta,\phi)$ indicate which sign is being used in the exponential term. (The factor $\sqrt{2}$ is merely an additional normalizing factor.) Thus

$$Y'(\theta,\phi) = \left(\frac{15}{4\pi}\right)^{1/2} \sin\theta\cos\theta\cos\phi$$

$$Y''(\theta,\phi) = \left(\frac{15}{4\pi}\right)^{1/2} \sin\theta\cos\theta\sin\phi$$

Figure 12-2(a) is a polar plot of $|Y'(\theta,\phi)|$ in the xz-plane, where $|\cos\phi| = 1$. The algebraic sign of $Y'(\theta,\phi)$ is indicated beside each lobe of the curve. Figure 12-2(b) shows $[Y'(\theta,\phi)]^2$, the scale being the same as in Fig. 12-2(a). A separate figure for $Y''(\theta,\phi)$ is not needed, as $Y''(\theta,\phi)$ is just $Y'(\theta,\phi)$ rotated 90° about the z-axis, i.e. $Y''(\theta,\phi)$ lies in the yz-plane.

Because $Y'(\theta,\phi)$ has its peak values along 45°-lines within the xz-plane and because the value of ℓ is 2, this orbital is known as the d_{xz} orbital.

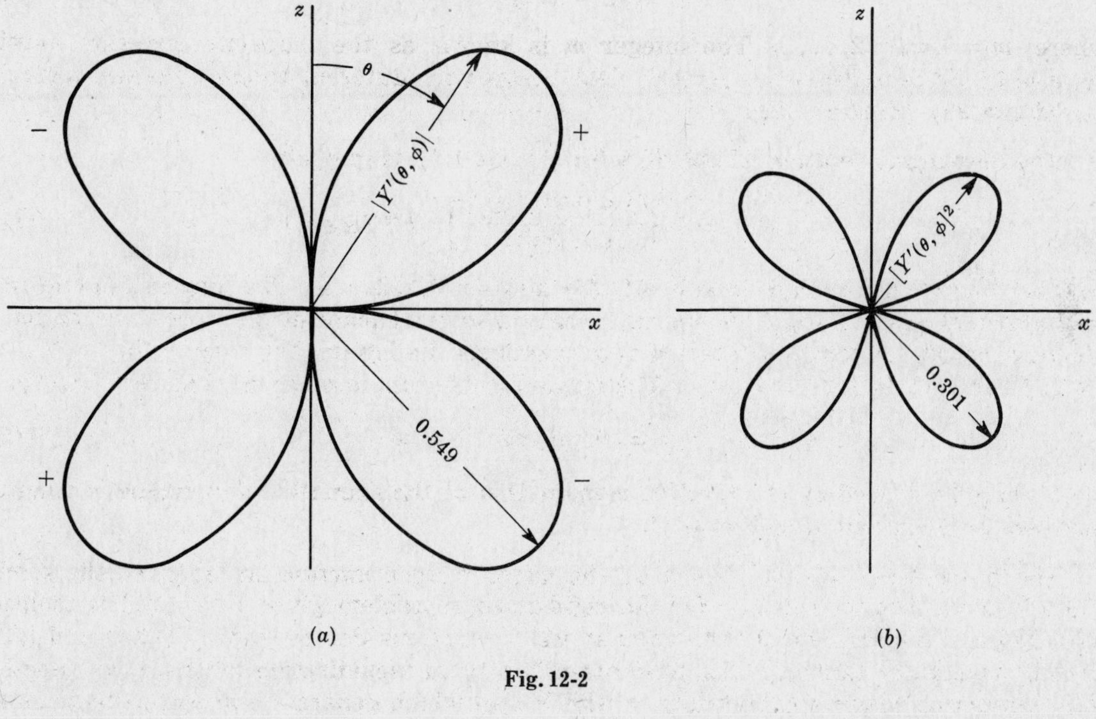

Fig. 12-2

12.3 THE RADIAL FUNCTION

The normalized solution of (*12.3a*) is

$$R_{n,\ell}(r) = -\left\{\frac{(2Z/na_0)^3(n-\ell-1)!}{2n[(n+\ell)!]^3}\right\}^{1/2} e^{-\rho/2}\rho^{\ell}L_{n+\ell}^{2\ell+1}(\rho) \qquad (12.7)$$

where $n = 1, 2, 3, \ldots,$

$$\rho = \left(\frac{2Z}{na_0}\right)r \qquad (12.8)$$

$$a_0 = \frac{4\pi\epsilon_0\hbar^2}{\mu e^2} \tag{12.9}$$

and the *associated Laguerre polynomials* are defined as

$$L_q^s(x) = \frac{d^s}{dx^s}\left[e^x \frac{d^q}{dx^q}(x^q e^{-x})\right] \tag{12.10}$$

The integer n is known as the *principal quantum number* and is related to the distance between the nucleus and electron. Equation (*12.7*) restricts ℓ to the values

$$\ell = 0, 1, 2, \ldots, n-1 \tag{12.11}$$

if $R(r)$ is to be defined.

The probability of finding an electron between r and $r+dr$ is given by $R(r)^* R(r) r^2\, dr$, where the factor r^2 appears from the volume element in the spherical coordinate system (see Problem 12.5).

EXAMPLE 12.2. Determine $R(r)$ for the 1*s* orbital.

Using (*12.10*) gives

$$L_1^1(\rho) = \frac{d}{d\rho}\left[e^\rho \frac{d}{d\rho}(\rho e^{-\rho})\right] = \frac{d}{d\rho}[1-\rho] = -1$$

for $n = 1$ and $\ell = 0$. Then (*12.7*) gives

$$R_{1,0}(r) = -\left(\frac{2Z}{a_0}\right)^{3/2}\left\{\frac{0!}{2(1!)^3}\right\}^{1/2} e^{-\rho/2}\rho^0(-1)$$

$$= 2\left(\frac{Z}{a_0}\right)^{3/2} e^{-\rho/2} = 2\left(\frac{Z}{a_0}\right)^{3/2} e^{-Zr/a_0}$$

12.4 ELECTRON POSITION

The probability of locating an electron within a volume V_0 is given by

$$\iiint_{V_0} \psi^* \psi\, dV$$

12.5 ENERGY VALUES

The energy eigenvalues for a hydrogenlike atom as determined by substituting (*12.2*), (*12.4*), (*12.5*) and (*12.7*) into (*12.1*) are

$$E = \frac{-\mu Z^2 e^4}{2n^2\hbar^2(4\pi\epsilon_0)^2} \tag{12.12}$$

This result is identical to that of the Bohr theory, (*11.11*). Hence the spectrum predicted by (*12.12*) will be identical to that described in Sections 11.4 and 11.5.

EXAMPLE 12.3. List the orbitals for hydrogenlike atoms in order of increasing energy.

Because (*12.12*) is a function of only n, all orbitals having the same value of n will have the same energy. Thus, $1s < 2s = 2p < 3s = 3p = 3d < 4s = 4p = 4d = 4f < 5s = 5p = 5d = 5f = 5g <$ etc.

Quantum Theory of Polyelectronic Atoms

12.6 ELECTRON SPIN WAVE FUNCTIONS

The coupling of the angular momenta of two or more electrons in an atom plays an important part in removing the degeneracy of the atomic orbitals having the same principal and azimuthal quantum numbers. The usual notation is α and β for the wave functions for electron spin, and $s = \pm\frac{1}{2}$ for the corresponding quantum numbers.

12.7 HAMILTONIAN OPERATOR AND WAVE FUNCTION

The Hamiltonian operator for a system containing n electrons is given by

$$\mathcal{H} = \frac{-\hbar^2}{2m_e}\sum_{i=1}^{n}\nabla_i^2 - \sum_{i=1}^{n}\frac{Ze^2}{4\pi\epsilon_0 r_i} + \sum_{j=2}^{n}\sum_{i<j}\frac{e^2}{4\pi\epsilon_0 r_{ij}} \qquad (12.13)$$

where r_{ij} is the distance between the ith and jth electrons. The Schrödinger equation cannot be solved exactly because of the r_{ij}-term, and approximate methods must be used: e.g. neglect the r_{ij}-term, self-consistent field theory, Hartree-Fock techniques, etc.

According to the *Pauli exclusion principle,* an acceptable wave function for electrons must change its algebraic sign when the coordinates (both spatial and spin) of any two particles are interchanged (antisymmetry). Such a wave function for the ground state of a polyelectronic atom is given by the *Slater determinant*

$$\psi = \frac{1}{\sqrt{n!}}\begin{vmatrix} \phi_{1s}(1)\alpha(1) & \phi_{1s}(2)\alpha(2) & \ldots & \phi_{1s}(n)\alpha(n) \\ \phi_{1s}(1)\beta(1) & \phi_{1s}(2)\beta(2) & \ldots & \phi_{1s}(n)\beta(n) \\ \phi_{2s}(1)\alpha(1) & \phi_{2s}(2)\alpha(2) & \ldots & \phi_{2s}(n)\alpha(n) \\ \vdots & \vdots & & \vdots \end{vmatrix} \qquad (12.14)$$

where $\phi_{1s}(1)\alpha(1)$ represents the product of the hydrogenlike $1s$ orbital containing electron number 1 and the α spin wave function for electron number 1, etc. Thus the n columns correspond to the n electrons, and the n rows to their n lowest quantum states. Interchanging the coordinates of two electrons means interchanging two columns, which reverses the sign of the determinant.

EXAMPLE 12.4. Using *(12.13)* and *(12.14)*, determine $\mathcal{H}$ and ψ for He. Verify that the expanded form of ψ is antisymmetric with respect to permutation of the electrons.

For two electrons the Hamiltonian given by *(12.13)* is

$$\mathcal{H} = \frac{-\hbar^2}{2m_e}(\nabla_1^2 + \nabla_2^2) - \frac{2e^2}{4\pi\epsilon_0}\left(\frac{1}{r_1} + \frac{1}{r_2}\right) + \frac{e^2}{4\pi\epsilon_0 r_{12}}$$

and the determinant given by *(12.14)* is

$$\psi = \frac{1}{\sqrt{2!}}\begin{vmatrix} \phi_{1s}(1)\alpha(1) & \phi_{1s}(2)\alpha(2) \\ \phi_{1s}(1)\beta(1) & \phi_{1s}(2)\beta(2) \end{vmatrix}$$

which upon expansion gives

$$\psi = 2^{-1/2}[\phi_{1s}(1)\alpha(1)\phi_{1s}(2)\beta(2) - \phi_{1s}(1)\beta(1)\phi_{1s}(2)\alpha(2)]$$

To demonstrate the antisymmetric behavior of ψ, exchanging electron number 2 for electron number 1 and electron number 1 for electron number 2 gives a new wave function ψ', where

$$\psi' = 2^{-1/2}[\phi_{1s}(2)\alpha(2)\phi_{1s}(1)\beta(1) - \phi_{1s}(2)\beta(2)\phi_{1s}(1)\alpha(1)] = -\psi$$

12.8 ENERGY LEVELS

The exact ordering of the atomic subshells with respect to energy depends on Z, but in general the filling order is $1s < 2s < 2p(3) < 3s < 3p(3) < 4s < 3d(5) < 4p(3) < 5s < 4d(5) < 5p(3) < 6s < 4f(7) < 5d(5) < 6p(3) < 7s < 5f(7) = 6d(5) < 7p(3) <$ etc., where the number in parentheses represents the number of orbitals comprising the subshell. Because of spin considerations, each orbital can hold two electrons. In the accepted notation for subshells a superscript is used to indicate the number of electrons in that subshell, e.g. $3d^3$ implies that there are three electrons with $n = 3$ and $\ell = 2$.

The Pauli exclusion principle can be restated as: *no two electrons can have identical values for all four quantum numbers in the same atom.* Thus, in the $3d^3$ subshell the three electrons must have three different combinations of $m = \pm 2, \pm 1, 0$ and $s = \pm\frac{1}{2}$.

The rule of maximum multiplicity (*Hund's first rule*) states that *the most stable state for a configuration will be the one having the most nonpaired electrons;* so, by convention, electrons with parallel spins are placed singly in the various degenerate orbitals until it is necessary to add a second electron. By convention, the orbitals having the most positive values of m and of s are lowest in energy and are used first. For example, the $3d^3$ configuration would correspond to $m = +2,\ s = +\frac{1}{2};\ m = +1,\ s = +\frac{1}{2}$ and $m = 0,\ s = +\frac{1}{2}$.

EXAMPLE 12.5. Predict the electronic configuration for the ground state of Cr and suggest possible oxidation states for the element.

The predicted configuration for the 24 electrons in Cr would be

$$1s^2 2s^2 2p^6 3s^2 3p^6 4s^2 3d^4$$

One major exception to the rules for filling subshells is that filled and half-filled d and f subshells are definitely favored, and slight rearrangements of predicted configurations will occur to give a more energetically favorable configuration. Thus, in Cr, the attainment of the d^5 configuration changes the predicted configuration to

$$1s^2 2s^2 2p^6 3s^2 3p^6 4s^1 3d^5$$

The possible oxidation states of an atom will correspond to the number of electrons that can easily be removed—seldom more than seven—and the number of electrons needed to complete a shell—seldom more than four. The order of removing electrons is more like the reverse of the order of filling hydrogenlike atoms than of filling polyelectron atoms. The configuration for Cr would suggest the possible oxidation states as 0, +1 (loss of the $4s$ electron), +2 (loss of the $4s$ electron and the $3d$ electron that was supposed to be a $4s$ electron), and +6 (loss of the $4s$ electron and the $3d$ electrons). The common +3 oxidation state corresponds to the loss of the $4s$ and two of the $3d$ electrons.

Atomic Term Symbols

12.9 RUSSELL-SAUNDERS COUPLING

The coupling of the angular momenta of two atomic orbitals, known as *ℓ-ℓ coupling*, gives rise to a quantum number L, where

$$L = \ell_1 + \ell_2,\ \ell_1 + \ell_2 - 1,\ \ldots,\ |\ell_1 - \ell_2| \tag{12.15}$$

The coupling of the angular momenta of two electrons, known as *s-s coupling*, gives rise to a quantum number S, where

$$S = 0 \text{ or } 1 \tag{12.16}$$

The *Russell-Saunders coupling* between L and S gives rise to a quantum number J, where

$$J = L + S,\ L + S - 1,\ \ldots,\ |L - S| \tag{12.17}$$

The atomic term symbol has the general form ${}^{2S+1}X_J$, where the leading superscript represents the degeneracy of the term, the subscript is the value of J as determined by (*12.17*), and X represents a letter symbol for the value of L; i.e. S (not to be confused with the spin quantum number) for $L = 0$, P for $L = 1$, D for $L = 2$, F for $L = 3$, G for $L = 4$, etc.

EXAMPLE 12.6. Determine the values of L for the interaction between a p and a d electron.

The values of ℓ for p and d electrons are 1 and 2, respectively. Using (*12.15*) gives

$$L = 1+2 = 3,$$
$$1+2-1 = 2,$$
$$1+2-2 = |1-2| = 1$$

which correspond to the letters F, D and P, respectively.

12.10 POLYELECTRONIC ATOM TERM SYMBOLS

For polyelectronic systems,

$$M_L = \sum m_i \quad \text{where} \quad M_L = L, L-1, \ldots, -L \tag{12.18}$$

$$M_S = \sum s_i \quad \text{where} \quad M_S = S, S-1, \ldots, -S \tag{12.19}$$

As can be seen from these equations, the only contributions to M_L and M_S are from nonfilled subshells.

To determine the possible term symbols for an atom, the following steps are used: (1) prepare a list of microstates that correspond to the possible combinations of wave functions that are permitted by the Pauli exclusion principle (see Example 12.7); (2) determine M_L and M_S for these microstates; (3) determine the term symbol for the microstate having the largest values of M_L and M_S, using $L = M_L$ and $S = M_S$; (4) to that same term symbol assign all microstates whose M_L and M_S values are related to the above L and S by (*12.18*) and (*12.19*); (5) repeat steps (3) and (4) for the largest remaining M_L-M_S combination until all microstates have been assigned. Table 12-1 lists the results of these steps for various electronic configurations for electrons having identical values of n and ℓ.

The ground state for the atom will correspond to the term symbol having the highest value of $2S+1$, according to the rule of maximum multiplicity (Hund's first rule). For terms of equal multiplicity, the ground state will have the highest value of M_L (*Hund's second rule*). The value of J for a given level is usually lowest for less-than-half-filled subshells and greatest for more-than-half-filled subshells.

Table 12-1

Configuration	Term Symbols
s^1	^2S
s^2	^1S
p^1 or p^5	^2P
p^2 or p^4	^3P, ^1D, ^1S
p^3	^4S, ^2D, ^2P
p^6	^1S
d^1 or d^9	^2D
d^2 or d^8	^3F, ^3P, ^1G, ^1D, ^1S
d^3 or d^7	^4F, ^4P, ^2H, ^2G, ^2F, ^2D (2), ^2P
d^4 or d^6	^5D, ^3H, ^3G, ^3F (2), ^3D, ^3P (2), ^1I, ^1G (2), ^1F, ^1D (2), ^1S (2)
d^5	^6S, ^4G, ^4F, ^4D, ^4P, ^2I, ^2H, ^2G (2), ^2F (2), ^2D (3), ^2P, ^2S
d^{10}	^1S

EXAMPLE 12.7. Determine the term symbol for C which has the configuration $\ldots 2p^2$.

The wave functions that are used for this configuration are $\phi_{2p,m}\gamma$ where $m = \pm 1, 0$ and $\gamma = \alpha$ or β. Thus there are $3 \times 2 = 6$ choices of wave function for each electron, or $6 \times 6 = 36$ choices for the pair. Of these, 6 give the same wave function to both electrons and so are ruled out by the Pauli principle; of the remaining 30, half must be eliminated because there is no way of distinguishing between "the first electron" and "the second electron." We are left with 15 microstates, which, using the notation $m\gamma$ instead of $\phi_{2p,m}\gamma$, can be indicated as follows: $(+1\alpha, +1\beta)$, $(+1\alpha, 0\alpha)$, $(+1\alpha, 0\beta)$, $(+1\beta, 0\alpha)$, $(+1\beta, 0\beta)$, $(+1\alpha, -1\alpha)$, $(+1\alpha, -1\beta)$, $(+1\beta, -1\alpha)$, $(+1\beta, -1\beta)$, $(0\alpha, 0\beta)$, $(0\alpha, -1\alpha)$, $(0\alpha, -1\beta)$, $(0\beta, -1\alpha)$, $(0\beta, -1\beta)$ and $(-1\alpha, -1\beta)$. The respective values of M_L and M_S for these microstates are $(2, 0)$, $(1, 1)$, $(1, 0)$, $(1, 0)$, $(1, -1)$, $(0, 1)$, $(0, 0)$, $(0, 0)$, $(0, -1)$, $(0, 0)$, $(-1, 1)$, $(-1, 0)$, $(-1, 0)$, $(-1, -1)$ and $(-2, 0)$.

Beginning with $M_L = L = 2$ and $M_S = S = 0$, the corresponding term symbol is ${}^1D$, and that term symbol is assigned to the five microstates $(2, 0)$, $(1, 0)$, $(0, 0)$, $(-1, 0)$ and $(-2, 0)$. The value of J for this term symbol is

$$J = 2 + 0 = |2 - 0| = 2$$

giving the complete term symbol ${}^1D_2$.

Working with the ten remaining microstates—$(1, 1)$, $(1, 0)$, $(1, -1)$, $(0, 1)$, $(0, 0)$, $(0, -1)$, $(0, 0)$, $(-1, 1)$, $(-1, 0)$ and $(-1, -1)$—the values of $M_L = L = 1$ and $M_S = S = 1$ define the term ${}^3P$ for nine of these microstates—$(1, 1)$, $(0, 1)$, $(-1, 1)$, $(1, 0)$, $(0, 0)$, $(-1, 0)$, $(1, -1)$, $(0, -1)$ and $(-1, -1)$—leaving only the microstate $(0, 0)$. The values of J for ${}^3P$ are

$$J = 1 + 1 = 2,$$
$$1 + 1 - 1 = 1,$$
$$1 + 1 - 2 = |1 - 1| = 0$$

giving the terms ${}^3P_0$, ${}^3P_1$ and ${}^3P_2$. The remaining microstate, $(0, 0)$, corresponds to ${}^1S$ with $J = 0$, or ${}^1S_0$.

Of the possible term symbols—${}^1D_2$, ${}^3P_0$, ${}^3P_1$, ${}^3P_2$ and ${}^5S_0$—Hund's first rule suggests that the ${}^3P$ state is the correct ground state for C and because the subshell is less than half-filled, the complete symbol is ${}^3P_0$.

The same ground state term symbol can be derived using a method that does not require the writing of all the permitted microstates. Substituting the values of m and s for the electrons, ($n = 2$, $\ell = 1$, $m = +1$, $s = +\frac{1}{2}$) and ($n = 2$, $\ell = 0$, $m = 0$, $s = \frac{1}{2}$), into (*12.18*) and (*12.19*) gives

$$M_L = 1 + 0 = 1 \qquad M_S = \frac{1}{2} + \frac{1}{2} = 1$$

which are assumed to be L and S, respectively, neglecting signs. The value of $L = 1$ gives a P for the term, the value of S gives the multiplicity as $2S + 1 = 3$, and the values of $L = 1$ and $S = 1$ gives the permitted values of J as 2, 1 and 0, using (*12.17*). Choosing the lowest value for J because the subshell is less than half-filled gives ${}^3P_0$. The reverse of this shorter technique is very useful in determining electronic configurations from experimental term symbols.

Spectra of Polyelectronic Atoms

12.11 SELECTION RULES

Only the transitions that are allowed by the selection rules

$$\Delta S = 0 \tag{12.20a}$$

$$\Delta L = 0, \pm 1, \text{ but } L = 0 \nleftrightarrow L = 0 \tag{12.20b}$$

$$\Delta J = 0, \pm 1, \text{ but } J = 0 \nleftrightarrow J = 0 \tag{12.20c}$$

$$\Delta \ell = \pm 1 \tag{12.20d}$$

will be observed in the spectra of complex atoms. The symbol $\nleftrightarrow$ represents a forbidden transition.

EXAMPLE 12.8. The principal series of sodium corresponds to electronic transitions between the 3*s* ground electronic state and the various *p* excited states. Prepare energy diagrams for the series showing both the transitions and the doublet structure that is observed.

The ground state, having a $3s^1$ configuration, corresponds to $\ell = 0$ and $s = +\frac{1}{2}$, giving $L = 0$ and $S = \frac{1}{2}$. The multiplicity of the ground state is $2S + 1 = 2$ and

$$J = 0 + \frac{1}{2} = \left|0 - \frac{1}{2}\right| = \frac{1}{2}$$

giving the term symbol for the ground state as $^2S_{1/2}$. For one electron in a *p* orbital, $\ell = +1$ and $s = +\frac{1}{2}$, giving $L = 1$ and $S = \frac{1}{2}$. The multiplicity is still 2 and the values of *J* are

$$J = 1 + \frac{1}{2} = \frac{3}{2},$$

$$1 + \frac{1}{2} - 1 = \left|1 - \frac{1}{2}\right| = \frac{1}{2}$$

giving the term symbols as $^2P_{3/2}$ and $^2P_{1/2}$, with the $^2P_{1/2}$ being lower in energy.

The spectra should consist of transitions between the ^2P states and the ^2S state, which are allowed by the selection rules, (*12.20*): (*12.20a*) is satisfied because the transitions are occurring between "doublets"; (*12.20b*) is satisfied because $P \leftrightarrow S$ is a change in *L* of ± 1; (*12.20c*) is satisfied because the $\frac{3}{2} \leftrightarrow \frac{1}{2}$ is a change of ± 1 and the $\frac{1}{2} \leftrightarrow \frac{1}{2}$ is a change of 0; and (*12.20d*) is satisfied because ℓ is changing by ± 1. Figure 12-3(*a*) shows the overall transitions in this series and Fig. 12-3(*b*) shows the two-line doublet that is observed.

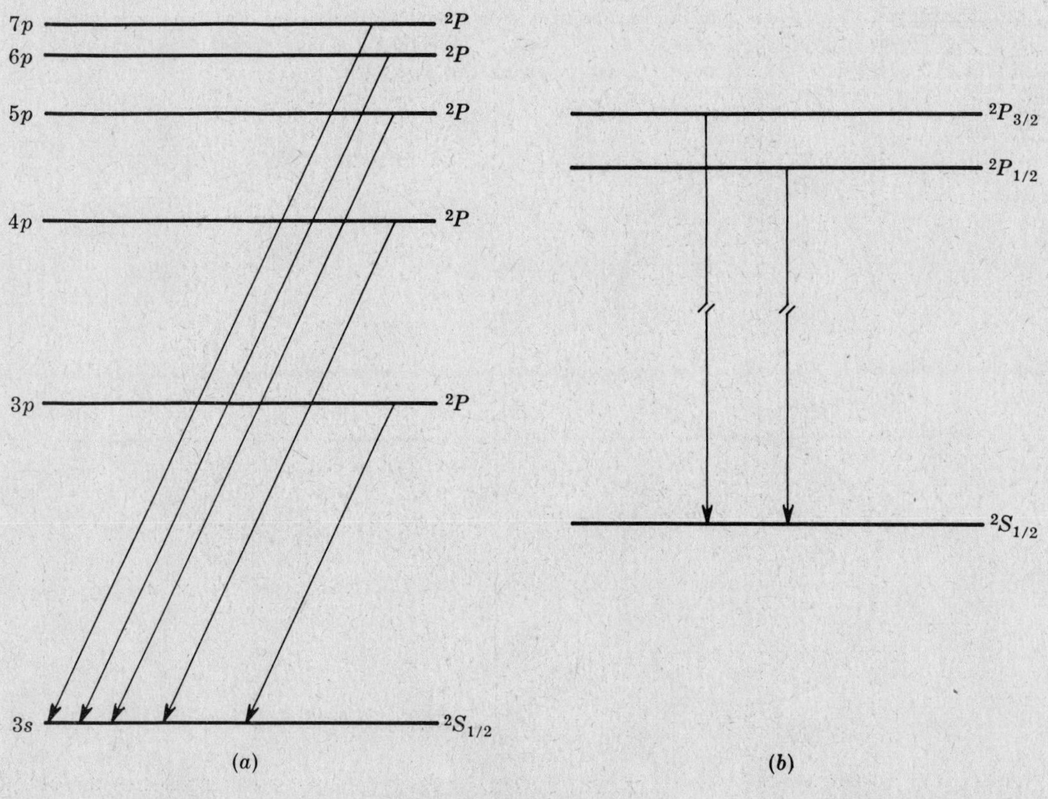

Fig. 12-3

12.12 THE NORMAL ZEEMAN EFFECT

If an atom with $S = 0$ is placed in a magnetic field parallel to the z-axis of the atom, the multiplets are split into $2L+1$ components corresponding to the quantum number M_L described in (*12.18*). The allowed transitions obey the additional rule

$$\Delta M_L = 0, \pm 1 \qquad (12.21)$$

For atoms with $S \neq 0$, the Zeeman effect is much more complicated.

Solved Problems

Hydrogenlike Atoms

12.1. The angular wave function for $\ell = 1$ and $m = 0$ is $Y(\theta, \phi) = (3/4\pi)^{1/2} \cos\theta$. Prepare two-dimensional sketches for $Y(\theta, \phi)$ and $Y(\theta,\phi)^* Y(\theta, \phi)$ in an arbitrary plane through the z-axis. Describe the three-dimensional sketches.

For $\theta = 0$, the value of the wave function is

$$Y(\theta, \phi) = \left(\frac{3}{4\pi}\right)^{1/2} \cos 0 = 0.489$$

and, noting that $Y(\theta, \phi)^* Y(\theta, \phi) = [Y(\theta, \phi)]^2$ because the function is real,

$$Y(\theta, \phi)^* Y(\theta, \phi) = (0.489)^2 = 0.239$$

Repeating the above calculations for 10°-intervals in θ generates the curves shown in Fig. 12-4. The algebraic signs given in Fig. 12-4(*a*) are those of $Y(\theta, \phi)$ in the four quadrants.

The three-dimensional figures commonly shown in textbooks are the surfaces generated by rotating the curves of Fig. 12-4 about the z-axis. Because the surfaces are extended along the z-axis and because $\ell = 1$, this orbital is known as the p_z orbital.

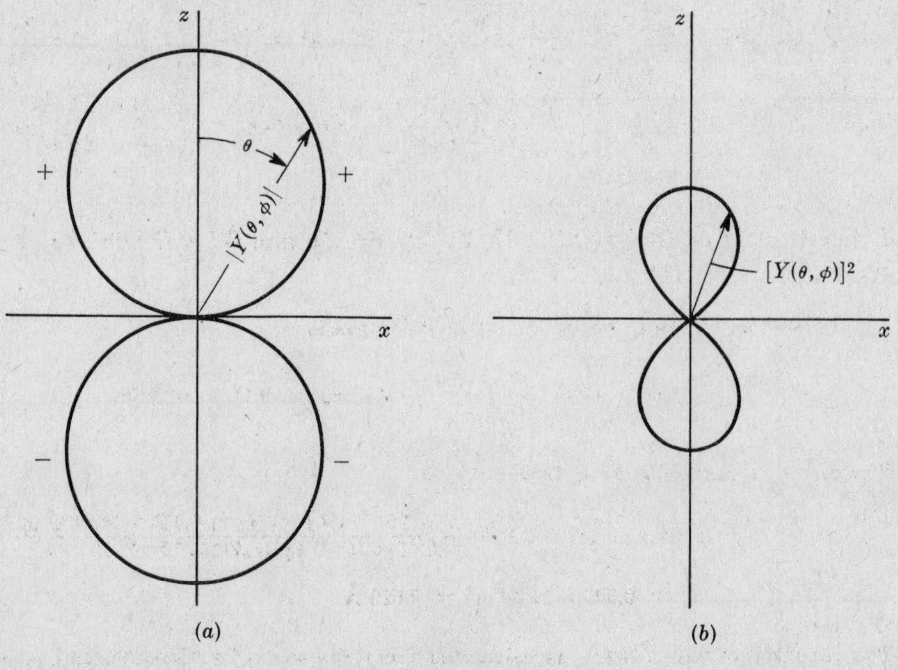

Fig. 12-4

12.2. Show that the angular wave functions for $\ell = 2$, $m = 0$ and for $\ell = 1$, $m = 1$,

$$Y(\theta,\phi) = \left(\frac{5}{16\pi}\right)^{1/2}(3\cos^2\theta - 1) \quad \text{and} \quad Y(\theta,\phi) = \left(\frac{3}{4\pi}\right)^{1/2}\sin\theta\cos\phi$$

are orthogonal.

To meet the criterion of (*11.13*), the angular part of $\langle\psi_i \mid \psi_j\rangle$ must be shown to be zero. Performing the integration gives

$$\int_{\theta=0}^{\pi}\int_{\phi=0}^{2\pi}\left(\frac{15}{64\pi^2}\right)^{1/2}(3\cos^2\theta - 1)(\sin\theta\cos\phi)\sin\theta\, d\theta\, d\phi$$

$$= \frac{\sqrt{15}}{8\pi}\int_0^{\pi}(3\cos^2 2\theta - 1)\sin^2\theta\, d\theta \int_0^{2\pi}\cos\phi\, d\phi$$

The integral over ϕ is clearly zero. (The integral over θ also vanishes.)

12.3. Determine $R(r)$ for the 2*s* and 2*p* subshells, where $n=2$, $\ell=0$ and $n=2$, $\ell=1$ respectively.

Using (*12.10*) gives

$$L_2^1(\rho) = \frac{d}{d\rho}\left[e^{\rho}\frac{d^2}{d\rho^2}(\rho^2 e^{-\rho})\right] = \frac{d}{d\rho}\left[e^{\rho}\frac{d}{d\rho}(2\rho - \rho^2)e^{-\rho}\right] = \frac{d}{d\rho}(2 - 4\rho + \rho^2) = 2\rho - 4$$

for $n = 2$ and $\ell = 0$, and

$$L_3^3(\rho) = \frac{d^3}{d\rho^3}\left[e^{\rho}\frac{d^3}{d\rho^3}(\rho^3 e^{-\rho})\right] = \frac{d^3}{d\rho^3}\left[e^{\rho}\frac{d^2}{d\rho^2}(3\rho^2 - \rho^3)e^{-\rho}\right]$$

$$= \frac{d^3}{d\rho^3}\left[e^{\rho}\frac{d}{d\rho}(6\rho - 6\rho^2 + \rho^3)e^{-\rho}\right] = \frac{d^3}{d\rho^3}(6 - 18\rho + 9\rho^2 - \rho^3) = -6$$

for $n = 2$ and $\ell = 1$. Using (*12.7*) and (*12.8*) gives for these subshells

$$R_{2,0}(r) = -\left(\frac{Z}{a_0}\right)^{3/2}\left[\frac{1!}{4(2!)^3}\right]^{1/2} e^{-\rho/2}\rho^0(2\rho - 4) = \left(\frac{Z}{a_0}\right)^{3/2}\left(\frac{1}{2}\right)^{1/2}\left(1 - \frac{Zr}{2a_0}\right)e^{-Zr/2a_0}$$

and

$$R_{2,1}(r) = -\left(\frac{Z}{a_0}\right)^{3/2}\left[\frac{0!}{4(3!)^3}\right]^{1/2} e^{-\rho/2}\rho^1(-6) = \left(\frac{Z}{a_0}\right)^{5/2}\left(\frac{1}{2\sqrt{6}}\right)re^{-Zr/2a_0}$$

12.4. Prepare plots of $R(r)$ for the 1*s*, 2*s*, 2*p*, 3*s*, 3*p* and 3*d* subshells for hydrogen, using values of r between 0 and $10a_0$.

The reduced mass given by (*11.10*) for hydrogen is

$$\mu = \frac{m_{\text{nucleus}} m_e}{m_{\text{nucleus}} + m_e} \approx m_e = 9.11 \times 10^{-31}\ \text{kg}$$

The corresponding value of a_0 from (*12.9*) is

$$a_0 = \frac{4\pi\epsilon_0\hbar^2}{\mu e^2} = \frac{(1.11265 \times 10^{-10}\ \text{C}^2\ \text{N}^{-1}\ \text{m}^{-2})(1.055 \times 10^{-34}\ \text{J s})^2}{(9.11 \times 10^{-31}\ \text{kg})(1.602 \times 10^{-19}\ \text{C})^2}$$

$$= 0.529 \times 10^{-10}\ \text{m} = 0.529\ \text{Å}$$

The required values of $R(r)$, as calculated from the wave functions determined in Example 12.2 and Problem 12.3, are plotted in Fig. 12-5.

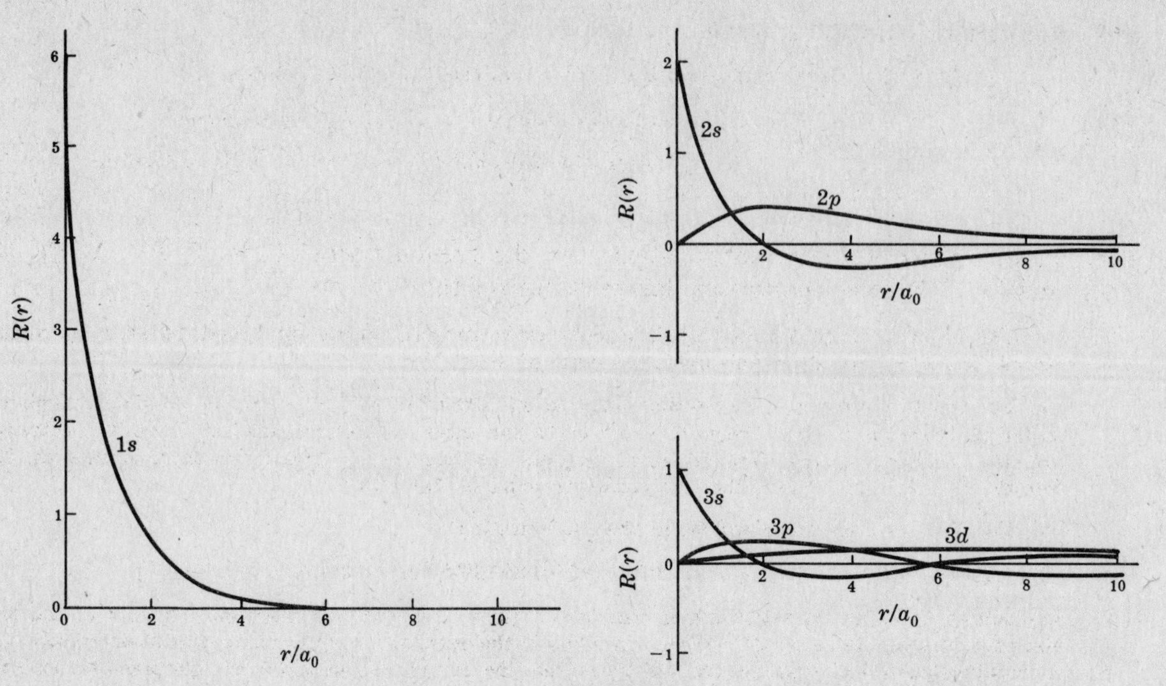

Fig. 12-5

12.5. What is the probability of finding a 1s electron for hydrogen in a sphere having $r = 0.5$ Å?

The normalization factors in (*12.14*), (*12.15*) and (*12.7*) have been chosen such that

$$\langle\psi\,|\,\psi\rangle \;=\; \iiint\limits_{\text{all space}} \psi^*\psi\,dV \;=\; \int_0^\infty R^*Rr^2\,dr \int_0^\pi \Theta^*\Theta\sin\theta\,d\theta \int_0^{2\pi}\Phi^*\Phi\,d\phi$$
$$= (1)(1)(1) \;=\; 1$$

This means that the (marginal) probability density functions for the r-coordinate, θ-coordinate and ϕ-coordinate are R^*Rr^2, $\Theta^*\Theta\sin\theta$ and $\Phi^*\Phi$, respectively. Thus, the probability of finding a 1s electron ($R = R_{1,0}$) within 0.5 Å of the nucleus is

$$\int_0^{0.5} R_{1,0}^* R_{1,0} r^2\,dr \;=\; 4\left(\frac{1}{0.529}\right)^3 \int_0^{0.5} e^{-2r/0.529} r^2\,dr$$

where we have used Example 12.2 and Problem 12.4 to evaluate $R_{1,0}$. Using integration by parts (twice) or tables to evaluate the integral, we obtain

$$\int_0^{0.5} R_{1,0}^* R_{1,0} r^2\,dr \;=\; 0.295$$

12.6. Determine the degeneracy of the hydrogenlike energy level corresponding to $n = 2$.

For $n = 2$, (*12.12*) predicts that the 2s orbital and the three 2p orbitals will have the same energy in a one-electron system, giving a degeneracy of 4.

Quantum Theory of Polyelectronic Atoms

12.7. Determine $\mathcal{H}$ and ψ for Li.

$$\mathcal{H} \;=\; \left(\frac{-\hbar^2}{2m_e}\right)(\nabla_1^2 + \nabla_2^2 + \nabla_3^2) \;-\; \frac{3e^2}{4\pi\epsilon_0}\left(\frac{1}{r_1} + \frac{1}{r_2} + \frac{1}{r_3}\right) \;+\; \frac{e^2}{4\pi\epsilon_0}\left(\frac{1}{r_{12}} + \frac{1}{r_{13}} + \frac{1}{r_{23}}\right)$$

and (*12.14*) gives, upon expansion,

$$\begin{aligned}\psi = 6^{-1/2}[&\phi_{1s}(1)\alpha(1)\phi_{1s}(2)\beta(2)\phi_{2s}(3)\alpha(3) - \phi_{1s}(1)\alpha(1)\phi_{2s}(2)\alpha(2)\phi_{1s}(3)\beta(3)\\ &- \phi_{1s}(1)\beta(1)\phi_{1s}(2)\alpha(2)\phi_{2s}(3)\alpha(3) + \phi_{1s}(1)\beta(1)\phi_{2s}(2)\alpha(2)\phi_{1s}(3)\alpha(3)\\ &+ \phi_{2s}(1)\alpha(1)\phi_{1s}(2)\alpha(2)\phi_{1s}(3)\beta(3) - \phi_{2s}(1)\alpha(1)\phi_{1s}(2)\beta(2)\phi_{1s}(3)\alpha(3)]\end{aligned}$$

12.8. Predict the electronic configurations for the ground states of Mg, P, P^{5+}, Y, Ce, O and O^{2-}. Predict possible oxidation states for the elements.

The 12 electrons in Mg fill according to $1s^2 2s^2 2p^6 3s^2$. In addition to 0, both $3s$ electrons could be lost to give a second possible oxidation state of +2.

For the 15 electrons in P, the configuration will be $1s^2 2s^2 2p^6 3s^2 3p^3$, giving possible oxidation states of +5, +3 and −3 as, respectively, both $3s$ and three $3p$ electrons are lost, three $3p$ electrons are lost, and three electrons are gained to complete the $3p$ subshell. In addition there is the state 0. For the 10 electrons in P^{5+}, the configuration would be $1s^2 2s^2 2p^6$.

For Y, the 39 electrons will be in the configuration

$$1s^2 2s^2 2p^6 3s^2 3p^6 4s^2 3d^{10} 4p^6 5s^2 4d^1$$

In addition to 0, the oxidation states will be +2 (loss of the $5s$ electrons) and +3 (loss of the $5s$ electrons and the $4d$ electron). When considering the removal of electrons in transition metals, it is important to recall that the order is more like the reverse of the filling of hydrogenlike atoms. Thus the $5s$ electrons are removed before the $4d$ electron and a +1 oxidation state is not observed.

The 58 electrons in Ce will have the configuration

$$1s^2 2s^2 2p^6 3s^2 3p^6 4s^2 3d^{10} 4p^6 5s^2 4d^{10} 5p^6 6s^2 4f^2$$

which predicts Ce^{4+} by loss of the $4f$ and $6s$ electrons, in addition to the oxidation state of 0. The $4f$ and $5d$ orbitals are very close in energy and the following configuration is also possible for Ce:

$$1s^2 2s^2 2p^6 3s^2 3p^6 4s^2 3d^{10} 4p^6 5s^2 4d^{10} 5p^6 6s^2 4f^1 5d^1$$

which predicts the common +3 oxidation state by loss of the $6s$ electrons and the $5d$ electron.

The 8 electrons in oxygen will be in $1s^2 2s^2 2p^4$, suggesting oxidation states of +6, +4, 0 and −2, where the configuration for O^{2-} is $1s^2 2s^2 2p^6$.

12.9. What are the quantum numbers for the 58th electron in Ce and the eighth electron in O?

Assuming the $\ldots 6s^2 4f^2$ configuration determined in Problem 12.8 for Ce, the last electron is the second one to enter the $4f$ subshell, thus $n = 4$ and $\ell = 3$. The first electron in the f subshell will be assigned $m = +3$ by convention; the second, $m = +2$; etc. The spins on the first five will be $+\frac{1}{2}$, giving the four quantum numbers as $n = 4$, $\ell = 3$, $m = +2$, $s = +\frac{1}{2}$. The eighth electron in oxygen is the fourth one to enter the $2p$ subshell, giving $n = 2$, $\ell = 1$, $m = +1$, $s = -\frac{1}{2}$.

Atomic Term Symbols

12.10. Determine the term symbols for two electrons such that $L = 2$ and $S = 1$.

The value of $L = 2$ is equivalent to a D term. The leading superscript given by

$$2S + 1 = (2)(1) + 1 = 3$$

Using (*12.17*) gives

$$\begin{aligned} J &= 2 + 1 = 3,\\ &\quad 2 + 1 - 1 = 2,\\ &\quad 2 + 1 - 2 = |2 - 1| = 1\end{aligned}$$

The term symbols are ${}^3D_3$, ${}^3D_2$ and ${}^3D_1$.

12.11. Determine the term symbol for the ground state of atomic O.

Assuming the ground state electronic configuration to be that given in Problem 12.8, Table 12-1 gives ^3P, ^1D and ^1S as possibilities for the equivalent electrons. Hund's first rule predicts that the ^3P is the preferred state. The value of L for this state is 1. Substituting $L = 1$ and $S = 1$ into (*12.17*) gives

$$J = 1 + 1 = 2,$$
$$1 + 1 - 1 = 1,$$
$$1 + 1 - 2 = |1 - 1| = 0$$

Choosing the largest value of J because the subshell is over half-filled, the complete term symbol is $^3P_2$.

12.12. The ground state term of Cr is $^7S_3$. Does this term symbol correspond to the $\ldots 4s^2 3d^4$ configuration or the $\ldots 4s^1 3d^5$ configuration as presented in Example 12.5?

The d^4 configuration gives

$$M_L = L = 2 + 1 + 0 + (-1) = 2 \qquad M_S = S = \frac{1}{2} + \frac{1}{2} + \frac{1}{2} + \frac{1}{2} = 2$$

which lead to the incorrect symbol ^5D. The $s^1 d^5$ configuration gives $M_L = L = 0$ and $M_S = S = 6/2$ (assuming parallel spins), whence $2S + 1 = 7$ and $J = 0 + 3 = |0 - 3| = 3$, for a total symbol of $^7S_3$.

Spectra of Polyelectronic Atoms

12.13. Is the transition between the 3s and 4s atomic orbitals allowed for Na?

The s atomic orbitals correspond to $^2S_{1/2}$ states, so that a $^2S_{1/2} \leftrightarrow {}^2S_{1/2}$ transition is in question. Condition (*12.20a*) is met by this transition, but condition (*12.20b*) is not met, because this is an $L = 0 \leftrightarrow L = 0$ transition. Thus this transition is not permitted.

12.14. Sketch the transitions that would occur between a $^1S_0$ and a $^1P_1$ level in the absence and in the presence of a magnetic field.

For the $^1S_0$ level, (*12.18*) gives $M_L = 0$, and for the $^1P_1$ level, $M_L = 1, 0, -1$. As shown in Fig. 12-6, what is normally a single spectral line becomes a triplet in the presence of a magnetic field.

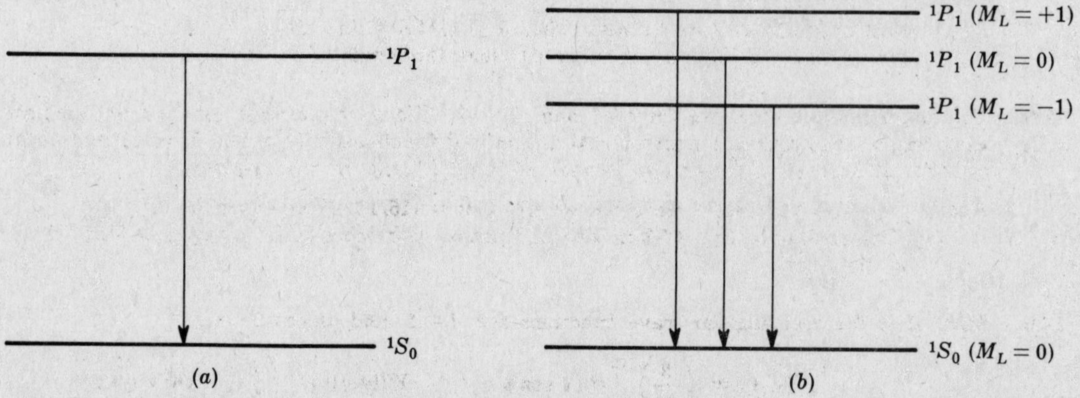

Fig. 12-6

Supplementary Problems

Hydrogenlike Atoms

12.15. The angular wave function for $\ell = 0$ and $m = 0$ is $Y(\theta, \phi) = (1/4\pi)^{1/2}$. Describe plots of $Y(\theta, \phi)$ and $Y(\theta, \phi)^* Y(\theta, \phi)$ in the xz-plane and the three-dimensional figure for an s orbital.

Ans. Wave function is independent of θ and ϕ, so in two dimensions plots are circles of radii 0.282 and 0.0796 and three-dimensional figure is spherical.

12.16. The angular wave function for the d_{z^2} orbital ($\ell = 2$ and $m = 0$) is $Y(\theta, \phi) = (5/16\pi)^{1/2}(3\cos^2\theta - 1)$. Graph in the xz-plane (*a*) $Y(\theta, \phi)$ and (*b*) $Y(\theta, \phi)^* Y(\theta, \phi)$. (*c*) Describe the three-dimensional figures.

Ans. (*a*) See Fig. 12-7(*a*). (*b*) See Fig. 12-7(*b*). (*c*) Rotate curves of Fig. 12-7 about z-axis.

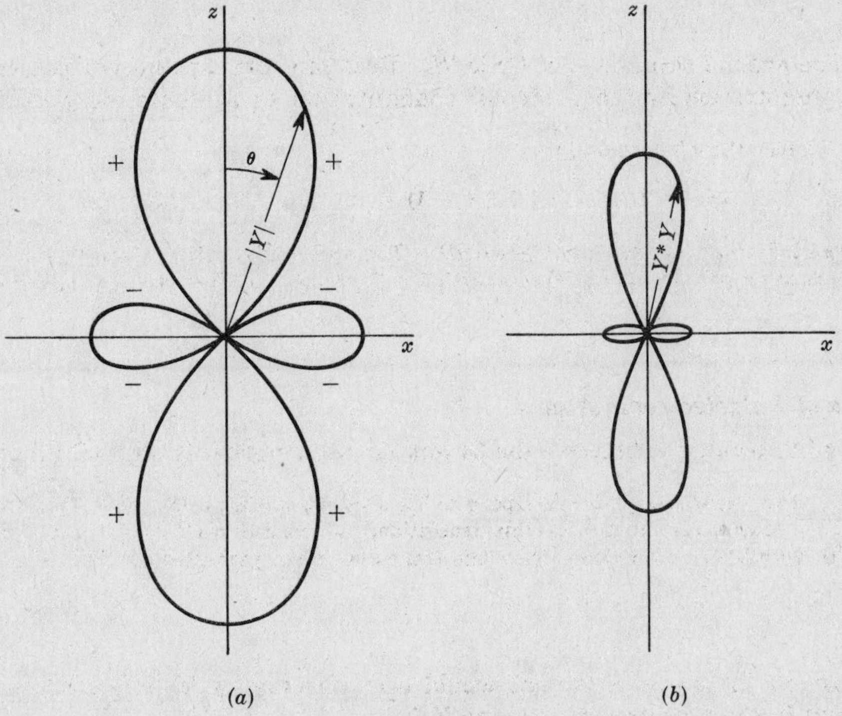

Fig. 12-7

12.17. The angular wave functions for $\ell = 1$ and $m = \pm 1$, $Y(\theta, \phi) = (3/8\pi)^{1/2} \sin\theta \; e^{\pm i\phi}$, contain imaginary terms. Construct two normalized real wave functions from these and prepare two-dimensional plots of the new wave functions, $Y'(\theta, \phi)$ and $Y''(\theta, \phi)$, and of $Y'(\theta, \phi)^* Y'(\theta, \phi)$ and $Y''(\theta, \phi)^* Y''(\theta, \phi)$.

Ans. $Y'(\theta, \phi) = (3/4\pi)^{1/2} \sin\theta \cos\phi$, $Y''(\theta, \phi) = (3/4\pi)^{1/2} \sin\theta \sin\phi$;
plots similar to Fig. 12-4 but located along the x-axis and y-axis respectively

12.18. The angular wave functions for $\ell = 2$ and $m = \pm 2$, $Y(\theta, \phi) = (15/32\pi)^{1/2} \sin^2\theta \; e^{\pm 2i\phi}$, contain imaginary terms. From these construct real normalized functions, $Y'(\theta, \phi)$ and $Y''(\theta, \phi)$, and prepare plots of $Y'(\theta, \phi)$, $Y''(\theta, \phi)$, $Y'(\theta, \phi)^* Y'(\theta, \phi)$ and $Y''(\theta, \phi)^* Y''(\theta, \phi)$ in the xy-plane.

Ans. $Y'(\theta, \phi) = (15/16\pi)^{1/2} \sin^2\theta \cos 2\phi$, $Y''(\theta, \phi) = (15/16\pi)^{1/2} \sin^2\theta \sin 2\phi$;
plots similar to Fig. 12-2 in size and shape, with lobes of Y' along, and lobes of Y'' at 45° to, the axes

12.19. Show that the real angular wave functions for $\ell = 1$ and $m = \pm 1$,

$$Y'(\theta, \phi) = \left(\frac{3}{4\pi}\right)^{1/2} \sin\theta \cos\phi \qquad Y''(\theta, \phi) = \left(\frac{3}{4\pi}\right)^{1/2} \sin\theta \sin\phi$$

are orthogonal.

12.20. Find $R(r)$ for the $3s$, $3p$ and $3d$ subshells.

Ans. $$R_{3,0} = \left(\frac{Z}{a_0}\right)^{3/2}\left(\frac{2}{3\sqrt{3}}\right)e^{-Zr/3a_0}\left(1 - \frac{2Zr}{3a_0} + \frac{2Z^2r^2}{27a_0^2}\right)$$

$$R_{3,1} = \left(\frac{Z}{a_0}\right)^{5/2}\left(\frac{8}{27\sqrt{6}}\right)e^{-Zr/3a_0}\left(r - \frac{Zr^2}{6a_0}\right)$$

$$R_{3,2} = \left(\frac{Z}{a_0}\right)^{7/2}\left(\frac{4}{81\sqrt{30}}\right)e^{-Zr/3a_0}r^2$$

12.21. Prepare plots of $R(r)^* R(r)r^2$ for the $1s$, $2s$, $2p$, $3s$, $3p$, and $3d$ subshells for hydrogen, using values of r between 0 and $10a_0$. *Ans.* See Fig. 12-8.

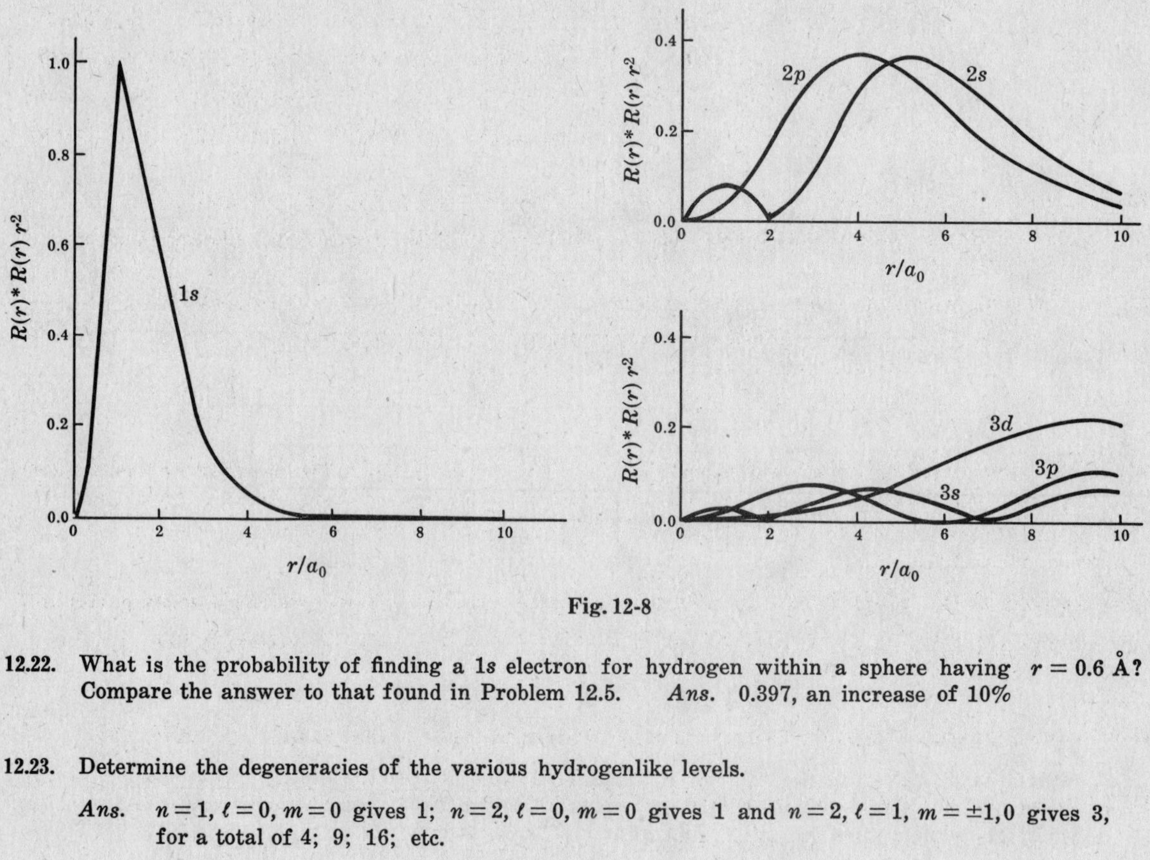

Fig. 12-8

12.22. What is the probability of finding a $1s$ electron for hydrogen within a sphere having $r = 0.6$ Å? Compare the answer to that found in Problem 12.5. *Ans.* 0.397, an increase of 10%

12.23. Determine the degeneracies of the various hydrogenlike levels.

Ans. $n = 1$, $\ell = 0$, $m = 0$ gives 1; $n = 2$, $\ell = 0$, $m = 0$ gives 1 and $n = 2$, $\ell = 1$, $m = \pm 1, 0$ gives 3, for a total of 4; 9; 16; etc.

12.24. Find the most probable value of r for the hydrogen $1s$ wave function.

Ans. $\frac{d}{dr}[R_{1,0}(r)^* R_{1,0}(r)r^2] = 0$ gives $r = a_0 = 0.529$ Å

12.25. Assume $\psi = e^{-ar}$ as a trial wave function for atomic hydrogen. Find $\langle\psi|\mathcal{H}|\psi\rangle$ and $\langle\psi|\psi\rangle$ and calculate E. Minimize E with respect to a, solve for the constant a, and find the minimum value of E. Compare with the actual energy of the ground state.

Ans. $$\int_0^\infty x^n e^{-ax}\,dx = \frac{n!}{a^{n+1}}; \quad \mathcal{H}\psi = \left[\frac{a\hbar^2}{2\mu}\left(\frac{2}{r} - a\right) - \frac{e^2}{4\pi\epsilon_0 r}\right]e^{-ar}, \quad \langle\psi|\mathcal{H}|\psi\rangle = \frac{\pi}{a}\left(\frac{\hbar^2}{2\mu} - \frac{e^2}{4\pi\epsilon_0 a}\right);$$

$$\langle\psi|\psi\rangle = \frac{\pi}{a^3}; \quad E = \frac{\hbar^2a^2}{2\mu} - \frac{e^2a}{4\pi\epsilon_0}; \quad a = \mu e^2/4\pi\epsilon_0\hbar^2;$$

$$E_{\text{min}} = \frac{-\mu e^4}{2\hbar^2(4\pi\epsilon_0)^2} = E_{\text{actual}} \quad (\text{because } \psi \propto \psi_{\text{actual}})$$

Quantum Theory of Polyelectronic Atoms

12.26. Write the Hamiltonian and the Slater wave function for C.

Ans.
$$\mathcal{H} = \left(\frac{-\hbar^2}{2m_e}\right)(\nabla_1^2+\nabla_2^2+\nabla_3^2+\nabla_4^2+\nabla_5^2+\nabla_6^2) - \frac{6e^2}{4\pi\epsilon_0}\left(\frac{1}{r_1}+\frac{1}{r_2}+\frac{1}{r_3}+\frac{1}{r_4}+\frac{1}{r_5}+\frac{1}{r_6}\right)$$
$$+\frac{e^2}{4\pi\epsilon_0}\left(\frac{1}{r_{12}}+\frac{1}{r_{13}}+\frac{1}{r_{14}}+\frac{1}{r_{15}}+\frac{1}{r_{16}}+\frac{1}{r_{23}}+\frac{1}{r_{24}}+\frac{1}{r_{25}}+\frac{1}{r_{26}}\right.$$
$$\left.+\frac{1}{r_{34}}+\frac{1}{r_{35}}+\frac{1}{r_{36}}+\frac{1}{r_{45}}+\frac{1}{r_{46}}+\frac{1}{r_{56}}\right)$$

$$\psi = \sqrt{\frac{1}{6!}}\begin{vmatrix} \phi_{1s}(1)\alpha(1) & \phi_{1s}(2)\alpha(2) & \phi_{1s}(3)\alpha(3) & \phi_{1s}(4)\alpha(4) & \phi_{1s}(5)\alpha(5) & \phi_{1s}(6)\alpha(6) \\ \phi_{1s}(1)\beta(1) & \phi_{1s}(2)\beta(2) & \phi_{1s}(3)\beta(3) & \phi_{1s}(4)\beta(4) & \phi_{1s}(5)\beta(5) & \phi_{1s}(6)\beta(6) \\ \phi_{2s}(1)\alpha(1) & \phi_{2s}(2)\alpha(2) & \phi_{2s}(3)\alpha(3) & \phi_{2s}(4)\alpha(4) & \phi_{2s}(5)\alpha(5) & \phi_{2s}(6)\alpha(6) \\ \phi_{2s}(1)\beta(1) & \phi_{2s}(2)\beta(2) & \phi_{2s}(3)\beta(3) & \phi_{2s}(4)\beta(4) & \phi_{2s}(5)\beta(5) & \phi_{2s}(6)\beta(6) \\ \phi_{2p,+1}(1)\alpha(1) & \phi_{2p,+1}(2)\alpha(2) & \phi_{2p,+1}(3)\alpha(3) & \phi_{2p,+1}(4)\alpha(4) & \phi_{2p,+1}(5)\alpha(5) & \phi_{2p,+1}(6)\alpha(6) \\ \phi_{2p,0}(1)\alpha(1) & \phi_{2p,0}(2)\alpha(2) & \phi_{2p,0}(3)\alpha(3) & \phi_{2p,0}(4)\alpha(4) & \phi_{2p,0}(5)\alpha(5) & \phi_{2p,0}(6)\alpha(6) \end{vmatrix}$$

12.27. Predict the electronic configurations for U, U^{3+}, U^{4+}, U^{5+}, U^{6+}, Cu, Cu^{+} and Cu^{2+}.

Ans. (Rn)$7s^2 6d^1 5f^3$ or (Rn)$7s^2 5f^4$, (Rn)$5f^3$, (Rn)$5f^2$, (Rn)$5f$, (Rn), (Ar)$4s^1 3d^{10}$, (Ar)$3d^{10}$, (Ar)$3d^9$

12.28. What are the quantum numbers for the 92nd electron in U and the 15th electron in P?

Ans. For U: $(n=5, \ell=3, m=+1, s=+\frac{1}{2})$ for (Rn)$7s^2 6d^1 5f^3$ and
$(n=5, \ell=3, m=0, s=+\frac{1}{2})$ for (Rn)$7s^2 5f^4$.
For P: $(n=3, \ell=1, m=-1, s=+\frac{1}{2})$.

12.29. Calculate the first ionization potential for He if the ground state of He is -78.98 eV and if *(12.12)* is valid for He^+. *Ans.* He^+ ground state is -8.715×10^{-18} J = 54.40 eV, IP = 24.58 eV

Atomic Term Symbols

12.30. Determine the values of L for the interactions between an s with an s, a p with a p, and a p with an f.

Ans. $L = 0+0 = |0-0| = 0$, giving S; $L = 1+1 = 2$ to $|1-1| = 0$, giving D, P, S;
$L = 1+3 = 4$ to $|1-3| = 2$, giving G, F, D

12.31. Determine the term symbol for two electrons such that $L = 2$ and $S = 0$. *Ans.* $^1D_2$

12.32. Determine the ground state term for Ti using Table 12-1 for the equivalent electrons.

Ans. (Ar)$4s^2 3d^2$; ^3F is preferred choice; $2S+1 = 3$ gives $S = 1$, F gives $L = 3$;
$J = 3+1 = 4$ to $|3-1| = 2$, d^2 is less than half-filled; $^3F_2$

12.33. The ground state of Cu is $^2S_{1/2}$. Determine the electronic configuration from this information.

Ans. $2S+1 = 2$ gives $S = M_S = \frac{1}{2}$, 1 unpaired electron; S term gives $L = M_L = 0$, s^1d^{10} gives $M_L = L = 0$ and s^2d^9 gives $M_L = -2$ and $L = 2$; $J = \frac{1}{2}$ agrees with S and L; structure is $1s^2 2s^2 2p^6 3s^2 3p^6 4s^1 3d^{10}$

12.34. The ground state for Nb is $^6D_{1/2}$; Pd, $^1S_0$; La, $^2D_{3/2}$; Ce, $^3H_4$; and Pr, $^4I_{9/2}$. Determine the electronic configurations.

Ans. $L = 2$, 5 unpaired electrons, $\ldots 4s^2 4p^6 5s^1 4d^4$; $L = 0$, no unpaired electrons, $\ldots 4s^2 4p^6 4d^{10}$;

$L = 2$, 1 unpaired electron, $\ldots 4s^2 4p^6 5s^2 4d^{10} 5p^6 6s^2 5d^1$;

$L = 5$, 2 unpaired electrons, $\ldots 4s^2 4p^6 5s^2 4d^{10} 5p^6 6s^2 5d^1 4f^1$ or $\ldots 4f^2$;

$L = 6$, 3 unpaired electrons, $\ldots 4s^2 4p^6 5s^2 4d^{10} 5p^6 6s^2 4f^3$

12.35. What are the quantum numbers of the 66th electron in Dy, assuming it to be the $4f^{10}$ electron? Write the term symbol for the ground state of this element.

Ans. $n = 4$, $\ell = 3$, $m = +1$, $s = -\frac{1}{2}$; $M_L = 0 + (-1) + (-2) + (-3) = -6$, $L = 6$, giving I, $M_S = 4(\frac{1}{2}) = 2$, $S = 2$, $2S + 1 = 5$, $J = 8$ to 4, ${}^5I_8$.

12.36. Using the microstate technique shown in Example 12.7, determine the term symbols for the interaction of three equivalent p electrons.

Ans. The twenty microstates are $(2, \frac{1}{2})$, $(1, \frac{1}{2})$, $(2, -\frac{1}{2})$, $(1, -\frac{1}{2})$, $(-1, \frac{1}{2})$, $(-1, -\frac{1}{2})$, $(1, \frac{1}{2})$, $(1, -\frac{1}{2})$, $(-1, \frac{1}{2})$, $(-2, \frac{1}{2})$, $(-1, -\frac{1}{2})$, $(-2, -\frac{1}{2})$, $(0, \frac{3}{2})$, $(0, \frac{1}{2})$, $(0, \frac{1}{2})$, $(0, -\frac{1}{2})$, $(0, \frac{1}{2})$, $(0, -\frac{1}{2})$, $(0, -\frac{1}{2})$, $(0, -\frac{3}{2})$; ${}^2D$ accounts for 10 of these, ${}^2P$ accounts for 6 and ${}^4S$ accounts for 4.

Spectra of Polyelectronic Atoms

12.37. The *diffuse series* of Na corresponds to electronic transitions between the d excited states and the $3p$ electronic state. Prepare energy diagrams for this series showing both the transitions and compound doublet structure that are observed.

Ans. ${}^2D_{3/2}$ and ${}^2D_{5/2}$ to ${}^2P_{1/2}$ and ${}^2P_{3/2}$, see Fig. 12-9.

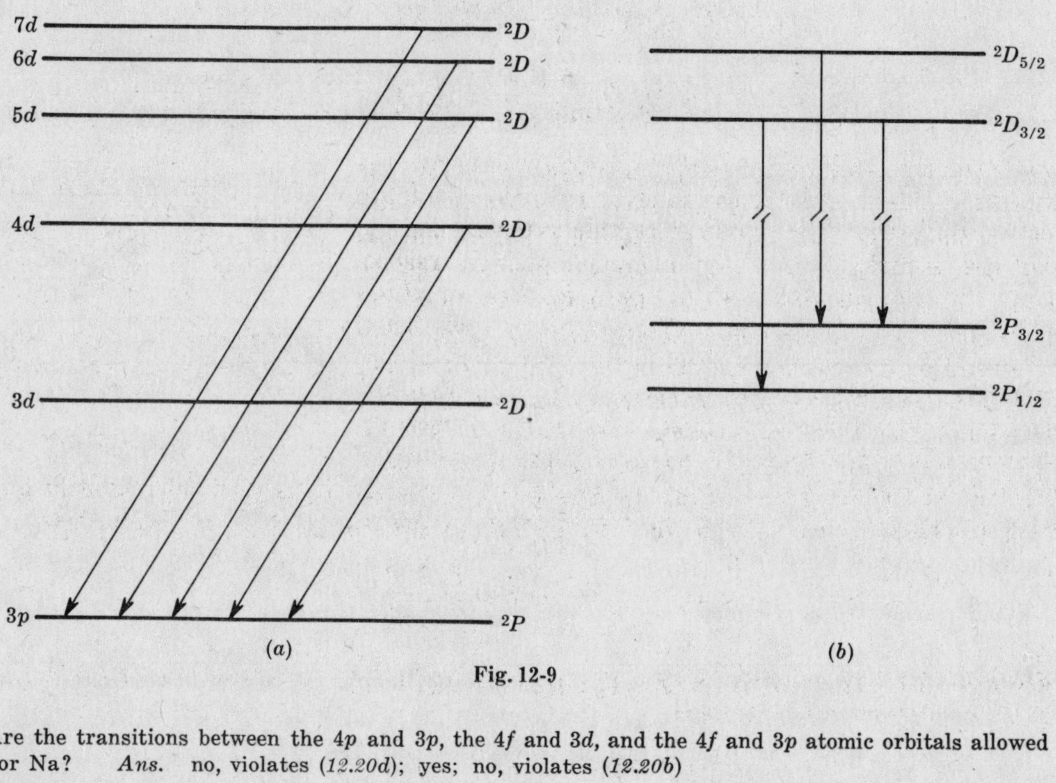

Fig. 12-9

12.38. Are the transitions between the $4p$ and $3p$, the $4f$ and $3d$, and the $4f$ and $3p$ atomic orbitals allowed for Na? *Ans.* no, violates (*12.20d*); yes; no, violates (*12.20b*)

12.39. How many transitions and how many spectral lines will occur for a transition between a ${}^1D_2$ and a ${}^1P_1$ level in the presence of a magnetic field?

Ans. Nine transitions (2 to 1, 1 to 1 or 0, 0 to ± 1 or 0, -1 to -1 or 0, -2 to -1), giving three lines because all similar ΔM_L values have the same energy splitting.

12.40. The low-resolution spectrum of He shows that two distinct sets of principal, sharp, diffuse and fundamental series exist. These result from orthohelium having $S = 1$ and parahelium having $S = 0$. (*a*) Are these types of helium allowed to interchange energy? (*b*) Describe the low-resolution spectra for parahelium and orthohelium.

Ans. (*a*) No, $\Delta S = 0$ must be obeyed. (*b*) Except that the spectra will consist of singlets and triplets instead of doublets, the spectra will be similar to that for Na, with the lowest energy levels being the $1s$ and $2s$, respectively.

Chapter 13

Electronic Structure of Diatomic Molecules

Quantum Theory of Diatomic Molecules

13.1 HAMILTONIAN OPERATOR

The complete Hamiltonian operator for a polyatomic molecule is

$$\mathcal{H} = \frac{-\hbar^2}{2}\sum_{\alpha}^{\text{all nuclei}}\frac{1}{m_\alpha}\nabla_\alpha^2 + \frac{-\hbar^2}{2m_e}\sum_{i}^{\text{all electrons}}\nabla_i^2$$

$$+ \sum_{\beta}\sum_{\alpha<\beta}\frac{Z_\alpha Z_\beta e^2}{4\pi\epsilon_0 r_{\alpha\beta}} - \sum_i\sum_\alpha\frac{Z_\alpha e^2}{4\pi\epsilon_0 r_{i\alpha}} + \sum_j\sum_{i<j}\frac{e^2}{4\pi\epsilon_0 r_{ij}} \qquad (13.1)$$

where the terms represent the nuclear kinetic energy, the electronic kinetic energy, the nuclear repulsion potential energy, the nuclear-electronic attraction potential energy, and the electronic repulsion potential energy, respectively. The *Born-Oppenheimer approximation* simplifies (*13.1*) by setting the nuclear kinetic energy term equal to zero and the nuclear repulsion term equal to a constant, because the nuclei are moving much slower than the electrons. Thus, for a two-nucleus system, the nuclear repulsion term is $Z_a Z_b e^2/4\pi\epsilon_0 r_{ab}$, where r_{ab}, the internuclear distance, is considered constant. The electronic energy, E, is then calculated in terms of the parameter r_{ab}, whereupon the total energy of the molecule, E', is obtained as

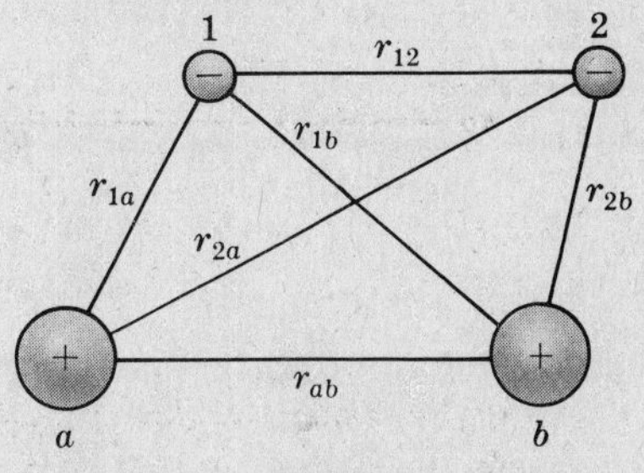

Fig. 13-1

$$E' = E + \frac{Z_a Z_b e^2}{4\pi\epsilon_0 r_{ab}}$$

EXAMPLE 13.1. The H_2 molecule ($Z_a = Z_b = 1$) is indicated in Fig. 13-1. Equation (*13.1*) becomes, under the Born-Oppenheimer approximation,

$$\mathcal{H} = \frac{-\hbar^2}{2m_e}(\nabla_1^2 + \nabla_2^2) + \frac{e^2}{4\pi\epsilon_0}\left(\frac{1}{r_{ab}} - \frac{1}{r_{1a}} - \frac{1}{r_{2a}} - \frac{1}{r_{1b}} - \frac{1}{r_{2b}} + \frac{1}{r_{12}}\right)$$

13.2 WAVE FUNCTIONS

The wave function, ϕ, is usually the product of the wave functions for the individual electrons:

$$\phi = \phi_1\phi_2\cdots \qquad (13.2)$$

where the ϕ_i are produced by taking linear combinations of hydrogenlike atomic orbitals (LCAO):

$$\phi_i = a_{ia}\psi_a(i) + a_{ib}\psi_b(i) + \cdots \qquad (13.3)$$

In (*13.3*) the $a_{i\alpha}$ are constants and the notation $\psi_\alpha(i)$ means a hydrogenlike atomic wave function describing electron i in terms of position with respect to nucleus α. Terms in ϕ which are of the form $\psi_a(1)\psi_a(2)$ are ionic terms, and terms which are of the form $\psi_a(1)\psi_b(2)$ are covalent terms. Depending on the actual construction of ϕ, these types of terms may be weighted differently or the same. A wave function for a diatomic molecule having unshared pairs of electrons usually consists of terms involving only the bonding electrons.

EXAMPLE 13.2. Determine a trial wave function using (*13.2*) and (*13.3*) for the H_2 molecule. Assuming that the $a_{i\alpha}$ are all equal and that identical normalized hydrogenlike wave functions are chosen, show that the normalization constant is $a = (2+2S)^{-1}$, where $S = S_{ab} = S_{ba}$ as defined in (*11.27*).

Applying (*13.3*) to each electron and using a single-subscript notation for the a's gives

$$\phi_1 = a_1\psi_a(1) + a_2\psi_b(1) \qquad \phi_2 = a_3\psi_a(2) + a_4\psi_b(2)$$

and (*13.2*) gives

$$\begin{aligned}\phi &= [a_1\psi_a(1) + a_2\psi_b(1)][a_3\psi_a(2) + a_4\psi_b(2)] \\ &= a_1a_3\psi_a(1)\psi_a(2) + a_2a_4\psi_b(1)\psi_b(2) + a_1a_4\psi_a(1)\psi_b(2) + a_2a_3\psi_b(1)\psi_a(2)\end{aligned}$$

Assuming that identical normalized hydrogenlike wave functions are being used to describe the electrons and that

$$a_1 = a_2 = a_3 = a_4 = a$$

gives

$$\langle\phi\,|\,\phi\rangle = \langle\phi_1\phi_2\,|\,\phi_1\phi_2\rangle = \langle\phi_1\,|\,\phi_1\rangle\langle\phi_2\,|\,\phi_2\rangle = \langle\phi_1\,|\,\phi_1\rangle^2$$

where

$$\begin{aligned}\langle\phi_1\,|\,\phi_1\rangle &= \langle a\psi_a(1) + a\psi_b(1)\,|\,a\psi_a(1) + a\psi_b(1)\rangle \\ &= a^2[\langle\psi_a(1)\,|\,\psi_a(1)\rangle + \langle\psi_b(1)\,|\,\psi_b(1)\rangle + \langle\psi_a(1)\,|\,\psi_b(1)\rangle + \langle\psi_b(1)\,|\,\psi_a(1)\rangle] \\ &= a^2(S_{aa} + S_{bb} + S_{ab} + S_{ba}) = a^2(1+1+S+S) = a^2(2+2S)\end{aligned}$$

Substituting these results into (*11.12*) gives

$$1 = \langle\phi\,|\,\phi\rangle = \langle\phi_1\,|\,\phi_1\rangle^2 = [a^2(2+2S)]^2$$

whence

$$a = (2+2S)^{-1}$$

Application of the Variation Method

13.3 ENERGY

The electronic contribution E (see Section 13.1) is calculated as a function of r_{ab} using (*11.23*) or the secular equation (*11.28*). Some integrals that are encountered in the solution to the H_2^-, H_2 and H_2^+ problems using hydrogenlike 1s atomic orbitals are:

$$S = \langle\psi_a(1)\,|\,\psi_b(1)\rangle = e^{-\rho}\left(1+\rho+\frac{\rho^2}{3}\right) \tag{13.4a}$$

$$J = \langle\psi_a(1)\,|\,(-e^2/4\pi\epsilon_0 r_{1b})\,|\,\psi_a(1)\rangle = \frac{e^2}{4\pi\epsilon_0 a_0}\left[\frac{-1}{\rho} + e^{-2\rho}\left(1+\frac{1}{\rho}\right)\right] \tag{13.4b}$$

$$K = \langle\psi_b(1)\,|\,(-e^2/4\pi\epsilon_0 r_{1b})\,|\,\psi_a(1)\rangle = \frac{-e^2}{4\pi\epsilon_0 a_0}e^{-\rho}(1+\rho) \tag{13.4c}$$

$$J' = \langle\psi_a(1)\psi_b(2)\,|\,(e^2/4\pi\epsilon_0 r_{12})\,|\,\psi_a(1)\psi_b(2)\rangle$$

$$= \frac{e^2}{4\pi\epsilon_0 a_0}\left[\frac{1}{\rho} - e^{-2\rho}\left(\frac{1}{\rho} + \frac{11}{8} + \frac{3\rho}{4} + \frac{\rho^2}{6}\right)\right] \tag{13.4d}$$

$$K' = \langle\psi_a(1)\psi_b(2)\,|\,(e^2/4\pi\epsilon_0 r_{12})\,|\,\psi_b(1)\psi_a(2)\rangle$$

$$= \frac{e^2}{4\pi\epsilon_0(5a_0)}\left\{-e^{-2\rho}\left(\frac{-25}{8} + \frac{23\rho}{4} + 3\rho^2 + \frac{\rho^3}{3}\right) + \frac{6}{\rho}\left[S^2(0.57722 + \log\rho)\right.\right.$$

$$\left.\left. + e^{2\rho}\left(1 - \rho + \frac{\rho^2}{3}\right)^2 W(-4\rho) - 2Se^{\rho}\left(1 - \rho + \frac{\rho^2}{3}\right)W(-2\rho)\right]\right\} \tag{13.4e}$$

$$L = \langle\psi_a(1)\psi_a(2)\,|\,(e^2/4\pi\epsilon_0 r_{12})\,|\,\psi_a(1)\psi_b(2)\rangle = \frac{e^2}{4\pi\epsilon_0 a_0}\left[e^{-\rho}\left(\rho + \frac{1}{8} + \frac{5}{16\rho}\right) + e^{-3\rho}\left(-\frac{1}{8} - \frac{5}{16\rho}\right)\right] \tag{13.4f}$$

$$C = \langle\psi_a(1)\psi_a(2)\,|\,(e^2/4\pi\epsilon_0 r_{12})\,|\,\psi_a(1)\psi_a(2)\rangle = \frac{e^2}{4\pi\epsilon_0 a_0}\left(\frac{5}{8}\right) \tag{13.4g}$$

where

$$\rho = \frac{r_{ab}}{a_0} \tag{13.5}$$

$$W(-x) = -\int_x^\infty \frac{e^{-t}}{t}\,dt \quad (x > 0) \tag{13.6}$$

$$a_0 = 0.52917706\ \text{Å}$$

EXAMPLE 13.3. Using the Hamiltonian and trial wave function for the H_2 molecule as determined in Examples 13.1 and 13.2, find the energy of the molecule in terms of the integrals given by (*13.4*).

The electronic energy is obtained from the normalized wave function via (*11.23*):

$$E = \langle\phi\,|\,\mathcal{H}\,|\,\phi\rangle = \left\langle\phi\,\middle|\,\mathcal{H}_1 + \mathcal{H}_2 + \frac{e^2}{4\pi\epsilon_0 r_{12}}\,\middle|\,\phi\right\rangle$$

$$= \langle\phi\,|\,\mathcal{H}_1\,|\,\phi\rangle + \langle\phi\,|\,\mathcal{H}_2\,|\,\phi\rangle + \left\langle\phi\,\middle|\,\frac{e^2}{4\pi\epsilon_0 r_{12}}\,\middle|\,\phi\right\rangle$$

where

$$\mathcal{H}_i = \frac{-\hbar^2}{2m_e}\nabla_i^2 - \frac{e^2}{4\pi\epsilon_0 r_{ia}} - \frac{e^2}{4\pi\epsilon_0 r_{ib}}$$

Note that the r_{ab}-term has been omitted from $\mathcal{H}$. Because the two electrons have identical wave functions, $\langle\phi\,|\,\mathcal{H}_1\,|\,\phi\rangle$ and $\langle\phi\,|\,\mathcal{H}_2\,|\,\phi\rangle$ are equal, so that

$$E = 2\langle\phi\,|\,\mathcal{H}_1\,|\,\phi\rangle + \left\langle\phi\,\middle|\,\frac{e^2}{4\pi\epsilon_0 r_{12}}\,\middle|\,\phi\right\rangle$$

The first integral on the right has the value

$$\langle\phi\,|\,\mathcal{H}_1\,|\,\phi\rangle = (2+2S)^{-2}\langle[\psi_a(1)+\psi_b(1)][\psi_a(2)+\psi_b(2)]\,|\,\mathcal{H}_1\,|\,[\psi_a(1)+\psi_b(1)][\psi_a(2)+\psi_b(2)]\rangle$$

$$= (2+2S)^{-2}\langle\psi_a(1)+\psi_b(1)\,|\,\mathcal{H}_1\,|\,\psi_a(1)+\psi_b(1)\rangle\langle\psi_a(2)+\psi_b(2)\,|\,\psi_a(2)+\psi_b(2)\rangle$$

The integral involving electron 2 was shown in Example 13.2 to be equal to $2+2S$, giving

$$
\begin{aligned}
(2+2S)\langle\phi|\mathcal{H}_1|\phi\rangle &= \left\langle \psi_a(1)+\psi_b(1)\left|\frac{-\hbar^2}{2m_e}\nabla_1^2 - \frac{e^2}{4\pi\epsilon_0 r_{1a}} - \frac{e^2}{4\pi\epsilon_0 r_{1b}}\right|\psi_a(1)+\psi_b(1)\right\rangle \\
&= \left\langle \psi_a(1)\left|\frac{-\hbar^2}{2m_e}\nabla_1^2 - \frac{e^2}{4\pi\epsilon_0 r_{1a}}\right|\psi_a(1)\right\rangle + \left\langle \psi_b(1)\left|\frac{-\hbar^2}{2m_e}\nabla_1^2 - \frac{e^2}{4\pi\epsilon_0 r_{1a}}\right|\psi_a(1)\right\rangle \\
&\quad + \left\langle \psi_a(1)\left|\frac{-\hbar^2}{2m_e}\nabla_1^2 - \frac{e^2}{4\pi\epsilon_0 r_{1b}}\right|\psi_b(1)\right\rangle \\
&\quad + \left\langle \psi_a(1)\left|-\frac{e^2}{4\pi\epsilon_0 r_{1a}}\right|\psi_b(1)\right\rangle \\
&\quad + \left\langle \psi_b(1)\left|\frac{-\hbar^2}{2m_e}\nabla_1^2 - \frac{e^2}{4\pi\epsilon_0 r_{1b}}\right|\psi_b(1)\right\rangle \\
&\quad + \left\langle \psi_b(1)\left|-\frac{e^2}{4\pi\epsilon_0 r_{1a}}\right|\psi_b(1)\right\rangle \\
&\quad + \left\langle \psi_a(1)\left|-\frac{e^2}{4\pi\epsilon_0 r_{1b}}\right|\psi_a(1)\right\rangle + \left\langle \psi_b(1)\left|-\frac{e^2}{4\pi\epsilon_0 r_{1b}}\right|\psi_a(1)\right\rangle \\
&= E_H + E_H S + E_H S + K + E_H + J + J + K \\
&= E_H(2+2S) + 2(J+K)
\end{aligned}
$$

where the first, second, third, and fifth integrals have been evaluated by use of the Schrödinger equation. Here $E_H = -13.60$ eV is the energy of the ground state of the hydrogen atom.

For the second integral in the equation for E, a similar calculation (see Problem 13.17) gives

$$\left\langle \phi\left|\frac{e^2}{4\pi\epsilon_0 r_{12}}\right|\phi\right\rangle = \frac{K' + 2L + (J'/2) + (C/2)}{(1+S)^2}$$

Hence the electronic energy is

$$E = 2\left(E_H + \frac{J+K}{1+S}\right) + \frac{K' + 2L + (J'/2) + (C/2)}{(1+S)^2}$$

and the overall energy (see Section 13.1) is $E' = E + (e^2/4\pi\epsilon_0 r_{ab})$.

13.4 MOLECULAR ORBITALS

The variation method predicts that upon combining two atomic orbitals, two molecular orbitals are generated. One orbital has an energy lower than that of the separated atoms; hence it is known as *bonding*. The other orbital has an energy higher than that of the separated atoms; it is known as *antibonding*. Each orbital can hold a maximum of two electrons.

The molecular orbitals formed from hydrogenlike atomic orbitals for homonuclear molecules with four or fewer electrons are shown in Fig. 13-2(*a*), and for homonuclear molecules with between four and twenty-one electrons in Fig. 13-2(*b*). The diagram for homonuclear molecules with up to 36 electrons would be similar to Fig. 13-2(*b*) with an additional set of higher-energy orbitals, 3*s* and 3*p*, at the top of the diagram.

For heteronuclear diatomic molecules, the molecular orbital diagrams are not symmetrical and differ for each molecule. The atomic orbitals for each atom are drawn at the approximate energy on the diagram and the proper atomic orbitals are allowed to combine to form the molecular orbitals. Often the diagram will contain the same orbitals as shown in Fig. 13-2(*b*).

Those molecular orbitals having a cross section perpendicular to the internuclear axis (usually the *z*-axis) consisting of a circle are called σ *orbitals*; of two lobes (180° apart),

π *orbitals*; of four lobes (90° apart), δ *orbitals*; etc. In Fig. 13-2 an asterisk indicates an antibonding orbital; in parentheses is the symbol of the atomic orbitals composing the molecular orbital. The subscripts g and u refer to the symmetry of the orbital (Section 13.8).

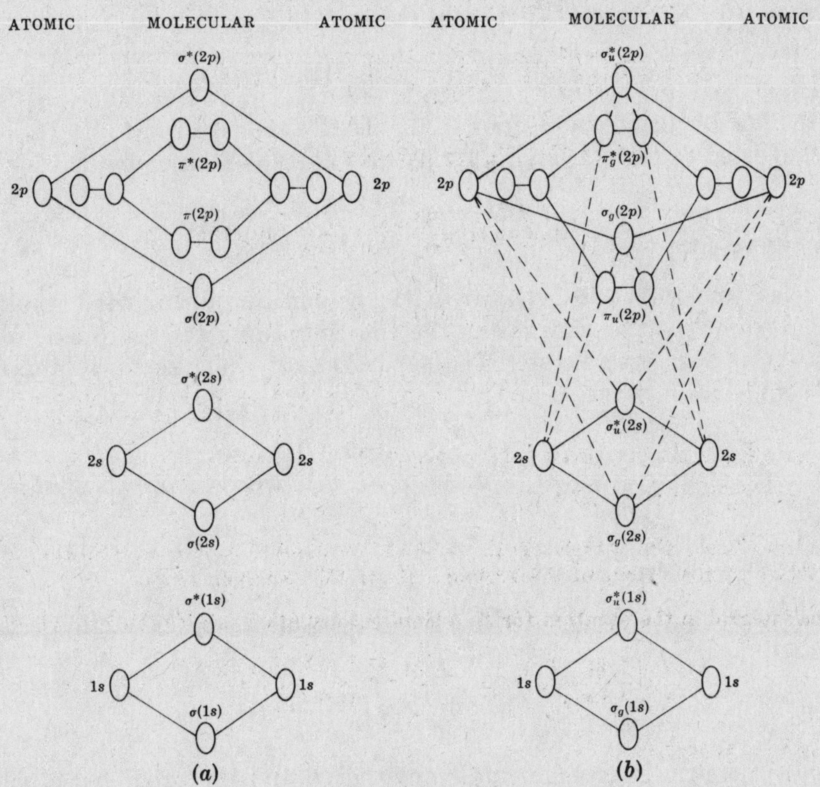

Fig. 13-2

EXAMPLE 13.4. Use Fig. 13-2 to write electronic configurations for the following diatomic molecules and discuss the bonding (if any): (*a*) H_2^+, H_2 and H_2^-; (*b*) N_2; (*c*) F_2.

(*a*) From Fig. 13-2(*a*) the configurations are $\sigma(1s)$ for H_2^+, $\sigma(1s)^2$ for H_2 and $\sigma(1s)^2\sigma^*(1s)$ for H_2^-, indicating stable molecules having $\frac{1}{2}$ of a σ bond, a σ bond and $\frac{1}{2}$ of a σ bond, respectively.

(*b*) Using Fig. 13-2(*b*) for the 14 electrons gives the configuration as

$$\sigma_g(1s)^2\sigma_u^*(1s)^2\sigma_g(2s)^2\sigma_u^*(2s^2)\pi_u(2p)^4\sigma_g(2p)^2$$

which is a triple bond consisting of a σ and two π bonds.

(*c*) For the 18 electrons Fig. 13-2(*b*) gives the configuration as a single σ bond:

$$\sigma_g(1s)^2\sigma_u^*(1s)^2\sigma_g(2s)^2\sigma_u^*(2s)^2\pi_u(2p)^4\sigma_g(2p)^2\pi_g^*(2p)^4$$

Bond Description

13.5 ELECTRONEGATIVITY

The quantitative measure of the unequal attraction of the atoms in a heteronuclear diatomic molecule for the bonding electrons is known as the *electronegativity*. Mulliken defined the electronegativity for an element, EN_i, as

$$EN_i = \frac{1}{2}(I_i + E_i) \qquad (13.7)$$

where I_i is the ionization potential and E_i is the electron affinity of the element. Pauling defined the difference in electronegativities for two elements as

$$\mathrm{EN_X} - \mathrm{EN_Y} = 0.102\,\Delta^{1/2} \tag{13.8}$$

where the constant 0.102 converts $\Delta^{1/2}$ from $(\mathrm{kJ\ mol^{-1}})^{1/2}$ to eV and

$$\Delta = \mathrm{BE_{XY}} - (\mathrm{BE_{X_2}BE_{Y_2}})^{1/2} \tag{13.9}$$

where BE_i is the bond energy, see Section 3.11. If $\mathrm{EN_H}$ is assumed to be 2.20, the Mulliken scale can be converted to the Pauling scale by dividing the former by 3.15.

13.6 DIPOLE MOMENT

A heteronuclear molecule will be polar, with the end containing the less electronegative element having a slight positive charge and the end containing the more electronegative element having a slight negative charge. The separation of charges $\pm q$ by a distance r gives rise to a *dipole moment*, μ, where

$$\mu = qr \tag{13.10}$$

Dipole moments are often expressed in units of *debyes*, where $1\ \mathrm{D} = 3.335641 \times 10^{-30}\ \mathrm{C\ m}$.

13.7 IONIC CHARACTER

The *percent ionic character*, %IC, of a chemical bond can be calculated from the dipole moment by

$$\%\mathrm{IC} = 100\frac{\mu_{\mathrm{actual}}}{\mu_{\mathrm{predicted}}} \tag{13.11}$$

The actual dipole moment is experimentally measured and the predicted dipole moment is calculated from (*13.10*) with $q = e$ and $r = r_{ab}$. The percent ionic character can also be estimated as

$$\%\mathrm{IC} = 16(\mathrm{EN}_i - \mathrm{EN}_j) + 3.5\,(\mathrm{EN}_i - \mathrm{EN}_j)^2 \tag{13.12}$$

Molecular Term Symbols

13.8 CLASSIFICATION OF ELECTRONIC STATES

The component of electronic angular momentum along the z-axis has the value $M_L\hbar$, where M_L is defined in (*12.18*). Electronic states are classified according to the value of the quantum number Λ given by

$$\Lambda = |M_L| \tag{13.13}$$

In analogy to atomic orbitals the symbol Σ is used for $\Lambda = 0$, Π for $\Lambda = 1$, Δ for $\Lambda = 2$, Φ for $\Lambda = 3$, Γ for $\Lambda = 4$, etc. The symbol for a Σ state carries as a following superscript a minus sign if the wave function changes sign when reflected across the xz-plane and a plus sign if there is no change in sign. The term symbol for a homonuclear diatomic molecule carries a following subscript of g (German: *gerade* = even) or u (*ungerade* = odd) depending on whether an inversion operation through the origin leaves the wave function unchanged or changed in sign, respectively.

A leading superscript on the symbol is $2S+1$, where S is found by s-s coupling techniques, see Section 12.9. An optional numerical following subscript on the term symbol, Ω, represents the total angular momentum. It is found by combining the value of $\mathcal{S}$ given by

$$\mathcal{S} = S, S-1, \ldots, -S \tag{13.14}$$

with Λ, yielding

$$\Omega = |\Lambda + \mathcal{S}| \tag{13.15}$$

EXAMPLE 13.5. Identify the term symbols that correspond to $\Lambda = 2$ and $S = 1$.

The symbol for $\Lambda = 2$ is Δ. The multiplicity is $2S+1 = 3$, giving $^3\Delta$. Equation (*13.14*) gives the values of $\mathcal{S}$ as 1, 0, −1, whence $\Omega = |2+1| = 3$, $|2+0| = 2$ and $|2-1| = 1$. The term symbols are $^3\Delta_3$, $^3\Delta_2$ and $^3\Delta_1$.

13.9 TERM SYMBOLS FOR ELECTRONIC CONFIGURATIONS

For various molecular orbital configurations, the major part of the term symbol can be found in Table 13-1. The *parity* or symmetry for the homonuclear diatomic molecules can be found by multiplying the parities of the orbitals being used, according to the usual laws of odd and even:

$$(g)(g) = (u)(u) = (g) \quad \text{and} \quad (g)(u) = (u)(g) = (u)$$

The term symbol for a heteronuclear diatomic molecule does not contain the g or u subscript. Electrons in partially filled atomic orbitals that are not involved in bonding also contribute to Λ.

Table 13-1

Configuration	Term Symbols
σ	$^2\Sigma^+$
σ^2	$^1\Sigma^+$
π	$^2\Pi$
π^2	$^1\Sigma^+$, $^1\Delta$, $^3\Sigma^-$
$\pi^2\sigma$	$^2\Sigma^+$, $^2\Sigma^-$, $^2\Delta$, $^4\Sigma$
$\pi^2\pi$	$^2\Pi$ (3), $^2\Phi$, $^4\Pi$
$\pi^2\delta$	$^2\Sigma^+$, $^2\Sigma^-$, $^2\Delta$ (2), $^2\Gamma$, $^4\Delta$
π^3	$^2\Pi$
$\pi^3\sigma$	$^1\Pi$, $^3\Pi$
$\pi^3\pi$	$^1\Sigma^+$, $^1\Sigma^-$, $^1\Delta$, $^3\Sigma^+$, $^3\Sigma^-$, $^3\Delta$
$\pi^3\delta$	$^1\Pi$, $^1\Phi$, $^3\Pi$, $^3\Phi$
π^4	$^1\Sigma^+$
δ	$^2\Delta$
δ^2	$^1\Sigma^+$, $^3\Sigma^-$, $^1\Gamma$
δ^3	$^2\Delta$
δ^4	$^1\Sigma^+$

EXAMPLE 13.6. For the ground state of H_2^+ the electronic configuration is $\sigma(1s)$, which gives rise to a $^2\Sigma^+$ symbol from Table 13-1. The parity is g, giving $^2\Sigma_g{}^+$.

Solved Problems

Quantum Theory of Diatomic Molecules

13.1. Determine $\mathcal{H}$ and a trial wave function for H_2^+.

The expression for $\mathcal{H}$ for the system composed of nuclei a and b and electron 1 is given by *(13.1)* as

$$\mathcal{H} = \frac{-\hbar^2}{2m_e}\nabla_1^2 + \frac{e^2}{4\pi\epsilon_0}\left(\frac{1}{r_{ab}} - \frac{1}{r_{1a}} - \frac{1}{r_{1b}}\right)$$

The trial wave function is, from *(13.2)* and *(13.3)*,

$$\phi = \phi_1 = a_1\psi_a(1) + a_2\psi_b(1)$$

where a_1 and a_2 have been written for a_{1a} and a_{1b}.

13.2. Construct a trial wave function for the bond between hydrogen and chlorine in HCl.

The electrons forming the bond are a $1s$ electron from the hydrogen and a $3p$ electron from the chlorine. Assuming identical wave functions for the two electrons, *(13.3)* gives

$$\phi_1 = a_1\psi_{1s\mathrm{H}}(1) + a_2\psi_{3p\mathrm{Cl}}(1) \qquad \phi_2 = a_1\psi_{1s\mathrm{H}}(2) + a_2\psi_{3p\mathrm{Cl}}(2)$$

and then *(13.2)* gives

$$\phi = a_1^2[\psi_{1s\mathrm{H}}(1)\,\psi_{1s\mathrm{H}}(2)] + a_1a_2[\psi_{1s\mathrm{H}}(1)\,\psi_{3p\mathrm{Cl}}(2) + \psi_{1s\mathrm{H}}(2)\,\psi_{3p\mathrm{Cl}}(1)] + a_2^2[\psi_{3p\mathrm{Cl}}(1)\,\psi_{3p\mathrm{Cl}}(2)]$$

Note that the covalent terms are of equal weight, but that the ionic terms have different weights from the covalent terms and from each other.

Application of the Variation Method

13.3. Prepare a plot of E' against r_{ab} for the bonding orbital of the H_2^+ molecule-ion, where

$$E' = E_{\mathrm{H}} + \frac{J+K}{1+S} + \frac{e^2}{4\pi\epsilon_0 r_{ab}}$$

Determine the dissociation energy, D_e, and the value of r_{ab} at which the lowest energy occurs.

Values of r_{ab} from 0.01 Å to 8.00 Å were used to calculate E', giving the solid curve in Fig. 13-3. A sample calculation follows for $r_{ab} = 1.00$ Å.

Equation *(13.5)* gives $\rho = 1.00\text{ Å}/0.529\text{ Å} = 1.89$, which upon substitution into *(13.4a)*, *(13.4b)* and *(13.4c)* gives

$$S = e^{-1.89}\left[1 + 1.89 + \frac{(1.89)^2}{3}\right] = (0.151)(4.08) = 0.616$$

$$J = \frac{e^2}{4\pi\epsilon_0 a_0}\left[\frac{-1}{1.89} + e^{-3.78}\left(1 + \frac{1}{1.89}\right)\right] = \frac{e^2}{4\pi\epsilon_0 a_0}(-0.494)$$

$$K = \frac{-e^2}{4\pi\epsilon_0 a_0}e^{-1.89}(1+1.89) = \frac{e^2}{4\pi\epsilon_0 a_0}(-0.437)$$

The expression for E' becomes

$$E' = (-13.60\text{ eV}) + \frac{e^2}{4\pi\epsilon_0 a_0}\left(\frac{-0.494 - 0.437}{1 + 0.616}\right) + \frac{e^2}{4\pi\epsilon_0 r_{ab}}$$

$$= (-13.60\text{ eV}) + \frac{e^2}{4\pi\epsilon_0}\left(\frac{-0.576}{a_0} + \frac{1}{r_{ab}}\right)$$

which upon substitution of numerical values of e, $4\pi\epsilon_0$, a_0 and r_{ab} gives

$$E' = (-13.60\text{ eV}) + \frac{(1.6022\times10^{-19}\text{ C})^2}{1.11265\times10^{-10}\text{ C}^2\text{ N}^{-1}\text{ m}^{-2}}(6.24145\times10^{18}\text{ eV N}^{-1}\text{ m}^{-1})\left(\frac{-0.576}{0.529\times10^{-10}\text{ m}} + \frac{1}{1.00\times10^{-10}\text{ m}}\right)$$

$$= (-13.60) + (-15.68) + (14.40) = -14.88\text{ eV}$$

The depth of the well is 1.76 eV ($= D_e$) at $r_{ab} = 1.32$ Å. The accepted values for these parameters are 2.791 eV and 1.06 Å.

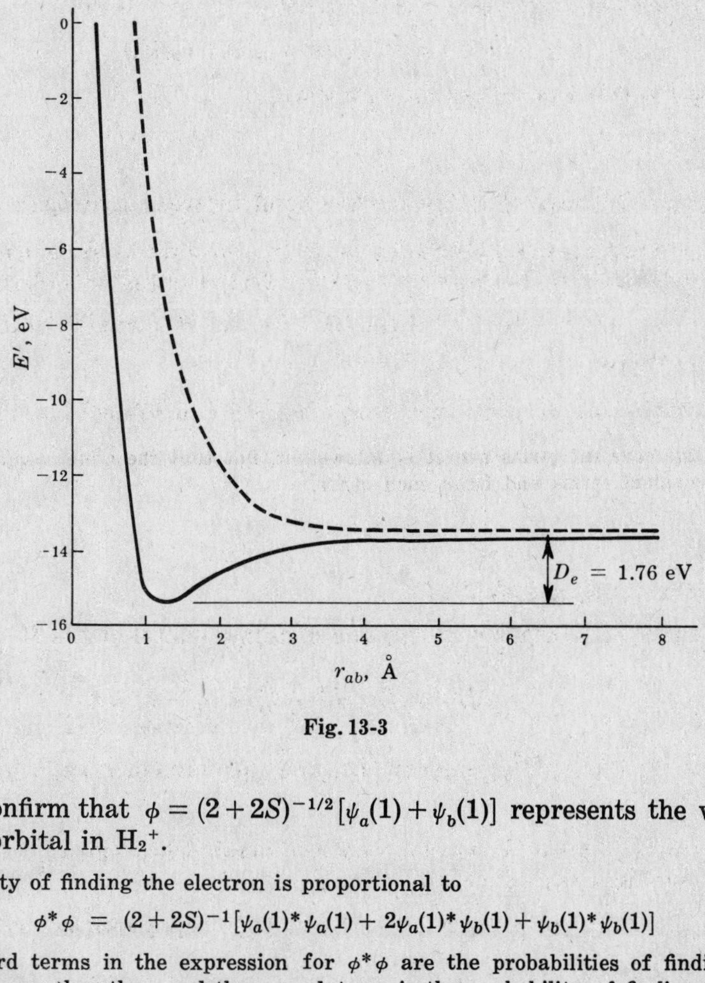

Fig. 13-3

13.4. **Qualitatively confirm that $\phi = (2+2S)^{-1/2}[\psi_a(1)+\psi_b(1)]$ represents the wave function for a bonding orbital in H_2^+.**

The probability of finding the electron is proportional to

$$\phi^*\phi = (2+2S)^{-1}[\psi_a(1)^*\psi_a(1) + 2\psi_a(1)^*\psi_b(1) + \psi_b(1)^*\psi_b(1)]$$

The first and third terms in the expression for $\phi^*\phi$ are the probabilities of finding the electron around one nucleus or the other, and the second term is the probability of finding the electron between the nuclei. A qualitative plot is shown in Fig. 13-4(*a*).

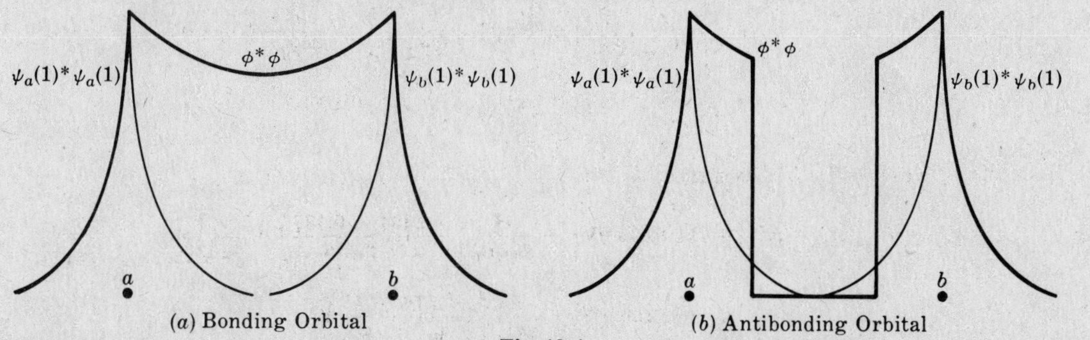

Fig. 13-4

13.5. With $\mathcal{H}$ and the trial wave function as determined in Problem 13.1, use the variation method to obtain the wave functions and the energies of the bonding and antibonding orbitals in the H_2^+ molecule-ion.

The secular equation for the system is given by (*11.28*) as

$$\begin{vmatrix} H_{aa} - ES_{aa} & H_{ab} - ES_{ab} \\ H_{ba} - ES_{ba} & H_{bb} - ES_{bb} \end{vmatrix} = 0$$

In view of the symmetry of the problem, (*11.26*) and (*11.27*) give $H_{aa} = H_{bb}$, $H_{ab} = H_{ba}$, $S_{ab} = S_{ba} = S$, where S is evaluated in (*13.4a*). Moreover, since $\psi_a(1)$ and $\psi_b(1)$ are assumed normalized, $S_{aa} = S_{bb} = 1$. The secular equation thus reduces to

$$\begin{vmatrix} H_{aa} - E & H_{ab} - ES \\ H_{ab} - ES & H_{aa} - E \end{vmatrix} = 0$$

whose roots are (see Problem 11.27):

$$E_1 = \frac{H_{aa} + H_{ab}}{1+S} \qquad E_2 = \frac{H_{aa} - H_{ab}}{1-S}$$

Using these values of E in (*11.25*),

$$a_1(H_{aa} - E) + a_2(H_{ab} - ES) = 0$$
$$a_1(H_{ab} - ES) + a_2(H_{aa} - E) = 0$$

we solve for a_1/a_2, obtaining

$$\frac{a_1}{a_2} = +1 \quad \text{for} \quad E = E_1, \qquad \frac{a_1}{a_2} = -1 \quad \text{for} \quad E = E_2$$

Using (*11.12*) for E_1 gives

$$1 = \langle\phi\,|\,\phi\rangle = \langle a_1\psi_a(1) + a_1\psi_b(1)\,|\,a_1\psi_a(1) + a_1\psi_b(1)\rangle = a_1^2(2+2S)$$

see Example 13.2. Solving for a_1 gives $a_1 = (2+2S)^{-1/2}$. Likewise for E_2, where $a_1 = -a_2$,

$$1 = \langle a_1\psi_a(1) - a_1\psi_b(1)\,|\,a_1\psi_a(1) - a_1\psi_b(1)\rangle = a_1^2(2-2S)$$

which gives $a_1 = (2-2S)^{-1/2}$. The normalized wave functions are thus

$$\psi_1 = (2+2S)^{-1/2}[\psi_a(1) + \psi_b(1)] \quad \text{for } E_1$$
$$\psi_2 = (2-2S)^{-1/2}[\psi_a(1) - \psi_b(1)] \quad \text{for } E_2$$

All that remains is to find the values of E_1 and E_2. The evaluations of H_{aa} and H_{ab} are as follows (omitting the r_{ab}-term in $\mathcal{H}$):

$$\begin{aligned} H_{aa} &= \langle\psi_a(1)|\mathcal{H}|\psi_a(1)\rangle = \left\langle\psi_a(1)\left|\frac{-\hbar^2}{2m_e}\nabla^2 - \frac{e^2}{4\pi\epsilon_0 r_{1a}} - \frac{e^2}{4\pi\epsilon_0 r_{1b}}\right|\psi_a(1)\right\rangle \\ &= \left\langle\psi_a(1)\left|\frac{-\hbar^2}{2m_e}\nabla^2 - \frac{e^2}{4\pi\epsilon_0 r_{1a}}\right|\psi_a(1)\right\rangle + \left\langle\psi_a(1)\left|\frac{-e^2}{4\pi\epsilon_0 r_{1b}}\right|\psi_a(1)\right\rangle \\ &= E_H + J \end{aligned}$$

$$\begin{aligned} H_{ab} &= \left\langle\psi_a(1)\left|\frac{-\hbar^2}{2m_e}\nabla^2 - \frac{e^2}{4\pi\epsilon_0 r_{1a}} - \frac{e^2}{4\pi\epsilon_0 r_{1b}}\right|\psi_b(1)\right\rangle \\ &= \left\langle\psi_a(1)\left|\frac{-\hbar^2}{2m_e}\nabla^2 - \frac{e^2}{4\pi\epsilon_0 r_{1a}}\right|\psi_b(1)\right\rangle + \left\langle\psi_a(1)\left|\frac{-e^2}{4\pi\epsilon_0 r_{1b}}\right|\psi_b(1)\right\rangle \\ &= E_H S + K \end{aligned}$$

Substituting these results into the expressions for E_1 and E_2 gives

$$E_1 = E_H + \frac{J+K}{1+S}$$

$$E_2 = E_H + \frac{J-K}{1-S}$$

which are respectively the electronic energies for the bonding and antibonding orbitals. The total energies, E_1' and E_2', are obtained by adding $e^2/4\pi\epsilon_0 r_{ab}$.

13.6. Consider the overlap of two *s* atomic orbitals, an *s* with a *p*, and two *p* atomic orbitals. Construct sketches of the newly formed molecular bonding orbitals.

As shown in Fig. 13-4, the bonding orbitals are characterized by a higher probability of finding the electrons between the nuclei than in the separated-atoms case. This is borne out by the sketches in the left half of Fig. 13-5. Thus, for an *s* overlapping with an *s*, the molecular orbital will fill in the gap between the atomic orbitals. The cross section perpendicular to the internuclear axis is circular, so that a σ orbital is formed. For the overlap of an *s* with a *p*, either a σ bond or a nonbonding arrangement will occur. For the overlap of two *p* orbitals, a head-on overlap will produce a σ bond and parallel overlap will produce a π bond.

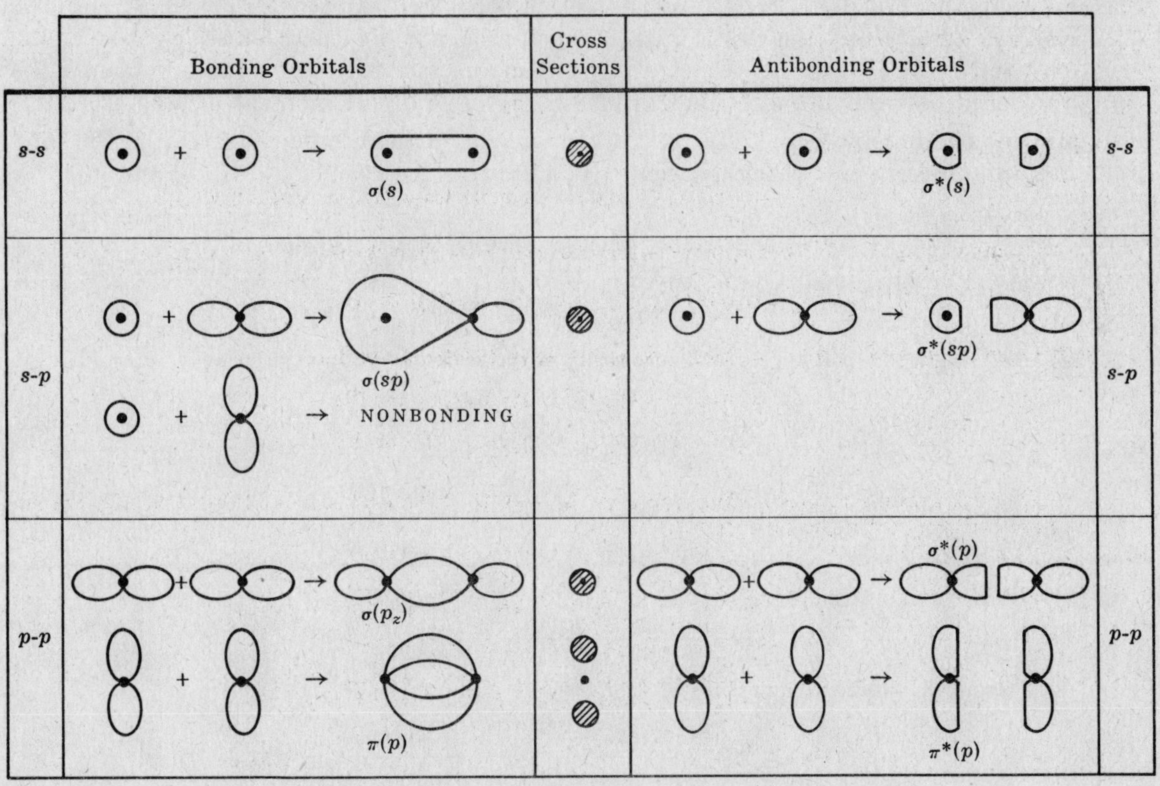

Fig. 13-5

13.7. Prepare a molecular energy diagram to represent the bonding in HCl.

Assuming that the 1*s* hydrogen orbital combines with the $3p_z$ chlorine orbital gives the bonding and antibonding orbitals shown in Fig. 13-6(*a*). The remainder of the electrons on the chlorine are nonbonding.

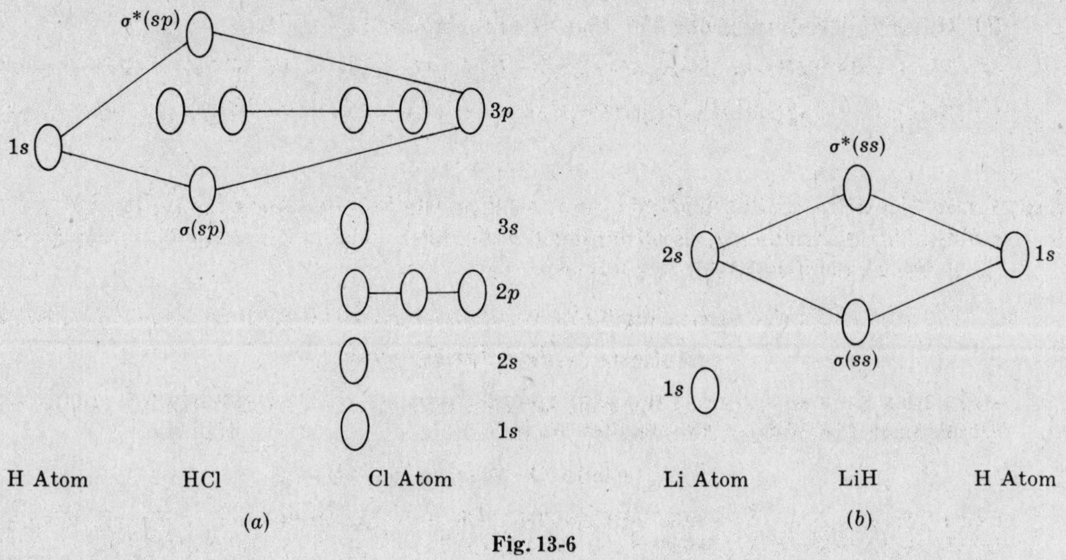

Fig. 13-6

Bond Description

13.8. (*a*) The bond energies for F_2, Br_2 and BrF are 159.0, 192.9 and 233.5 kJ mol^{-1}, respectively. Calculate the difference in electronegativities between F and Br. (*b*) The electron affinity and the first ionization potential are 3.45 and 17.418 eV for F and 3.37 and 11.84 eV for Br. Calculate the electronegativities from these data and the difference between the electronegativities. (*c*) The dipole moment of BrF is 1.29 D and the bond distance is 1.7555 Å. Calculate the percent ionic character of BrF and the difference in electronegativities. (*d*) Compare the results of (*a*), (*b*) and (*c*).

(*a*) Using (*13.9*) gives

$$\Delta = 233.5 - [(192.9)(159.0)]^{1/2} = 58.4 \text{ kJ mol}^{-1}$$

and (*13.8*) gives

$$EN_F - EN_{Br} = (0.102)(58.4)^{1/2} = 0.78 \text{ eV}$$

(*b*) Applying (*13.7*) to F and Br and converting to the scale of (*a*) gives

$$EN_F = \frac{17.418 + 3.45}{(2)(3.15)} = 3.31 \text{ eV}$$

$$EN_{Br} = \frac{11.84 + 3.37}{(2)(3.15)} = 2.41 \text{ eV}$$

whence

$$EN_F - EN_{Br} = 3.31 - 2.41 = 0.90 \text{ eV}$$

(*c*) Using (*13.11*) gives

$$\%IC = 100\,\frac{(1.29 \text{ D})(3.34\times10^{-30}\text{ C m D}^{-1})}{(1.6022\times10^{-19}\text{ C})(1.7555\times10^{-10}\text{ m})} = 15.3\%$$

Solving the quadratic equation (*13.12*) gives

$$EN_F - EN_{Br} = \frac{-16 + \sqrt{(16)^2 - 4(3.5)(-15.3)}}{2(3.5)} = 0.81 \text{ eV}$$

(*d*) The three theories predict essentially the same value for the electronegativity difference.

Molecular Term Symbols

13.9. Determine the term symbol for the ground state of (*a*) H_2, (*b*) H_2^-, (*c*) N_2 and (*d*) N_2^+.

(*a*) The ground state of H_2 is $\sigma_g(1s)^2$ which gives a $^1\Sigma^+$ term (see Table 13-1) having a parity of $(g)(g) = g$, or a complete term symbol of $^1\Sigma_g{}^+$.

(b) H_2^- is $\sigma_g(1s)^2\sigma_u^*(1s)$ giving $^2\Sigma^+$ with $(g)(g)(u) = u$ parity, or $^2\Sigma_u^+$.

(c) N_2 is $\sigma_2(1s)^2\sigma_u^*(1s)^2\sigma_g(2s)^2\sigma_u^*(2s)^2\pi_u(2p)^4\sigma_g(2p)^2$ giving $^1\Sigma^+$ with $(g)^6(u)^8 = g$ parity, or $^1\Sigma_g^+$.

(d) N_2^+ is $\sigma_g(1s)^2\sigma_u^*(1s)^2\sigma_g(2s)^2\sigma_u^*(2s)^2\pi_u(2p)^4\sigma_g(2p)$ giving $^2\Sigma^+$ with $(g)^5(u)^8 = g$ parity, or $^2\Sigma_g^+$.

13.10. Write electronic configurations for C_2 using the orbitals shown in Fig. 13-2. Which configuration predicts a paramagnetic molecule? If the term for the ground state is $^1\Sigma_g^+$, which configuration is correct?

Placing the 12 electrons in the orbitals given in Fig. 13-2(a) predicts the configuration as

$$\sigma(1s)^2\sigma^*(1s)^2\sigma(2s)^2\sigma^*(2s)^2\sigma(2p)^2\pi(2p)^2$$

which incorrectly gives $^3\Sigma^-$ as the term symbol (based on maximum multiplicity). Using the orbitals given in Fig. 13-2(b), the configuration is

$$\sigma(1s)^2\sigma^*(1s)^2\sigma(2s)^2\sigma^*(2s)^2\pi(2p)^4$$

which correctly gives $^1\Sigma^+$ as the term symbol. The first configuration incorrectly predicts the molecule to be paramagnetic because of the two unpaired electrons in the $\pi(2p)$ orbitals.

13.11. Determine the term symbol for the ground state of (a) NO, (b) HCl and (c) CH.

(a) Because the atomic electronic configurations and electronegativities of N and O are not greatly different, the molecular orbital diagram for this substance will resemble that given in Fig. 13-2(b). For the electronic configuration

$$\sigma(1s)^2\sigma^*(1s)^2\sigma(2s)^2\sigma^*(2s)^2\pi(2p)^4\sigma(2p)^2\pi^*(2p)^1$$

Table 13-1 gives $^2\Pi$ as the predicted term symbol for NO.

(b) As described in Problem 13.7, the bonding in HCl involves the molecular orbitals formed by the 1s orbital of hydrogen interacting with the $3p_z$ orbital of chlorine. Two of the 3p orbitals on chlorine are not involved in bonding, giving the electronic configuration as

$$1s_{\mathrm{Cl}}^2\,2s_{\mathrm{Cl}}^2\,2p_{\mathrm{Cl}}^6\,3s_{\mathrm{Cl}}^2\,\sigma(1s, 3p_z)^2\,3p_{\mathrm{Cl}}^4$$

Because all the atomic orbitals are filled, there is no contribution to the angular momentum from this source [$M_L = (+1) + (-1) + (+1) + (-1) = 0$ for the $3p_{\mathrm{Cl}}^4$ electrons] and Table 13-1 gives $^1\Sigma^+$ for the σ^2 configuration.

(c) The bonding in CH is similar to HCl in that the 1s orbital of hydrogen interacts with the $2p_z$ orbital of carbon, forming two molecular orbitals, $\sigma(1s, 2p_z)$ and $\sigma^*(1s, 2p_z)$, which have the remaining 2p orbitals of the carbon between them. The electronic configuration for CH is $1s_{\mathrm{C}}^2 2s_{\mathrm{C}}^2\sigma(1s, 2p_z)^2 2p_{\mathrm{C}}^1$. The only contribution to the angular momentum is from the $2p_{\mathrm{C}}$ electron, giving $M_L = +1$ and $S = +\frac{1}{2}$. Thus $\Lambda = 1$ and $S = +\frac{1}{2}$, giving $^2\Pi$ as the term for CH.

Supplementary Problems

Quantum Theory of Diatomic Molecules

13.12. Determine $\mathcal{H}$ and a trial wave function for the H_2^- molecule-ion.

Ans. $$\mathcal{H} = \frac{-\hbar^2}{2m_e}(\nabla_1^2 + \nabla_2^2 + \nabla_3^2) + \frac{e^2}{4\pi\epsilon_0}\left(\frac{1}{r_{ab}} - \frac{1}{r_{1a}} - \frac{1}{r_{2a}} - \frac{1}{r_{3a}} - \frac{1}{r_{1b}} - \frac{1}{r_{2b}} - \frac{1}{r_{3b}} + \frac{1}{r_{12}} + \frac{1}{r_{13}} + \frac{1}{r_{23}}\right);$$

$\phi = \phi_1\phi_2\phi_3$ where $\phi_1 = a_1\psi_a(1) + a_2\psi_b(1)$, $\phi_2 = a_3\psi_a(2) + a_4\psi_b(2)$, $\phi_3 = a_5\psi_a(3) + a_6\psi_b(3)$

13.13. Construct a trial wave function for the bond in ClF.

Ans. $\phi = \phi_1\phi_2$ where $\phi_1 = a_1\psi_{2p\mathrm{F}}(1) + a_2\psi_{3p\mathrm{Cl}}(1)$, $\phi_2 = a_1\psi_{2p\mathrm{F}}(2) + a_2\psi_{3p\mathrm{Cl}}(2)$

Application of the Variation Method

13.14. Prepare a plot of E' against r_{ab} for the antibonding orbital in the H_2^+ molecule-ion, where

$$E' = E_H + \frac{J-K}{1-S} + \frac{e^2}{4\pi\epsilon_0 r_{ab}}$$

Qualitatively discuss the plot.

Ans. See dashed curve in Fig. 13-3. The curve has no minimum and the values of $E' > -13.60$ eV indicate a nonbonding system.

13.15. Qualitatively demonstrate that $\phi = (2-2S)^{-1/2}\{\psi_a(1) - \psi_b(1)\}$ represents the wave function for an antibonding orbital. *Ans.* See Fig. 13-4(*b*).

13.16. (*a*) The trial wave function used by Heitler and London to describe the H_2 molecule in terms of hydrogenlike wave functions is

$$\phi = c_1\psi_a(1)\psi_b(2) + c_2\psi_a(2)\psi_b(1)$$

Note that the ionic terms in the trial wave function determined in Example 13.2 for this same system are eliminated in this wave function. Using the variation method, find the expressions for the energies of the bonding and antibonding orbitals and evaluate c_1 and c_2. (*b*) A plot of E' against r_{ab} has a minimum at 0.869 Å and -3.140 eV using the Heitler-London function, and for the wave function including the ionic terms the minimum is at 0.85 Å and -2.68 eV. What can be said about the inclusion of ionic terms if the accepted value is 0.740 Å and -4.747 eV?

Ans. (*a*) For bonding: $c_1 = c_2 = (2+2S^2)^{-1/2}$, $E = 2E_H + \dfrac{2(J+SK) + J' + K'}{1+S^2}$.

For antibonding: $c_1 = -c_2 = (2-2S^2)^{-1/2}$, $E = 2E_H + \dfrac{2(J-SK) + J' - K'}{1-S^2}$.

For both orbitals, $E' = E + \dfrac{e^2}{4\pi\epsilon_0 r_{ab}}$.

(*b*) Including ionic terms with equal weight to covalent terms gives poorer results.

13.17. Show that if $\phi \propto [\psi_a(1)+\psi_b(1)][\psi_a(2)+\psi_b(2)]$ and $\langle\phi|\phi\rangle = 1$, then

$$\left\langle \phi \left| \frac{e^2}{4\pi\epsilon_0 r_{12}} \right| \phi \right\rangle = \frac{K' + 2L + (J'/2) + (C/2)}{(1+S)^2}$$

13.18. Sketch the molecular antibonding orbitals formed by the overlap of (*a*) two *s* atomic orbitals, (*b*) an *s* and a *p* atomic orbital, (*c*) two *p* atomic orbitals.

Ans. See right half of Fig. 13-5.

13.19. Arrange the following molecules in order of increasing bond length: O_2, O_2^+, O_2^- and O_2^{2-}. Which molecule will have the greater bond dissociation energy: O_2 or O_2^+?

Ans. Configurations are $\ldots\pi^*(2p)^2$, $\ldots\pi^*(2p)^1$, $\ldots\pi^*(2p)^3$ and $\ldots\pi^*(2p)^4$, giving net bonding of $\sigma+\pi$, $\sigma+(3/2)\pi$, $\sigma+(1/2)\pi$ and σ; assuming bond length inversely proportional to net bonding gives $O_2^+ < O_2 < O_2^- < O_2^{2-}$. Assuming dissociation energy directly proportional to net bonding gives $O_2^+ > O_2$.

13.20. Using Fig. 13-2(*b*), write electronic configurations for the following diatomic molecules and discuss the bonding, if any: (*a*) He_2^+; (*b*) He_2; (*c*) O_2; (*d*) Ne_2.

Ans. (*a*) $\sigma(1s)^2\sigma^*(1s)$ giving net effect of $\frac{1}{2}$ of a σ bond

(*b*) $\sigma(1s)^2\sigma^*(1s)^2$ giving no net bonding

(*c*) $\sigma(1s)^2\sigma^*(1s)^2\sigma(2s)^2\sigma^*(2s)^2\pi(2p)^4\sigma(2p)^2\pi^*(2p)^2$ giving a net effect of one double bond consisting of a one σ bond and two half π-bonds [the $\pi^*(2p)$ electrons have parallel spins according to the rule of maximum multiplicity]

(*d*) $\sigma(1s)^2\sigma^*(1s)^2\sigma(2s)^2\sigma^*(2s)^2\pi(2p)^4\sigma(2p)^2\pi^*(2p)^4\sigma^*(2p)^2$ giving no net bonding

13.21. Prepare a molecular energy diagram to represent the bonding in LiH, neglecting any contribution from the vacant $2p$ atomic orbitals of Li. *Ans.* See Fig. 13-6(*b*).

Bond Description

13.22. If the bond energies for HCl, H_2 and Cl_2 are 431.96, 436.0 and 242.3 kJ mol^{-1}, respectively, calculate $EN_{Cl} - EN_H$ and infer the dipole moment if $r_{ab} = 1.2746$ Å. Compare with the measured value, 1.08 D. Ans. $EN_{Cl} - EN_H = 1.05$ eV; 1.26 D (12% high)

13.23. The dipole moments of HF, HCl, HBr and HI are 1.82, 1.08, 0.82 and 0.44 D, respectively. If the bond lengths are 0.9168, 1.2746, 1.414 and 1.608 Å, respectively, calculate the percent ionic character for these molecules and comment.

Ans. 41.3%, 17.7%, 12.1% and 5.7%, respectively; less ionic character as halogen gets larger

13.24. If an ionic bond is defined as one having at least 50% ionic character, what minimum difference in electronegativities will be defined by (*13.12*)? *Ans.* 2.13 eV

Molecular Term Symbols

13.25. Identify the term symbol that corresponds to $\Lambda = 1$ and $S = 0$. *Ans.* $^1\Pi_1$

13.26. Using Table 13-1, determine the term symbol for the ground state of (*a*) He_2^+, (*b*) O_2 and (*c*) O_2^+.

Ans. (*a*) $^2\Sigma_u{}^+$, (*b*) $^3\Sigma_g{}^-$ ($^3\Sigma^-$ has maximum multiplicity over $^1\Sigma^+$ and $^1\Delta$), (*c*) $^2\Pi_g$

13.27. Using Table 13-1, determine the term symbol for the ground state of (*a*) LiH and (*b*) CN^-, NO^+ and CO. *Ans.* (*a*) $^1\Sigma^+$, (*b*) $^1\Sigma^+$ for the isoelectronic species

13.28. Using Table 13-1, determine the molecular term symbols for the molecules OH^-, OH and OH^+.

Ans. $^1\Sigma^+$, $^2\Pi$, $^3\Sigma^-$

13.29. Write the predicted electronic configuration for the ground state of BN and determine the term symbol for this state. If the actual term is $^3\Pi$, determine the correct ground state electronic configuration.

Ans. $\sigma(1s)^2\sigma^*(1s)^2\sigma(2s)^2\sigma^*(2s)^2\pi(2p)^4$, $^1\Sigma$; $\sigma(1s)^2\sigma^*(1s)^2\sigma(2s)^2\sigma^*(2s)^2\pi(2p)^3\sigma(2p)^1$

Chapter 14

Spectroscopy of Diatomic Molecules

Rotational and Vibrational Spectra

14.1 ROTATIONAL SPECTRA

A diatomic molecule undergoing only rotational motion will be acting, to the first approximation, as a two-particle rigid rotator, see Problem 11.22, having an energy

$$E_J = B^* J(J+1) \tag{14.1}$$

where

$$B^* = \frac{\hbar^2}{2I} = \frac{\hbar^2}{2\mu r_{ab}^2} \tag{14.2}$$

see (*11.50*) and (*11.51*). Most spectroscopists express energy in units of cm^{-1} and write (*14.1*) and (*14.2*) as

$$F(J) = B_e J(J+1) \tag{14.3}$$

$$B_e = \frac{\hbar 10^{-2}}{4\pi c \mu r_{ab}^2} = \frac{B^* 10^{-2}}{hc} = \frac{2.7993 \times 10^{-46}}{\mu r_{ab}^2} \tag{14.4}$$

where B_e will be given in cm^{-1} and the normal SI units of kg and m are used for μ and r_{ab}, respectively, in (*14.4*).

If the molecule has a permanent dipole moment, it can absorb or emit microwave radiation corresponding to the rotational transitions that obey the selection rule $\Delta J = \pm 1$. For these transitions the wave numbers are

$$\bar{\nu} = F(J) - F(J-1) = 2B_e J \tag{14.5a}$$

Thus the spectrum will consist of a series of evenly spaced lines separated by

$$\Delta\bar{\nu} = 2B_e(J+1) - 2B_e J = 2B_e \tag{14.5b}$$

Because the energy differences between the rotational levels are quite small, several levels are populated under normal temperatures, giving rise to several intense lines. The degeneracy of any level is $2J+1$.

EXAMPLE 14.1. The microwave spectrum of CN shows a series of lines separated by $3.7978\ \text{cm}^{-1}$. Find the internuclear distance in the molecule.

Substituting $B_e = 3.7978/2 = 1.8989\ \text{cm}^{-1}$ into (*14.4*) gives

$$\mu r_{ab}^2 = \frac{2.7993 \times 10^{-46}}{1.8989} = 1.4742 \times 10^{-46}\ \text{kg m}^2$$

The reduced mass of the molecule is found from the molecular weights as

$$\mu = \frac{M_C M_N}{(M_C + M_N)L} = \frac{(12.011)(14.0067)}{(26.018)(6.022045 \times 10^{23})}$$

$$= 1.0737 \times 10^{-23}\ \text{g} = 1.0737 \times 10^{-26}\ \text{kg}$$

and so

$$r_{ab} = \left(\frac{1.4742 \times 10^{-46}}{1.0737 \times 10^{-26}}\right)^{1/2} = 1.1717 \times 10^{-10}\ \text{m} = 1.1717\ \text{Å}$$

14.2 VIBRATIONAL SPECTRA

The diatomic molecule undergoing only vibrational motion will be acting, to the first approximation, as a simple harmonic oscillator, see Problem 11.5, having an energy

$$E_v = \omega^*\left(v + \frac{1}{2}\right) \tag{14.6}$$

where

$$\omega^* = h\nu_0 = \hbar\left(\frac{k}{\mu}\right)^{1/2} \tag{14.7}$$

see (*11.39*). If the energy is expressed in units of cm^{-1}, (*14.6*) and (*14.7*) become

$$G(v) = \omega_e\left(v + \frac{1}{2}\right) \tag{14.8}$$

$$\omega_e = \frac{10^{-2}}{2\pi c}\left(\frac{k}{\mu}\right)^{1/2} = (5.3088 \times 10^{-12})\left(\frac{k}{\mu}\right)^{1/2} \tag{14.9}$$

where ω_e will be given in cm^{-1} and the normal SI units of kg and N m^{-1} are used for μ and k, respectively, in (*14.9*).

Vibrational transitions can occur only if $\Delta v = \pm 1$ and only in molecules having an oscillating dipole moment. Under these conditions,

$$\bar{\nu} = G(v) - G(v-1) = \omega_e \tag{14.10}$$

which means the spectrum will consist of one line having wave number ω_e. Because the energy difference between vibrational levels is quite high, most of the molecules will be in the $v=0$ level. Thus the major contribution to the spectrum will be the transition between the $v=0$ and $v=1$ levels.

The value of k, the force constant for the chemical bond, is such that ω_e will be in the infrared region of the spectrum. Homonuclear diatomic molecules will not be infrared active, i.e. the vibrational spectrum is not observable, while heteronuclear diatomic molecules will show an infrared spectrum. Vibrational data for homonuclear diatomics can be obtained from the Raman spectrum.

14.3 ANHARMONIC OSCILLATOR

The potential-energy well describing an electronic state (solid curve in Fig. 13-3) does not look like that for a simple harmonic oscillator (Fig. 11-8), except at very low values of v. Experimentally it is found that

$$G(v) = \omega_e\left(v + \frac{1}{2}\right) - \omega_e x_e\left(v + \frac{1}{2}\right)^2 + \omega_e y_e\left(v + \frac{1}{2}\right)^3 + \cdots \tag{14.11}$$

where x_e and y_e are molecular constants which are usually given only in the combinations $\omega_e x_e$ and $\omega_e y_e$. In (*14.11*) the cubic and higher terms are usually neglected. The separation between levels v and $v+1$ is given by

$$\Delta G(v) = \omega_e - \omega_e x_e(2v+2) \tag{14.12}$$

EXAMPLE 14.2. The dissociation energy predicted by equations similar to (*14.11*) is denoted D_e, whereas the experimental dissociation energy is denoted D_0. What is the relation between these dissociation energies?

Because D_e is measured from the bottom of the potential well to the top, while D_0 is measured from the ground level ($v=0$ and $J=0$) to the top, $D_e = D_0 + (\omega_e/2)$.

14.4 VIBRATIONAL-ROTATIONAL SPECTRA

Because a real molecule is simultaneously undergoing both rotational and vibrational motion, the energy will be

$$T(v,J) = \omega_e\left(v+\frac{1}{2}\right) - \omega_e x_e\left(v+\frac{1}{2}\right)^2 + \cdots + B_e J(J+1)$$

$$- \bar{D}_e J^2(J+1)^2 + \cdots - \alpha_e\left(v+\frac{1}{2}\right)J(J+1) \qquad (14.13)$$

where the first term represents the harmonic vibration contribution, see (*14.8*); the second term represents the anharmonic vibration contribution, see (*14.11*); the third term represents the rotational contribution, see (*14.3*); the fourth term represents the centrifugal stretching of the chemical bond; and the fifth term accounts for rotational-vibrational interaction. Usually the terms involving the centrifugal distortion constant, $\bar{D}_e$, and the vibrational-rotation coupling constant, α_e, are small for low values of J.

The selection rules for the vibrational-rotational transitions in heteronuclear diatomic molecules with $\Lambda = 0$ are $\Delta J = \pm 1$ and $\Delta v = \pm 1$. Because of the order-of-magnitude difference between the rotational and vibrational contributions, the spectrum will appear as a series of bands corresponding to different values of v, which under high resolution give lines corresponding to different values of J. As mentioned in Section 14.2, homonuclear diatomic molecules will be infrared inactive, while heteronuclear diatomic molecules will show an infrared spectrum.

The rotational fine structure having $\Delta J = +1$ is known as the *R branch* and that having $\Delta J = -1$ as the *P branch.* If the upper state is designated with a prime and the lower state with a double prime, it can be shown that

$$\bar{\nu}_R = \bar{\nu}_0 + (2B'_e - 3\alpha_e) + (3B'_e - B''_e - 4\alpha_e)J + (B'_e - B''_e - \alpha_e)J^2 \qquad (14.14)$$

where $J = 0, 1, 2, 3, \ldots,$ and

$$\bar{\nu}_P = \bar{\nu}_0 - (B'_e + B''_e - 2\alpha_e)J + (B'_e - B''_e - \alpha_e)J^2 \qquad (14.15)$$

where $J = 1, 2, 3, \ldots,$ and the wave number of the "forbidden" transition between $v' = 0$, $J' = 0$ and $v'' = 0$, $J'' = 0$ is given by

$$\bar{\nu}_0 = \omega_e - 2\omega_e x_e \qquad (14.16)$$

if $\bar{D}_e$ is assumed to be zero. If $B'_e = B''_e$,

$$\bar{\nu}_R = \bar{\nu}_0 + (2B_e - 3\alpha_e) + (2B_e - 4\alpha_e)J - \alpha_e J^2 \qquad (14.17)$$

$$\bar{\nu}_P = \bar{\nu}_0 - (2B_e - 2\alpha_e)J - \alpha_e J^2 \qquad (14.18)$$

If m is defined as $J+1$ for the R branch and as $-J$ for the P branch, (*14.17*) and (*14.18*) can be written as

$$\bar{\nu} = \bar{\nu}_0 + (2B_e - 2\alpha_e)m - \alpha_e m^2 \qquad (14.19)$$

and the separation between the lines will be given by

$$\Delta\bar{\nu} = (2B_e - 3\alpha_e) - 2\alpha_e m \qquad (14.20)$$

The selection rules for vibrational-rotational interactions with $\Lambda \neq 0$ are $\Delta J = 0, \pm 1$ and $\Delta v = \pm 1$. The rotational fine structure having $\Delta J = 0$ is known as the ***Q branch,*** given by

$$\bar{\nu}_Q = \bar{\nu}_0 + (B'_e - B''_e)J + (B'_e - B''_e)J^2 \qquad (14.21)$$

where $J = 0, 1, 2, 3, \ldots,$ if α_e and $\bar{D}_e$ are assumed to be zero.

14.5 THE RAMAN EFFECT

Various rotational and vibrational transitions may occur within the ground electronic state as a result of the scattering of incident radiation on a sample, provided the energy, $\bar{\nu}_{\text{incident}}$, is greater than the vibrational energies and less than the electronic energies. Information concerning homonuclear diatomic molecules can be obtained because a permanent dipole is not required as in infrared spectroscopy. Because of the population of vibrational levels, the most intense contributions to the Raman spectrum will be $\Delta v = \pm 1$ and, in particular, $v = 0 \rightarrow v = 1$.

The spectrum will contain a band centered at $\bar{\nu}_{\text{incident}}$ resulting from Rayleigh scattering, a very weak *Antistokes band* centered at $\bar{\nu}_{\text{incident}} + \bar{\nu}_0$, and an intense *Stokes band* centered at $\bar{\nu}_{\text{incident}} - \bar{\nu}_0$. Under high resolution these bands give rotational information corresponding to the selection rules $\Delta J = 0, \pm 2$. The lines in the Q branch (usually unresolved), corresponding to $\Delta J = 0$, are separated from the center line by

$$\Delta\bar{\nu}_Q = (B'_e - B''_e)J + (B'_e - B''_e)J^2 \qquad (14.22)$$

where $J = 0, 1, 2, 3, \ldots$; those in the S branch, corresponding to $\Delta J = +2$, by

$$\Delta\bar{\nu}_S = 6B'_e + (5B'_e - B''_e)J + (B'_e - B''_e)J^2 \qquad (14.23)$$

where $J = 0, 1, 2, 3, \ldots$; and those in the O branch, corresponding to $\Delta J = -2$, by

$$\Delta\bar{\nu}_O = 2B'_e - (3B'_e + B''_e)J + (B'_e - B''_e)J^2 \qquad (14.24)$$

where $J = 2, 3, 4, \ldots$. Equations (*14.22*)-(*14.24*) do not include α_e- or $\bar{D}_e$-terms.

EXAMPLE 14.3. Describe the rotational fine structure in a Raman spectrum if $B'_e = B''_e = B_e$.

Substituting B_e for B'_e and B''_e in (*14.22*) gives $\Delta\bar{\nu}_Q = 0$. Thus the Q branch would be predicted to consist of one line located at the center. Similarly, (*14.23*) becomes

$$\Delta\bar{\nu}_S = 6B_e + (5B_e - B_e)J + (B_e - B_e)J^2 = 6B_e + 4B_eJ$$

which predicts that the first line ($J = 0$) of the S branch would be $6B_e$ above the center line and the rest of the lines would be separated by $4B_e$. For the O branch, (*14.24*) becomes

$$\Delta\bar{\nu}_O = 2B_e - (3B_e + B_e)J + (B_e - B_e)J^2 = 2B_e - 4B_eJ$$

which predicts that the first line ($J = 2$) would be $6B_e$ below the center line and the rest of the lines would be separated by $4B_e$.

Electronic Spectra

14.6 SELECTION RULES

The selection rules describing interacting electronic states are very complicated. However, the selection rule for the vibrational transitions between permitted electronic states is quite simple: Δv is arbitrary. The vibrational transitions will also include the rotational structure, but unless a very high resolution instrument is used, meaningful data are difficult to obtain; they are best found from infrared or Raman spectra.

EXAMPLE 14.4. The intensities of the observed bands will depend on the value of $\psi(r_{ab})^*\psi(r_{ab})$ at the same value of r_{ab} for the two levels in the transition. Consider the interacting electronic states shown in Fig. 14-1(*a*). Will the interactions indicated by vertical lines from a'' to a' and to b', and from b'' to a' and to b', be observed?

The transition from a'' to a' will not be observed, because the positions of $\psi^*\psi$ are such that there is very little overlap. The line from a'' to b' will be observed, because the $\psi^*\psi$'s indicate high population of both levels at this value of r_{ab}. The line from b'' to both a' and b' passes through high population values of these levels, so both of these transitions will be observed.

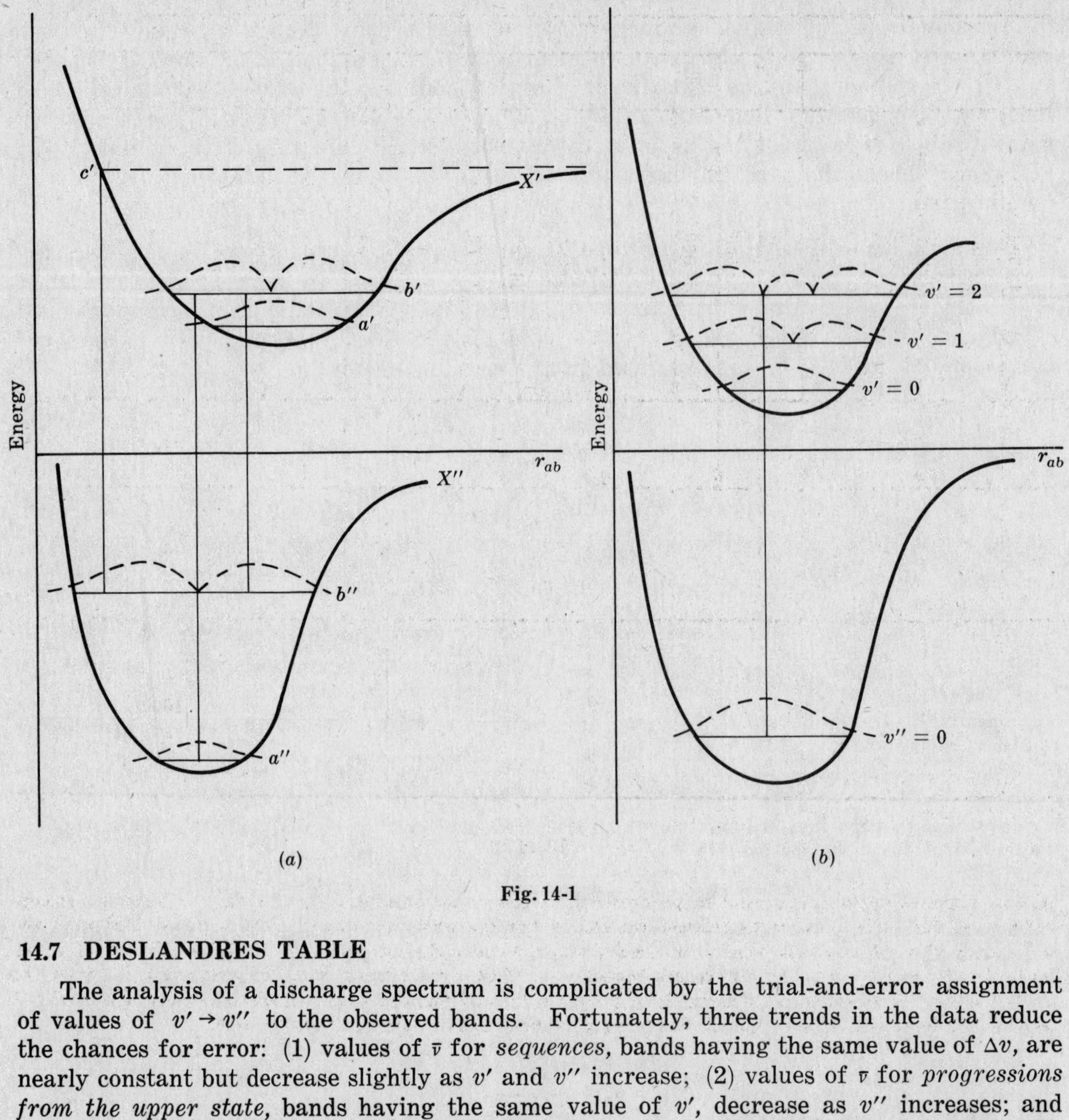

Fig. 14-1

14.7 DESLANDRES TABLE

The analysis of a discharge spectrum is complicated by the trial-and-error assignment of values of $v' \rightarrow v''$ to the observed bands. Fortunately, three trends in the data reduce the chances for error: (1) values of $\bar{\nu}$ for *sequences,* bands having the same value of Δv, are nearly constant but decrease slightly as v' and v'' increase; (2) values of $\bar{\nu}$ for *progressions from the upper state,* bands having the same value of v', decrease as v'' increases; and (3) values of $\bar{\nu}$ for *progressions to the lower state,* bands having the same value of v'', increase as v' increases. Once the correct assignments are made, (*14.12*) can be used to determine ω_e and $\omega_e x_e$ for each state by plotting the differences between the values of $\bar{\nu}$ for the various progressions against $2v+2$, giving ω_e as the intercept and $\omega_e x_e$ as the slope. The value of $\bar{\nu}_{00}$, for the $v'=0 \rightarrow v''=0$ transition, is usually calculated from

$$\bar{\nu}_{00} = \bar{\nu} - [(\omega_e' - \omega_e' x_e')v' - \omega_e' x_e'(v')^2] + [(\omega_e'' - \omega_e'' x_e'')v'' - \omega_e'' x_e''(v'')^2] \tag{14.25}$$

using several of the observed frequencies rather than relying on only one observed value.

EXAMPLE 14.5. Prepare a Deslandres table summarizing the (hypothetical) transitions shown in Fig. 14-2.

The table consists of entries of $\bar{\nu}$ corresponding to the values of v' and v'', see Table 14-1. Note that the three trends discussed above are present: (1) values of $\bar{\nu}$ along diagonals, which correspond to sequences (e.g. $0 \rightarrow 0$, $1 \rightarrow 1$, etc.), decrease as v' and v'' increase; (2) values of $\bar{\nu}$ in rows, which correspond to progressions from the upper state (e.g., $0 \rightarrow 0$, $0 \rightarrow 1$, $0 \rightarrow 2$, etc.), decrease as v'' increases; and (3) values

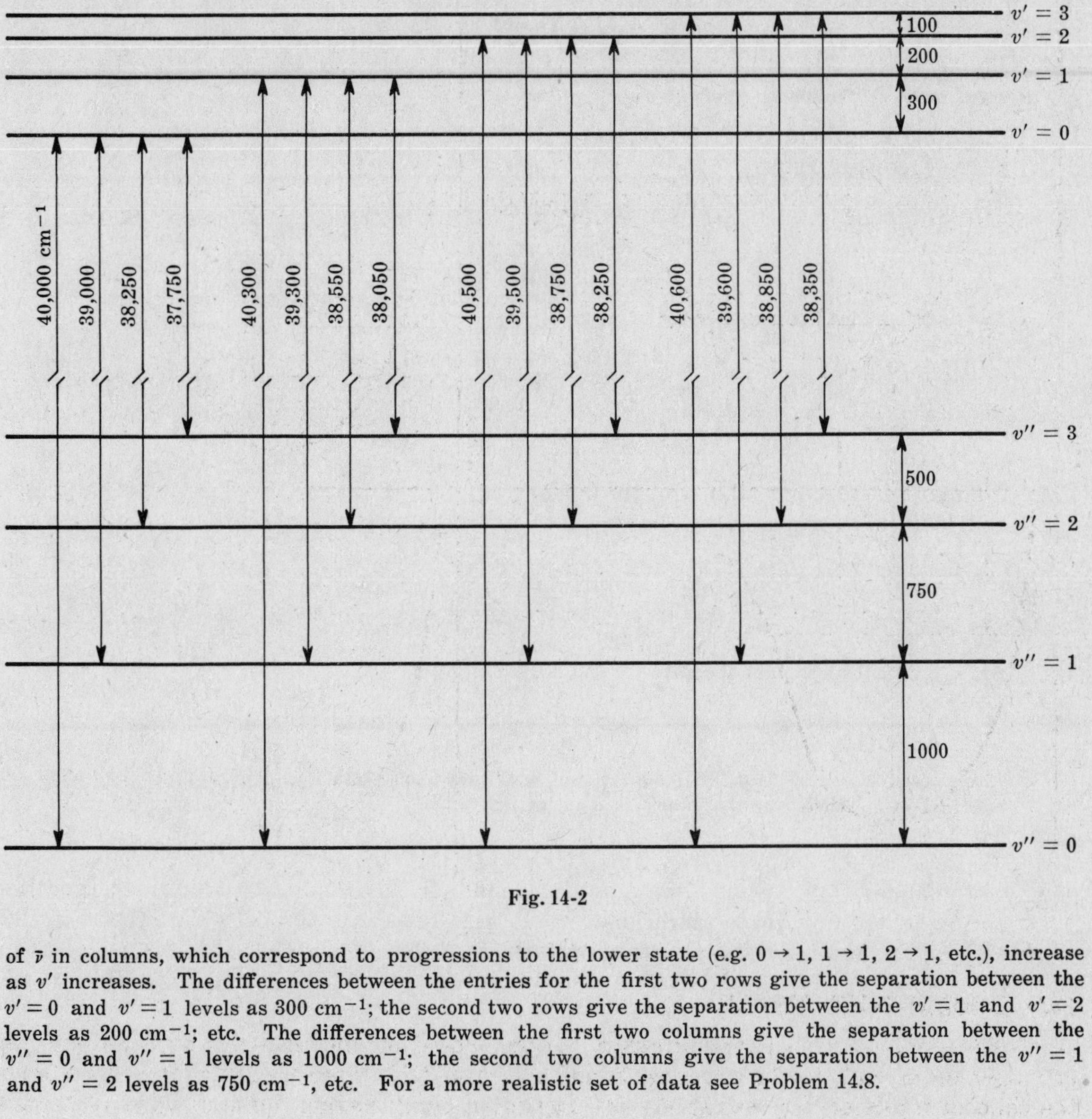

Fig. 14-2

of $\bar{\nu}$ in columns, which correspond to progressions to the lower state (e.g. $0 \to 1$, $1 \to 1$, $2 \to 1$, etc.), increase as v' increases. The differences between the entries for the first two rows give the separation between the $v' = 0$ and $v' = 1$ levels as 300 cm^{-1}; the second two rows give the separation between the $v' = 1$ and $v' = 2$ levels as 200 cm^{-1}; etc. The differences between the first two columns give the separation between the $v'' = 0$ and $v'' = 1$ levels as 1000 cm^{-1}; the second two columns give the separation between the $v'' = 1$ and $v'' = 2$ levels as 750 cm^{-1}, etc. For a more realistic set of data see Problem 14.8.

Table 14-1

Upper State, $v' =$	Lower State: $v'' = 0$		$v'' = 1$		$v'' = 2$		$v'' = 3$	Average separation in upper state
0	40000	1000	39000	750	38250	500	37750	
	300		300		300		300	300
1	40300	1000	39300	750	38550	500	38050	
	200		200		200		200	200
2	40500	1000	39500	750	38750	500	38250	
	100		100		100		100	100
3	40600	1000	39600	750	38850	500	38350	
Average separation in lower state		1000		750		500		

Solved Problems

Rotational and Vibrational Spectra

14.1. The bond length in CN^+ is 1.29 Å. Predict the position of the first four lines in the microwave spectrum.

Substituting $\mu = 1.0737 \times 10^{-26}$ kg, see Example 14.1, into (*14.4*) gives

$$B_e = \frac{2.7993 \times 10^{-46}}{(1.0737 \times 10^{-26})(1.29 \times 10^{-10})^2} = 1.567 \text{ cm}^{-1}$$

The first four lines as predicted by (*14.5*) are

$$\bar{\nu}_1 = 2(1.567 \text{ cm}^{-1})(1) = 3.133 \text{ cm}^{-1}$$

$\bar{\nu}_2 = 6.267 \text{ cm}^{-1}$, $\bar{\nu}_3 = 9.400 \text{ cm}^{-1}$ and $\bar{\nu}_4 = 12.534 \text{ cm}^{-1}$.

14.2. Compare the force constants for the bond strengths in CN and CN^+ if $\omega_e = 2068.61 \text{ cm}^{-1}$ and 1580 cm^{-1}, respectively. The reduced mass for both molecules is 1.0737×10^{-26} kg.

Upon rearrangement, (*14.9*) gives

$$k = \frac{\omega_e^2 \mu}{(5.3088 \times 10^{-12})^2}$$

which upon substitution of the data for the molecules gives

$$k_{CN} = \frac{(2068.61)^2(1.0737 \times 10^{-26})}{(5.3088 \times 10^{-12})^2} = 16.302 \times 10^2 \text{ N m}^{-1}$$

and $k_{CN^+} = 9.51 \times 10^2 \text{ N m}^{-1}$. There is one fewer bonding electron in CN^+ than in CN; thus the weaker bond predicted by the values of k is correct.

14.3. If the anharmonicity constant, $\omega_e x_e$, is 49 cm^{-1} for BH and $\omega_e = 2368 \text{ cm}^{-1}$, find the energy of the first three vibrational levels with respect to the bottom of the potential well and determine the separation between these levels.

Using (*14.11*) gives

$$G(0) = (2368)\left(0 + \frac{1}{2}\right) - (49)\left(0 + \frac{1}{2}\right)^2 = 1172 \text{ cm}^{-1}$$

$G(1) = 3442 \text{ cm}^{-1}$ and $G(2) = 5614 \text{ cm}^{-1}$. We then have for the separation between the $v = 0$ and $v = 1$ levels

$$\Delta G(0) = 3442 - 1172 = 2270 \text{ cm}^{-1}$$

and for the separation between the $v = 1$ and $v = 2$ levels, $\Delta G(1) = 2172 \text{ cm}^{-1}$.

14.4. The contributions of the harmonic oscillator, $G(v)$, and the rigid rotator, $F(J)$, are the largest terms in (*14.13*). For lack of complete data, $T(v, J)$ may be estimated fairly well by $T = G(v) + F(J)$. Compare values of T and $T(v, J)$ for $v = 0$, $J = 2$ and for $v = 1$, $J = 10$, if $\omega_e = 2068.1 \text{ cm}^{-1}$, $\omega_e x_e = 13.114 \text{ cm}^{-1}$, $B_e = 1.8989 \text{ cm}^{-1}$ and $\alpha_e = 0.0172 \text{ cm}^{-1}$.

Using (*14.13*) gives

$$T(0,2) = (2068.1)\left(0 + \frac{1}{2}\right) - (13.114)\left(0 + \frac{1}{2}\right)^2 + (1.8989)(2)(2+1)$$
$$+ 0 - (0.0172)\left(0 + \frac{1}{2}\right)(2)(2+1) = 1042.1 \text{ cm}^{-1}$$

while using *(14.3)* and *(14.8)*, which ignores the anharmonicity, rotational-vibrational coupling and centrifugal distortion, gives

$$T = (1.8989)(2)(2+1) + (2068.1)\left(0+\frac{1}{2}\right) = 1045.4\ \text{cm}^{-1}$$

which differs by 3.3 cm^{-1} or 0.32%. Similarly, $T(1, 10) = 3278.7\ \text{cm}^{-1}$ and $T = 3311.0\ \text{cm}^{-1}$, a difference of 32.3 cm^{-1} or 0.99%.

14.5. Using the Boltzmann distribution given in Problem 14.10, determine J_{max} as a function of temperature, where J_{max} is the quantum number of the most intensely populated rotational state. Using the data from Problem 14.1, find J_{max} for CN^+ at 298 K and 1000 K.

Substituting *(14.1)* into the expression for N_J found in Problem 14.10 gives

$$N_J = (2J+1)N_0 e^{-B^*J(J+1)/kT}$$

For a maximum (treating J as a continuous variable):

$$\frac{\partial N_J}{\partial J} = 2N_0 e^{-B^*J(J+1)/kT} + (2J+1)N_0\left(\frac{-B^*}{kT}\right)(2J+1)e^{-B^*J(J+1)/kT} = 0$$

Solving for J_{max} gives

$$J_{\text{max}} = \frac{(2kT/B^*)^{1/2} - 1}{2}$$

where the right-hand side is to be rounded off to the nearest integral value.

In terms of B_e, the above result becomes

$$J_{\text{max}} = \frac{(2kT/10^2 B_e hc)^{1/2} - 1}{2}$$

which upon substitution of the data for CN^+ gives

$$J_{\text{max}} = \frac{1}{2}\left\{\left[\frac{2(1.3807\times10^{-23}\ \text{J K}^{-1})T}{(10^2\ \text{cm m}^{-1})(1.566\ \text{cm}^{-1})(6.626\times10^{-34}\ \text{J s})(2.9979\times10^{8}\ \text{m s}^{-1})}\right]^{1/2} - 1\right\}$$

$$= \frac{(0.8877\,T)^{1/2} - 1}{2}$$

At 298 K, J_{max} is 8 and at 1000 K the value is 14.

Electronic Spectra

14.6. Consider the interacting electronic states shown in Fig. 14-1(*b*). Will the $v=0 \rightarrow 0$, $v=0 \rightarrow 1$ and $v=0 \rightarrow 2$ absorptions be observed?

Because the values of $\psi^*\psi$ are large, large and small, respectively, these transitions will be strong, strong and very weak, respectively.

14.7. What will happen if the transition between b'' and c' in Fig. 14-1(*a*) takes place?

Because the upper state c' is above D_e, the molecule will dissociate.

14.8. Using the following wavelengths (in Å) obtained by Tilford and Simmons for the $^1\Pi \rightarrow {}^1\Sigma^+$ electronic transition of $^{12}C^{16}O$, determine ω_e and $\omega_e x_e$ for both states and find $\bar{\nu}_{00}$: 1115.10, 1130.34, 1139.69, 1161.15, 1173.15, 1185.99, 1199.67, 1214.21, 1216.91, 1229.65, 1246.04, 1246.65, 1262.93, 1263.41, 1280.22, 1281.83, 1298.56, 1301.37, 1318.03, 1322.10, 1338.74, 1344.13, 1360.66, 1367.56, 1384.00, 1392.46, 1408.85, 1418.97, 1435.29, 1447.26, 1463.47, 1477.46, 1493.58, 1509.65, 1525.76, 1544.31, 1560.21 and 1597.16.

The wave numbers (in cm^{-1}) corresponding to the data are, by *(11.2)*, 89677.7, 88469.3, 87743.2, 86121.1, 85240.3, 84318.0, 83356.2, 82357.9, 82175.3, 81324.0, 80215.0, 80254.5, 79181.0, 79150.9, 78111.6, 78013.3, 77008.4, 76842.2, 75870.8, 75637.1, 74697.1, 74397.3, 73493.7, 73122.8, 72254.3, 71815.5, 70979.9, 70473.3, 69672.3, 69095.9, 68330.7, 67683.9, 66953.2, 66240.6, 65541.1, 64754.0, 64093.9 and 62611.1. If the lower-energy data are analyzed by taking differences, values near 2140 and 1500 cm^{-1} appear several times, and a similar analysis of the high-energy data gives values near 2140 and 1000 cm^{-1}. Assuming the 2140 cm^{-1} value to correspond to the $v''=1 \rightarrow v''=0$ change (because it appears in both the high- and low-energy emissions) and the 1500 to 1000 cm^{-1} values to correspond to changes in v' (which decrease as v' increases), the Deslandres table, Table 14-2, can be constructed.

To find ω_e and $\omega_e x_e$ for the $^1\Pi$ state, values of the average energy difference between the v'-states were plotted against $2(v+1)$, see Fig. 14.3. Equation *(14.12)* indicates that the intercept of this line is $\omega_e' = 1516$ cm^{-1} and the slope is $\omega_e' x_e' = 17.3$ cm^{-1}. Using the value of the $0 \rightarrow 0$ assigned transition as $\bar{\nu}_{00}$ gives $\bar{\nu}_{00} = 64754.0$ cm^{-1}. Because only one $\Delta G(v'')$ was obtained, ω_e'' and $\omega_e'' x_e''$ cannot be determined, but for $v''=0$, *(14.12)* indicates that ω_e'' should be about 2143 cm^{-1} if $\omega_e'' x_e''$ is not too large.

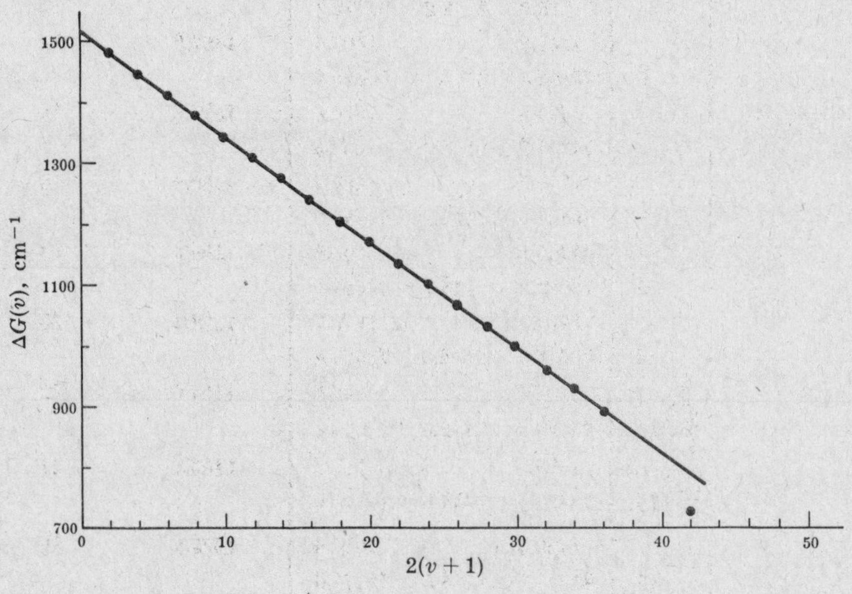

Fig. 14-3

Supplementary Problems

Rotational and Vibrational Spectra

14.9. If it is assumed that $r_{ab} = 1.275$ Å for $H^{35}Cl$, $D^{35}Cl$, $H^{37}Cl$ and $D^{37}Cl$, what will be the respective spacings for the rotational spectra? Assume atomic weights of 1.007825, 2.0140, 34.96885 and 36.959 for H, D, ^{35}Cl and ^{37}Cl, respectively. The change in the spacings of the rotational lines resulting from isotopic substitution is known as the *isotopic shift effect.* In which spectra will this effect be greater: (*a*) $H^{35}Cl$ with $H^{37}Cl$ or $D^{35}Cl$ with $D^{37}Cl$ and (*b*) $H^{35}Cl$ with $D^{35}Cl$ or $H^{37}Cl$ with $D^{37}Cl$?

Ans. (*a*) HCl change is 0.028 cm^{-1}, DCl change is 0.032 cm^{-1}; greater effect in $D^{35}Cl$ with $D^{37}Cl$;
(*b*) Both changes are 10.280 cm^{-1}; same effect.

14.10. The Boltzmann distribution, see *(6.18)*, describing the population of the various rotational states is

$$N_J/N_0 = (g_J e^{-E_J/kT})/(g_0 e^{-E_0/kT})$$

Table 14-2

Upper State $v' =$	Lower State $v'' = 0$		$v'' = 1$	Average separation in upper state	$2(v'+1)$
0	64754.0	2142.9	62611.1		
	1486.6		1482.8	1484.7	2
1	66240.6	2146.7	64093.9		
	1443.3		1447.2	1445.3	4
2	67683.9	2142.8	65541.1		
	1412.0		1412.1	1412.1	6
3	69095.9	2142.7	66953.2		
	1377.8		1377.5	1377.7	8
4	70473.7	2143.0	68330.7		
	1341.8		1341.6	1341.7	10
5	71815.5	2143.2	69672.3		
	1307.3		1307.6	1307.5	12
6	73122.8	2142.9	70979.9		
	1274.5		1274.4	1274.5	14
7	74397.3	2143.0	72254.3		
	1239.8		1239.4	1239.6	16
8	75637.1	2143.4	73493.7		
	1205.1		1203.4	1204.3	18
9	76842.2	2145.1	74697.1		
	1171.1		1173.7	1172.4	20
10	78013.3	2142.5	75870.8		
	1137.6		1137.6	1137.6	22
11	79150.9	2142.5	77008.4		
	1103.6		1103.2	1103.4	24
12	80254.5	2142.9	78111.6		
	1069.5		1069.4	1069.5	26
13	81324.0	2143.0	79181.0		
	1033.9		1034.0	1034.0	28
14	82357.9	2142.9	80215.0		
	998.3			998.3	30
15	83356.2				
	961.8			961.8	32
16	84318.0	2142.7	82175.3		
	922.3			922.3	34
17	85240.3				
	880.8			880.8	36
18	86121.1				
19					
20	87743.2				
	726.1			726.1	42
21	88469.3				
22					
23	89677.7				

Average separation in lower state 2143.3

where g_J and g_0 are the degeneracies of the levels.

(a) Show that

$$N_J = (2J+1)N_0 e^{-E_J/kT}$$

(b) If $N_0 = 100$, find N_J for $J = 1$ to $J = 15$ at 25 °C for $D^{35}Cl$, if $I = 5.08 \times 10^{-47}$ kg m^2.

(c) The intensity of a peak for a given transition is proportional to the number of molecules in that state. Calculate the theoretical relative intensities of the first 15 peaks by dividing N_J by the maximum value of N_J.

(d) Compare the theoretical values to the experimental values calculated from observed intensities of 55, 66, 73, 75, 75, 73, 70, 64, 58, 49, 40, 31, 24, 18, 11, and 7 by dividing the observed intensity by the maximum observed intensity.

Ans. (b) $E_J = 1.095 \times 10^{-22} J(J+1)$ joule;
$N_J = 100, 285, 426, 508, 530, 494, 426, 338, 250, 173, 113, 69, 39, 22, 10, 5.$

(c) 0.19, 0.54, 0.80, 0.96, 1, 0.93, 0.80, 0.64, 0.47, 0.33, 0.21, 0.13, 0.07, 0.04, 0.02, 0.01.

(d) 0.73, 0.88, 0.97, 1, 1, 0.97, 0.93, 0.85, 0.77, 0.65, 0.53, 0.41, 0.32, 0.24, 0.15, 0.09; same general shape with same maximum peaks, theoretical drops off faster from the maximum than does the experimental.

14.11. Compare the force constants for the bond strengths in $H^{35}Cl$ and $D^{35}Cl$ if $\omega_e = 2888$ cm^{-1} and 2092 cm^{-1}, respectively. The reduced masses for these molecules are 1.6266×10^{-27} kg and 3.1622×10^{-27} kg, respectively.

Ans. 4.81×10^2 N m^{-1} and 4.91×10^2 N m^{-1}; essentially the same

14.12. What is the energy separation between the 23rd and 24th vibrational levels for BH, assuming the system to be described by (a) the anharmonic oscillator model (see Problem 14.3 for pertinent data)? (b) the harmonic oscillator model? *Ans.* (a) 16 cm^{-1}, (b) 2368 cm^{-1}

14.13. The *Morse potential,* given by

$$V(r) = D_e[1 - e^{-a(r-r_e)}]^2$$

generates the first two terms of (*14.11*) if

$$\omega_e = 10^{-1} a \left(\frac{\hbar D_e}{\pi c \mu} \right)^{1/2} \qquad \omega_e x_e = 10^{-2} \frac{\hbar a^2}{4\pi c \mu}$$

Here, D_e, ω_e and $\omega_e x_e$ are in cm^{-1}, while the other quantities are in normal SI units. If $r_e = 0.7417$ Å, $D_e = 38{,}318$ cm^{-1}, $\omega_e = 4405.3$ cm^{-1} and $\omega_e x_e = 125.325$ cm^{-1} for H_2, plot $U(r) \equiv V(r) - D_e$ against r, showing the first eleven vibrational levels.

Ans. potential well like solid curve in Fig. 13-3, with minimum at 0.7417 Å and −38,318 cm^{-1}; vibrational lines at −36,147, −31,922, −28,088, −24,435, −21,032, −17,880, −14,979, −12,328, −9928, −7778, −5879 cm^{-1}

14.14. The ground state for NO is $^2\Pi$. (a) In addition to the P and R branches of the infrared spectrum, what else will be observed? (b) If $B_e' = B_e''$ for the molecule, describe the spectrum.

Ans. (a) Q branch will be present. (b) (*14.20*) suggests that the R-branch lines get closer together as J increases and the P-branch lines get farther apart as J increases; (*14.21*) suggests that the Q branch is one line at $\bar{\nu}_0$.

14.15. What will be the separation of the lines for $J = 10$ in the P and R branches of HN if the spectroscopic data are $\omega_e = 3315$ cm^{-1}, $\omega_e x_e = 94.7$ cm^{-1}, $B_e = 16.6684$ cm^{-1} and $\alpha_e = 0.646$ cm^{-1}?

Ans. $m = -10$ for P branch giving $\Delta\bar{\nu} = 44.32$ cm^{-1};
$m = 11$ for R branch giving $\Delta\bar{\nu} = 17.19$ cm^{-1}

14.16. The high-resolution infrared spectrum of $D^{35}Cl$ shows the following fine structure: 2244.7, 2238.7, 2232.0, 2225.2, 2218.5, 2211.0, 2203.5, 2195.5, 2187.2, 2179.0, 2170.2, 2161.5, 2152.5, 2143.0, 2133.2, 2123.2, 2113.2, 2103.0, 2081.5, 2070.2, 2059.2, 2047.7, 2035.7, 2024.0, 2012.0, 1997.2, 1985.0, 1972.2, 1959.7, 1946.7, 1933.2, 1920.2, 1906.5, 1892.7, 1879.0, and 1864.2 cm^{-1}. Assign values of m to these lines. Prepare a plot of $\Delta\bar{\nu}$ against m as suggested by (*14.20*) to obtain α_e and B_e. Use (*14.19*) for values of m from -5 to $+5$ to determine an average value of $\bar{\nu}_0$. If $\mu = 3.1622 \times 10^{-27}$ kg, find r_e.

Ans. $\alpha_e = 0.121\ cm^{-1}$, $B_e = 5.46\ cm^{-1}$, $\bar{\nu}_0 = 2092.3\ cm^{-1}$, $r_e = 1.274$ Å

14.17. If $B_e' = B_e'' = B_e$, where will the first lines of the O and S branches be located with respect to $\bar{\nu}_0$?

Ans. The first line of the O branch is $J = 2$, which is $-6B_e$ from $\bar{\nu}_0$, and the first line of the S branch is $J = 0$, which is $6B_e$ from $\bar{\nu}_0$.

14.18. Assume that the rotational spectrum is described by

$$F(J) = B_e J(J+1) - \bar{D}_e J^2(J+1)^2$$

where the $\bar{D}_e$-term corrects for a centrifugal distortion effect. Show that

$$\bar{\nu} = 2B_e J - 4\bar{D}_e J^3$$

If $\bar{D}_e = 10^{-4}B_e$ and $J = 4$, find $\bar{\nu}$ for CN^+ using the data in Problem 14.1.

Ans. 12.488 cm^{-1}

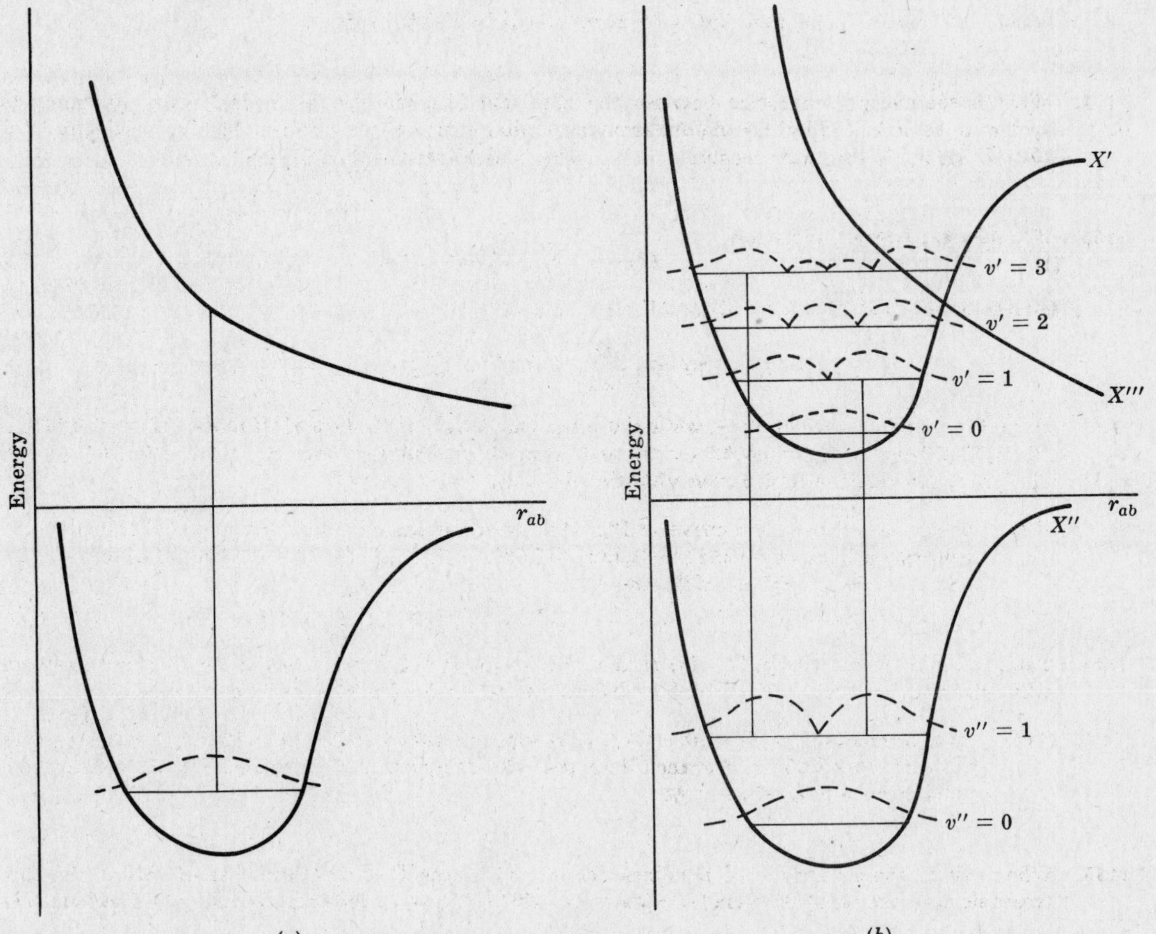

Fig. 14-4

14.19. If the electronic potential-energy well is approximated by an empirical function $V(r)$, then the values for ω_e and $\omega_e x_e$ in (*14.11*) can be determined from (*14.9*) with

$$k = 10^2 hcV''(r_e)$$

and from

$$\omega_e x_e = \frac{1}{24}\left\{5\left[\frac{V'''(r_e)}{V''(r_e)}\right]^2 - 3\,\frac{V^{(\mathrm{iv})}(r_e)}{V''(r_e)}\right\}\frac{10^{-2}\hbar}{4\pi c\mu}$$

where $V'(r) = dV(r)/dr$, etc. Show that the expressions for ω_e and $\omega_e x_e$ given in Problem 14.13 indeed follow from the Morse potential.

Ans. $V^{(n)}(r) = 2a^n D_e(-1)^{n-1}[e^{-a(r-r_e)} - 2^{n-1}e^{-2a(r-r_e)}]$

Electronic Spectra

14.20. (*a*) Describe the absorption spectrum for the system shown in Fig. 14-4(*a*). (*b*) Describe the spectrum for the system shown in Fig. 14-4(*b*) for $v'' = 1$ to $v' = 0, 1, 2$. (*c*) Describe the spectrum for the system shown in Fig. 14-4(*b*) for $v'' = 1$ to $v' = 3$.

Ans. (*a*) no bands (continuum); (*b*) normal bands; (*c*) continuum if crossing over to X''' occurs

14.21. Using the following data reported by Tilford and Simmons for the $^1\Pi \rightarrow {}^1\Sigma^+$ electronic transition of $^{13}C^{16}O$, determine ω_e' and $\omega_e'x_e'$: 1478.68, 1449.05, 1421.25, 1395.15, 1370.61, 1347.51, 1325.76, 1305.25, 1285.95, 1267.64, 1250.40, 1234.12, 1218.74, 1204.24, and 1190.57 Å. All data are for a $v'' = 0$ progression, and the $v' = 1$ and $v' = 0$ lines are not resolvable from the spectrum of $^{12}C^{16}O$.

Ans. 1418 cm^{-1}, 15.8 cm^{-1}

14.22. The following bands were observed as part of the discharge spectrum of N_2: 31678.65, 29698.27, 28600.03, 28270.95, 27991.60, 26959.99, 26638.25, 26297.10, 25700.99, 25361.40, 25028.16 and 24642.07 cm^{-1}. Assign these bands in sequences between v' and v'', prepare a Deslandres table, determine the average vibrational level separation in each state, find ω_e and $\omega_e x_e$ for both states, and calculate $\bar{\nu}_{00}$.

Ans. Band assignments are $v' \rightarrow v''$ as follows: $1 \rightarrow 0$, $0 \rightarrow 0$, $2 \rightarrow 3$, $1 \rightarrow 2$, $0 \rightarrow 1$, $2 \rightarrow 4$, $1 \rightarrow 3$, $0 \rightarrow 2$, $3 \rightarrow 6$, $2 \rightarrow 5$, $1 \rightarrow 4$, $0 \rightarrow 3$. Separations are: $v' = 0$ to 1, 1983.47; $v' = 1$ to 2, 1946.81 cm^{-1}; $v'' = 0$ to 1, 1706.67; $v'' = 1$ to 2, 1694.50; $v'' = 2$ to 3, 1643.87; $v'' = 3$ to 4, 1625.07; and $v'' = 4$ to 5, 1598.59 cm^{-1}. Plots of $\Delta\bar{\nu}$ against $2(v+1)$ give intercepts $\omega_e' = 2020.13$ and $\omega_e'' = 1739$ cm^{-1} and slopes $\omega_e'x_e' = 18.33$ and $\omega_e''x_e'' = 14.2$ cm^{-1}. Average value of $\bar{\nu}_{00}$ is 29676.6 cm^{-1}.

Chapter 15

Electronic Structure of Polyatomic Molecules

Hybridization

15.1 ANGULAR WAVE FUNCTIONS

The concept of localized bonds around an atom in its ground electronic state, as presented for diatomic molecules, often fails to predict the correct formula or geometrical structure for a polyatomic molecule. This difficulty can be overcome by assuming localized bonds to be formed between atoms that have been excited to the extent of allowing the partially filled and unfilled atomic orbitals to mix to form the proper number of *hybrid atomic orbitals* having the correct geometrical arrangement.

Although various combinations of *s*, *p*, *d*, etc., wave functions could be used to construct the wave functions for the hybrid orbitals, only the *s* and *p* angular wave functions are necessary to describe most bonding between the representative elements. These functions are given by (*12.4*), (*12.5*) and (*11.49*) as

$$Y_s = \left(\frac{1}{4\pi}\right)^{1/2}, \quad Y_{p_z} = \left(\frac{3}{4\pi}\right)^{1/2} \cos\theta, \quad Y_{p_x} = \left(\frac{3}{4\pi}\right)^{1/2} \sin\theta\cos\phi, \quad Y_{p_y} = \left(\frac{3}{4\pi}\right)^{1/2} \sin\theta\sin\phi$$

The angular part of the ith hybrid orbital is then expressed as

$$X_i = a_i Y_s + b_i Y_{p_z} + c_i Y_{p_x} + d_i Y_{p_y} \tag{15.1}$$

where, by requirements of normalization and orthogonality,

$$a_i^2 + b_i^2 + c_i^2 + d_i^2 = 1 \tag{15.2a}$$

$$a_i a_j + b_i b_j + c_i c_j + d_i d_j = 0 \quad (i \neq j) \tag{15.2b}$$

Additional restraints on the coefficients are determined by the amounts of s and p "character" desired in the hybrid orbital; e.g. $a_i^2 = b_i^2$ for sp, etc.

EXAMPLE 15.1. The bond angles between hydrogens in H_2O, H_2S, H_2Se and H_2Te are 104.45°, 92.2°, 91.0° and 89.5°, respectively. What can be said about the importance of sp^3 hybridization, which predicts bonding angles of 109°28′, in describing all these molecules?

The importance decreases as the period number increases. The concept of hybridization approaches the notion of localized bonds around atoms in the ground states as the period number increases.

EXAMPLE 15.2. Give a molecular orbital description for NH_x.

The molecular orbital diagram in Fig. 15-1(*a*) predicts that three equivalent N—H bonds will be formed between the $2p$ atomic orbitals on the N and the $1s$ atomic orbitals on the H's. Even though the correct formula is predicted, these bonds would form H—N—H angles of 90°, which does not agree with the experimental value of 106.67°.

The molecular orbital diagram in Fig 15-1(*b*) shows the N atom undergoing sp^3 hybridization before interacting with H atomic orbitals. Again three equivalent N—H bonds will be formed, but the H—N—H bond angles will be predicted as 109°28′ (see Problem 15.2), which agrees with the experimental value fairly well.

In diagrams like Fig. 15-1 the notation $n(\ )$ is used for nonbonding atomic orbitals.

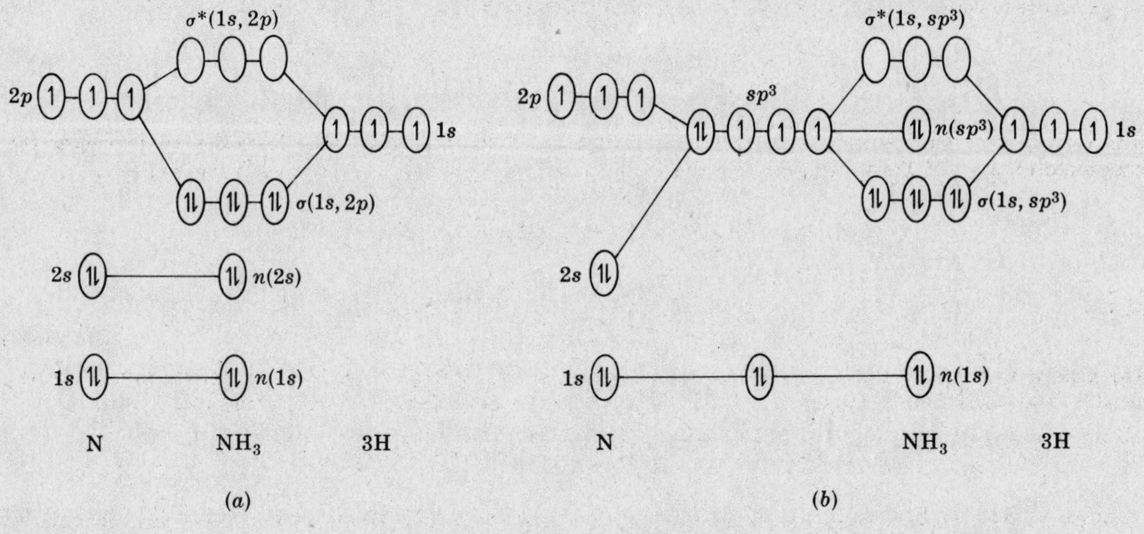

Fig. 15-1

15.2 RELATIVE BOND STRENGTH

The *relative bond strength*, rbs, of an orbital can be defined as

$$\text{rbs} \equiv \frac{\max X_i}{Y_s} = \frac{\max X_i}{(1/4\pi)^{1/2}} \tag{15.3}$$

where the numerator is the maximum value of X_i for that orbital. For an unmixed s atomic orbital, $X_i = Y_s$ and rbs = 1.

EXAMPLE 15.3. Determine the angular wave functions describing sp hybridization. Determine the relative bond strengths of these wave functions and the angle between the orbitals. Assume the bonding axis to be the x-axis, i.e. contributions from p_y and p_z need not be considered.

From *(15.1)*,

$$X_1 = a_1 Y_s + b_1 Y_{p_x} = a_1\left(\frac{1}{4\pi}\right)^{1/2} + b_1\left(\frac{3}{4\pi}\right)^{1/2} \sin\theta\cos\phi$$

For sp hybridization, the ratio of "p character" to "s character" must be unity; thus

$$\frac{\langle b_1 Y_{p_x} \mid b_1 Y_{p_x}\rangle}{\langle a_1 Y_s \mid a_1 Y_s\rangle} = \frac{b_1^2\langle Y_{p_x} \mid Y_{p_x}\rangle}{a_1^2\langle Y_s \mid Y_s\rangle} = \frac{b_1^2}{a_1^2} = 1$$

or $a_1^2 = b_1^2$. A second relation between a_1 and b_1 is given by *(15.2a)* as

$$a_1^2 + b_1^2 = 1$$

Solving simultaneously gives $a_1 = \pm 2^{-1/2}$ and $b_1 = \pm 2^{-1/2}$. The positive value for a_1 is always chosen when determining the maximum value for X_1. The expression for X_1 becomes

$$X_1 = \left(\frac{1}{8\pi}\right)^{1/2}(1 \pm 3^{1/2}\sin\theta\cos\phi)$$

By inspection, the maximum value of X_1 occurs at $\theta = 90°$ and $\phi = 0°$ (along the positive x-axis) if the plus sign is chosen or at $\theta = 90°$ and $\phi = 180°$ (along the negative x-axis) if the minus sign is chosen. Equation (*15.3*) then gives

$$\text{rbs} = \frac{(1/8\pi)^{1/2}[1 \pm 3^{1/2}(1)(\pm 1)]}{(1/4\pi)^{1/2}} = 1.932$$

The coefficients for X_2 are found in a similar manner using

$$\frac{\langle b_2 Y_{p_x} \mid b_2 Y_{p_x}\rangle}{\langle a_2 Y_s \mid a_2 Y_s\rangle} = \frac{b_2^2}{a_2^2} = 1 \qquad a_2^2 + b_2^2 = 1$$

which give $a_2 = \pm 2^{-1/2}$ and $b_2 = \pm 2^{-1/2}$. Similarly, the positive value of a_2 is chosen to determine the maximum of X_2, but the value of b_2 for these choices of a_1, a_2 and b_1 is restricted by (*15.2b*) as

$$b_2 = -\frac{a_1 a_2}{b_1} = -\frac{(2^{-1/2})(2^{-1/2})}{\pm 2^{-1/2}} = \mp 2^{-1/2}$$

giving

$$X_2 = \left(\frac{1}{8\pi}\right)^{1/2}(1 \mp 3^{1/2}\sin\theta\cos\phi)$$

The maximum for X_2 occurs at $\theta = 90°$ and $\phi = 180°$ (along the negative x-axis) if the minus sign is chosen, or at $\theta = 90°$ and $\phi = 0°$ (along the positive x-axis) if the plus sign is chosen. Hence

$$\text{rbs} = \frac{(1/8\pi)^{1/2}[1 \mp 3^{1/2}(1)(\mp 1)]}{(1/4\pi)^{1/2}} = 1.932$$

The identity $\cos(\phi + 180°) = -\cos\phi$ shows that X_1 and X_2 are identical wave functions 180° apart. Usually X_1 is written using only the positive sign between the terms and X_2 using the negative sign.

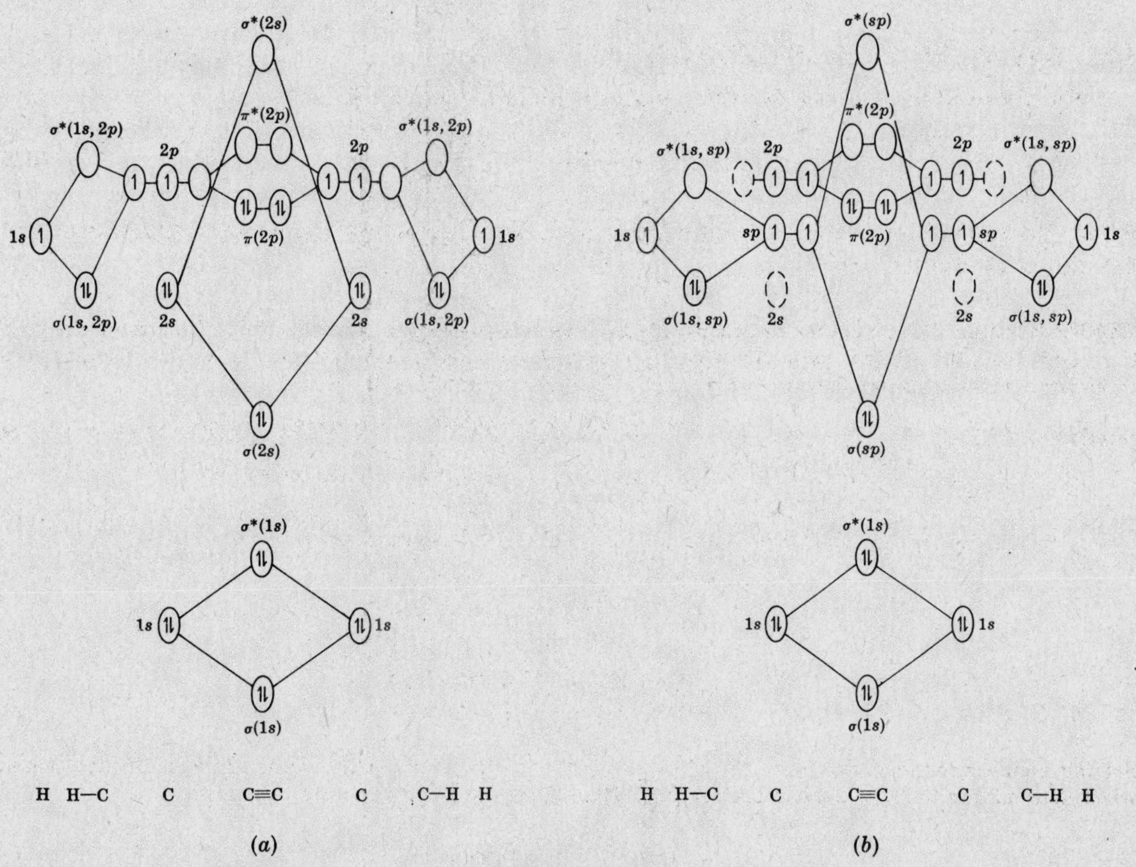

Fig. 15-2

Localized Multiple Bonds

The molecular orbital theory predicts that for every two atomic orbitals used, two molecular orbitals will be generated. For head-on overlap these are σ and σ^* orbitals; for parallel overlap, they are π and π^* orbitals. See Fig. 13-5.

EXAMPLE 15.4. Prepare a molecular orbital energy diagram similar to Fig. 15-1 representing the bonding in C_2H_2 and predict the types of electronic transitions that could occur.

The molecular orbitals shown in Fig. 15-2(*a*) are generated by using carbon atoms in their ground state and hydrogen atoms. If the carbon atoms are assumed to be *sp*-hybridized, the molecular orbitals shown in Fig. 15-2(*b*) are formed. The dashed circles in Fig. 15-2(*b*) represent the original carbon orbitals used in hybridization. The hybridization steps in the diagram, see Fig. 15-1(*b*), have been omitted for clarity.

Both diagrams predict a $\sigma^2\pi^4$ configuration for the triple bond. The two lowest electronic transitions that can take place will be from the uppermost filled orbital, π, to the nearest unfilled orbitals, π^* and σ^*, giving the predicted spectrum as $\pi \to \pi^*$ and $\pi \to \sigma^*$ (weak). The $\sigma \to \sigma^*$ transitions for the C—H bonds could also be observed (weak). Both diagrams predict a linear molecule.

Conjugated Bonds

15.3 CHAIN MOLECULES

For conjugated chain molecules the *free-electron molecular orbital treatment* (FEMO) assumes the π electrons to be moving in a one-dimensional box, see Examples 11.4 and 11.7. No more than two electrons are allowed in a molecular orbital, whose energy is given by (*11.19*), so in the ground state the π electrons fill the lowest $n_\pi/2$ orbitals, where n_π is the number of π electrons. For this simple theory it can be shown that the transition from the highest occupied to the lowest vacant molecular orbital has an energy given (in cm^{-1}) by

$$\bar{\nu} = \frac{h(n_\pi + 1)}{8m_e c a^2} \tag{15.4}$$

where a is the length of the carbon chain. Better agreement between (*15.4*) and experiment is realized if a is defined as the zigzag distance along the carbon chain and allowance is made for the molecular orbitals to extend past the end carbons. This gives

$$\bar{\nu} = \frac{153{,}000\ \text{cm}^{-1}}{n_c + 1} \tag{15.5}$$

where $n_\pi = n_c$, the number of conjugated carbon atoms in the chain. An improved FEMO theory uses a sinusoidal potential-energy function with a minimum at the center of each double bond, giving

$$\bar{\nu} = \frac{153{,}000\ \text{cm}^{-1}}{n_c + 1} + (16{,}000\ \text{cm}^{-1})\left(1 - \frac{1}{n_c}\right) \tag{15.6}$$

For polymethine ions having the formula

$$R\overset{+}{\text{N}}{=}\text{CH}(\text{—CH}{=}\text{CH})_k\text{—}\ddot{\text{N}}R$$

(*15.4*) can be shown to give

$$\bar{\nu} = \frac{(2k+5)(155{,}000\ \text{cm}^{-1})}{(2k+4)^2} \tag{15.7}$$

The *Hückel molecular orbital method*, HMO, assumes that the π-bonding for n_c conjugated carbons is described by a secular equation of the form

$$\begin{vmatrix} x & 1 & 0 & 0 & \ldots & 0 & 0 & 0 \\ 1 & x & 1 & 0 & \ldots & 0 & 0 & 0 \\ 0 & 1 & x & 1 & \ldots & 0 & 0 & 0 \\ \vdots & & & & & & & \vdots \\ 0 & 0 & 0 & 0 & \ldots & 1 & x & 1 \\ 0 & 0 & 0 & 0 & \ldots & 0 & 1 & x \end{vmatrix} = 0 \tag{15.8}$$

The determinant has n_c rows and columns, and

$$x = \frac{\alpha - E}{\beta} \tag{15.9}$$

In obtaining (*15.8*) from (*11.28*) it is assumed that the overlap integrals are $S_{jj} = 1$ and $S_{jk} = 0$; the coulombic integrals are $H_{jj} = \alpha$; and the resonance integrals are, for atoms bonded together, $H_{jk} = \beta$, and for nonbonded atoms, $H_{jk} = 0$. The solution to (*15.8*) is

$$x = -2\cos\left(\frac{j\pi}{n_c + 1}\right) \tag{15.10}$$

where $j = 1, 2, \ldots, n_c$, and from (*15.9*)

$$E_j = \alpha + 2\beta\cos\left(\frac{j\pi}{n_c + 1}\right) \tag{15.11}$$

Because β is negative, E_1 will be the lowest energy level and the predicted absorption will be at

$$\bar{\nu} = \frac{-4\beta}{kc}\sin\left(\frac{\pi}{2n_c + 2}\right) \tag{15.12}$$

where k has the same significance as in (*15.7*).

EXAMPLE 15.5. Calculate the energy levels for the conjugated bonding in 1,3-butadiene. Prepare an energy diagram showing the ground and first excited states.

Using (*15.11*) with $n_c = 4$ gives

$$\begin{aligned} E_1 &= \alpha + 2\beta\cos\frac{\pi}{5} \\ &= \alpha + 2\beta\cos 36^\circ \\ &= \alpha + 1.618\,\beta \\ E_2 &= \alpha + 2\beta\cos 72^\circ \\ &= \alpha + 0.618\,\beta \\ E_3 &= \alpha - 0.618\,\beta \\ E_4 &= \alpha - 1.618\,\beta \end{aligned}$$

If the midline of Fig. 15-3 is α, then E_1 and E_2 lie below α, and E_3 and E_4 lie above. In the ground state the four electrons occupy the lowest two orbitals, see Fig. 15-3(a), and one electron is promoted to E_3 for the first excited state, see Fig. 15-3(b).

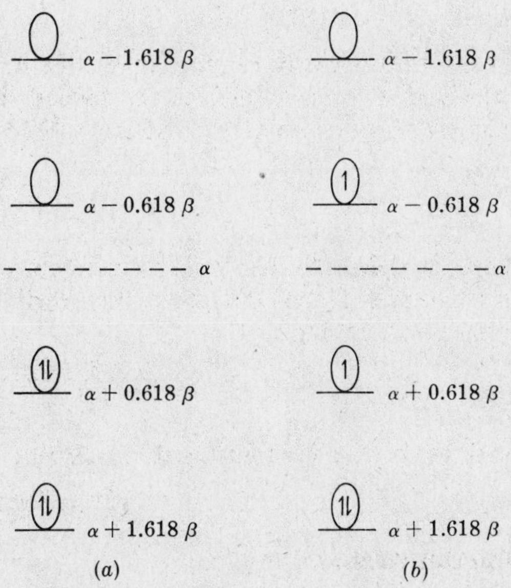

Fig. 15-3

15.4 CYCLIC MOLECULES

The FEMO theory for a cyclic molecule assumes the π electrons to have energies given by

$$E_n = \frac{h^2 n^2}{2m_e a^2} \tag{15.13}$$

where a is the circumference of a circle drawn through the conjugated nuclei and $n = 0, \pm 1, \pm 2, \ldots$. Note that the energy levels above the ground state are doubly degenerate.

The HMO theory for a cyclic conjugated molecule uses a secular equation of the form

$$\begin{vmatrix} x & 1 & 0 & 0 & \ldots & 0 & 0 & 1 \\ 1 & x & 1 & 0 & \ldots & 0 & 0 & 0 \\ 0 & 1 & x & 1 & \ldots & 0 & 0 & 0 \\ \vdots & & & & & & & \vdots \\ 0 & 0 & 0 & 0 & \ldots & 1 & x & 1 \\ 1 & 0 & 0 & 0 & \ldots & 0 & 1 & x \end{vmatrix} = 0 \tag{15.14}$$

whose solutions are

$$E_k = \alpha + 2\beta \cos\left(\frac{2\pi k}{n_c}\right) \tag{15.15}$$

where $k = 0, 1, 2, \ldots, n_c - 1$. Because of the cyclic nature of the cosine term, values of E_k as given by (*15.15*) may be degenerate. A mnemonic device is available to determine the energies of the HMO's for C_nH_n. A vertex of the regular polygon of $n = n_c$ sides inscribed in a circle of radius 2β is placed at the bottom of the sketch and an energy state drawn beside it. Additional energy states are drawn corresponding to the other corners of the polygon, creating n energy states. The value of α in the diagram corresponds to the center of the polygon and the value of $\alpha + 2\beta$ corresponds to the lowest energy level.

To have the extra stability associated with aromatic compounds, the number of π electrons must be

$$n_\pi = 4m + 2 \tag{15.16}$$

where $m = 0, 1, 2, 3, \ldots$. If $n_\pi = 4m \pm 1$, the compound is a free radical with a singlet ground state and if $n_\pi = 4m$, the compound is a diradical with a triplet ground state.

15.5 BOND ORDER AND LENGTH

The *total bond order* between two atoms, r and s, including a bond order of 1 for the σ bond, is given by

$$P_{rs} = 1 + p_{rs} \tag{15.17}$$

where the *π-electron bond order*, p_{rs}, is given by

$$p_{rs} = \sum_j \frac{n_j}{2}(C_{jr}^* C_{js} + C_{js}^* C_{jr}) \tag{15.18}$$

where n_j represents the number of electrons in the jth orbital and the sum is over all the π-molecular orbitals. The values of C_{jr} are determined from

$$C_{jr} = \left(\frac{2}{n_c + 1}\right)^{1/2} \sin\left(\frac{jr\pi}{n_c + 1}\right) \tag{15.19a}$$

for chain molecules and from

$$C_{jr} = \left(\frac{1}{n_c}\right)^{1/2} e^{i2\pi jr/n_c} \tag{15.19b}$$

for cyclic molecules. The bond length in Å is given by

$$r_{rs} = 1.707 - 0.186\, P_{rs} \tag{15.20}$$

Coordination Compounds

15.6 VALENCE BOND THEORY

The *valence bond theory* assumes the formation of coordinate-covalent bonds between the ligands and the central atom, with the central atom making available the proper number of orbitals (equal to the coordination number). *Inner-orbital complexes* are those in which incompletely filled d orbitals are used for bonding, forming *inert complexes* (those which undergo slow ligand substitution); *outer-orbital complexes* use outer d orbitals for bonding, forming *labile complexes* (those which undergo rapid ligand substitution). The shape of the complex is determined by the orbitals used: sp^3 is tetrahedral, sp^2d is square planar, sp^3d or spd^3 is trigonal bipyramidal, sp^2d^2 or sd^4 is square pyramidal, and sp^3d^2 is octahedral. The major contribution of the valence bond theory is in predicting shapes of molecules and the number of unpaired electrons.

EXAMPLE 15.6. The ligands F^- and CN^- are quite different in their abilities to form labile and inert complexes. The F^- is a weak ligand and the CN^- a strong ligand, forming outer- and inner-orbital complexes, respectively. Prepare a diagram showing the configuration of CoF_6^{3-} and $Co(CN)_6^{3-}$ and predict the number of unpaired electrons.

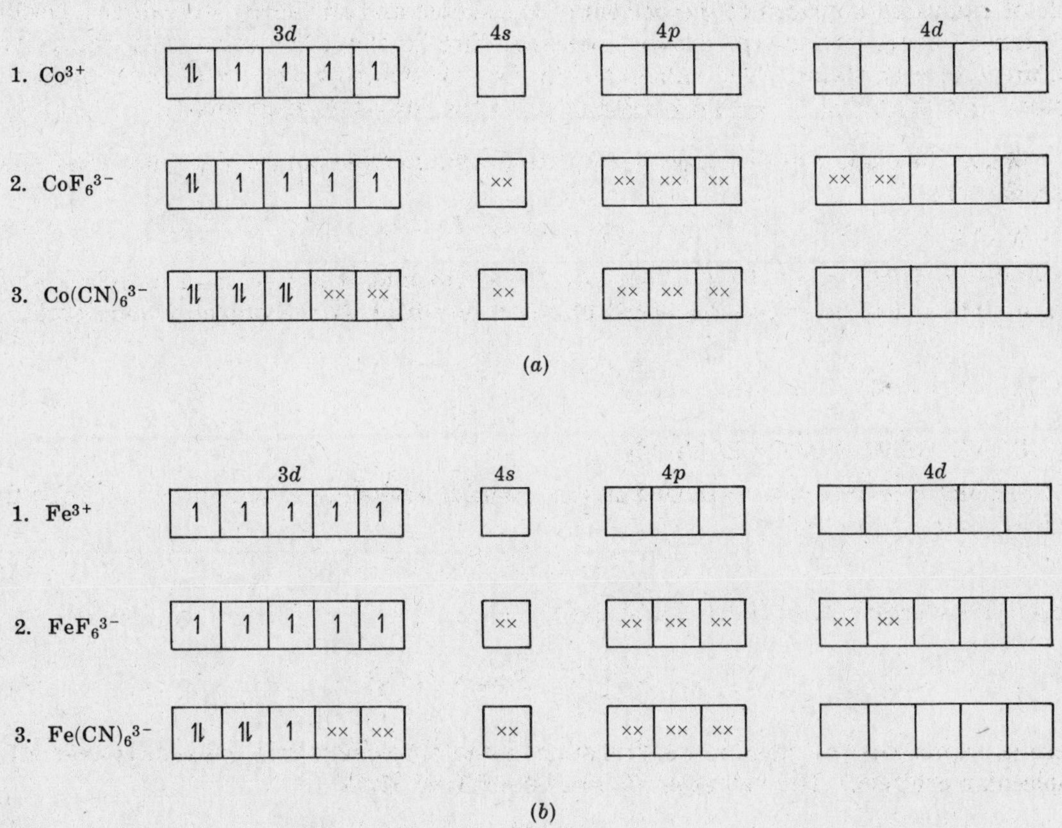

Fig. 15-4

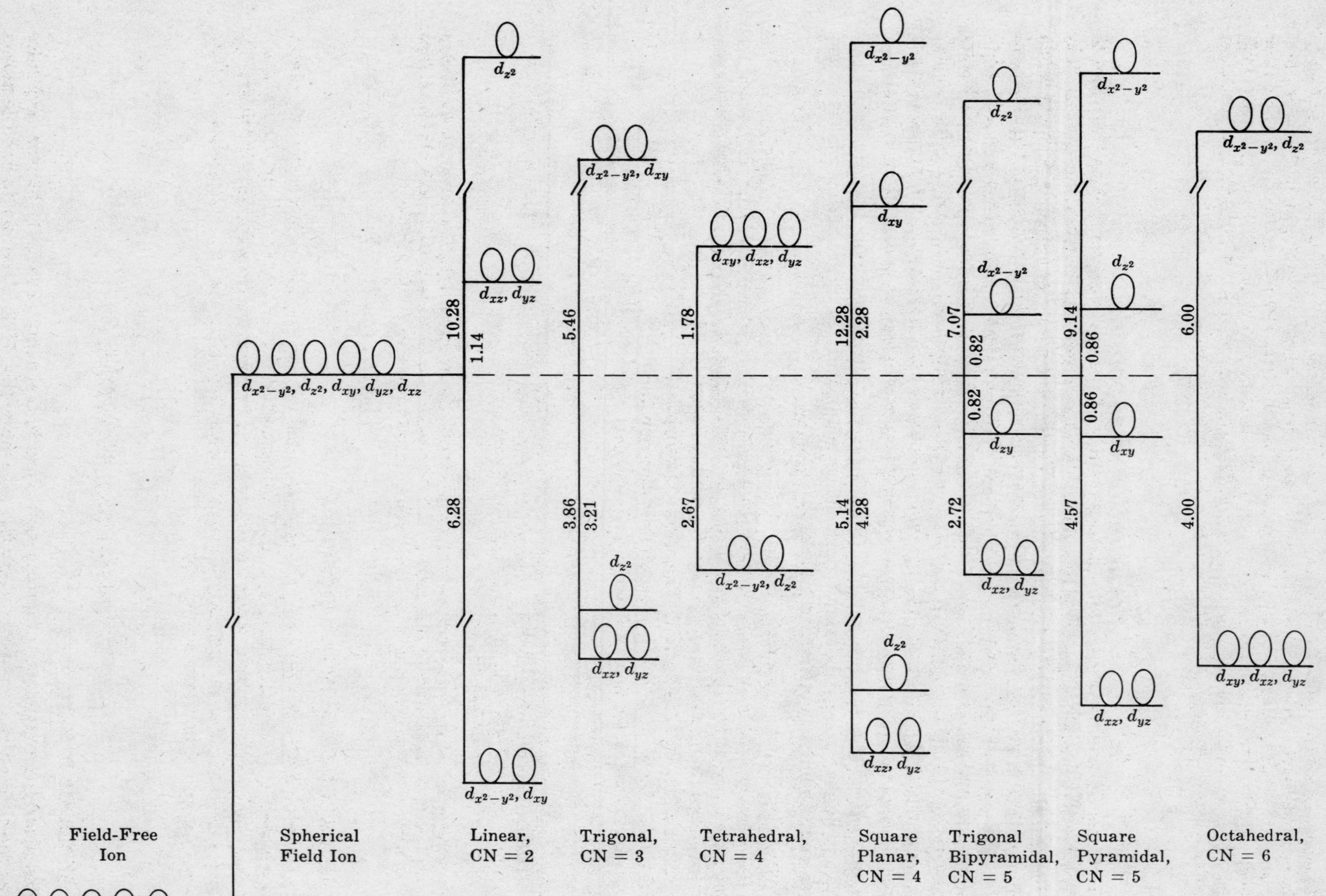

d_{z^2}
d_{xz}, d_{yz}
$d_{x^2-y^2}, d_{xy}$
10.28
1.14
6.28
$d_{x^2-y^2}, d_{xy}$
5.46
3.86
3.21
d_{z^2}
d_{xz}, d_{yz}
d_{xy}, d_{xz}, d_{yz}
1.78
2.67
$d_{x^2-y^2}, d_{z^2}$
$d_{x^2-y^2}$
d_{xy}
12.28
2.28
5.14
4.28
d_{z^2}
d_{xz}, d_{yz}
d_{z^2}
$d_{x^2-y^2}$
7.07
0.82
0.82
d_{zy}
2.72
d_{xz}, d_{yz}
$d_{x^2-y^2}$
d_{z^2}
9.14
0.86
0.86
d_{xy}
4.57
d_{xz}, d_{yz}
$d_{x^2-y^2}, d_{z^2}$
6.00
4.00
d_{xy}, d_{xz}, d_{yz}
$d_{x^2-y^2}, d_{z^2}, d_{xy}, d_{yz}, d_{xz}$
Field-Free Ion
Spherical Field Ion
Linear, CN = 2
Trigonal, CN = 3
Tetrahedral, CN = 4
Square Planar, CN = 4
Trigonal Bipyramidal, CN = 5
Square Pyramidal, CN = 5
Octahedral, CN = 6

Fig. 15-5

The electronic configuration of Co^{3+} is such that the outer orbitals can be illustrated as in Fig. 15-4(*a*1). The six pairs of bonding electrons from the weak ligand simply fill the 4*s*, 4*p*(3) and 4*d*(2) orbitals, producing an outer-orbital complex, see Fig. 15-4(*a*2), with four unpaired electrons on the Co. The six pairs of bonding electrons and the strong ligand pair up the 3*d* electrons of Co^{3+} and fill the 3*d*(2), 4*s* and 4*p*(3) orbitals, producing an inner-orbital complex, see Fig. 15-4(*a*3), with no unpaired electrons. In both cases sp^3d^2 orbitals are being used by the ligands, giving an octahedral shape.

15.7 CRYSTAL FIELD THEORY

The basis of this theory is that the degeneracy of the *d* orbitals on the central atom is removed as the ligands are placed on the molecule. Figure 15-5 gives the crystal field splitting for several geometric configurations. Though the actual separations between levels depend on the strength of the ligand, the separations between the orbitals and the spherical field ion always have the relative magnitudes indicated by the vertical numbers in Fig. 15-5. If a strong ligand is used, the magnitude of the CF splitting will be large and the lower-lying orbitals will fill first, giving rise to "low-spin" complexes. If a weak ligand is used, the magnitude of the splitting will be small, giving rise to "high-spin" complexes because all orbitals will fill with parallel spins before a second electron is placed in an orbital.

The differences between these energy levels lie near the visible region of the spectrum and many of these compounds are highly colored. For a d^1 configuration in an octahedral field, the CF splitting is shown in Fig. 15-6. The ^2D on the vertical axis is the Russell-Saunders term for the free ion and at the right are the permitted components in the octahedral field—namely, E_g (doubly degenerate) and T_{2g} (triply degenerate). The allowed absorption transition is $^2T_{2g} \rightarrow {^2E_g}$. The corresponding diagram for a d^6 configuration is similar to Fig. 15-6 except that the terms are ^5D, ^5E_g and $^5T_{2g}$.

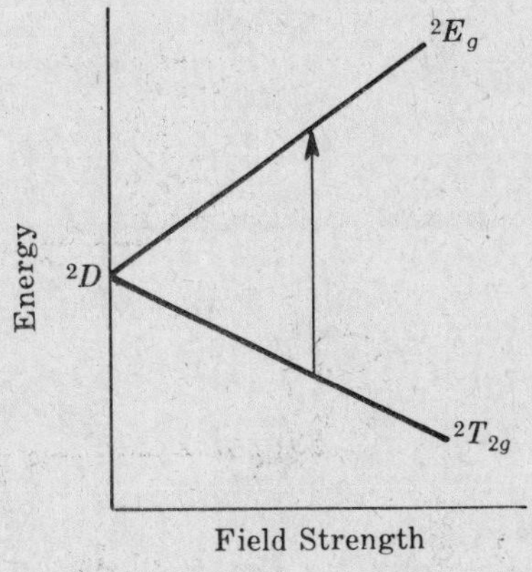

Fig. 15-6

EXAMPLE 15.7. $Cu(NH_3)_4 \cdot 2H_2O^{2+}$ absorbs at the wavelength 600 mμ (orange) and $Cu(H_2O)_4 \cdot 2H_2O^{2+}$ absorbs at 800 mμ (red). Compare the relative strengths of the ligands and predict the colors of the solutions containing these ions.

Because energy is inversely proportional to λ, see (*11.1*) and (*11.3*), the NH_3 has separated the energy levels on Cu^{2+} more than the H_2O has, making it the stronger ligand. A substance which absorbs orange light will appear as blue-purple, and red light absorption will result in a blue solution.

15.8 MOLECULAR ORBITAL THEORY

By combining atomic orbitals of the central atom and the bonding orbitals of the ligands, the molecular orbitals shown in Fig. 15-7 for an octahedral complex can be constructed. Note that the MO theory allows for π bonding using another energy diagram. The energy separation between the nonbonding T_{2g} and antibonding E_g^* levels will determine whether high- or low-spin complexes will result.

Spatial Relationships

15.9 INTRODUCTION

The spatial arrangement of atoms and electrons in many covalently bonded molecules or ions can be predicted correctly using the scheme in Fig. 15-8. In order to find the molecular geometry, the number of available electrons, AE, and the number of electrons needed to construct a molecule containing only single bonds, NE, are calculated. Depending on the relationship of AE to NE, one of the three major procedures shown in Fig. 15-8 will determine the correct Lewis structure(s) (Section 15.10); the structure number, SN_X, for each atom; the correct three-dimensional sketch; and the molecular geometry.

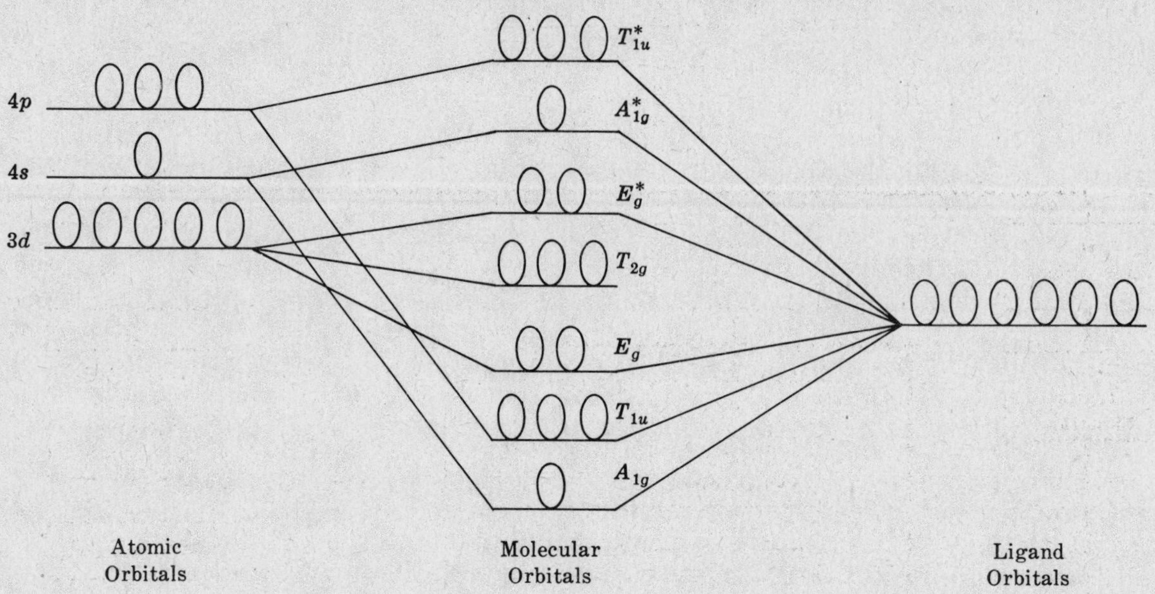

Fig. 15-7

In calculating AE, only the valence electrons are considered, not the lower-lying kernel electrons. Thus,

$$\text{AE} = \sum_X (\text{group number})_X - (\text{charge on species}) \qquad (15.21)$$

where the summation of the periodic table group number for atom X is carried out for every atom present. The group number for transition metals in complexes is rather loosely interpreted as the oxidation state for the metal rather than the actual group number.

Assuming each hydrogen present in the species to need two valence electrons and each nonhydrogen to need eight valence electrons, the number of needed electrons is given by

$$\text{NE} = 2(\text{number of H atoms}) + 8(\text{number of non-H atoms}) - 2(\text{number of atoms} - 1) \qquad (15.22)$$

where the last term corrects for the number of shared electrons assuming the entire molecule (ion) to contain only single bonds.

15.10 LEWIS STRUCTURES

The *Lewis structure* for the species under consideration is drawn as an aid in determining the structure number for each atom in the species. The kernel of the atom (including the nucleus and inner electrons is represented by the elemental symbol for the atom. Dots, circles, or crosses are used to represent the electrons in the outermost orbital, with a dash commonly representing a pair of electrons.

If AE = NE, the species is said to be *saturated.* In such a species, all bonds are single bonds and all "octets" are completely filled.

If AE < NE, an electron deficiency exists in the species. There are three ways in which an electron deficiency can be satisfied: (1) formation of a cyclic or ring structure;

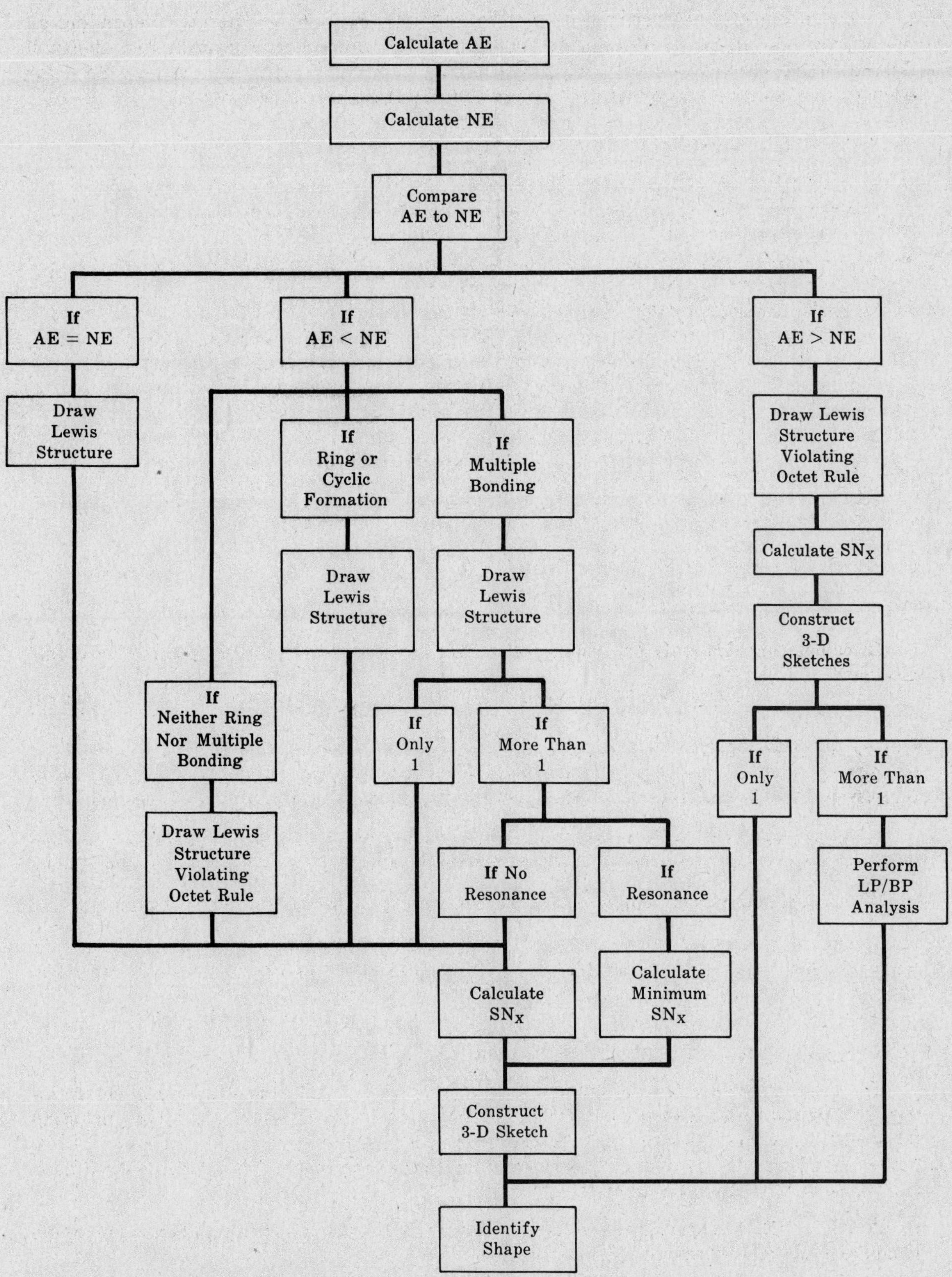

Fig. 15-8 (*after Metz, STRC-056*, Modular Laboratory Program, *Willard Grant Press, Inc.*)

(2) multiple bonding; or (3) violation of the "octet" rule for one or more atoms in the bond, with the proper choice depending on the information known for the species. Some elements, particularly C, N, O and S, will form double bonds to eliminate a two-electron deficiency and triple bonds to eliminate a four-electron deficiency. These multiple bonds are formed using hybridized orbitals to create a σ bond, and unhybridized atomic orbitals with parallel overlap to create one or two π bonds, between the atoms.

For some substances more than one Lewis structure can be drawn which satisfies the data for AE and NE. To determine whether the various structures all contribute to the molecular geometry, the *formal charge*, FC_X, given by

$$FC_X = (\text{group number})_X - [2(\text{LP}) + \tfrac{1}{2}(\text{number of shared electrons})]_X \qquad (15.23)$$

is calculated for each atom in the proposed structures, where LP is the number of lone or unshared pairs of electrons around atom X. The structures for which the sum of the absolute values of the FC_X is small are usually the important structures to consider and those with higher formal charge are discarded. In case more than one Lewis structure having the same skeleton is acceptable based on values of FC_X, the contributing forms are drawn with double-headed arrows placed between them to indicate that the bonding and spatial arrangement is somewhere between the limiting structures (*resonance*).

If $AE > NE$, the Lewis structure is drawn showing only saturated bonding and the "octet" rule for one or more of the atoms is violated.

15.11 STRUCTURE NUMBER AND SHAPE

The structure number for atom X, SN_X, is given by

$$SN_X = (\text{number of bonds})_X + LP_X \qquad (15.24)$$

An unpaired electron or a multiple bond in the Lewis structure counts as one in (*15.24*).

The value of SN_X corresponds to a particular geometrical arrangement of the electron pairs around atom X as shown in Table 15-1. After preparing a three-dimensional sketch, the shape of the species is determined by the arrangement of the atoms in the molecule.

In those cases where $AE < NE$ and resonance has been determined to exist, SN_X is calculated for each atom in each structure and the minimum value is used. The three-dimensional sketch is then drawn using these minimum SN_X's and the remaining electrons are assumed to be in the parallel overlapping orbitals forming extended π bonding.

In those cases where $AE > NE$ and it is possible to have more than one three-dimensional isomer, an analysis of the lone-lone pair, lone-bonded pair and bonded-bonded pair interactions of electrons for angles up to and including 90° can often predict the correct shape. This qualitative analysis is based on the assumption that LP-LP interactions are less favored than LP-BP interactions, which, in turn, are less favored than BP-BP interactions.

Solved Problems

Hybridization

15.1. Give a molecular orbital description for H_2O.

The molecular orbital diagram shown in Fig. 15-9(*a*) predicts two equivalent H—O bonds at 90° apart if direct overlap of atomic hydrogen and oxygen orbitals occurs. Although predicting the correct formula of the compound, the predicted bond angle does not agree with the experimental value

Table 15-1
(*after Metz, STRC-056,* Modular Laboratory Program, *Willard Grant Press, Inc.*)

Structure Number, SN_X	Geometric Shape for X	Hybridization	Sketch of Shape	Molecular Shape Possibilities
1	spherical	....	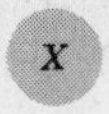	
2	linear	sp	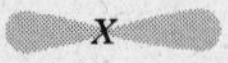	LP = 0, BP = 2 linear LP = 1, BP = 1 linear
3	triangular	sp^2	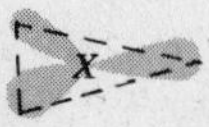	LP = 0, BP = 3 triangular LP = 1, BP = 2 bent (angle ~ 120°) LP = 2, BP = 1 linear
4	tetrahedral	sp^3	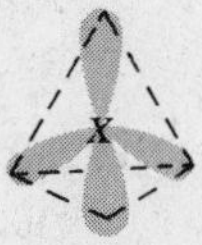	LP = 0, BP = 4 tetrahedral LP = 1, BP = 3 trigonal pyramidal LP = 2, BP = 2 bent (angle ~ 109°) LP = 3, BP = 1 linear
4 (not common)	square planar	dsp^2 or sp^2d	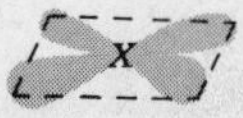	LP = 0, BP = 4 square planar
5	trigonal bipyramidal	dsp^3 or sp^3d	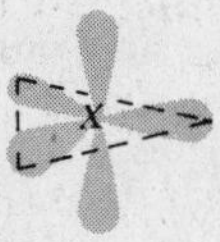	LP = 0, BP = 5 trigonal bipyramidal LP = 1, BP = 4 seesaw LP = 2, BP = 3 T-shaped LP = 3, BP = 2 linear LP = 4, BP = 1 linear
6	octahedral	d^2sp^3 or sp^3d^2	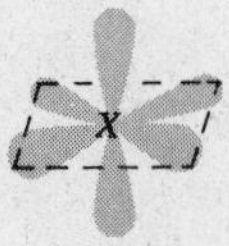	LP = 0, BP = 6 octahedral LP = 1, BP = 5 square pyramidal LP = 2, BP = 4 square planar
7	pentagonal bipyramidal	....	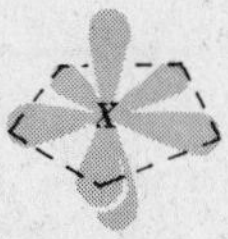	
8	cubic	....	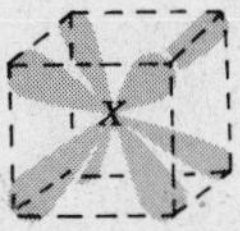	
8	square antiprismal	....	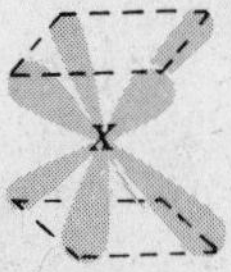	

of 104.45°. If the oxygen is assumed to undergo sp^3 hybridization before interacting with the hydrogens, see Fig. 15-9(*b*), two equivalent bonds are again predicted but at an approximate angle of 109°28′, which agrees fairly well with the experimental value.

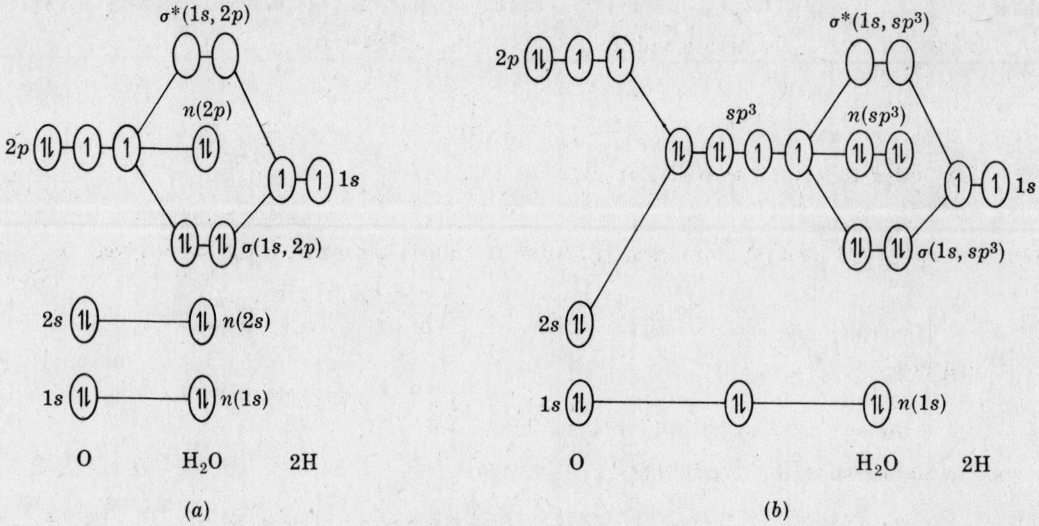

Fig. 15-9

15.2. Determine the angular wave functions describing the four hybrid orbitals representing sp^3 hybridization. Determine the relative bond strengths of these wave functions and the angles between the orbitals.

Assuming the first hybrid orbital to lie along the z-axis, (*15.1*) gives

$$X_1 = a_1 Y_s + b_1 Y_{p_z} = a_1\left(\frac{1}{4\pi}\right)^{1/2} + b_1\left(\frac{3}{4\pi}\right)^{1/2} \cos\theta$$

because Y_{p_x} and Y_{p_y} are zero along this axis. Recognizing that the ratio of "p character" to "s character" requires that

$$\frac{\langle b_1 Y_{p_z} \mid b_1 Y_{p_z}\rangle}{\langle a_1 Y_s \mid a_1 Y_s\rangle} = \frac{b_1^2}{a_1^2} = 3$$

or $b_1^2 = 3a_1^2$, and that normalization, (*15.2a*), requires that

$$a_1^2 + b_1^2 = 1$$

the values of the coefficients are $a_1 = \pm 1/2$ and $b_1 = \pm 3^{1/2}/2$. Choosing the positive value for a_1 so that the maximum of X_1 can be considered,

$$X_1 = \frac{1}{2}\left(\frac{1}{4\pi}\right)^{1/2} (1 \pm 3\cos\theta)$$

The maximum of X_1 will lie along the z-axis (where $\theta = 0°$ or $180°$), giving

$$\text{rbs} = \frac{(1/2)(1/4\pi)^{1/2}[1 \pm 3(\pm 1)]}{(1/4\pi)^{1/2}} = 2.000$$

It is possible to retain the $\pm$ sign in X_1 as in Example 15.3, but traditionally only the positive sign is used (i.e. $b_1 = +3^{1/2}/2$), thus assigning X_1 to lie along the positive z-axis. This assignment is then reflected in the choice of other coefficients and the extraneous coefficients are discarded.

Choosing the second hybrid orbital to lie in the xz-plane, (*15.1*) gives

$$X_2 = a_2 Y_s + b_2 Y_{p_z} + c_2 Y_{p_x} = a_2\left(\frac{1}{4\pi}\right)^{1/2} + b_2\left(\frac{3}{4\pi}\right)^{1/2} \cos\theta + c_2\left(\frac{3}{4\pi}\right)^{1/2} \sin\theta\cos\phi$$

The amount of p character requires that

$$\frac{\langle (b_2 Y_{p_z} + c_2 Y_{p_x}) \mid (b_2 Y_{p_z} + c_2 Y_{p_x}) \rangle}{\langle a_2 Y_s \mid a_2 Y_s \rangle} = 3$$

which because of the orthogonality of Y_{p_z} and Y_{p_x} simplifies to

$$\frac{b_2^2 + c_2^2}{a_2^2} = 3$$

Combining this result with *(15.2a)* gives

$$a_2^2 + 3a_2^2 = 1$$

or $a_2 = \pm 1/2$ and $b_2^2 + c_2^2 = 3/4$. Because X_1 and X_2 are orthogonal, *(15.2b)* gives

$$b_2 = -\frac{a_1 a_2}{b_1} = -\frac{(1/2)(1/2)}{+3^{1/2}/2} = -\frac{1}{2(3)^{1/2}}$$

and hence

$$c_2 = \pm\left[\frac{3}{4} - b_2^2\right]^{1/2} = \pm\left(\frac{2}{3}\right)^{1/2}$$

The second wave function is then

$$X_2 = \left(\frac{1}{4\pi}\right)^{1/2}\left(\frac{1}{2} - \frac{1}{2}\cos\theta \pm 2^{1/2}\sin\theta\cos\phi\right)$$

The orientation of the maximum of the orbital can be found from

$$0 = \frac{\partial X_2}{\partial \theta} = \left(\frac{1}{4\pi}\right)^{1/2}\left(0 + \frac{1}{2}\sin\theta \pm 2^{1/2}\cos\theta\cos\phi\right)$$

which upon rearrangement gives

$$\tan\theta = \mp 2^{3/2}\cos\phi$$

For $\phi = 0°$ (towards the positive x-axis), $\tan\theta = \mp 2^{3/2}$, giving $\theta = \mp 70°32'$ or $\pm 109°28'$; and for $\phi = 180°$ (towards the negative x-axis), $\tan\theta = \pm 2^{3/2}$, giving $\theta = \pm 70°32'$ or $\mp 109°28'$. The negative values for θ are discarded because $0° \leq \theta \leq 180°$ and the values of $70°32'$ are discarded because they are too near X_1. Thus $\theta = 109°28'$. Depending on the choice of the sign for c_2, the maximum will lie at an angle of $109°28'$ from the maximum of X_1, either at $\phi = 0$ or $\phi = 180°$. Normally c_2 is chosen as positive, giving

$$X_2 = \left(\frac{1}{4\pi}\right)^{1/2}\left(\frac{1}{2} - \frac{1}{2}\cos\theta + 2^{1/2}\sin\theta\cos\phi\right)$$

which has an rbs of

$$\text{rbs} = \frac{(1/4\pi)^{1/2}[(1/2) - (1/2)\cos 109°28' + 2^{1/2}\sin 109°28'\cos 0°]}{(1/4\pi)^{1/2}} = 2.000$$

Likewise it can be shown that

$$X_3 = \left(\frac{1}{4\pi}\right)^{1/2}\left[\frac{1}{2} - \frac{1}{2}\cos\theta + \left(\frac{3}{2}\right)^{1/2}\sin\theta\cos\phi - \left(\frac{1}{2}\right)^{1/2}\sin\theta\sin\phi\right]$$

$$X_4 = \left(\frac{1}{4\pi}\right)^{1/2}\left[\frac{1}{2} - \frac{1}{2}\cos\theta - \left(\frac{3}{2}\right)^{1/2}\sin\theta\cos\phi - \left(\frac{1}{2}\right)^{1/2}\sin\theta\sin\phi\right]$$

each with an rbs of 2.000.

15.3. Prepare a plot in the xz-plane of $X = (1/2)(1/4\pi)^{1/2}(1 + 3\cos\theta)$, the sp^3 orbital along the z-axis.

Figure 15-10(*a*) is the polar plot of $|X|$ as a function of θ. On the larger lobe X is positive; on the smaller it is negative.

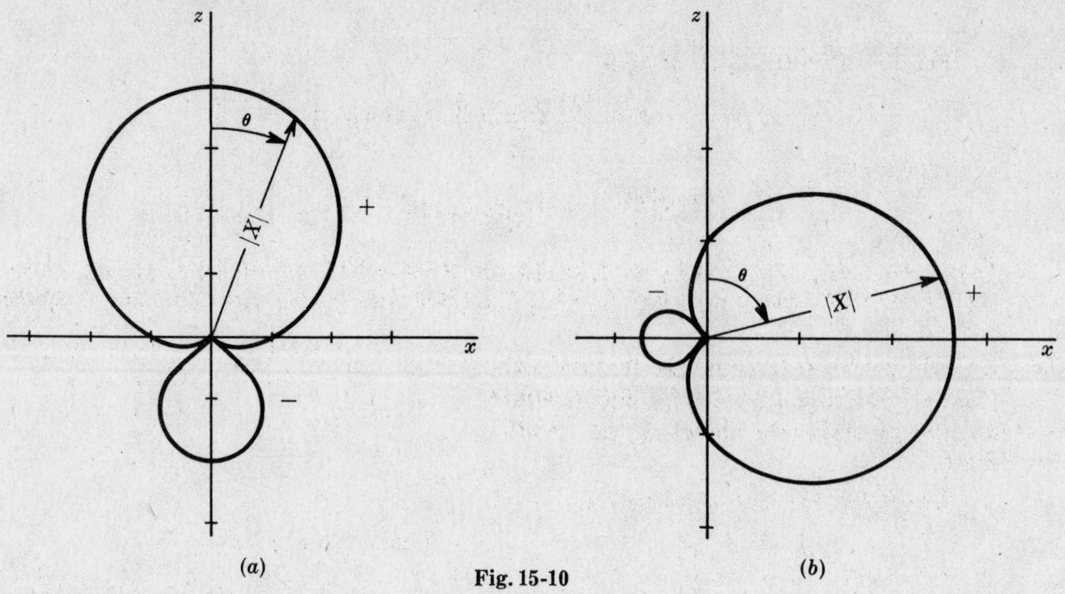

Fig. 15-10

Localized Multiple Bonds

15.4. Prepare a molecular orbital energy diagram representing the bonding in C_2H_4 and predict the types of electronic transitions that could occur.

See Fig. 15-11 for diagrams based (*a*) on a ground-state carbon atom and (*b*) on an sp^2 hybridized carbon atom. The most probable transitions are $\pi \rightarrow \pi^*$ and $\pi \rightarrow \sigma^*$(weak) within the C═C double bond and $\sigma \rightarrow \sigma^*$(weak) within the C—H bond. Figure 15-11(*a*) incorrectly predicts H—C—C angles of 90° and Fig. 15-11(*b*) correctly predicts H—C—C angles of 120°.

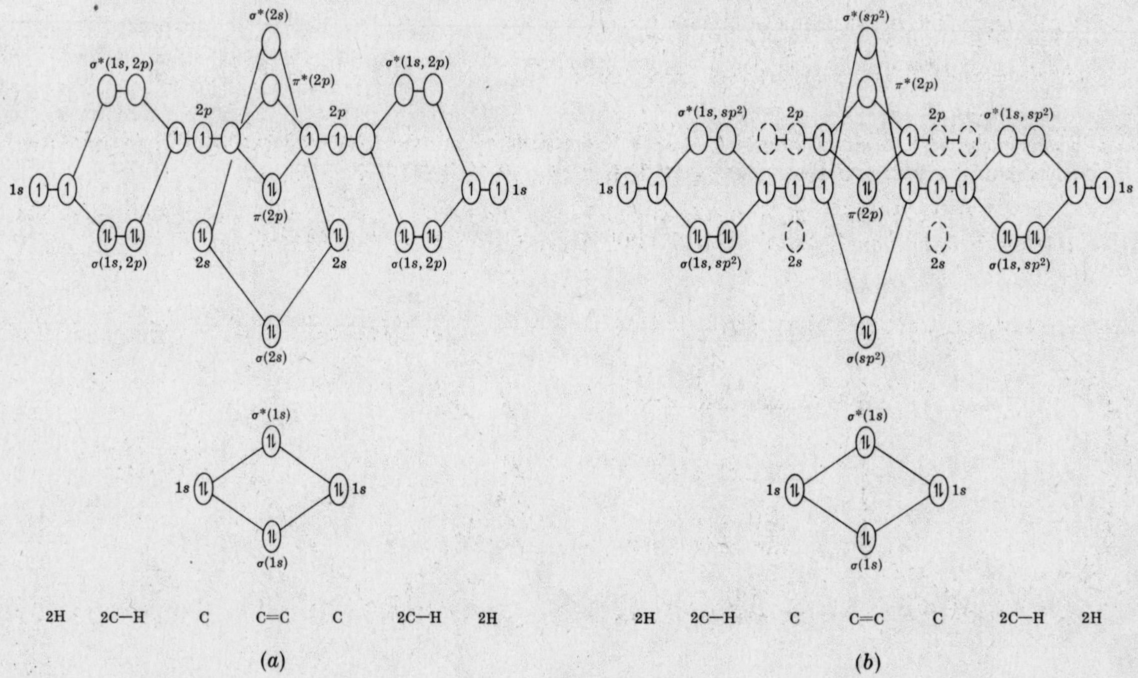

Fig. 15-11

Conjugated Bonds

15.5. Calculate $\bar{\nu}$ for the absorption band of H—(CH═CH—)$_k$—H for $k = 1$ and 10 using the FEMO and improved FEMO theories.

For H—CH=CH—H, (*15.5*) gives

$$\bar{\nu} = \frac{153{,}000\ \text{cm}^{-1}}{2+1} = 51{,}000\ \text{cm}^{-1}$$

and (*15.6*) gives

$$\bar{\nu} = \frac{153{,}000\ \text{cm}^{-1}}{2+1} + (16{,}000\ \text{cm}^{-1})\left(1 - \frac{1}{2}\right) = 59{,}000\ \text{cm}^{-1}$$

The observed value is 61,500 cm^{-1}. Likewise for H—(CH=CH—)$_{10}$—H, (*15.5*) gives 7300 cm^{-1} and (*15.6*) gives 22,500 cm^{-1}, the latter agreeing quite well with the experimental value of 22,400 cm^{-1}.

15.6. Calculate the energy levels for the conjugated bonding in benzene and prepare an energy diagram showing the ground state.

Equation (*15.14*) becomes for six atoms

$$\begin{vmatrix} x & 1 & 0 & 0 & 0 & 1 \\ 1 & x & 1 & 0 & 0 & 0 \\ 0 & 1 & x & 1 & 0 & 0 \\ 0 & 0 & 1 & x & 1 & 0 \\ 0 & 0 & 0 & 1 & x & 1 \\ 1 & 0 & 0 & 0 & 1 & x \end{vmatrix} = 0$$

and using (*15.15*) gives

$$E_0 = \alpha + 2\beta\cos(0) = \alpha + 2\beta$$
$$E_1 = \alpha + 2\beta\cos(2\pi/6) = \alpha + \beta$$

$E_2 = \alpha - \beta$, $E_3 = \alpha - 2\beta$, $E_4 = \alpha - \beta$ and $E_5 = \alpha + \beta$. These are sketched in Fig. 15-12(*a*). Because E_1 and E_5, as well as E_2 and E_4, is degenerate, only four energy levels are present.

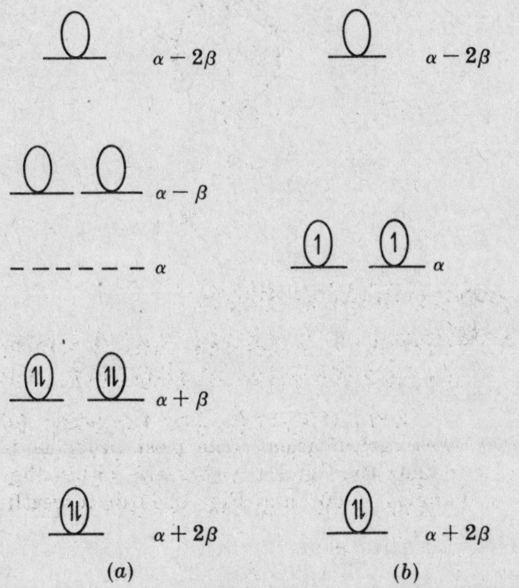

Fig. 15-12

15.7. Determine the energy levels in C_6H_6 for the conjugated bonding using the mnemonic device and compare the results to those found in Problem 15.6.

Placing the hexagon on a vertex and drawing energy levels parallel to each atom gives the system shown in Fig. 15-13(*a*). The spacings are the same as in Fig. 15-12(*a*).

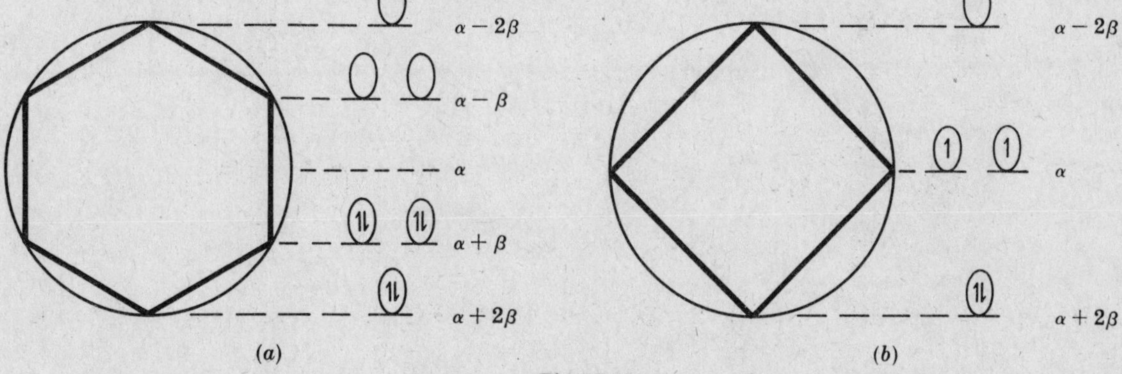

Fig. 15-13

15.8. Predict the aromaticity of C_6H_6.

Benzene satisfies (*15.16*) with $m = 1$, so C_6H_6 is predicted to have extra stability resulting from "resonance energy" associated with aromatic compounds.

15.9. Find P_{rs} and r_{rs} for the 1—2 and 3—4 bonds in 1,3-butadiene.

Using (*15.19a*) gives for atom 1

$$C_{11} = \left(\frac{2}{5}\right)^{1/2} \sin\left[\frac{(1)(1)\pi}{5}\right] = (0.633)\sin(36°) = 0.371$$

$$C_{21} = (0.633)\sin\left[\frac{(2)(1)\pi}{5}\right] = 0.601$$

$C_{31} = 0.601$ and $C_{41} = 0.371$. Likewise for atom 2,

$$C_{12} = (0.633)\sin\left[\frac{(1)(2)\pi}{5}\right] = 0.601$$

$C_{22} = 0.371$, $C_{32} = -0.371$ and $C_{42} = -0.601$. Using the electronic distribution shown in Fig. 15-3(*a*), (*15.18*) gives

$$p_{12} = \frac{2}{2}[(0.371)(0.601) + (0.601)(0.371)] + \frac{2}{2}[(0.601)(0.371) + (0.371)(0.601)]$$
$$+ \frac{0}{2}[(0.601)(-0.371) + (-0.371)(0.601)] + \frac{0}{2}[(0.371)(-0.601) + (-0.601)(0.371)]$$
$$= 0.893$$

and (*15.17*) gives $$P_{12} = 1 + 0.893 = 1.893$$

The bond length for this value of P_{12} is given by (*15.20*) as

$$r_{12} = 1.707 - (0.186)(1.893) = 1.355 \text{ Å}$$

The observed value is 1.34 Å.

Coordination Compounds

15.10. Prepare sketches of the electronic configurations of CoF_6^{3-}, $Co(CN)_6^{3-}$ and $CoCl_4^{2-}$ (tetrahedral) using the crystal field splittings shown in Fig. 15-5.

The six electrons in Co^{3+} will be arranged as shown in Fig. 15-14(*a*) for the weak octahedral complex formed by the F^- and as shown in Fig. 15-14(*b*) for the strong octahedral complex formed by the CN^-. The seven *d* electrons in Co^{2+} will be arranged as shown in Fig. 15-14(*c*) for the weak tetrahedral complex.

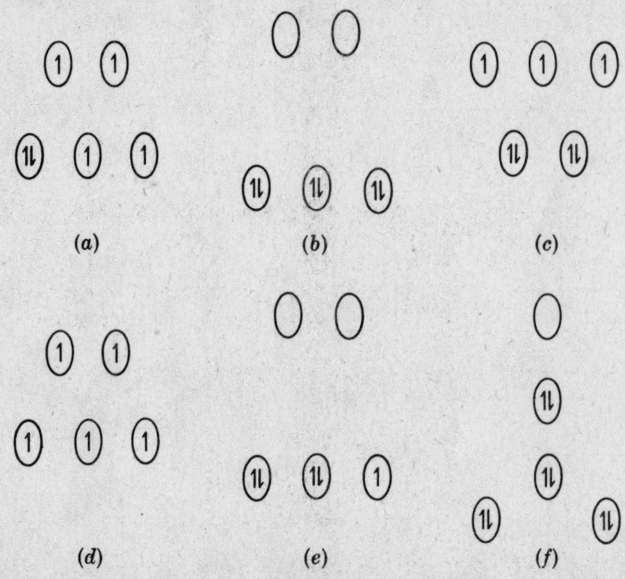

Fig. 15-14

15.11. $Fe(H_2O)_6^{2+}$ is a high-spin complex which absorbs light at about 1000 nm corresponding to a transition between the $^5T_{2g}$ and ^5E_g levels. What is the energy between these levels? Predict the color of this ion.

Using *(11.2)* gives

$$\bar{\nu} = \frac{1}{1000 \times 10^{-9}\ \text{m}}(10^{-2}\ \text{cm}^{-1}/\text{m}^{-1}) = 10{,}000\ \text{cm}^{-1}$$

The 1000 nm (= 10,000 Å) absorption peak is in the very near-infrared region and part of the absorption peak falls into the red visible region. Thus the ion will absorb some red, giving a pale, blue-green color.

15.12. Sketch the molecular orbital diagram for CoF_6^{3-}.

The F^-, a weak ligand, will not separate the T_{2g} and E_g^* levels sufficiently to produce electron pairing, so the high-spin complex shown in Fig. 15-15(*a*) results.

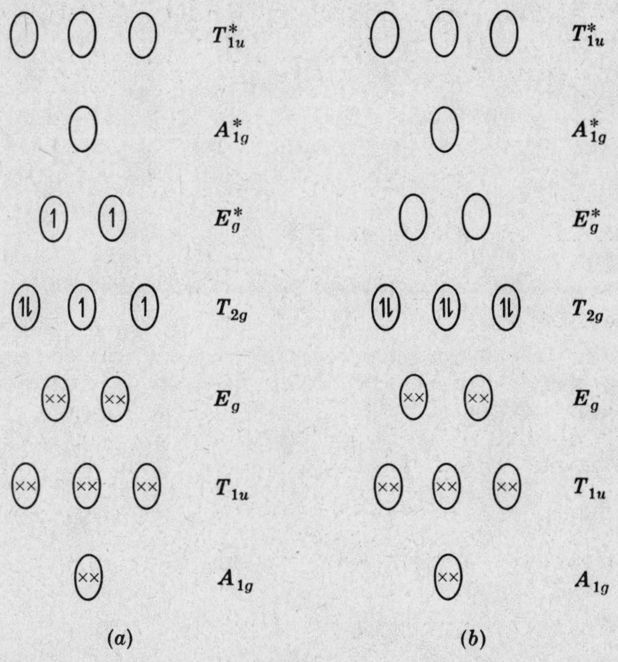

Fig. 15-15

Spatial Relationships

15.13. Determine the shapes of the following species: (*a*) n-C_8H_{18}, (*b*) BCl_3, (*c*) S_8, (*d*) C_2H_4, (*e*) C_2H_2, (*f*) HCNO, (*g*) N_2O, (*h*) $CrCl_6^{3-}$ and (*i*) XeF_4.

The Lewis diagrams are given in Fig. 15-16 and the three-dimensional sketches are given in Fig. 15-17. The information used to determine the structures is given below.

(*a*)

$$\begin{aligned}
\text{AE} &= [(8)(4) + (18)(1)] - (0) = 50 \\
\text{NE} &= 2(18) + 8(8) - 2(26 - 1) = 50 \\
\text{AE} &= \text{NE} \\
\text{SN}_\text{H} &= (1) + (0) = 1 \\
\text{SN}_\text{C} &= (4) + (0) = 4
\end{aligned}$$

There are four bonded pairs of electrons located tetrahedrally around each C atom, giving the entire molecule many shapes depending on rotation of the tetrahedrons with respect to each other.

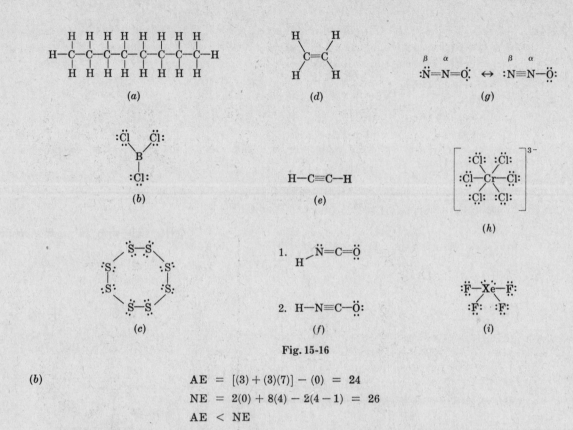

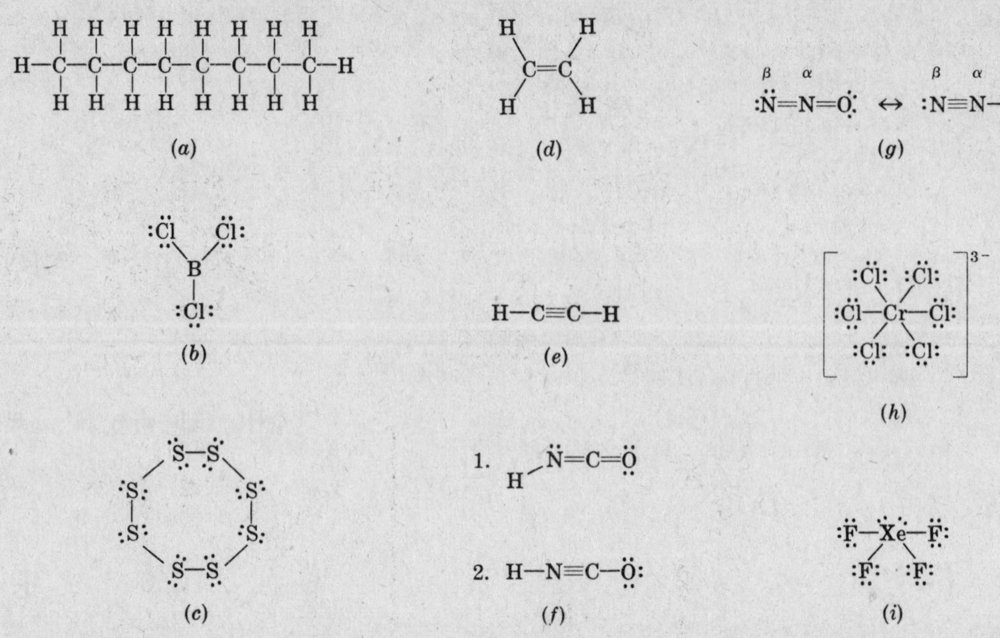

Fig. 15-16

(*b*)

$$\begin{aligned} AE &= [(3) + (3)(7)] - (0) = 24 \\ NE &= 2(0) + 8(4) - 2(4-1) = 26 \\ AE &< NE \end{aligned}$$

BCl_3 is experimentally known not to contain significant multiple bonding nor to be cyclic; it is known to have three equivalent B—F bonds. Based on the electronegativities of F and B the electron deficiency is assigned to the B.

$$SN_B = (3) + (0) = 3 \qquad SN_{Cl} = (1) + (3) = 4$$

This is a triangular molecule.

(*c*)

$$\begin{aligned} AE &= [(8)(6)] - (0) = 48 \\ NE &= 2(0) + 8(8) - 2(8-1) = 50 \\ AE &< NE \end{aligned}$$

As only one type of bonding is present, multiple bonding and branching are not present.

$$SN_S = (2) + (2) = 4$$

This is a puckered ring with four atoms in one plane and four in another plane.

(*d*)

$$\begin{aligned} AE &= [(2)(4) + (4)(1)] - (0) = 12 \\ NE &= 2(4) + 8(2) - 2(6-1) = 14 \\ AE &< NE \end{aligned}$$

A triple bond between the C's eliminates the deficiency of four electrons.

$$\begin{aligned} SN_H &= (1) + (0) = 1 \\ SN_C &= (3) + (0) = 3 \end{aligned}$$

This is a planar molecule because of the required parallel overlap of the p atomic orbitals used for the π bonding.

(*e*)

$$\begin{aligned} AE &= [(2)(4) + (2)(1)] - (0) = 10 \\ NE &= 2(2) + 8(2) - 2(4-1) = 14 \\ AE &< NE \end{aligned}$$

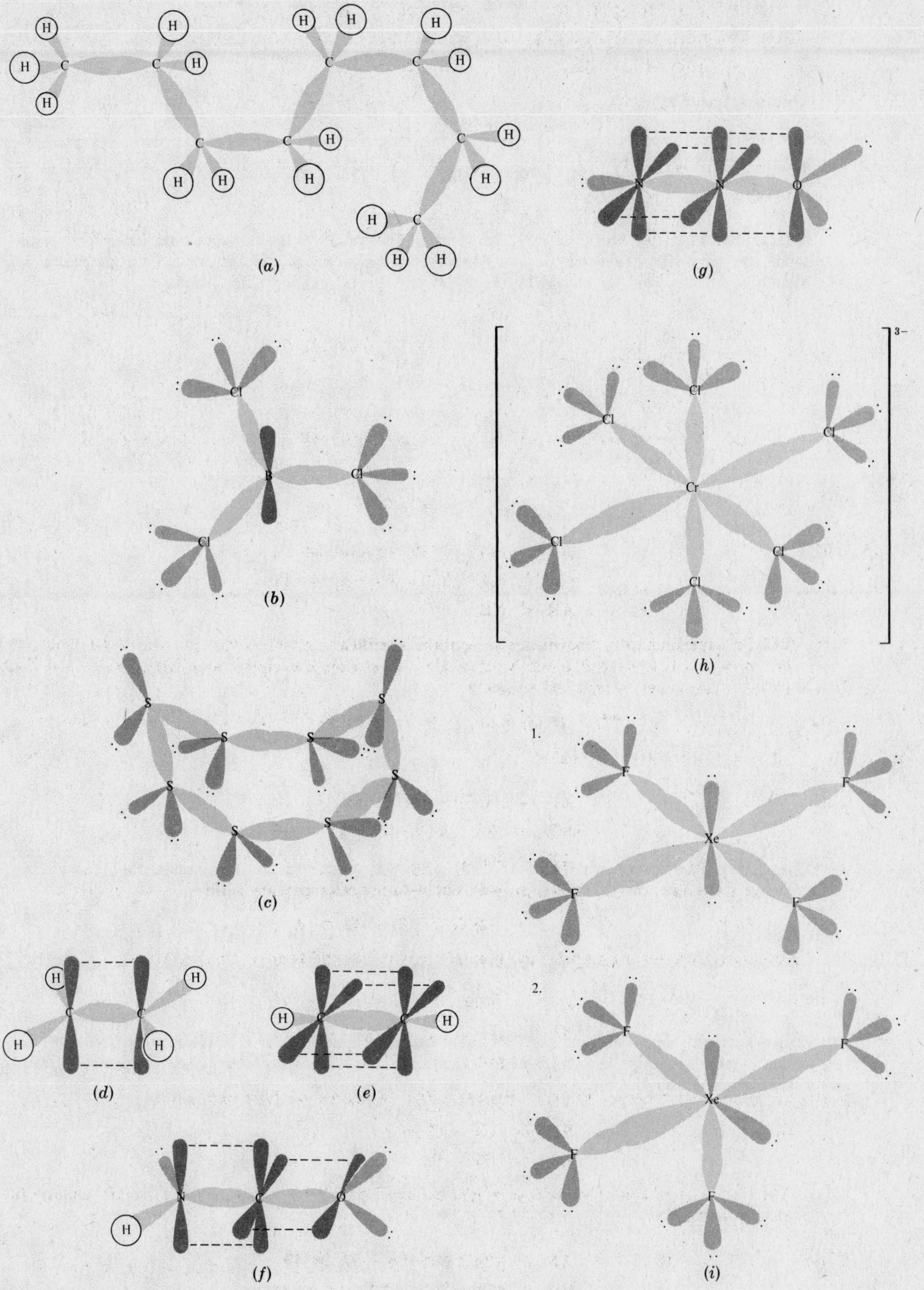

Fig. 15-17

A triple bond between the C's eliminates the deficiency of four electrons.

$$SN_H = (1) + (0) = 1$$
$$SN_C = (2) + (0) = 2$$

This is a linear molecule.

(*f*)

$$AE = [(1)+(5)+(4)+(6)] - (0) = 16$$
$$NE = 2(1) + 8(3) - 2(4-1) = 20$$
$$AE < NE$$

A triple bond between the C and N (based on additional formal charge calculations, C—O triple bonds are very little favored) or two double bonds eliminates the deficiency of four electrons. Structure 1 is favored, as shown by the following formal charge calculations:

structure 1

$$FC_H = (1) - [2(0) + \tfrac{1}{2}(2)] = 0$$
$$FC_N = (5) - [2(1) + \tfrac{1}{2}(6)] = 0$$
$$FC_C = (4) - [2(0) + \tfrac{1}{2}(8)] = 0$$
$$FC_O = (6) - [2(2) + \tfrac{1}{2}(4)] = 0$$
$$\text{sum of absolute values} = 0$$

structure 2

$$FC_H = (1) - [2(0) + \tfrac{1}{2}(2)] = 0$$
$$FC_N = (5) - [2(0) + \tfrac{1}{2}(8)] = 1$$
$$FC_C = (4) - [2(0) + \tfrac{1}{2}(8)] = 0$$
$$FC_O = (6) - [2(3) + \tfrac{1}{2}(2)] = -1$$
$$\text{sum of absolute values} = 2$$

$$SN_H = (1) + (0) = 1$$
$$SN_N = (2) + (1) = 3$$
$$SN_C = (2) + (0) = 2$$
$$SN_O = (1) + (2) = 3$$

The preferred Lewis structure shown in Fig. 15-16(*f*1) predicts a nonlinear molecule. The atomic ordering HCNO can be eliminated by additional formal charge calculations.

(*g*)

$$AE = [(2)(5) + (6)] - (0) = 16$$
$$NE = 2(0) + 8(3) - 2(3-1) = 20$$
$$AE < NE$$

Either a triple bond between the N's (again, triple bonds using O's are not favored) or two double bonds eliminates the deficiency of four electrons. Both structures have the same formal charge content and therefore contribute as resonance forms.

$$\text{minimum } SN_{\alpha N} = (1) + (1) = 2$$
$$\text{minimum } SN_{\beta N} = (2) + (0) = 2$$
$$\text{minimum } SN_O = (1) + (2) = 3$$

This is a linear molecule with extended π bonding.

(*h*)

$$AE = [(3) + (6)(7)] - (-3) = 48$$
$$NE = 2(0) + 8(7) - 2(7-1) = 44$$
$$AE > NE$$

The "octet" rule is to be violated for the central Cr atom.

$$SN_{Cr} = (6) - (0) = 6$$
$$SN_{Cl} = (1) + (3) = 4$$

This is an octahedral molecule.

(*i*)
$$AE = [(8) + (4)(7)] - (0) = 36$$
$$NE = 2(0) + 8(5) - 2(5-1) = 32$$
$$AE > NE$$

The "octet" rule is to be violated for Xe.

$$SN_{Xe} = (4) + (2) = 6$$
$$SN_F = (1) + (3) = 4$$

There are two corresponding three-dimensional figures, see Fig. 15-17(*i*). In the first structure there are 8 LP-BP and 4 BP-BP interactions at 90° on the central atom and in the second structure there are 1 LP-LP, 6 LP-BP and 5 BP-BP interactions at 90° on the central atom. On the basis of the LP-LP interaction the first structure, square planar, is favored.

Supplementary Problems

Hybridization

15.14. Give a molecular orbital description for CH_x.

Ans. Figure 15-18(*a*) predicts CH_2 with H—C—H angle of 90°; Fig. 15-18(*b*) predicts CH_4 with one C—H bond of different energy and angles of 90° and 125°; Fig. 15-18(*c*) predicts (correctly) tetrahedral CH_4 with four equivalent bonds.

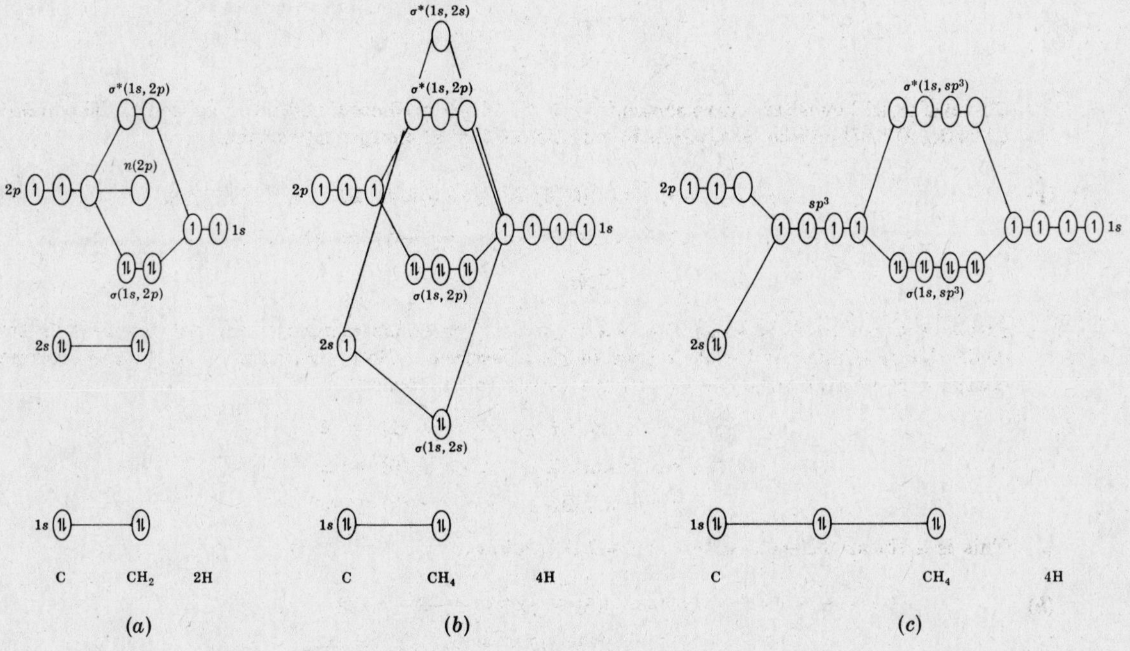

Fig. 15-18

15.15. Represent sp^2 hybridization by means of three hybrid orbitals in the xy-plane. Determine the relative bond strengths and the angles between the orbitals.

Ans. $a_1 = +(1/3)^{1/2}$, $b_1 = +(2/3)^{1/2}$, $c_1 = 0$; $a_2 = +(1/3)^{1/2}$, $b_2 = -(1/6)^{1/2}$, $c_2 = +(1/2)^{1/2}$; $a_3 = +(1/3)^{1/2}$, $b_3 = -(1/6)^{1/2}$, $c_3 = -(1/2)^{1/2}$; 1.992; 120°

15.16. Besides the set found in Problem 15.2, the following set of hybrid atomic orbitals can be written to describe the sp^3 orientation:

$$X_1 = \frac{1}{2}(Y_s + Y_{p_x} + Y_{p_y} + Y_{p_z}) \qquad X_3 = \frac{1}{2}(Y_s - Y_{p_x} + Y_{p_y} - Y_{p_z})$$

$$X_2 = \frac{1}{2}(Y_s + Y_{p_x} - Y_{p_y} - Y_{p_z}) \qquad X_4 = \frac{1}{2}(Y_s - Y_{p_x} - Y_{p_y} + Y_{p_z})$$

Show that these wave functions predict a relative bond strength of 2.000. Show that X_1 is normalized. Show that X_1 and X_2 are orthogonal.

15.17. Prepare a plot in the xz-plane of $X = (1/8\pi)^{1/2}[1 + 3^{1/2} \sin\theta \cos\phi]$, the sp orbital along the positive x-axis, and compare the plot to Fig. 15-10(a). *Ans.* See Fig. 15-10(b).

Localized Multiple Bonds

15.18. Prepare molecular orbital energy diagrams for the carbonyl group

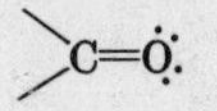

assuming the bonding to consist of a carbon atom that is sp^2-hybridized with (a) an O atom in its ground state and (b) an sp^2-hybridized O atom. If $\pi \rightarrow \pi^*$, $n \rightarrow \pi^*$ and $n \rightarrow \sigma^*$ transitions are observed, which assumption correctly describes the bonding? Assume that the only contributions to the spectrum are from electrons making angles with the bonding axis of from 0° to 90°.

Ans. Nonhybridized oxygen, because $n(2p)$ is 90° from bonding axis and $n(sp^2)$ are 120° from bonding axis (see Fig. 15-19).

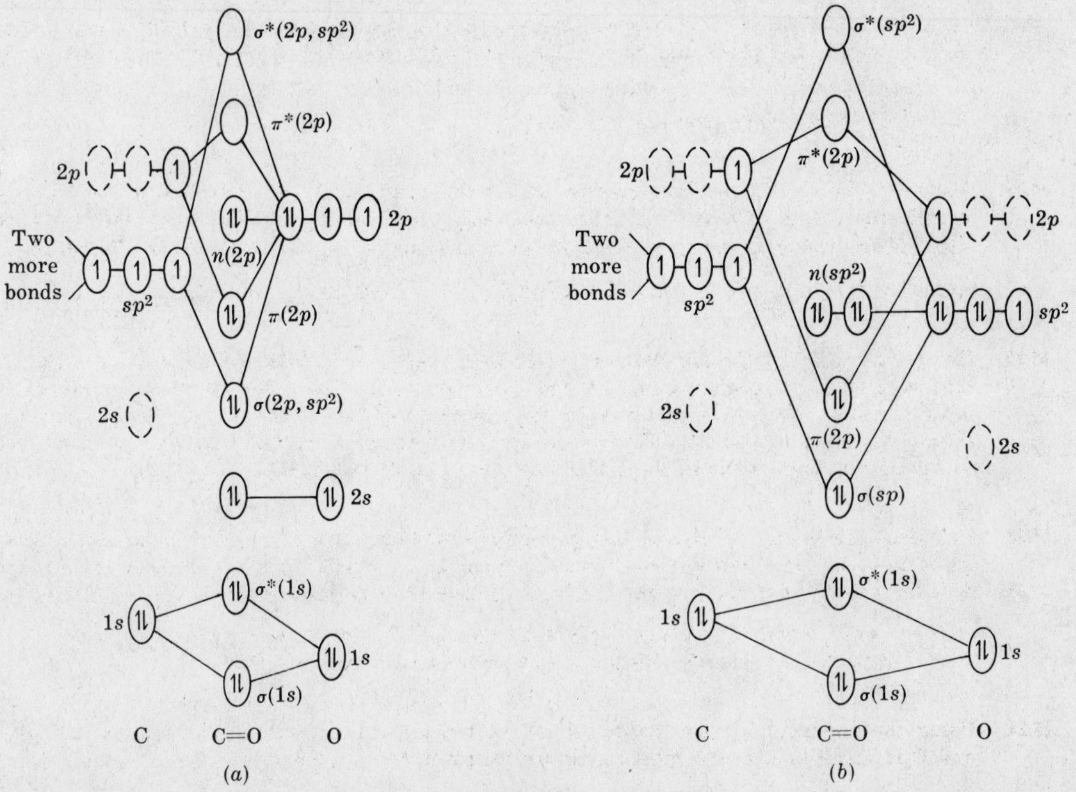

Fig. 15-19

Conjugated Bonds

15.19. An important compound for the sight process in animals is β-carotene, which has the formula

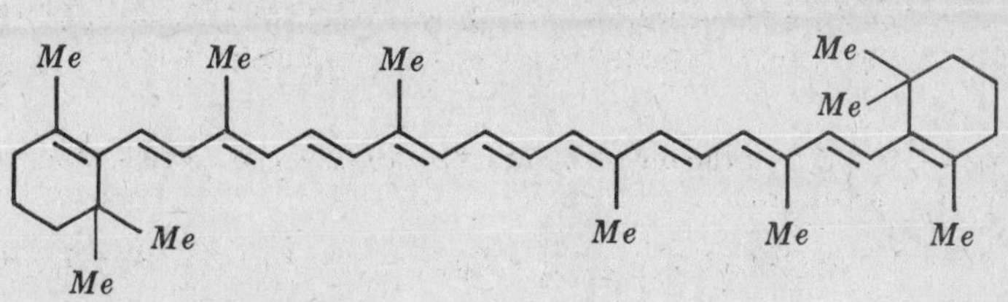

Predict the color of this compound.

Ans. $n_c = 22$ gives $\bar{\nu} = 21{,}900\ \text{cm}^{-1}$ using the improved FEMO theory, $\lambda = 4566$ Å; orange (coloring in carrots)

15.20. The three polymethine dyes 1,1′-diethyl-2,2′-cyanine iodide, 1,1′-diethyl-2,2′carbocyanine iodide and 1,1′-diethyl-2,2′-dicarbocyanine iodide have the structural formulas

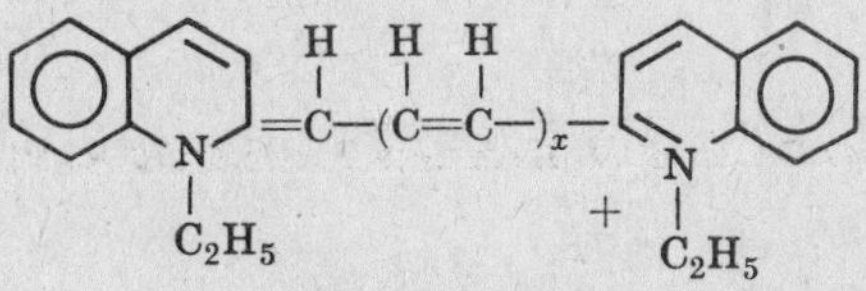

where $x = 0$, 1 and 2, respectively. (*a*) Predict the frequency of light at which the maximum absorbancy should occur. (*b*) Predict the color of the solutions of the substances if the actual frequencies are 520, 601 and 701 nm respectively.

Ans. (*a*) For the shortest path (direct movement between nitrogens) $k = x + 1$ in (*15.7*) giving 30,100, 21,800 and 17,100 cm^{-1}, which are too high; $k = x + 3$ for the intermediate path (movement between one nitrogen and around one inner ring) giving 17,100, 14,000 and 11,900 cm^{-1}, which are a little low; $k = x + 5$ for the longest path (movement between the nitrogens via both outer rings) giving 11,900, 10,300 and 9,100 cm^{-1}, which are too low.

(*b*) Red-orange, red-violet and green.

15.21. Assume the FEMO theory to correctly predict the energies of the conjugated π electrons in benzene. Predict the values of λ at which absorption will occur for the transition between $n = 1$ and $n = 2$, which corresponds to the $(\alpha + \beta) \rightarrow (\alpha - \beta)$ transition. Assume the C—C bond length to be 1.397 Å.

Ans. $a = 6(1.397)$, $\lambda = 2m_e a^2 c/3h = 1930$ Å; $a = 2\pi(1.397)$, $\lambda = 2120$ Å; observed is 2038 Å

15.22. The total energy of the six electrons in Fig. 15-13(*a*) is $2(\alpha + 2\beta) + 4(\alpha + \beta) = 6\alpha + 8\beta$. If π orbitals were used, the energy would be $6(\alpha + \beta) = 6\alpha + 6\beta$. The difference between these descriptions is the "resonance energy" of the molecule, see Problem 3.31. Evaluate β. (This value is only an estimate because of additional energy required to make all C—C bond lengths the same and because of the assumptions made in the HMO theory.) *Ans.* -72.0 kJ mol^{-1}

15.23. Calculate the energy levels for the conjugated bonding in cyclobutadiene using (*15.15*) and prepare an energy diagram showing the ground state for C_4H_4. Repeat the calculations using the mnemonic device (Section 15.4) and compare results. Discuss the aromaticity of C_4H_4 using the $4m + 2$ rule.

Ans. $E_0 = \alpha + 2\beta$, $E_1 = E_3 = \alpha$, $E_2 = \alpha - 2\beta$, see Fig. 15-12(*b*); same results, see Fig. 15-13(*b*); diradical, which is very reactive

15.24. Using the mnemonic device (Section 15.4), sketch the ground state configurations of $C_5H_5^+$, $C_5H_5\cdot$ and $C_5H_5^-$. Which is the most stable according to the $4m + 2$ rule?

Ans. See Fig. 15-20. $C_5H_5^-$.

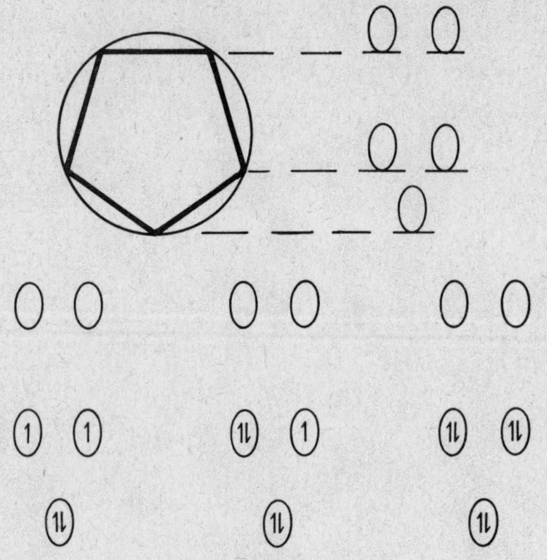

$C_5H_5^+$ $C_5H_5\cdot$ $C_5H_5^-$

Fig. 15-20

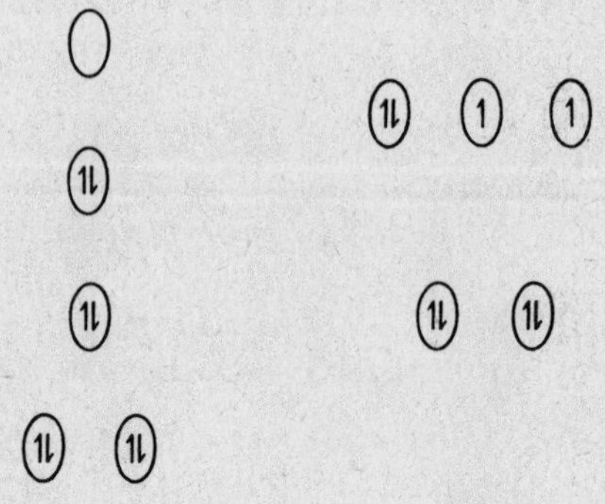

Square Planar Tetrahedral

Fig. 15-21

15.25. The bond order in naphthalene

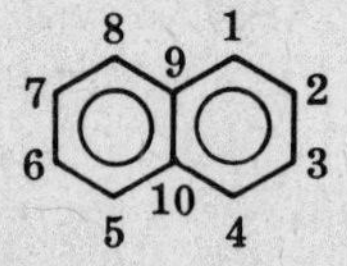

between the 1 and 2 carbons is 1.725; 2 and 3, 1.603; 1 and 9, 1.555; 9 and 10, 1.518. Determine these bond lengths. *Ans.* 1.386, 1.409, 1.418 and 1.425 Å

15.26. Find P_{rs} and r_{rs} for the 2—3 bond in 1,3-butadiene.

Ans. $C_{13} = C_{43} = 0.601$, $C_{23} = C_{33} = -0.371$, $p_{23} = 0.447, 1.447$; 1.438 Å

Coordination Compounds

15.27. Predict the configurations, the number of unpaired electrons, and the shapes of the molecules for FeF_6^{3-} and $Fe(CN)_6^{3-}$. *Ans.* See Fig. 15-4(*b*); 5 and 1; octahedral for both.

15.28. A coordination compound having a ligancy of four can be either square planar or tetrahedral. Using the CF splitting shown in Fig. 15-5, predict the configuration for $Ni(CN)_4^{2-}$ for both structures. If $Ni(CN)_4^{2-}$ is diamagnetic, which structure is correct?

Ans. See Fig. 15-21; square planar.

15.29. Prepare sketches of the electronic configurations of FeF_6^{3-}, $Fe(CN)_6^{3-}$ and $Ni(CN)_4^{2-}$ (square planar) using the crystal field splittings shown in Fig. 15-5. *Ans.* See Fig. 15-14(*d*), (*e*) and (*f*).

15.30. $Ti(H_2O)_6^{3+}$ absorbs light at 4900 Å (blue-green), corresponding to the $^2T_{2g} \rightarrow {}^2E_g$ transition shown in Fig. 15-6. Calculate the energy between these levels and predict the color of the solution containing this ion. *Ans.* 20,400 cm^{-1}; passes blue and red giving a red-violet solution

15.31. Is it possible for a sample of $Pt(NH_3)_2Cl_2$ to be polar and another sample to be nonpolar?

Ans. Yes, if the compound is square planar, the *cis*-isomer will be polar and the *trans*-isomer will be nonpolar.

15.32. Describe the bonding in a substance having the empirical formula $AgCN_2H_3$. The description should be consistent with the following properties: (1) the van't Hoff factor is 2; (2) AgCl will not precipitate if the substance is added to an aqueous solution of Cl^-; and (3) if Zn is added to a solution of this substance, two moles of Ag and one mole of $Zn(CN)_4^{2-}$ are formed for each mole of Zn added.

Ans. $Ag(NH_3)_2^+Ag(CN)_2^-$, first ion is linear with Ag—N bonds and second ion is linear with C—Ag bonds.

15.33. Sketch the molecular orbital diagram for $Co(CN)_6^{3-}$.

Ans. See the low-spin complex in Fig. 15-15(*b*).

Spatial Relationships

15.34. Identify the shapes of the following species: (*a*) H_2O_2; (*b*) $SnCl_2$; (*c*) Al_2Cl_6; (*d*) $COCl_2$; (*e*) cyanogen, NCCN; (*f*) CO_2; (*g*) NO_3^-; (*h*) PCl_5 and (*i*) $SeBr_4$.

Ans. Values of AE and NE are (*a*) 14, 14; (*b*) 18, 20; (*c*) 48, 50; (*d*) 24, 26; (*e*) 18, 26; (*f*) 16, 20; (*g*) 24, 26; (*h*) 40, 38 and (*i*) 34, 32. Lewis diagrams are given in Fig. 15-22. SN_X and shapes are (*a*) $SN_H = 1$, $SN_O = 4$, nonlinear; (*b*) $SN_{Sn} = 3$, $SN_{Cl} = 4$, bent; (*c*) $SN_{Cl} = 4$, $SN_{Al} = 4$, Al's and 4 Cl's planar with shared Cl's above and below the plane or Al's and shared Cl's planar with end Cl's above and below the plane; (*d*) $SN_C = 3$, $SN_O = 3$, $SN_{Cl} = 4$, planar and Y-shaped, (*e*) $SN_C = 2$, $SN_N = 2$, linear; (*f*) $SN_C = 2$, $SN_O = 3$, linear; (*g*) $SN_N = 3$, $SN_O = 3$ (minimum), planar and Y-shaped; (*h*) $SN_P = 5$, $SN_{Cl} = 4$, triangular bipyramidal; and (*i*) $SN_{Se} = 5$, $SN_{Br} = 4$, seesaw.

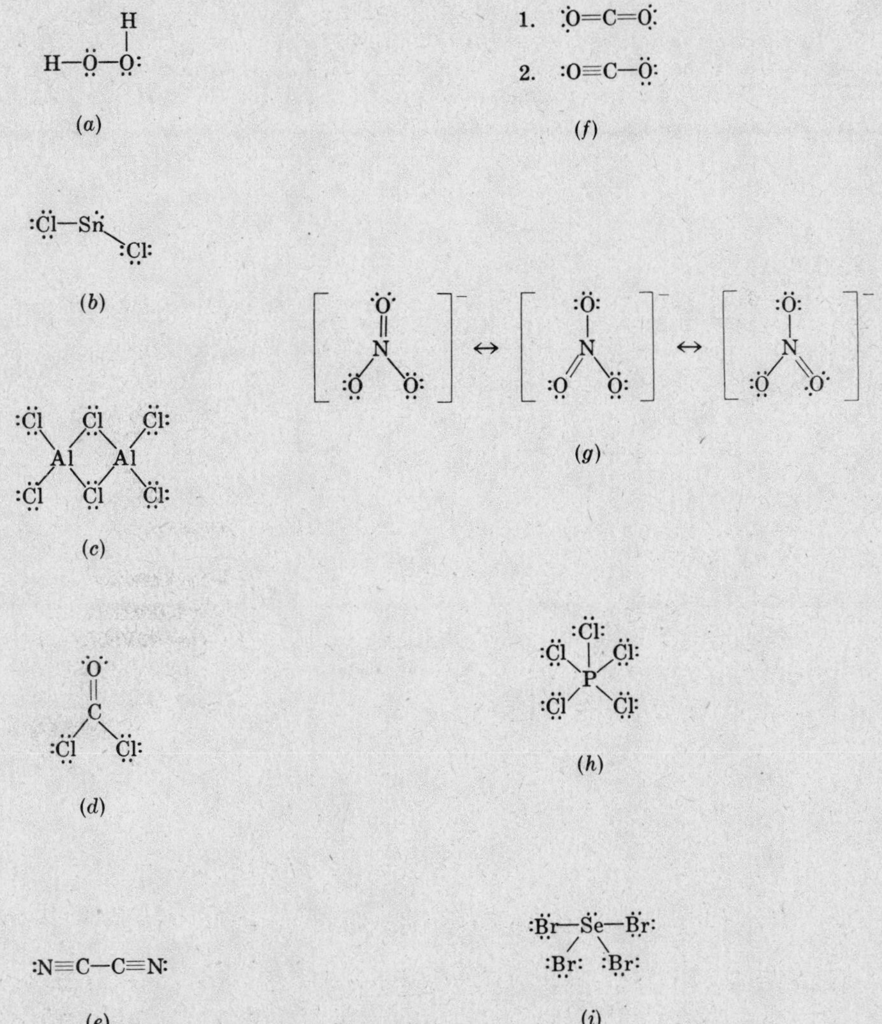

Fig. 15-22

15.35. Determine the change in the molecular geometry caused by adding a proton to NH_3 to form NH_4^+.

Ans. trigonal pyramidal to tetrahedral

15.36. Determine the molecular geometry for BrF_3 and ICl_4^-. *Ans.* T-shaped, square planar

15.37. The molecule B_2H_6 has a deficiency of two electrons from that needed for normal bonding. Experimentally the molecule is known to have two types of B—H bonding but neither can be a multiple bond. Four of the six H's may be replaced by methyl groups without breaking the molecule down. Write a Lewis structure consistent with these data and describe the geometrical shape of the molecule.

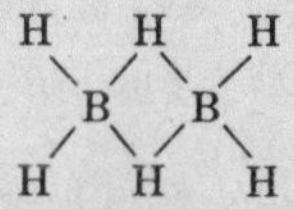

Fig. 15-23

Ans. See Fig. 15-23 and see answer to Problem 15.34(*c*).

15.38. (*a*) Determine the molecular geometry of $NO_2(g)$ assuming the unpaired electron to remain in an unhybridized atomic orbital or, alternatively, to occupy a hybrid orbital. (*b*) Which structure predicts the molecule to be paramagnetic? (*c*) Which structure predicts the molecule to be polar? (*d*) If three nondegenerate vibrational frequencies are observed, which structure is correct? (*e*) Because an unpaired electron system is very reactive, NO_2 dimerizes forming N_2O_4. Describe the molecular geometry of N_2O_4.

Ans. (*a*) linear and bent; (*b*) both; (*c*) bent; (*d*) bent; (*e*) N's bonded with very little change in N—O arrangements

15.39. Determine the molecular geometry for $Cu(H_2O)_6^{2+}$. Two of the waters of hydration (*trans* to each other) are farther from the Cu^{2+} than the other four, changing the formula to $Cu(H_2O)_4 \cdot 2H_2O^{2+}$ or $Cu(H_2O)_4^{2+}$. What is the molecular geometry for the $Cu(H_2O)_4 \cdot 2H_2O^{2+}$ and $Cu(H_2O)_4^{2+}$ ions?

Ans. octahedral; distorted octahedral or square bipyramidal; square planar

Chapter 16

Spectroscopy of Polyatomic Molecules

Rotational Spectra

16.1 MOMENTS OF INERTIA FOR A RIGID MOLECULE

The *principal moments of inertia, A, B* and *C*, for a molecule containing n atoms are the solutions for I of the determinantal equation

$$\begin{vmatrix} I_{xx}-I & -I_{xy} & -I_{xz} \\ -I_{xy} & I_{yy}-I & -I_{yz} \\ -I_{xz} & -I_{yz} & I_{zz}-I \end{vmatrix} = 0 \tag{16.1}$$

where by convention $C \geqq B \geqq A$ and

$$I_{xx} = \sum_{i=1}^{n} m_i(y_i^2 + z_i^2) \tag{16.2a}$$

$$\cdots\cdots\cdots\cdots\cdots\cdots \qquad \cdots$$

$$I_{xy} = \sum_{i=1}^{n} m_i x_i y_i \tag{16.2d}$$

$$\cdots\cdots\cdots\cdots\cdots\cdots \qquad \cdots$$

Calculations using (*16.1*) are greatly simplified if the Cartesian coordinate system used in (*16.2*) has its origin at the center of mass of the molecule. The coordinates of the center of mass of the molecule with respect to an arbitrary Cartesian coordinate system are

$$x_{\text{cm}} = \frac{\sum_{i=1}^{n} m_i x_i}{\sum_{i=1}^{n} m_i} \qquad y_{\text{cm}} = \frac{\sum_{i=1}^{n} m_i y_i}{\sum_{i=1}^{n} m_i} \qquad z_{\text{cm}} = \frac{\sum_{i=1}^{n} m_i z_i}{\sum_{i=1}^{n} m_i} \tag{16.3}$$

The location of the principal axes of inertia can often be simplified by determining the symmetry elements present in a molecule, see Chapter 17. Usually a principal axis coincides with a higher-order axis of rotation, a mirror plane contains two principal axes and is perpendicular to the third, and a center of symmetry coincides with the origin of the principal axes.

Depending on the values of the principal moments of inertia, molecules are divided into three general classes: (1) *spherical tops* where $A = B = C$, (2) *symmetrical tops* where $A < B = C$ (prolate) or $A = B < C$ (oblate), and (3) *asymmetrical tops* where $A < B < C$.

EXAMPLE 16.1. Determine the principal moments of inertia for CH_4 and classify this molecule. The C—H bond length is 1.091 Å and the H—C—H bond angle is 109°28′.

The center of mass is located at the carbon atom. In the coordinate system shown in Fig. 16-1(*a*), the coordinates of the atoms are (0, 0, 0) for C, (0, 0, 1.091) for H_1, (1.028, 0, −0.364) for H_2, (−0.514, 0.890, −0.364) for H_3 and (−0.514, −0.890, −0.364) for H_4, giving

$$\begin{aligned} I_{xx} &= m_C[(0)^2+(0)^2] + m_H[(0)^2+(1.091)^2] + m_H[(0)^2+(-0.364)^2] \\ &\qquad + m_H[(0.890)^2+(-0.364)^2] + m_H[(-0.890)^2+(-0.364)^2] \\ &= 3.172\, m_H \end{aligned}$$

$$\begin{aligned} I_{xy} &= m_C[(0)(0)] + m_H[(0)(0) + (1.028)(0) + (-0.514)(0.890) + (-0.514)(-0.890)] \\ &= 0 \end{aligned}$$

$I_{yy} = I_{zz} = 3.172\, m_H$ and $I_{xz} = I_{yz} = 0$, in units of Å².

Using (*16.1*) gives

$$\begin{vmatrix} 3.172\, m_H - I & 0 & 0 \\ 0 & 3.172\, m_H - I & 0 \\ 0 & 0 & 3.172\, m_H - I \end{vmatrix} = 0$$

and solving gives $I = A = B = C = 3.172\, m_H$ Å² $= 5.318 \times 10^{-47}$ kg m², a spherical top molecule.

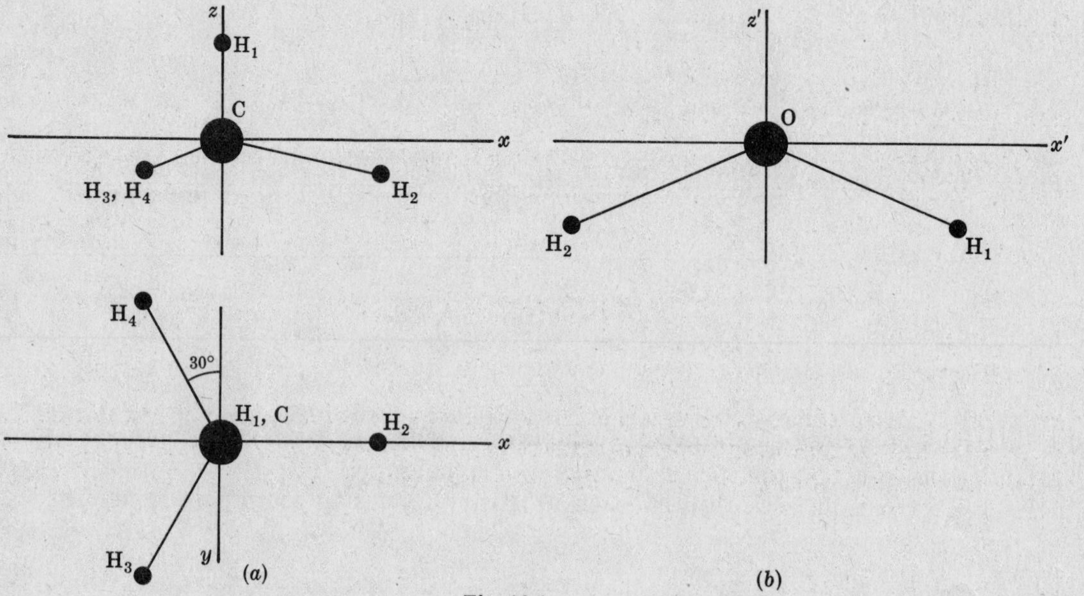

Fig. 16-1

16.2 SPHERICAL TOP MOLECULES

The rotational energy levels for a spherical top molecule are given by

$$E_J = \frac{J(J+1)\hbar^2}{2I} \tag{16.4}$$

where $J = 0, 1, 2, \ldots$. Because of the symmetry of the molecule, the rotational levels must be analyzed from Raman spectra and the infrared-active transitions.

16.3 SYMMETRICAL TOP MOLECULES

The rotational energy levels for an oblate symmetrical top are given by

$$E_{J,K} = \frac{J(J+1)\hbar^2}{2B} - K^2\hbar^2\left(\frac{1}{2B} - \frac{1}{2C}\right) \tag{16.5}$$

where $K = 0, \pm 1, \pm 2, \ldots, \pm J$. Equation (*16.5*) may be rewritten as

$$F(J,K) = B'J(J+1) - (B' - C')K^2 \tag{16.6}$$

Likewise for a prolate top

$$F(J,K) = B'J(J+1) + (A' - B')K^2 \tag{16.7}$$

In (*16.6*) and (*16.7*) the rotational constants A', B' and C' are defined, in units of s^{-1}, as

$$A' = \frac{h}{8\pi^2 A} \qquad B' = \frac{h}{8\pi^2 B} \qquad C' = \frac{h}{8\pi^2 C} \tag{16.8a}$$

and in units of cm^{-1} as

$$A' = \frac{h10^{-2}}{8\pi^2 Ac} \qquad B' = \frac{h10^{-2}}{8\pi^2 Bc} \qquad C' = \frac{h10^{-2}}{8\pi^2 Cc} \tag{16.8b}$$

The linear molecule is a special case of a prolate top with $A = 0$ and $B = C$ and will have a rotational spectrum only if it has a permanent dipole moment. The energy levels will be given by (*16.7*) where $K = 0$ and the energy diagram is similar to that given for the diatomic molecule, Fig. 11-10(*b*), with energy spacings (in Hz) of

$$\nu = 2B'(J+1) \tag{16.9}$$

16.4 ASYMMETRICAL TOP MOLECULES

The spectra and energy spacings for the rotational motion of an asymmetrical top molecule are too complex for treatment in this book.

Vibrational Spectra

16.5 DEGREES OF FREEDOM

A linear polyatomic molecule containing N atoms will have $3N - 5$ vibrational degrees of freedom and a nonlinear molecule will have $3N - 6$ degrees. These degrees of freedom can be assigned to normal modes of vibration, see Section 17.22.

16.6 INFRARED SPECTRA

Lines corresponding to

$$\bar{\nu} = G'(v_1, v_2, \ldots) - G''(v_1, v_2, \ldots) \tag{16.10}$$

where $\Delta v_i = 0, \pm 1, \pm 2, \ldots$, will be observed in the infrared only if the molecule has a permanent dipole moment or if the mode of vibration under consideration induces a dipole moment in the molecule. *Fundamental levels* are those in which all v_i are zero except one which is equal to unity. *Overtone levels* are those in which all v_i are zero except one which is greater than unity. *Combination levels* are those in which various combinations of v_i exist.

Rotational branches are present in the infrared spectra, but the analysis of the data is quite complicated.

EXAMPLE 16.2. A shorthand notation for the transitions uses a mathematical combination of the fundamentals corresponding to the transition. An advantage of this notation is that it is nearly numerically equal to the observed wave number. For example, the (000) → (010) transition in a molecule having three vibrational frequencies is represented by $\bar{\nu}_2$ and the (011) → (110) transition by $\bar{\nu}_1 - \bar{\nu}_3$. Find similar expressions for the (000) → (002), (000) → (211) and (110) → (002) transitions.

The notations for the transitions are $2\bar{\nu}_3$, $2\bar{\nu}_1 + \bar{\nu}_2 + \bar{\nu}_3$ and $2\bar{\nu}_3 - \bar{\nu}_1 - \bar{\nu}_2$, respectively.

Electron Magnetic Properties

16.7 MAGNETIC SUSCEPTIBILITY

The observed effects of a magnetic field on a material are related to the magnetic induction or flux density, B, given by

$$B = \mu H \tag{16.11}$$

where H is the magnetic field strength and μ is the magnetic permeability. The SI units of H are A m^{-1}, where 1 oersted = 79.577472 A m^{-1}; of B are T (tesla), where 1 T = 1 kg s^{-2} A^{-1} = 10^4 gauss; and of μ are H m^{-1} (henry per meter), where 1 H m^{-1} = 1 m kg s^{-2} A^{-2}. The magnetic permeability of a material is defined with reference to the permeability of a vacuum, μ_0, as

$$\mu = \mu_0(1 + X_v) \tag{16.12}$$

where $\mu_0 = 4\pi \times 10^{-7}$ m kg s^{-2} A^{-2} and X_v is the dimensionless parameter known as the *magnetic susceptibility* (or *susceptibility per unit volume* or *volume susceptibility*). Reported values of X_v having the units H m^{-1} are actually values of $\mu_0 X_v$.

Materials with negative values of X_v are called *diamagnetic*, and B in the material will be less than H in a vacuum. A diamagnetic material in a nonuniform field will move, if possible, toward the weakest region of the field and an elongated sample will have a tendency to orient itself at right angles to the the field. *Paramagnetic* materials have values of X_v greater than zero and B in these materials will be greater than H in a vacuum. A paramagnetic material in a nonuniform field will move, if possible, toward the strongest region of the field and an elongated sample will have a tendency to orient itself parallel to the field. *Ferromagnetic* materials have values of X_v that are about 1000 times the normal values for paramagnetic materials.

Although not included within the SI system, chemists still retain the quantities known as the *magnetic susceptibility per gram* (*mass magnetic susceptibility*), X_g, given by

$$X_g = \frac{X_v}{d} 10^{-3} \tag{16.13}$$

where d is the density expressed in kg m^{-3} and X_g has the units m^3 g^{-1}, and the *magnetic susceptibility per mole* (*molar magnetic susceptibility*), X_n, given by

$$X_n = X_g M \tag{16.14}$$

where M is the molecular weight expressed in g mol^{-1} and X_n has the units m^3 mol^{-1}.

The value of X_n is the sum of two terms, the *molar diamagnetic susceptibility*, $X_{n,d}$, and the *molar paramagnetic susceptibility*, $X_{n,p}$:

$$X_n = X_{n,d} + X_{n,p} \tag{16.15}$$

The value of $X_{n,d}$ for many ions is of the order of 10^{-11} to 10^{-12} m^3 mol^{-1} and it is negligible compared to $X_{n,p}$ for paramagnetic materials. For n unpaired electrons in a paramagnetic species and a Kelvin temperature T,

$$n = (1 + 7.998 \times 10^6 T X_{n,p})^{1/2} - 1 \tag{16.16}$$

Magnetic susceptibility measurements for a solute in a solution are usually made with a *Gouy balance*. The apparent mass of the sample (in g) is measured in the presence of the magnetic field of the earth, H_e, only, giving m'_e, and in the presence of an applied field of strength H_f, giving m'_f. It can be shown that

$$X_v = \frac{2g10^{-3}(m'_f - m'_e)}{A(H_f^2 - H_e^2)\mu_0} + X_{v,\text{air}} \qquad (16.17)$$

where g is the gravitational constant (in m s^{-2}) and A is the sample cross-sectional area (in m^2). Usually $X_{v,\text{air}}$ is neglected in (*16.17*) and the Gouy balance constant, $2g10^{-3}/A(H_f^2 - H_e^2)\mu_0$, is determined by standardization using $NiCl_2$(aq). The molar susceptibility of the solute is related to X_v by

$$X_n = \frac{X_v 10^{-3} + (7.20 \times 10^{-13})(d - CM)}{C} \qquad (16.18)$$

where C is the concentration in mol dm^{-3}.

16.8 ELECTRON SPIN (MAGNETIC OR PARAMAGNETIC) RESONANCE

In the presence of an external field, the degeneracy of the spin wave functions for an unpaired electron is removed, with the state having $s = -\frac{1}{2}$ taken, by convention, to be the lower energy state and the $s = +\frac{1}{2}$ state to be the higher state. Each of these states is split into $n+1$ components for each n equivalent nuclei having a nuclear spin present in the molecule. By convention, the nuclear spin states with positive spin are assumed lower than those having negative spin in the $s = -\frac{1}{2}$ state, and vice versa in the $s = +\frac{1}{2}$ state. The selection rule for allowed transitions is $\Delta M_I = 0$, where $M_I = I, I-1, \ldots, -I+1, -I$ and $I = n(1/2)$.

The intensities of the resonance peaks (as well as the nmr splittings, see Section 16.11) can be shown to be proportional to the number of combinations of nuclear spins which will create the value of M_I. An easy way to determine the relative intensities is to use Pascal's triangle of binomial coefficients, given by

n	*relative intensities*
0	1
1	1 1
2	1 2 1
3	1 3 3 1
4	1 4 6 4 1
5	1 5 10 10 5 1
6	1 6 15 20 15 6 1

(*16.19*)

where the coefficients in additional rows can be determined by adding the coefficients to the right and left of the desired coefficient in the previous row.

EXAMPLE 16.3. Describe the esr spectrum of $C_6H_6^-$.

In the presence of the field, the spin wave functions for the unpaired electron will split into two components as shown in Fig. 16-2. The six equivalent protons give $I = 6(1/2) = 3$, so that both levels are split into seven sublevels corresponding to $M_I = 3, 2, 1, 0, -1, -2$ and -3. The selection rule $\Delta M_I = 0$ gives seven equally spaced peaks having relative intensities of 1, 6, 15, 20, 15, 6 and 1 according to (*16.19*). The ^{12}C nuclei have no net nuclear spin and do not contribute to the spectrum.

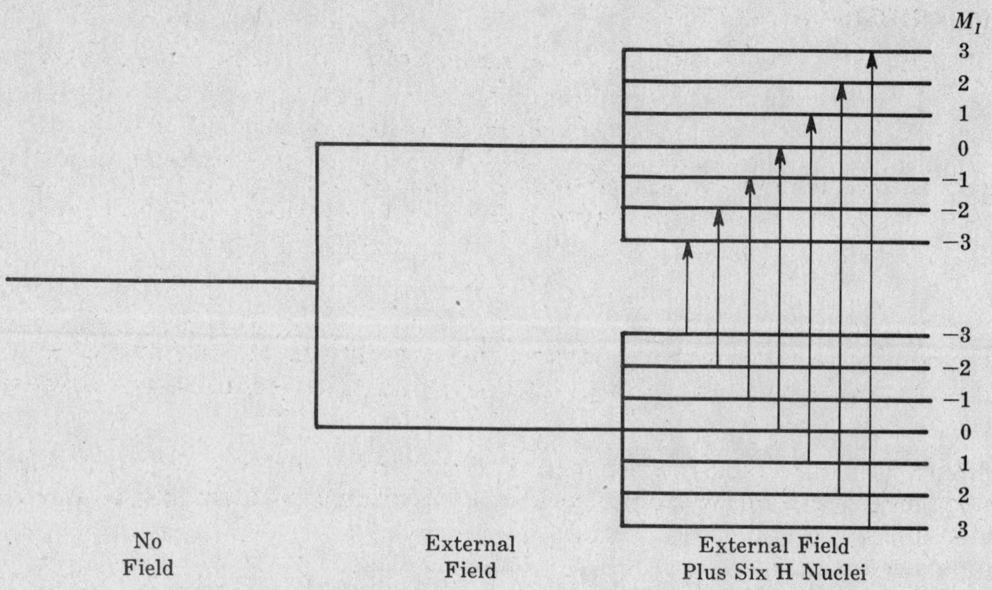

Fig. 16-2

Nuclear Magnetic Resonance

16.9 INTRODUCTION

The energy levels of an isolated nuclear magnetic moment in an applied magnetic field of flux density B_0 are given by

$$E = -g_N \beta B_0 M_I \tag{16.20}$$

where g_N is the nuclear "g factor" ($g_N = 5.5856$ for ^{1}H), $\beta = 5.050951 \times 10^{-27}$ J T^{-1}, and $M_I = I, I-1, \ldots, -I$, where I is the nuclear spin ($I = \frac{1}{2}$ for ^{1}H). The allowed transitions obey the selection rule $\Delta M_I = \pm 1$, giving for a proton

$$\nu = \frac{g_N \beta B_0}{h} \tag{16.21}$$

Sections 16.9 and 16.10 will be restricted to proton magnetic resonance, although other nuclei having nonzero spins are currently being used to identify molecular structure, e.g. ^{11}B, ^{13}C, ^{19}F.

EXAMPLE 16.4. Assuming a room temperature of 25 °C, find the ratio of protons having $-\frac{1}{2}$ spin to the number having $+\frac{1}{2}$ spin in a 14,100-gauss magnetic field (60 MHz).

Using (*16.20*) gives

$$\Delta E = -(5.5856)(5.051 \times 10^{-27}\text{ J T}^{-1})(14{,}100\text{ gauss})(10^{-4}\text{ T gauss}^{-1})\left[\left(-\frac{1}{2}\right) - \left(\frac{1}{2}\right)\right]$$
$$= 3.978 \times 10^{-26}\text{ J}$$

The Boltzmann distribution law, (*6.18*), then gives

$$\frac{N_-}{N_+} = e^{-(3.978 \times 10^{-26}\text{ J})/(1.3806 \times 10^{-23}\text{ J K}^{-1})(298\text{ K})} = e^{-9.67 \times 10^{-6}} = 0.99999033$$

where the exponential was evaluated by the approximation given in Problem 1.20. Thus, in a mole of protons, the number of protons in each level is very nearly 3.01×10^{23}. Because of the very small value of ΔE, very sensitive equipment and very low temperatures are required to obtain strong signals.

16.10 CHEMICAL SHIFTS

The magnetic flux density, B_i, at the nucleus of an atom in a chemical environment i is given by

$$B_i = B_0(1-\sigma_i) \tag{16.22}$$

where the *screening (shielding) constant* σ_i is the result of the electronic interaction of the chemical environment with the magnetic field. The frequencies of the nmr lines are given by

$$\nu = \frac{(g_N)_j(1-\sigma_i)\beta B_0}{h} \tag{16.23}$$

Thus the different values of g_N, corresponding to different nuclear species j, will produce well-separated frequencies which undergo small shifts as a result of the respective chemical environments i.

Chemical shifts occurring in organic proton nmr work are expressed relative to the absorption of a reference material such as TMS [tetramethylsilane, $Si(CH_3)_4$] by

$$\delta_i = (\sigma_{ref} - \sigma_i) \times 10^6 \text{ ppm} \tag{16.24}$$

or, in terms of an alternate scale, by

$$\tau = 10.000 - \delta_i \tag{16.25}$$

The area under each absorption peak in the spectrum is directly proportional to the number of protons having that type of chemical environment.

EXAMPLE 16.5. Predict the chemical shifts in the nmr spectrum for CH_3OH given that $\sigma_{OH} > \sigma_{CH_3}$ in a CCl_4 solution.

There will be two peaks observed, one for the proton in the OH-type environment, having a relative area of 1, and the second for the protons in the CH_3-type environment, having a relative area of 3. Because $\sigma_{OH} > \sigma_{CH_3}$, the shift will be farther away from the TMS reference for the OH than for the CH_3.

16.11 SPIN-SPIN SPLITTINGS

Under high resolution, the chemical shift peak for one type of nuclei often shows splittings resulting from magnetic fields from adjacent nuclei. For a molecule having m protons of type A and n protons of type X, generally a set of $n+1$ lines, centered about the frequency for proton type A, will appear with relative intensities as given by (*16.19*), and a set of $m+1$ lines, centered about the frequency for the proton type X, will appear with similar relative intensities.

Unless the spin-spin coupling constants are small compared to the chemical shifts, spectra of systems containing several nuclei are complex. Because chemical shifts are proportional to B_0 and spin-spin splittings are independent of B_0, a technique of simplifying the spectra is to use higher-frequency spectrometers. Changes in the coupling effected by using two radio-frequency magnetic fields superimposed on the sample (*decoupling*) or by isotopic substitution often aid in the identification of a spin-spin interaction.

EXAMPLE 16.6. Predict the splittings in the spectrum for CH_3OH.

The methyl group containing 3 protons will split the alcohol peak into 4 components, centered at the original frequency, with relative intensities of 1, 3, 3 and 1. The alcohol proton will split the methyl peak into 2 components of equal relative intensity, centered at the original methyl frequency.

Solved Problems

Rotational Spectra

16.1. Using the arbitrary Cartesian axes (x', y', z') in Fig. 16-1(*b*), determine the center of mass for water. Find the coordinates of the atoms with respect to the center of mass and calculate A, B and C. Classify the molecule. The O—H bond length is 0.9584 Å and the H—O—H bond angle is 104.45°.

The coordinates of the atoms shown in Fig. 16-1(*b*) are (in Å)

$$x'_{H_1} = (0.9584)\sin\frac{104.45°}{2} = 0.7575$$

$$y'_{H_1} = 0$$

$$z'_{H_1} = -(0.9584)\cos\frac{104.45°}{2} = -0.5871$$

$x'_{H_2} = -0.7575$, $y'_{H_2} = 0$, $z'_{H_2} = -0.5871$; and $x'_O = 0$, $y'_O = 0$, $z'_O = 0$. Substituting these into (*16.3*) gives

$$x'_{cm} = \frac{m_H(0.7575) + m_H(-0.7575) + m_O(0)}{m_H + m_H + m_O} = 0$$

$$y'_{cm} = \frac{m_H(0) + m_H(0) + m_O(0)}{m_H + m_H + m_O} = 0$$

$$z'_{cm} = \frac{m_H(-0.5871) + m_H(-0.5871) + m_O(0)}{m_H + m_H + m_O}$$

$$= \frac{2(-0.5871)(1.007825/L)}{2(1.007825/L) + 15.99491/L} = -0.0657$$

The coordinates (x, y, z) of the atoms relative to the center of mass are (in Å)

$$x_{H_1} = x'_{H_1} - x'_{cm} = 0.7575$$

$$y_{H_1} = y'_{H_1} - y'_{cm} = 0$$

$$z_{H_1} = z'_{H_1} - z'_{cm} = -0.5214$$

$x_{H_2} = -0.7575$, $y_{H_2} = 0$, $z_{H_2} = -0.5214$; and $x_O = 0$, $y_O = 0$, $z_O = 0.0657$. Substituting the latter set of coordinates into (*16.2*) gives

$$I_{xx} = (1.007825/L)[(0)^2 + (-0.5214)^2] + (1.007825/L)[(0)^2 + (-0.5214)^2] + (15.99491/L)[(0)^2 + (0.0657)^2] = (0.6168/L)\text{ g Å}^2 = 1.025 \times 10^{-47}\text{ kg m}^2$$

$$I_{yy} = 1.7736/L = 2.945 \times 10^{-47}\text{ kg m}^2$$

$$I_{zz} = 1.1566/L = 1.921 \times 10^{-47}\text{ kg m}^2$$

$$I_{xy} = m_H(0.7575)(0) + m_H(-0.7575)(0) + m_O(0)(0) = 0$$

$$I_{xz} = 0$$

$$I_{yz} = 0$$

Because the off-diagonal terms in (*16.1*) are zero, the principal moments of inertia are just I_{xx}, I_{yy} and I_{zz}; namely,

$$A = I_{xx} \qquad B = I_{zz} \qquad C = I_{yy}$$

The molecule is an asymmetrical top.

16.2. Sketch the energy levels for a prolate top molecule with $A' = 5B'$.

For the molecule *(16.7)* gives

$$F(J,K) = B'J(J+1) + 4B'K^2$$

The first few allowed terms are $F(0,0)$, $F(1,0)$, $F(1,\pm 1)$, $F(2,0)$, $F(2,\pm 1)$ and $F(2,\pm 2)$, which have values of

$$F(0,0) = B'(0)(0+1) + 4B'(0)^2 = 0$$

$$F(1,0) = B'(1)(1+1) + 4B'(0)^2 = 2B'$$

$$F(1,\pm 1) = B'(1)(1+1) + 4B'(\pm 1)^2 = 6B'$$

$6B'$, $10B'$ and $22B'$, respectively. These are plotted in Fig. 16-3(*a*) along with a few other low terms.

16.3. The rotational spectrum of HCN shows an absorption at 88,631.62 MHz and that of DCN at 72,414.61 MHz. Calculate the H—C and C—N bond lengths from these data.

Combining *(16.9)* with *(16.8)* gives

$$B = \frac{h(J+1)}{4\pi^2 \nu}$$

Thus, for the $J=0 \rightarrow J=1$ transition,

$$B_{\text{HCN}} = \frac{(6.626176 \times 10^{-34}\ \text{J s})(0+1)}{4\pi^2(8.863162 \times 10^{10}\ \text{Hz})} = 1.893715 \times 10^{-46}\ \text{kg m}^2$$

$$B_{\text{DCN}} = \frac{(6.626176 \times 10^{-34}\ \text{J s})(0+1)}{4\pi^2(7.241461 \times 10^{10}\ \text{Hz})} = 2.317806 \times 10^{-46}\ \text{kg m}^2$$

For a linear triatomic molecule it can be shown that

$$B = \frac{m_1 m_2 r_{12}^2 + m_1 m_3 r_{13}^2 + m_2 m_3 r_{23}^2}{m_1 + m_2 + m_3}$$

where $r_{13} = r_{12} + r_{23}$. Assuming that the substitution of D for H does not significantly change the H—C bond length, solving the simultaneous equations gives

$$r_{\text{HC}} = 1.068\ \text{Å} \qquad r_{\text{CN}} = 1.156\ \text{Å}$$

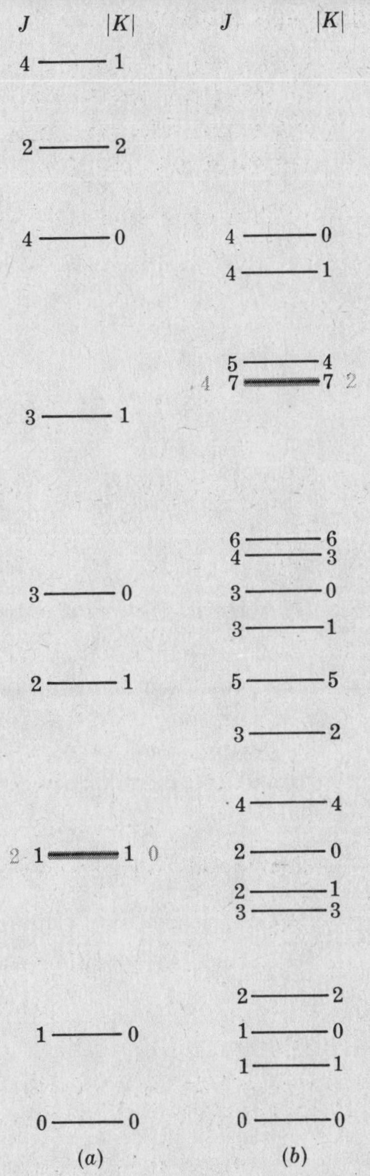

Fig. 16-3

Vibrational Spectra

16.4. Determine the number of vibrational degrees of freedom for linear and bent triatomic molecules.

For the linear molecule $3N - 5 = 4$ and for the bent molecule $3N - 6 = 3$.

16.5. Describe the structure of a triatomic molecule AB_2 which has three vibrational frequencies, two of which are in the infrared and the third of which is in the Raman spectrum.

The molecule will have four vibrational frequencies if linear and three if bent. If the molecule were *BAB* bent or *BBA* bent or linear, all three or four frequencies would be in the infrared, which is not the case; so these possibilities can be eliminated. The last possibility, linear *BAB*, will show the two infrared-active transitions for the three asymmetric modes (two are degenerate) and one Raman-active transition for the symmetric stretching mode. See Fig. 17.19.

16.6. The fundamental vibrational frequencies of H_2O are 3657.05, 1594.59 and 3755.79 cm^{-1}. Predict the energies of the absorption bands for (000) → (002), (020), (200), (021), (120), (121) and (111).

For the transition between (000) and (002), the predicted energy change is

$$\bar{\nu} = 2\bar{\nu}_3 = 2(3755.79) = 7511.58 \text{ cm}^{-1}$$

Likewise, for (000) → (121),

$$\bar{\nu} = \bar{\nu}_1 + 2\bar{\nu}_2 + \bar{\nu}_3 = 3657.05 + 2(1594.59) + 3755.79 = 10{,}602.02 \text{ cm}^{-1}$$

The remaining energy differences are 7511.58, 3189.18, 7314.10, 6944.97, 6846.23, 10,602.02 and 9007.43 cm^{-1}, respectively. These values will be high because of the anharmonicity of the potential-energy well, see Section 14.3.

Electron Magnetic Properties

16.7. A Gouy balance was calibrated at 25 °C using NiCl(aq) such that $2g10^{-3}/A(H_f^2 - H_e^2)\mu_0 = 1.05 \times 10^{-4}\text{ g}^{-1}$. A sample of 0.521 *M* $MnSO_4$ solution had an apparent mass of 10.2164 g in the magnetic field and 10.1480 g with the field removed. If the density of the solution was 1.070×10^3 kg m^{-3} and $M = 151.00$ g mol^{-1}, calculate the number of unpaired electrons on a Mn(II) ion.

If $X_{v,\text{air}}$ is neglected, (*16.17*) gives

$$X_v = (1.05 \times 10^{-4})(10.2164 - 10.1480) = 7.18 \times 10^{-6}$$

which upon substitution into (*16.18*) gives

$$X_n = \frac{(7.18 \times 10^{-6})(10^{-3}) + (7.20 \times 10^{-13})[(1.070 \times 10^3) - (0.521)(151.00)]}{0.521} = 1.515 \times 10^{-8} \text{ m}^3\text{ mol}^{-1}$$

Assuming $X_{n,d} \ll X_{n,p}$, $X_{n,p} = 1.515 \times 10^{-8}$ and (*16.16*) gives

$$n = [1 + (7.998 \times 10^6)(298)(1.515 \times 10^{-8})]^{1/2} - 1 = 5.09$$

Because n should be an integer, the answer is assumed to be 5.

16.8. The esr spectrum of a radical having the formula $C_3H_7\cdot$ showed 14 absorption peaks with relative intensities of 1, 1, 6, 6, 15, 15, 20, 20, 15, 15, 6, 6, 1 and 1. Is this an *n*-propyl or an isopropyl radical?

An *n*-propyl radical

$$CH_3—CH_2—CH_2\cdot$$

would show three peaks of intensities 1, 2 and 1, each split into three peaks of intensities 1, 2 and 1, each in turn split into 4 peaks of intensities 1, 3, 3 and 1, giving a total of 36 peaks, which does not agree with the experimental data. The isopropyl radical

$$CH_3—\dot{C}H—CH_3$$

would show two peaks of intensities 1 and 1, each split into 7 peaks of intensities 1, 6, 15, 20, 15, 6 and 1, giving a total of 14 peaks whose intensities fit the data.

Nuclear Magnetic Resonance

16.9. A low-resolution nmr spectrum of a compound having the formula $C_2H_3Cl_3$ showed two peaks, one area being twice the other. Another substance having the same formula showed only one nmr peak. Identify these substances.

The substance showing two peaks has two types of protons, giving the structure as

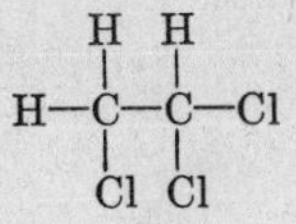

which agrees with the areas under the peaks. For the substance showing only one peak, only one type of proton is present, as indicated by the structure

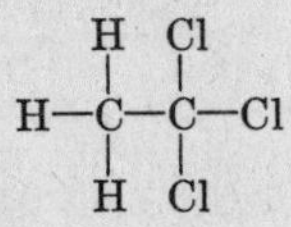

16.10. Describe the splittings in the spectrum for 1,1,1-trichloroethane.

As can be seen from the structure given in Problem 16.9, there are no protons on the carbon atom adjacent to the CH_3 group, so no splitting will occur.

Supplementary Problems

Rotational Spectra

16.11. The molecules C_6H_6 and CH_3Br are both symmetric tops. Classify these as oblate or prolate.

Ans. C_6H_6 is planar giving $A = B < C$, oblate;
CH_3Br is trigonal pyramidal giving $A < B = C$, prolate.

16.12. Determine the principal moments of inertia for H_2CO and classify this molecule. The C—H bond length is 1.12 Å, the C=O bond length is 1.21 Å, and the H—C—H angle is 118°.

Ans. $A = 3.09 \times 10^{-47}$ kg m^2, $B = 21.70 \times 10^{-47}$, $C = 24.79 \times 10^{-47}$; asymmetric top

16.13. Sketch the energy levels for an oblate top molecule with $B' = 5C'$.

Ans. See Fig. 16-3(*b*) for plot of $F(J,K) = B'J(J+1) - (4/5)B'K^2$.

16.14. The absorption spectrum of ^{16}OCS shows a peak at $24{,}325.92 \times 10^6$ Hz. Calculate B for this molecule. If $B = 147.03 \times 10^{-47}$ kg m^2 for ^{18}OCS, find r_{CO} and r_{CS}. Assume atomic weights of 15.99491 for ^{16}O, 17.9992 for ^{18}O, 12.01115 for C and 32.064 for S.

Ans. $B = 137.996 \times 10^{-47}$ kg m^2; $r_{CO} = 1.164$ Å, $r_{CS} = 1.558$ Å

Vibrational Spectra

16.15. Determine the number of vibrational degrees of freedom for CH_4. *Ans.* 9

16.16. Suppose the molecule in Problem 16.5 showed three strong infrared absorption bands. What would be the structure of AB_2? *Ans.* ABB bent or BAB bent.

16.17. The fundamental vibrational frequencies of SO_2 are 1151.38, 517.69 and 1361.76 cm^{-1}. Account for the absorption bands at 1875.55, 2295.88 and 2499.55 cm^{-1}. *Ans.* $\bar{\nu}_2 + \bar{\nu}_3$, $2\bar{\nu}_1$ and $\bar{\nu}_1 + \bar{\nu}_3$

Electron Magnetic Properties

16.18. A 0.1027 *M* solution of $KMnO_4$ had an apparent mass of 9.8059 g in a magnetic field and 9.8099 g out of the field, when placed in the Gouy balance described in Problem 16.7. Calculate the number of unpaired electrons for Mn(VII).

Ans. The sample is diamagnetic (for paramagnetic materials, $m'_f > m'_e$) and $n = 0$.

16.19. A 0.5070 *M* solution of $K_3Fe(CN)_6$ had an apparent mass of 8.0498 g both in and out of the field when placed in the Gouy balance described in Problem 16.7. The density of the solution was 1.085×10^3 kg m^{-3} and the molecular weight of the solute is 329.25 g mol^{-1}. Is CN^- a strong or weak ligand?

Ans. $X_v = 0$, $X_n = 1.304 \times 10^{-9}$ m^3 mol^{-1}, $n \approx 1$. A low-spin complex is formed by a strong ligand.

16.20. Describe the esr spectrum of $CH_3\cdot$.

Ans. four equally spaced peaks of relative intensities 1, 3, 3 and 1
($M_I = 3/2 \rightarrow 3/2$, $1/2 \rightarrow 1/2$, $-1/2 \rightarrow -1/2$ and $-3/2 \rightarrow -3/2$)

16.21. An esr spectrum for an organic radical containing two carbons consisted of 12 lines having relative intensities of 1, 2, 3, 1, 6, 3, 3, 6, 1, 3, 2 and 1. What is the radical?

Ans. $CH_3CH_2\cdot$ because CH_3-splitting gives 4 peaks with intensities 1 : 3 : 3 : 1 and CH_2-splitting gives 3(4) = 12 peaks with intensities (1 : 2 : 1)(1 : 3 : 3 : 1).

16.22. The esr spectrum of the naphthalene anion consists of 25 lines. Show that this corresponds to the structure given in Problem 15.25. What are the relative intensities of these peaks?

Ans. H's on the 4α carbons give 5 peaks and on the 4β carbons give 5 peaks, 25 peaks total; 4 at intensity 1, 8 at 4, 4 at 6, 4 at 16, 4 at 24, and 1 at 36.

Nuclear Magnetic Resonance

16.23. Given that magnetic field strength is directly proportional to applied frequency, repeat Example 16.4 at 100 MHz and liquid nitrogen temperatures (−195° C). *Ans.* $e^{-6.16 \times 10^{-5}} = 0.9999384$

16.24. Predict the major components of the nmr spectrum for CH_3CHO given that $\sigma_{CHO} > \sigma_{CH_3}$ in a CCl_4 solution.

Ans. Two groups of peaks, CHO farther from TMS with area 1 and CH_3 nearer to TMS with area 3.

16.25. Discuss the splittings in the nmr spectrum peaks described in Problem 16.24.

Ans. CH_3 is doublet (1 and 1 relative intensities) and CHO is quartet (1, 3, 3 and 1 relative intensities).

16.26. A compound having the formula $C_4H_{10}O$ gave an nmr spectrum consisting of two groups of lines with relative areas of 3 and 2. Another substance with the same formula gave an nmr spectrum consisting of two lines with relative areas of 9 and 1. Identify these substances.

Ans. diethyl ether, *t*-butyl alcohol

16.27. Describe the splittings in the spectrum for 1,1,2-trichloroethane.

Ans. triplet (1, 2, 1 intensities) and doublet (1 and 1 intensities)

16.28. In ethanol, σ_{CH_2} is between σ_{OH} and σ_{CH_3}. How many lines will be observed for each peak in the nmr spectrum? *Ans.* CH_3 peak is 3, OH peak is 3 and CH_2 peak is 8.

Chapter 17

Symmetry and Group Theory

Symmetry Operations and Elements

17.1 INTRODUCTION

Several types of *symmetry elements* are used to describe the symmetry present in molecules and crystals. These include the identity element, axes of proper rotation, a center of inversion, mirror planes, and axes of improper rotation (rotoreflection and rotoinversion)—although not all of these elements are necessarily present in a given case. Associated with each of these elements is a *symmetry operation* which transforms the molecule or crystal into a configuration indistinguishable from the original configuration. The additional operation of translation is permitted in crystallography, which upon combination with the operations of proper rotation or reflection across a mirror plane generates the operations corresponding to the screw axis and glide plane elements, respectively.

There are two systems of symbols for representing symmetry elements: the *Schönflies system,* which is used primarily for molecular geometry and group theory, and the *Hermann-Mauguin system,* which is used in crystallography. The basic symmetry operation corresponding to a symmetry element is represented by putting a caret over the Schönflies symbol for that element; a superscript 1, 2, 3, ... is added to denote the symmetry operation equivalent to 1, 2, 3, ... repetitions of the basic operation (the superscript 1 is seldom used). An operation is called *distinct* if the equivalent position generated for the molecule or crystal cannot be generated in another way which is less complicated.

EXAMPLE 17.1. Describe the symmetry elements found in the letter M.

There are four operations which generate a configuration that is indistinguishable from the original letter: (1) if the letter is rotated by 180° out of and into the plane of the paper around the axis shown in Fig. 17-1(*a*), an equivalent letter is formed—thus an axis of proper rotation is present, see Section 17.3; (2) if a plane is constructed perpendicular to the plane of the letter as shown in Fig. 17-1(*b*) and the various parts of the letter "reflected", an equivalent letter is formed—thus a mirror plane is present, see Section 17.5; (3) the plane of the letter [Fig. 17-1(*c*)] is, by the same reasoning, a mirror plane; (4) if the letter is simply left alone, an equivalent letter is certainly obtained—thus the identity element is present, see Section 17.2.

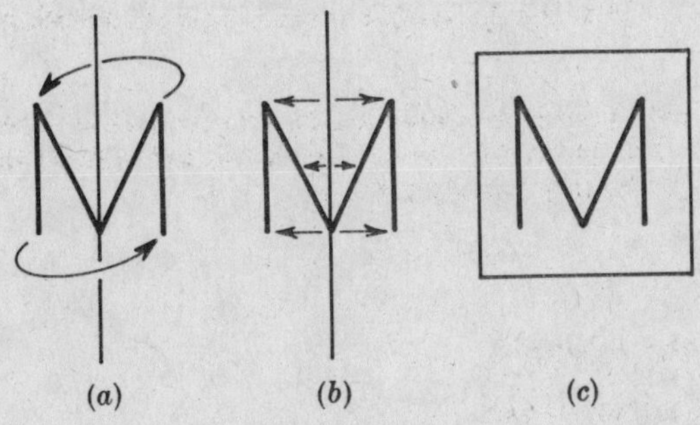

Fig. 17-1

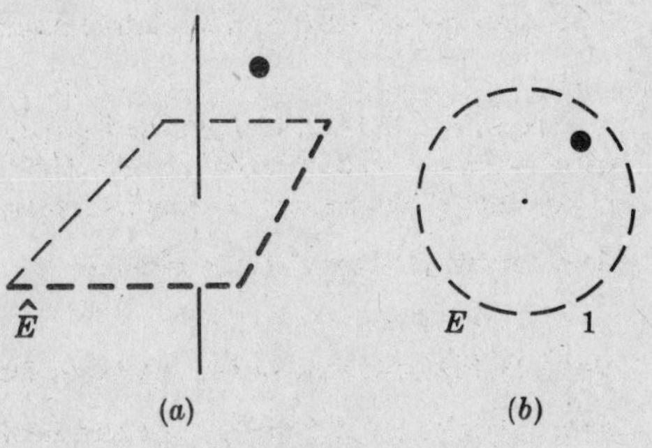

Fig. 17-2

17.2 IDENTITY

The identity element is always present in a molecule or crystal by virtue of the motif's being itself. The corresponding symmetry operation is the operation in which nothing is moved. The Schönflies symbols E and $\hat{E}$ represent the element and the operation, respectively, and the Hermann-Mauguin symbol for the element is 1. Although trivial in concept, the identity operation is important as a limit for the repetitions of a given operation (see Example 17.3).

EXAMPLE 17.2. To help in understanding an operation or to illustrate the relationship of crystal faces or atoms in a molecule around a symmetry element, perspective sketches and/or orthographic projections can be prepared. In a perspective sketch a rhombus represents a plane perpendicular to the page and a line represents an axis which is perpendicular to this plane (and lies in the plane of the page). The crystal face or atom is represented by a motif, usually a point or an asymmetrical figure like a 2, which is drawn in a general position above the plane and off the axis. The perspective sketch in Fig. 17-2(*a*) illustrates the identity operation.

The orthographic projection is essentially a top view of a perspective sketch with the axis shown as a dot and the plane as a dashed circle. A point or motif above the plane is indicated by a solid dot or solid motif, and below the plane by a cross or dashed motif. Figure 17-2(*b*) is an orthographic projection illustrating both the result of the identity operation and the distribution of points (in this case, one point) around the identity element.

17.3 AXIS OF PROPER ROTATION

The basic operation corresponding to the element C_n (Schönflies) or n (Hermann-Mauguin) consists in rotating the motif around the axis (by convention, counterclockwise as viewed in the orthographic projection) by an angle of $2\pi/n$ and generating the motif in the new location. The various operations are represented in the Schönflies notation by $\hat{C}_n^k$ and generate a total of n equivalent crystal faces or positions of atoms around the element. The axis for which n is largest is chosen as the z-axis of a Cartesian coordinate system and is known as the *principal rotation axis*.

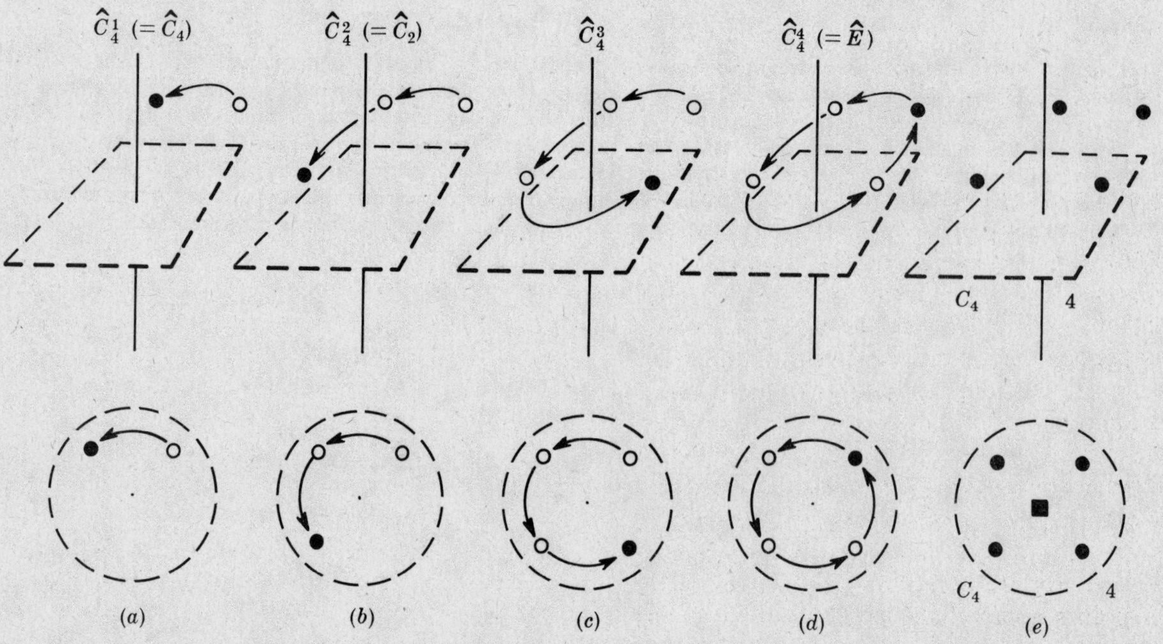

Fig. 17-3

EXAMPLE 17.3. Make perspective and orthographic drawings for $\hat{C}_4^k$. Identify the distinct operations. Prepare similar diagrams illustrating the complete set of equivalent positions for the C_4 (or 4) element.

The basic operation consists in rotating the motif around the axis by an angle of $2\pi/4 = 90°$ from the original point. The required sketches for $1 \leq k \leq 4$ are shown in Fig. 17-3. No new locations are generated for values of $k > 4$, so these values of k need not be considered. Because $\hat{C}_4^4 = \hat{C}_1 = \hat{E}$ and $\hat{C}_4^2 = \hat{C}_2^1$, these operations are not distinct; but the operations $\hat{C}_4^1$ and $\hat{C}_4^3$ generate points in locations that cannot be generated in a less complex manner and are distinct.

The symmetry element C_4 or 4 will have about it all four of the points generated by the above operations, see Fig. 17-3(*e*). Note that the planar shapes ●, ⬮, ▲, ■, etc., are used to describe the appropriate axes in the figures.

17.4 CENTER OF SYMMETRY AND INVERSION

The basic inversion operation corresponding to i (Schönflies) or $\bar{1}$ (Hermann-Mauguin) consists in projecting a motif equidistant through a center of symmetry located at the point of intersection between the plane and the axis used in the orthographic and perspective drawings, see Fig. 17-4(*a*). If this element appears in a molecule or crystal, the two equivalent points will be related as shown in Fig. 17-4(*b*).

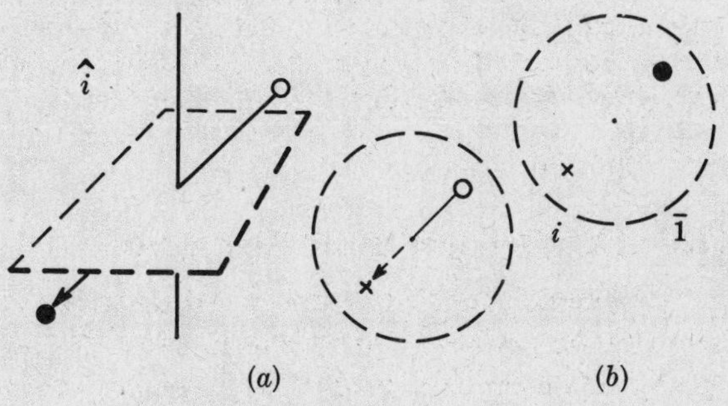

Fig. 17-4

17.5 MIRROR PLANE

The basic reflection operation corresponding to the element σ (Schönflies) or m (Hermann-Mauguin) consists in creating a mirror image of a motif equidistant from and perpendicular to a plane. If the mirror plane is perpendicular to or contains the principal axis of rotation, the respective Schönflies symbols are σ_h and σ_v. The drawings usually indicate the σ_h plane by a solid figure, see Fig. 17-5(*a*). If the mirror plane is perpendicular to or contains any n-fold axis of rotation, the respective Hermann-Mauguin symbols are n/m and m. The Schönflies symbol σ_d means a σ_v which bisects the angle formed by two C_2 axes which lie in a plane perpendicular to the axis. Figure 17-5(*b*) shows the operation $\hat{\sigma}_v$ and Fig. 17-5(*c*) shows the distribution of points about the σ_h $(= 1/m)$ and σ_v $(= m)$ elements.

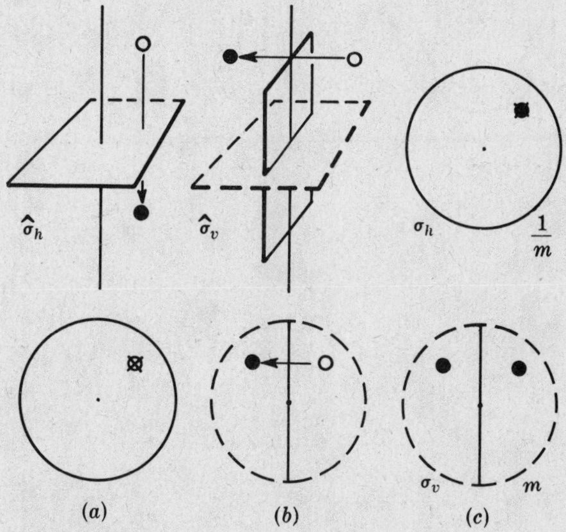

Fig. 17-5

17.6 ROTOREFLECTION

The basic operation corresponding to the element S_n (Schönflies) or $\tilde{n}$ (Hermann-Mauguin, pronounced "tilde-n") consists in a rotation about an axis through $2\pi/n$ (i.e. $\hat{C}_n$) and a reflection through a plane perpendicular to the axis (i.e. $\hat{\sigma}_h$), in either order. For some values of n, the operation $\hat{S}_n^k$ will not produce the same result as $\hat{E}$ until $k = 2n$. Rotoreflection operations are much used in describing molecular geometry, whereas a second method of generating the same distribution of points in space—rotoinversion—is used extensively by crystallographers. Unshaded geometrical figures are used to represent S_n axes. Combination figures may appear; e.g. ◩, which indicates coincident S_4 and C_2 axes.

EXAMPLE 17.4. Prepare perspective and orthographic drawings for $\hat{S}_1^k$, $\hat{S}_2^k$ and $\hat{S}_4^k$. Prepare orthographic projections for the equivalent positions found around the elements S_1, S_2 and S_4.

The basic operation for S_1 consists in rotating the point 360° and reflecting it through the orthographic plane, see Fig. 17-6(*a*). The operation performed twice, $\hat{S}_1^2$, generates the original point, see Fig. 17-6(*b*). Because $\hat{S}_1 = \hat{\sigma}_h$ and $\hat{S}_1^2 = \hat{E}$, these operations are not distinct.

The diagrams in Fig. 17-6(*c*) illustrate $\hat{S}_2^1$, $\hat{S}_2^2$ and $\hat{S}_4^1$, $\hat{S}_4^2$, $\hat{S}_4^3$, $\hat{S}_4^4$. Figure 17-6(*d*) illustrates the complete set of equivalent faces present in a crystal, or atoms found in a molecule, that contains the S_1, S_2 or S_4 element.

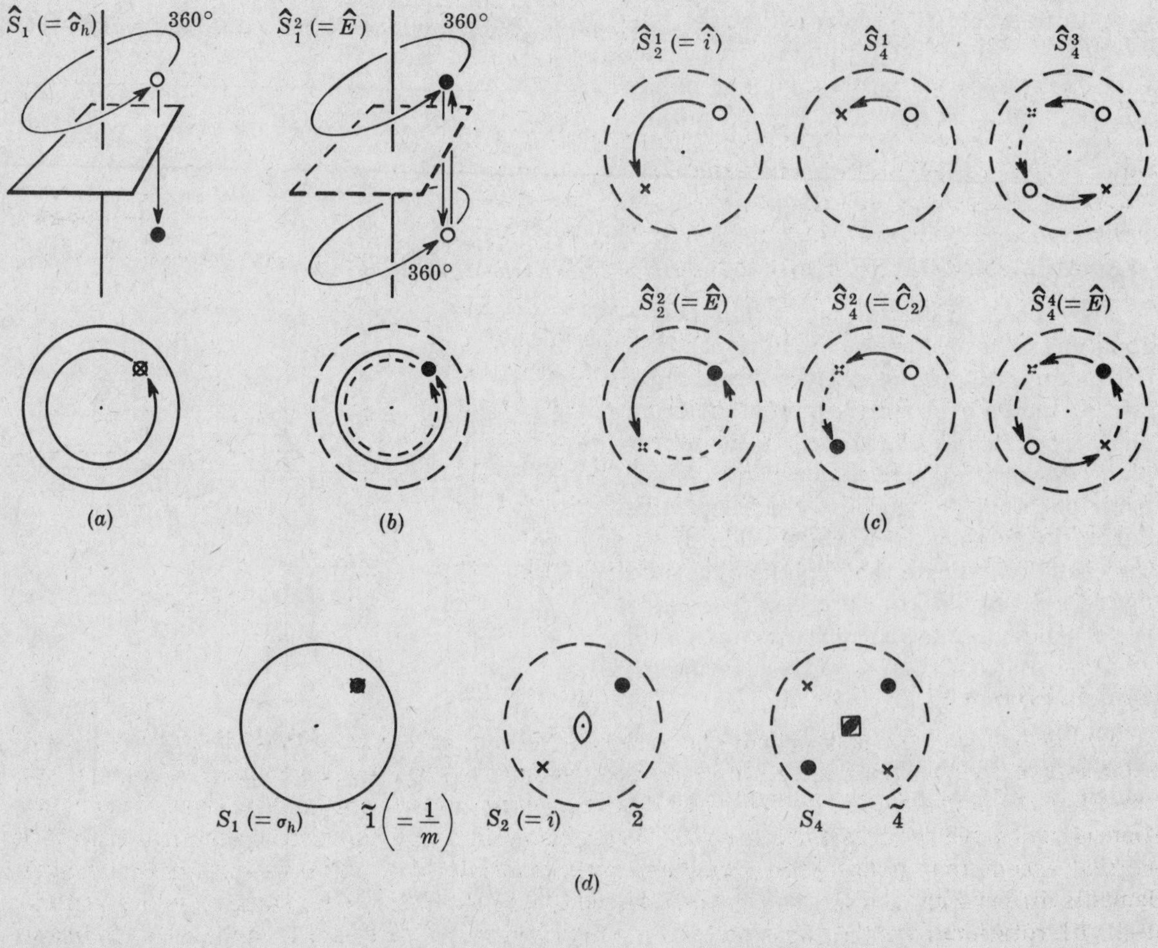

Fig. 17-6

17.7 ROTOINVERSION

The basic operation corresponding to $\bar{n}$ (Hermann-Mauguin only, pronounced "n-bar" or "bar-n") consists in a rotation about an axis through $2\pi/n$ (i.e. $\hat{C}_n$) and an inversion through the point of intersection between the plane and the axis used in the orthographic and perspective drawings (i.e. $\hat{i}$), in either order. For a system containing the $\bar{n}$ element, there will be n or $2n$ points alternating above and below the orthographic projection plane.

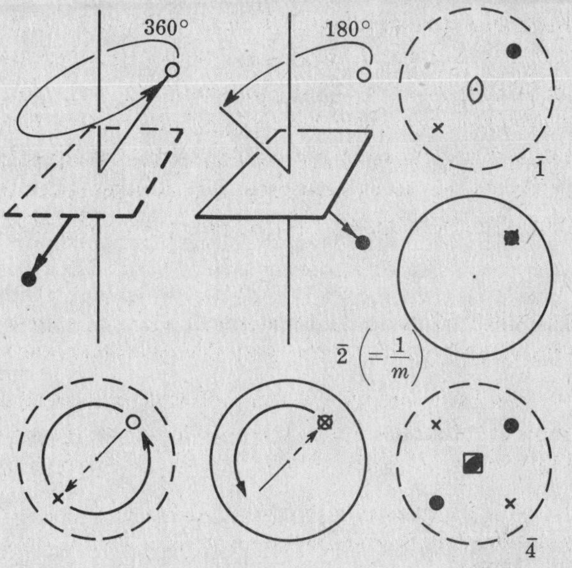

(a) (b)

Fig. 17-7

EXAMPLE 17.5. Prepare drawings for $\bar{1}$, $\bar{2}$ and $\bar{4}$ to determine the equivalences between $\bar{n}$ and $\tilde{n}$ where $n = 1, 2$ and 4.

The basic operations corresponding to $\bar{1}$ and $\bar{2}$ are shown in Fig. 17-7(*a*) and the complete sets of points for the three rotoinversion elements are shown in Fig. 17-7(*b*). Upon comparison of these latter figures with Fig. 17-6(*d*), it is obvious that $\bar{1} = \tilde{2}$, $\bar{2} = \tilde{1}$ and $\bar{4} = \tilde{4}$.

17.8 TRANSLATION

The translational operation is the movement of a motif along a straight line and the construction of its image at a distance t from the original position, see Fig. 17-8(*a*). If the operation is continued a large number of times, a one-dimensional array of points (commonly called a *row*) is generated. Just as the various rotation, reflection and inversion operations are performed until the result of $\hat{E}$ is generated, the various operations involving translation are continued until a motif in a position similar to the original at some multiple of the distance t is generated. The distance t is chosen (anticipating the discussion of unit cells given in Section 19.1) such that it contains the points necessary to generate the entire row of points by placing several of these line segments end to end, see Fig. 17-8(*b*).

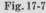

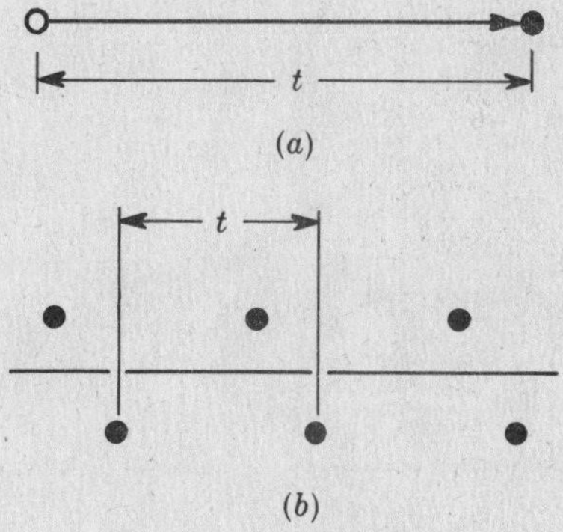

Fig. 17-8

17.9 SCREW AXIS

The basic operation corresponding to the element n_k (Hermann-Mauguin only), where k is an integer, consists in a rotation by $2\pi/n$ about an axis (by convention, clockwise as viewed in the orthographic projection) and a translation by kt/n, in either order. This operation is continued n times until a motif is generated in a position that is identical with the original except that it has been translated by a multiple of t. The permitted screw axis elements in crystals are 2_1; 3_1, 3_2; 4_1, 4_2, 4_3; and 6_1, 6_2, 6_3, 6_4, 6_5. The planar symbols associated with rotational axes in the drawings are modified with "tails" for screw axes to indicate the effective direction of rotation.

EXAMPLE 17.6. Prepare perspective and orthographic drawings for 4_1 and 4_2.

The basic operation associated with 4_1 is a rotation by $2\pi/4 = 90°$ and a translation by $t/4$. By continuing the operation four times, a motif is generated in a position similar to the original at a distance t; thus the set of points shown in Fig. 17-9(*a*) is generated. If the orthographic plane is placed at t, the projection shown in Fig. 17-9(*a*) results, where the fractions represent the distances in fractions of t between the points and the plane.

The basic operation corresponding to 4_2 is rotation by 90° and translation by $2t/4 = t/2$. This operation must be continued four times, covering a distance of $2t$, before generating a motif in a similar position to the original, see Fig. 17-9(*b*). Because all points must be contained within a distance t (i.e. must keep within the unit cell), the positions generated by the various operations are transformed to positions within the permitted length by subtraction of suitable integral multiples of t. This is shown by the double-headed arrows in Fig. 17-9(*b*). The rather messy working diagram is usually simplified to that shown on the right of Fig. 17-9(*b*), which apparently illustrates the operation 2_1 performed on a pair of points. Assuming the orthographic plane to pass through $t/2$, the projection shown in Fig. 17-9(*b*) results.

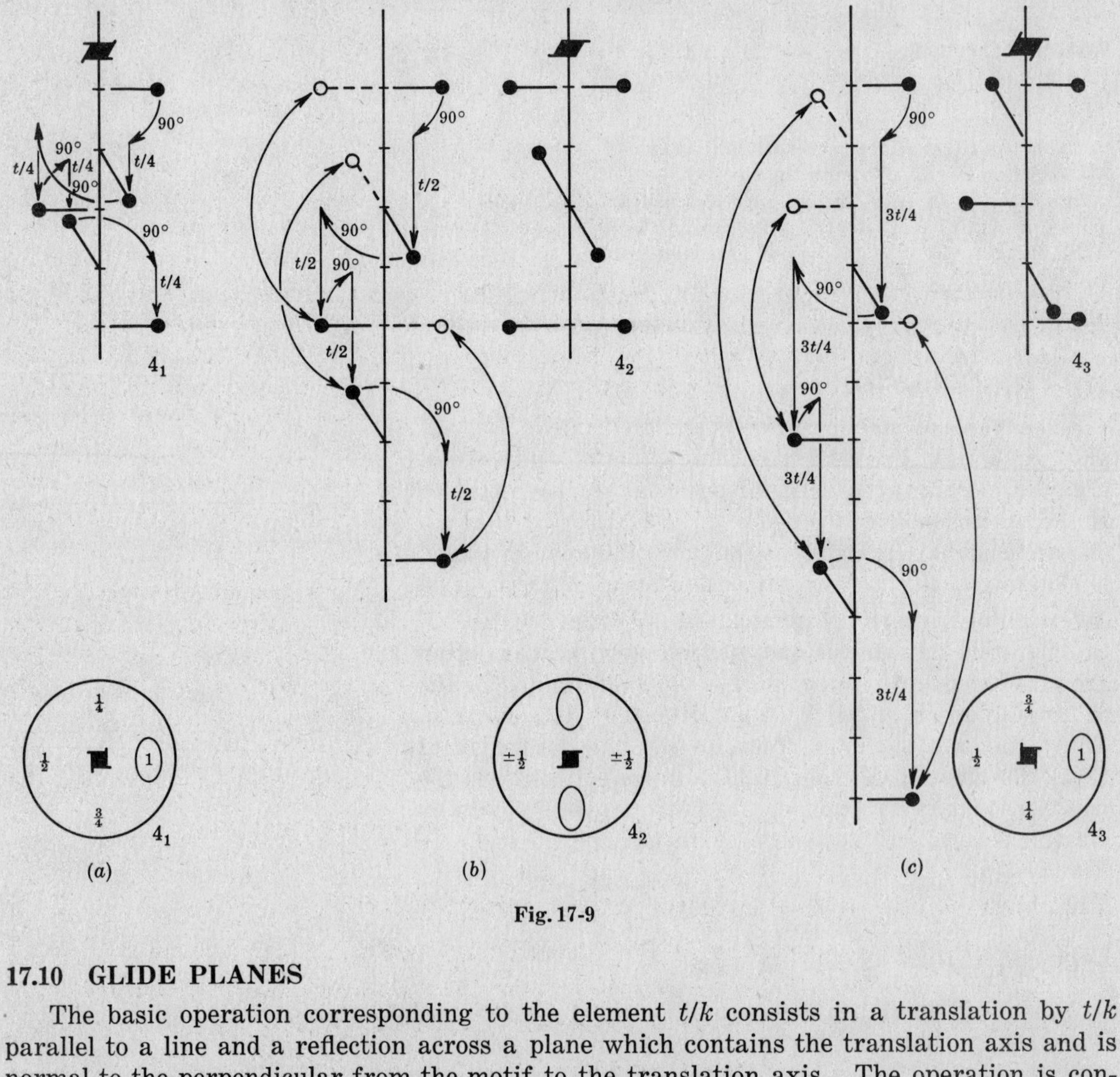

Fig. 17-9

17.10 GLIDE PLANES

The basic operation corresponding to the element t/k consists in a translation by t/k parallel to a line and a reflection across a plane which contains the translation axis and is normal to the perpendicular from the motif to the translation axis. The operation is continued until a motif is generated in a similar position to the original at some multiple of t. The three classifications of glide planes permitted in crystals are (1) an *axial glide* along an axis of the crystal, $t/2$; (2) a *diagonal glide*, which occurs in the plane containing two axes of the crystal, $t_1/2 + t_2/2$; and (3) a *diamond glide*, which is a three-dimensional operation, $t_1/4 + t_2/4$.

EXAMPLE 17.7. Find the relationship between $t/2$ and 2_1.

The perspective sketches of the location of all points around these elements are shown in Fig. 17-10. The symmetry operations used to generate these points are shown in dashed lines. Since the two elements have identical points, $t/2 = 2_1$.

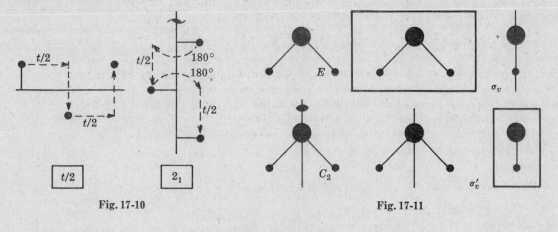

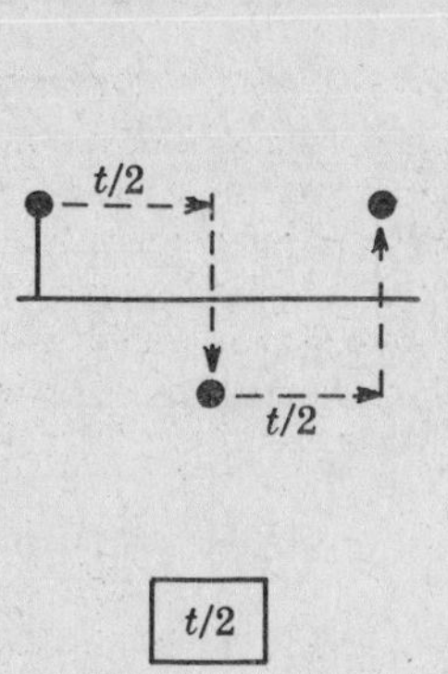

Fig. 17-10

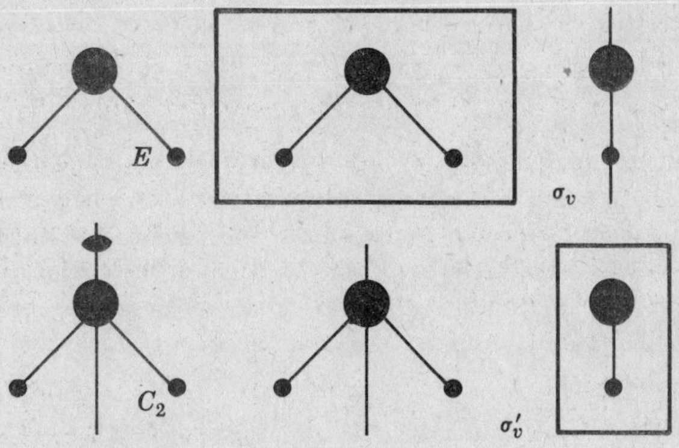

Fig. 17-11

Point Groups

17.11 CONCEPT

Usually more than one symmetry element is present in a molecule or crystal. The set of all symmetry elements (or their representative operations) present in a physical system is called a *group*. If the set includes no elements involving translation (namely t, n_k and t/k), a *point group* is formed. For crystals, only the rotational values $n = 1, 2, 3, 4$ and 6 are permitted, and 32 *crystallographic point groups* are generated. If all symmetry operations possible in crystals are considered, 230 *space groups* result. The Schönflies symbol for a group is a script or boldface letter similar to the notation for the symmetry elements and the Hermann-Mauguin representation is simply a combination of symbols (up to three) for the symmetry elements present in that group.

A number and a symbol in a listing of the various elements in a group represents the number of elements of that type that are related by other symmetry operations in the group, and if these elements need to be identified, alphanumeric subscripts are used. Similar elements that are not related by other symmetry operations in the group are listed separately and are differentiated by primes or parentheses containing orientation information.

EXAMPLE 17.8. Consider a molecule of water (nonlinear). Determine the symmetry elements present.

Figure 17-11 shows that the elements E, C_2 and two types of σ_v are present.

17.12 MATHEMATICAL PROPERTIES OF A POINT GROUP

1. If $\hat{A}$ and $\hat{B}$ are symmetry operations in the group, then $\hat{A} \times \hat{B} = \hat{F}$, where $\hat{F}$ is also a symmetry operation in the group. The product $\hat{A} \times \hat{B}$ means that operation $\hat{B}$ is performed and then operation $\hat{A}$ is performed on the result. In general, $\hat{A} \times \hat{B} \neq \hat{B} \times \hat{A}$.
2. The group contains an identity operation $\hat{E}$ such that $\hat{A} \times \hat{E} = \hat{E} \times \hat{A} = \hat{A}$ for every $\hat{A}$ in the group.
3. For every operation $\hat{A}$ in the group there exists an inverse operation $\hat{A}^{-1}$ in the group, such that $\hat{A}^{-1} \times \hat{A} = \hat{A} \times \hat{A}^{-1} = \hat{E}$.
4. The associative law, $\hat{A} \times (\hat{B} \times \hat{C}) = (\hat{A} \times \hat{B}) \times \hat{C}$, holds.

EXAMPLE 17.9. Prepare the multiplication table for the group of distinct symmetry operations in water: $\hat{E}$, $\hat{C}_2$, $\hat{\sigma}_v$ and $\hat{\sigma}_v'$. Find $\hat{C}_2^{-1}$.

The first step is to make projections of the known distinct operations, see Fig. 17-12. Always place the motif in a general position in these projections, so that a complete set of results can be obtained. The second step is to construct orthographic projections for the various multiplications, except for those involving $\hat{E}$, see Fig. 17-13. The third step is to prepare a table with the operations $\hat{A}$ listed at the left, the operations $\hat{B}$ listed at the top, and the products $\hat{F}$ listed within the table, see Table 17-1. By inspection of Table 17-1, $\hat{C}_2^{-1} = \hat{C}_2$ because $\hat{C}_2 \times \hat{C}_2 = \hat{E}$. The group specified by Table 17-1 is designated C_{2v} in the Schönflies system.

Table 17-1

C_{2v}	$\hat{E}$	$\hat{C}_2$	$\hat{\sigma}_v$	$\hat{\sigma}_v' = \hat{B}$
$\hat{A} = \hat{E}$	$\hat{E}$	$\hat{C}_2$	$\hat{\sigma}_v$	$\hat{\sigma}_v'$
$\hat{C}_2$	$\hat{C}_2$	$\hat{E}$	$\hat{\sigma}_v'$	$\hat{\sigma}_v$
$\hat{\sigma}_v$	$\hat{\sigma}_v$	$\hat{\sigma}_v'$	$\hat{E}$	$\hat{C}_2$
$\hat{\sigma}_v'$	$\hat{\sigma}_v'$	$\hat{\sigma}_v$	$\hat{C}_2$	$\hat{E}$

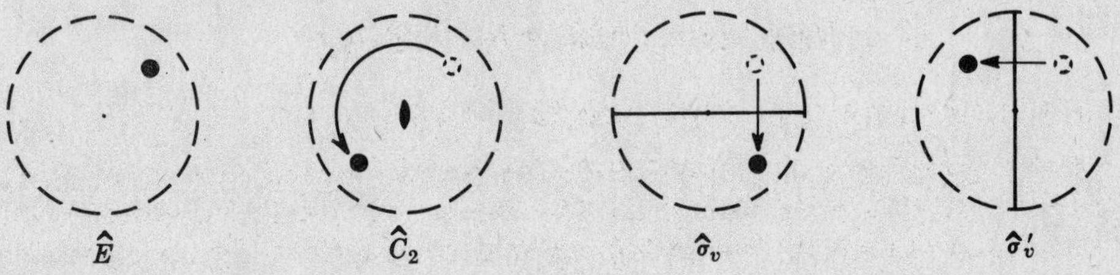

Fig. 17-12

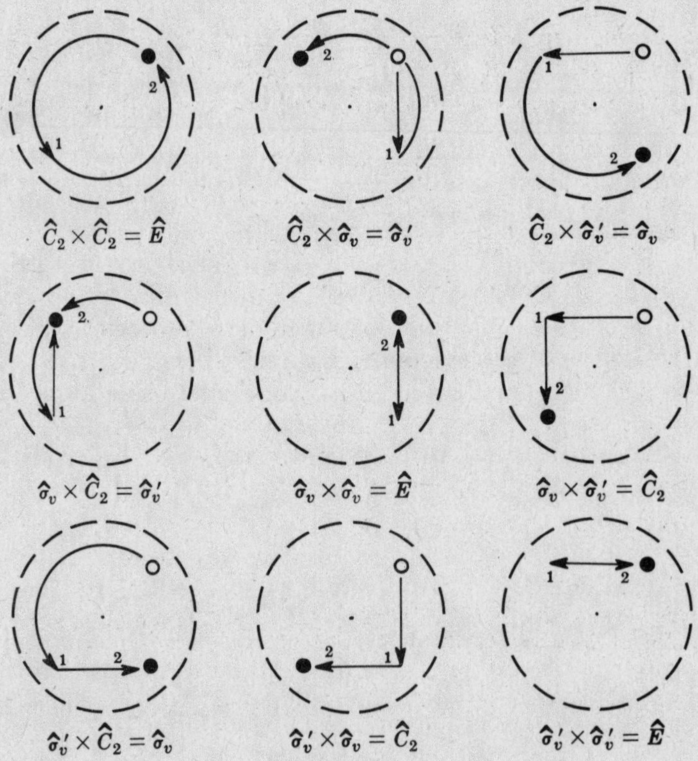

Fig. 17-13

17.13 DETERMINATION OF A POINT GROUP

Once the symmetry elements have been identified, the point group to which a molecule belongs can be determined using the flow chart given in Fig. 17-14. The symmetry elements contained in the point groups are summarized in Table 17-2. In a macroscopic crystal, screw axes and glide planes appear as axes of proper rotation and mirror planes, respectively, and Fig. 17-14 can be used to determine which of the 32 possible crystallographic point groups pertains. This assignment will agree with that for the unit cell of the crystal (Section 19.1) if the macroscopic crystal displays all the symmetry elements present in the unit cell.

EXAMPLE 17.10. Determine the point group for water (see Fig. 17-11).

Using Fig. 17-14, the following analysis can be made: (1) are there ∞ C_∞ axes present? no; (2) is there a pentagonal dodecahedron or icosahedron present? no; (3) are there four C_3 axes at 50°44′? no; (4) is there at least one C_n where $n \geq 2$? yes, C_2; (5) is there an S_{2n} present? no; (6) are there n C_2 axes perpendicular to C_n? no; (7) are there any σ_h planes present? no; (8) are there n σ_v planes present? yes, 2, therefore C_{2v}.

Representation of Groups

17.14 MATRIX EXPRESSIONS FOR OPERATIONS

If the distinct operations of a group are considered to form the point group, many results can be derived abstractly which are universally applicable to any molecule or crystalline unit cell that is found in that group. For example, all nonlinear molecules having the formula AB_2 (e.g. NO_2, H_2O, SO_2) can be shown to have identical modes of intramolecular vibration by using group theory.

Each operation contained in a point group can be expressed in matrix form, see Table 17-3, such that the matrix will serve as well as the original operator in performing coordinate transformations, producing a valid multiplication table for the group, etc.

Table 17-3

$$\hat{E} \longrightarrow \begin{pmatrix} 1 & 0 & 0 \\ 0 & 1 & 0 \\ 0 & 0 & 1 \end{pmatrix} \qquad \hat{C}_n(z)^m \longrightarrow \begin{pmatrix} \cos(2\pi m/n) & -\sin(2\pi m/n) & 0 \\ \sin(2\pi m/n) & \cos(2\pi m/n) & 0 \\ 0 & 0 & 1 \end{pmatrix}$$

$$\hat{i} \longrightarrow \begin{pmatrix} -1 & 0 & 0 \\ 0 & -1 & 0 \\ 0 & 0 & -1 \end{pmatrix} \qquad \hat{S}_n(z)^m \longrightarrow \begin{pmatrix} \cos(2\pi m/n) & -\sin(2\pi m/n) & 0 \\ \sin(2\pi m/n) & \cos(2\pi m/n) & 0 \\ 0 & 0 & -1 \end{pmatrix} \quad \text{for odd } m$$

$$\hat{\sigma}_h \longrightarrow \begin{pmatrix} 1 & 0 & 0 \\ 0 & 1 & 0 \\ 0 & 0 & -1 \end{pmatrix} \qquad \hat{\sigma}_v \longrightarrow \begin{pmatrix} \cos 2\beta & \sin 2\beta & 0 \\ \sin 2\beta & -\cos 2\beta & 0 \\ 0 & 0 & 1 \end{pmatrix} \quad \beta = \text{angle between } \sigma_v \text{ and the } x\text{-axis}$$

EXAMPLE 17.11. Consider the symmetry elements for the C_{2v} point group displayed in Fig. 17-15. Show that in the given coordinate system the matrix expression for $\hat{\sigma}_v$ is

$$\begin{pmatrix} 1 & 0 & 0 \\ 0 & -1 & 0 \\ 0 & 0 & 1 \end{pmatrix}$$

A point whose coordinates are x_1, y_1, z_1 is taken by $\hat{\sigma}_v$ into the point x_2, y_2, z_2 where

$$x_2 = \hat{\sigma}_v \times x_1 = x_1$$

$$y_2 = \hat{\sigma}_v \times y_1 = -y_1$$

$$z_2 = \hat{\sigma}_v \times z_1 = z_1$$

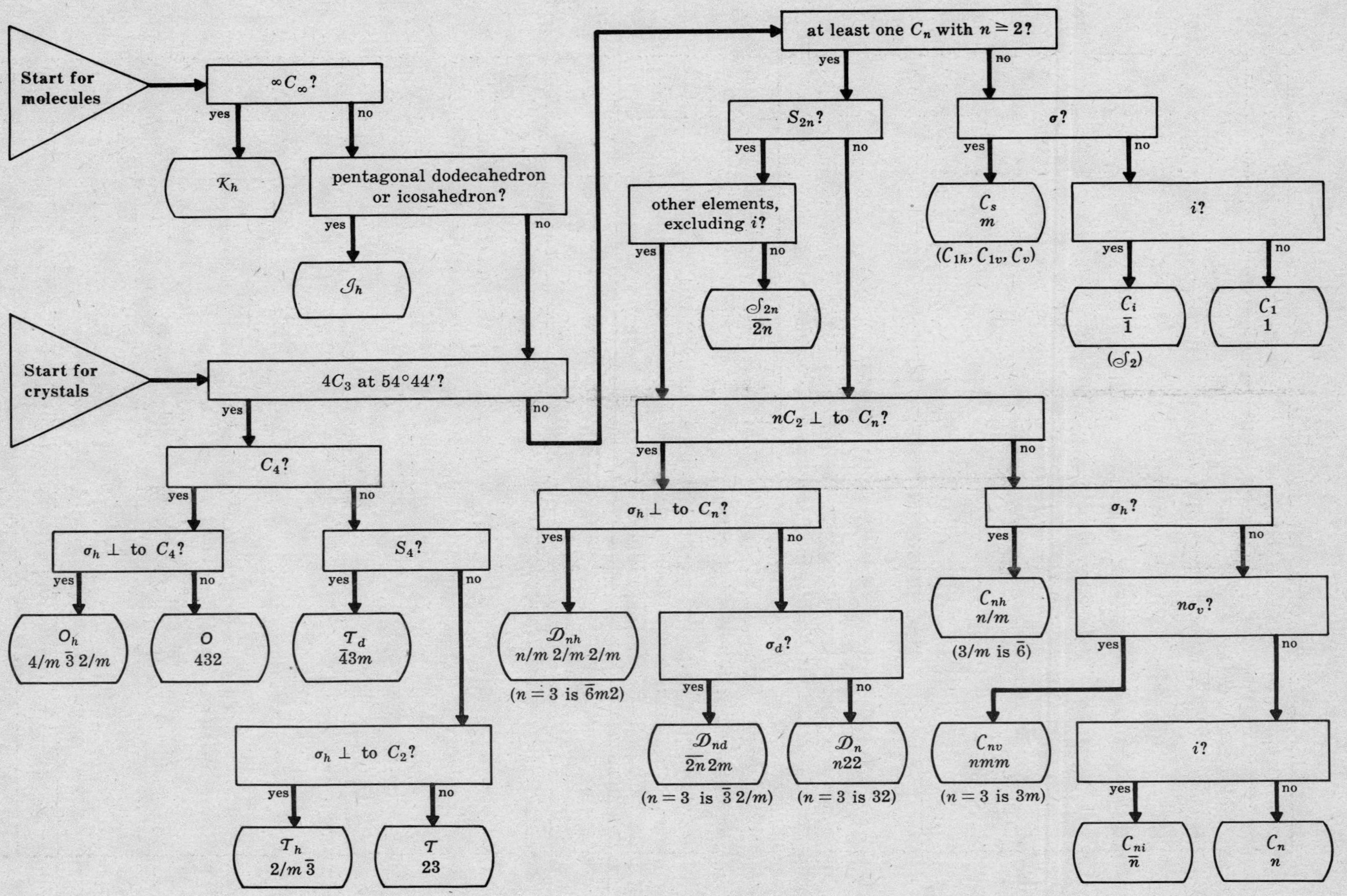

Start for molecules
∞C_∞?
yes
no
$\mathcal{K}_h$
pentagonal dodecahedron or icosahedron?
$\mathcal{I}_h$
Start for crystals
$4C_3$ at 54°44′?
C_4?
$\sigma_h \perp$ to C_4?
O_h
$4/m\,\bar{3}\,2/m$
O
432
S_4?
$\mathcal{T}_d$
$\bar{4}3m$
$\sigma_h \perp$ to C_2?
$\mathcal{T}_h$
$2/m\,\bar{3}$
$\mathcal{T}$
23
at least one C_n with $n \geq 2$?
S_{2n}?
other elements, excluding i?
$\mathcal{S}_{2n}$
$\overline{2n}$
σ?
C_s
m
(C_{1h}, C_{1v}, C_v)
i?
C_i
$\bar{1}$
$(\mathcal{S}_2)$
C_1
1
$nC_2 \perp$ to C_n?
$\sigma_h \perp$ to C_n?
$\mathcal{D}_{nh}$
$n/m\,2/m\,2/m$
$(n = 3$ is $\bar{6}m2)$
σ_d?
$\mathcal{D}_{nd}$
$\overline{2n}\,2m$
$(n = 3$ is $\bar{3}\,2/m)$
$\mathcal{D}_n$
$n22$
$(n = 3$ is 32)
σ_h?
C_{nh}
n/m
$(3/m$ is $\bar{6})$
$n\sigma_v$?
C_{nv}
nmm
$(n = 3$ is $3m)$
i?
C_{ni}
$\bar{n}$
C_n
n

Fig. 17-14

Table 17-2

Point Group	Special Comments	E	Axes of Rotation	σ_h	σ_v	i
$\mathcal{K}_h$	sphere	√	∞C_∞	√	$\infty\sigma_d$	√
$\mathcal{I}_h$	regular pentagonal dodecahedron (12 pentagons) or icosahedron (20 triangles)	√	$6C_5$ (S_{10}) $15C_2$ (S_4)		$15\sigma_d$	√
$\mathcal{O}_h$ $4/m\,\bar{3}\,2/m$	octahedron or cube	√	$4C_3$ (S_6) $3C_4$ (S_4) $6C_2$	√	$6\sigma_d$	√
$\mathcal{O}$ 432		√	$4C_3$ $3C_4$ $6C_2$			
$\mathcal{T}_d$ $\bar{4}3m$	tetrahedron	√	$4C_3$ $3C_2$ (S_4)		$6\sigma_d$	
$\mathcal{T}_h$ $2/m\,\bar{3}$		√	$4C_3$ (S_6) $3C_2$	√		√
$\mathcal{T}$ 23		√	$4C_3$ $3C_2$			
$\mathcal{S}_{2n}$ $\overline{2n}$	$n = 2, 3, 4, \ldots$ $\mathcal{S}_1$ is C_s, $\mathcal{S}_2$ is C_i $\mathcal{S}_n$ is C_{nh} if n odd	√	S_{2n} (C_n)			if n odd
$\mathcal{D}_{nh}$ $n/m\,2/m\,2/m$	$n = 2, 3, 4, \ldots$ $\mathcal{D}_{1h}$ is C_{2v}	√	C_n (S_n) nC_2	√	$n\sigma_v$	if n even
$\mathcal{D}_{nd}$ $\overline{2n}2m$	$n = 2, 3, 4, \ldots$ $\mathcal{D}_{1d}$ is C_{2h}	√	C_n (S_{2n}) nC_2		$n\sigma_d$	if n odd
$\mathcal{D}_n$ $n22$	$n = 2, 3, 4, \ldots$ $\mathcal{D}_1$ is C_2	√	C_n nC_2			
C_{nh} n/m	$n = 2, 3, 4, \ldots$ C_{1h} is C_s	√	C_n (S_n)	√		if n even
C_{nv} nmm	$n = 2, 3, 4, \ldots$ C_{1v} is C_s	√	C_n		$n\sigma_v$	
C_{ni} $\bar{n}$	$n = 3, 5, 7, \ldots$ C_{1i} is C_i For even values of n, C_{ni} is C_{nh} if $n/2$ is odd and $\mathcal{S}_{2n}$ if $n/2$ is even.	√	C_n (S_{2n})			√
C_n n	$n = 2, 3, 4, \ldots$	√	C_n			
C_s m		√		√		
C_i $\bar{1}$		√				√
C_1 1		√				

This can be stated alternatively as

$$x_2 = 1x_1 + 0y_1 + 0z_1$$
$$y_2 = 0x_1 - 1y_1 + 0z_1$$
$$z_2 = 0x_1 + 0y_1 + 1z_1$$

or in matrix form as

$$\begin{pmatrix} x_2 \\ y_2 \\ z_2 \end{pmatrix} = \begin{pmatrix} 1 & 0 & 0 \\ 0 & -1 & 0 \\ 0 & 0 & 1 \end{pmatrix} \begin{pmatrix} x_1 \\ y_1 \\ z_1 \end{pmatrix}$$

which is the desired result. Note that the matrix can also be obtained by substituting $\beta = 0$ in Table 17-3.

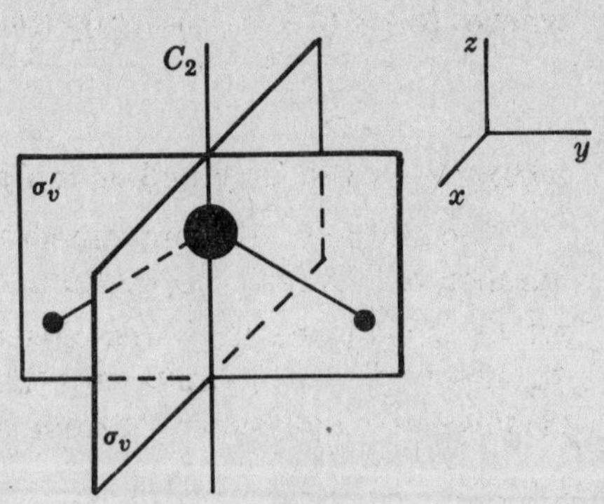

Fig. 17-15

EXAMPLE 17.12. Using matrix expressions for $\hat{C}_2$ and $\hat{E}$, show that $\hat{C}_2 \times \hat{C}_2 = \hat{E}$ as given in Table 17-1 for the C_{2v} point group.

Substituting $n = 2$ and $m = 1$ into the general expression given in Table 17-3 for $\hat{C}_n^m$ gives

$$\hat{C}_2 \longrightarrow \begin{pmatrix} \cos\pi & -\sin\pi & 0 \\ \sin\pi & \cos\pi & 0 \\ 0 & 0 & 1 \end{pmatrix} = \begin{pmatrix} -1 & 0 & 0 \\ 0 & -1 & 0 \\ 0 & 0 & 1 \end{pmatrix}$$

Thus

$$\hat{C}_2 \times \hat{C}_2 = \begin{pmatrix} -1 & 0 & 0 \\ 0 & -1 & 0 \\ 0 & 0 & 1 \end{pmatrix} \begin{pmatrix} -1 & 0 & 0 \\ 0 & -1 & 0 \\ 0 & 0 & 1 \end{pmatrix} = \begin{pmatrix} 1 & 0 & 0 \\ 0 & 1 & 0 \\ 0 & 0 & 1 \end{pmatrix} = \hat{E}$$

17.15 REPRESENTATIONS

A *representation*, V, for a point group is any set of square matrices that multiply as the symmetry operations of the group.

A *reducible representation* contains matrices all of which can be partitioned into the same block-diagonal form consisting of a series of submatrices which lie along the main diagonal, exclude only zero elements, and can be treated as single elements in obtaining a matrix product. Usually these submatrices are the matrices for the *irreducible representations*, V_i, which cannot be partitioned in the above fashion. In that case the representation V is said to be the *direct sum* (common notations are **+**, + and $\oplus$) of the irreducible representations V_i. For example, if a reducible representation V consists of the matrices (A), (B) and (C), each of which can be partitioned into the block-diagonal form

$$(X) = \left(\begin{array}{cc|c|c} x_{11} & x_{12} & 0 & 0 \\ x_{21} & x_{22} & 0 & 0 \\ \hline 0 & 0 & x_{33} & 0 \\ \hline 0 & 0 & 0 & x_{44} \end{array}\right) = \begin{pmatrix} x_1 & 0 & 0 \\ 0 & x_2 & 0 \\ 0 & 0 & x_3 \end{pmatrix}$$

where $(x_1) = \begin{pmatrix} x_{11} & x_{12} \\ x_{21} & x_{22} \end{pmatrix}$, $(x_2) = (x_{33})$ and $(x_3) = (x_{44})$, then

$$(A) \times (B) = \begin{pmatrix} a_1 & 0 & 0 \\ 0 & a_2 & 0 \\ 0 & 0 & a_3 \end{pmatrix} \times \begin{pmatrix} b_1 & 0 & 0 \\ 0 & b_2 & 0 \\ 0 & 0 & b_3 \end{pmatrix} = \begin{pmatrix} c_1 & 0 & 0 \\ 0 & c_2 & 0 \\ 0 & 0 & c_3 \end{pmatrix} = (C)$$

where $(a_1) \times (b_1) = (c_1)$, $(a_2) \times (b_2) = (c_2)$, $(a_3) \times (b_3) = (c_3)$ and

$$V = V_1 \oplus V_2 \oplus V_3$$

where V_i is the irreducible representation consisting of the matrices (a_i), (b_i) and (c_i).

The number of nonequivalent irreducible representations for a group is equal to the number of *classes of operations* in the group, where a class can be loosely defined as a subset of operations that are closely related (e.g. in C_{3v} the classes are $\hat{E}$, $\hat{C}_3$ and $\hat{C}_3^2$, and $\hat{\sigma}_{v1}$, $\hat{\sigma}_{v2}$ and $\hat{\sigma}_{v3}$). If ℓ_i represents the dimension of the ith irreducible representation (number of rows or columns in the square matrices),

$$\sum_{V_i} \ell_i^2 = h \tag{17.1}$$

where h is known as the *order* of the group and is equal to the number of distinct operations within the group.

EXAMPLE 17.13. Show that the representation for C_{2v} derived from Table 17-3 is reducible. Find the irreducible representations for this group.

The representation consisting of the expressions given by Table 17-3 is

$$V: \quad \hat{E} \longrightarrow \begin{pmatrix} 1 & 0 & 0 \\ 0 & 1 & 0 \\ 0 & 0 & 1 \end{pmatrix}, \qquad \hat{C}_2 \longrightarrow \begin{pmatrix} -1 & 0 & 0 \\ 0 & -1 & 0 \\ 0 & 0 & 1 \end{pmatrix},$$

$$\hat{\sigma}_v \longrightarrow \begin{pmatrix} 1 & 0 & 0 \\ 0 & -1 & 0 \\ 0 & 0 & 1 \end{pmatrix}, \qquad \hat{\sigma}'_v \longrightarrow \begin{pmatrix} -1 & 0 & 0 \\ 0 & 1 & 0 \\ 0 & 0 & 1 \end{pmatrix}$$

and has dimension 3. If this representation were one of the irreducible ones, its contribution to the left-hand side of *(17.1)* would be such that the sum over all the irreducible representations would be equal to 4, the number of distinct operations. But the contribution from this representation alone is $3^2 = 9$, so it must be reducible.

Three of the irreducible representations of this group can be found by converting all of the above matrices to the block-diagonal form as shown above. Each row of blocks provides an irreducible representation. In this case the blocks are 1 by 1 matrices. Labeling these representations using subscripts corresponding to entries in the character table for this group, see Table 17-4, we have $V = V_3 \oplus V_4 \oplus V_1$, where

$$V_3: \quad \hat{E} \longrightarrow (1) \quad \hat{C}_2 \longrightarrow (-1) \quad \hat{\sigma}_v \longrightarrow (1) \quad \hat{\sigma}'_v \longrightarrow (-1)$$

$$V_4: \quad \hat{E} \longrightarrow (1) \quad \hat{C}_2 \longrightarrow (-1) \quad \hat{\sigma}_v \longrightarrow (-1) \quad \hat{\sigma}'_v \longrightarrow (1)$$

$$V_1: \quad \hat{E} \longrightarrow (1) \quad \hat{C}_2 \longrightarrow (1) \quad \hat{\sigma}_v \longrightarrow (1) \quad \hat{\sigma}'_v \longrightarrow (1)$$

For the dimension of the fourth irreducible representation, V_2, *(17.1)* gives

$$1^2 + \ell_2^2 + 1^2 + 1^2 = 4$$

or $\ell_2 = 1$. Using methods not discussed here, it can be shown that

$$V_2: \quad \hat{E} \longrightarrow (1) \quad \hat{C}_2 \longrightarrow (1) \quad \hat{\sigma}_v \longrightarrow (-1) \quad \hat{\sigma}'_v \longrightarrow (-1)$$

Table 17-4

C_{2v} Representation	$\hat{E}$	$\hat{C}_2$	$\hat{\sigma}_v$	$\hat{\sigma}'_v$	Translation and Rotation
$V_1 = A_1$	1	1	1	1	z
$V_2 = A_2$	1	1	−1	−1	R_z
$V_3 = B_1$	1	−1	1	−1	x, R_y
$V_4 = B_2$	1	−1	−1	1	y, R_x

17.16 CHARACTER

Many applications of group theory can be treated thoroughly using the *characters* of the matrices making up the irreducible representations rather than the set of entire matrices. The *character* (or *trace*) for the operation $\hat{R}$, $\chi(V, \hat{R})$, is defined as

$$\chi(V, \hat{R}) = \sum r_{jj} \tag{17.2}$$

where the r_{jj} are the diagonal elements of the matrix corresponding to $\hat{R}$ in the representation V. Some properties of the characters of irreducible representations which are of interest include

$$\sum_{\hat{R}} \chi(V_i, \hat{R})\, \chi(V_j, \hat{R}) = h\delta_{ij} \tag{17.3}$$

where $\delta_{ij} = 0$ if $i \neq j$ and $\delta_{ij} = 1$ if $i = j$;

$$\sum_{V_i} [\chi(V_i, \hat{E})]^2 = h \tag{17.4}$$

and if $\hat{R}_1$ and $\hat{R}_2$ belong to the same class,

$$\chi(V_i, \hat{R}_1) = \chi(V_i, \hat{R}_2) \tag{17.5}$$

EXAMPLE 17.14. The characters of the irreducible representations of a group can be used to determine the number of times that the irreducible representation V_i occurs in a reducible representation V. If v_i represents this number,

$$v_i = \frac{1}{h} \sum_{\hat{R}} \chi(V, \hat{R})\, \chi(V_i, \hat{R}) \tag{17.6}$$

Show that the representation for C_{2v} given in Example 17.13 is the direct sum of V_1, V_3 and V_4.

Using (*17.2*), the characters of the reducible representation are

$$\chi(V, \hat{E}) = (1) + (1) + (1) = 3 \qquad \chi(V, \hat{C}_2) = (-1) + (-1) + (1) = -1$$

$$\chi(V, \hat{\sigma}_v) = (1) + (-1) + (1) = 1 \qquad \chi(V, \hat{\sigma}_v') = (-1) + (1) + (1) = 1$$

and those of the irreducible representations are

$$\chi(V_1, \hat{E}) = 1 \quad \chi(V_1, \hat{C}_2) = 1 \quad \chi(V_1, \hat{\sigma}_v) = 1 \quad \chi(V_1, \hat{\sigma}_v') = 1$$

$$\chi(V_2, \hat{E}) = 1 \quad \chi(V_2, \hat{C}_2) = 1 \quad \chi(V_2, \hat{\sigma}_v) = -1 \quad \chi(V_2, \hat{\sigma}_v') = -1$$

$$\chi(V_3, \hat{E}) = 1 \quad \chi(V_3, \hat{C}_2) = -1 \quad \chi(V_3, \hat{\sigma}_v) = 1 \quad \chi(V_3, \hat{\sigma}_v') = -1$$

$$\chi(V_4, \hat{E}) = 1 \quad \chi(V_4, \hat{C}_2) = -1 \quad \chi(V_4, \hat{\sigma}_v) = -1 \quad \chi(V_4, \hat{\sigma}_v') = 1$$

Applying (*17.6*) gives

$$v_1 = \frac{1}{h}[\chi(V, \hat{E})\chi(V_1, \hat{E}) + \chi(V, \hat{C}_2)\chi(V_1, \hat{C}_2) + \chi(V, \hat{\sigma}_v)\chi(V_1, \hat{\sigma}_v) + \chi(V, \hat{\sigma}_v')\chi(V_1, \hat{\sigma}_v')]$$

$$= \frac{1}{4}[(3)(1) + (-1)(1) + (1)(1) + (1)(1)] = 1$$

$$v_2 = \frac{1}{4}[(3)(1) + (-1)(1) + (1)(-1) + (1)(-1)] = 0$$

$$v_3 = \frac{1}{4}[(3)(1) + (-1)(-1) + (1)(1) + (1)(-1)] = 1$$

$$v_4 = \frac{1}{4}[(3)(1) + (-1)(-1) + (1)(-1) + (1)(1)] = 1$$

which means that V can be reduced to

$$V = 1V_1 \oplus 0V_2 \oplus 1V_3 \oplus 1V_4 = V_1 \oplus V_3 \oplus V_4$$

17.17 CHARACTER TABLES

The characters of the symmetry operations for each nonequivalent irreducible representation can be found in a character table for the group, e.g. Table 17-4. In many tables the first column lists the designations of the representations in the notation developed by Mulliken, see Table 17-5. The first column may include additional information such as equivalent spectroscopic designations.

Table 17-5. Mulliken Designation for Irreducible Representations

		INTERPRETATION
CAPITAL LETTER	A	1-dimensional and symmetric to rotation of $2\pi/n$ about the principal C_n axis as indicated by $\chi(V_i, \hat{C}_n) = 1$
	B	1-dimensional and antisymmetric to rotation of $2\pi/n$ about the principal C_n axis as indicated by $\chi(V_i, \hat{C}_n) = -1$
	E	2-dimensional
	T or F	3-dimensional
	G	4-dimensional
	H	5-dimensional
NUMERAL SUBSCRIPT	1	symmetric to rotation about a secondary C_2 axis as indicated by $\chi(V_i, \hat{C}_2) = 1$
	2	antisymmetric to rotation about a secondary C_2 axis as indicated by $\chi(V_i, \hat{C}_2) = -1$ (if a secondary C_2 axis does not exist, used for σ_v if present)
LETTER SUBSCRIPT	g	symmetric to inversion as indicated by $\chi(V_i, \hat{\imath}) = 1$
	u	antisymmetric to inversion as indicated by $\chi(V_i, \hat{\imath}) = -1$
SUPERSCRIPT	$'$	symmetric to σ_h as indicated by $\chi(V_i, \hat{\sigma}_h) = 1$
	$''$	antisymmetric to σ_h as indicated by $\chi(V_i, \hat{\sigma}_h) = -1$

The second group of columns gives the values of $\chi(V_i, \hat{R})$, although the entries are usually made according to classes of operations instead of individual operations. The number of operations in a given class is given by an integer before the symbol for that class and must be considered when performing summations of characters, e.g. in (*17.3*) and (*17.6*). The symbol $\hat{C}_\infty^\phi$ or $\hat{S}_\infty^\phi$ represents a rotation of ϕ about a C_∞ or S_∞ axis.

Many character tables have third and fourth columns which assign molecular rotational and translational modes and various vector products to given V_i.

Applications of Group Theory to Molecular Properties

17.18 OPTICAL ACTIVITY

The S_n operation transforms a molecule or crystalline unit cell into its mirror image and thus any potential optical activity vanishes. Because $\hat{S}_1 = \hat{\sigma}$ and $\hat{S}_2 = \hat{\imath}$, the presence of a mirror plane or center of symmetry also renders a system inactive.

EXAMPLE 17.15. Discuss the optical activity of SiO_2.

The molecular structure of SiO_2 in the gaseous, liquid or true solution phase is such that it contains a mirror plane and is optically inactive. However, SiO_4 tetrahedra are formed in the various solid forms of SiO_2 and depending on their arrangement, the substance may be active. The crystalline arrangement for SiO_2 as cristobalite is $4/m\,\bar{3}\,2/m$ and cannot be optically active; as tridymite, is $6/m\,2/m\,2/m$ and cannot be optically active; and as α-quartz, is 32 and is observed to be optically active.

17.19 DIPOLE MOMENT

The dipole moment of a molecule must lie along the principal axis of rotation and the molecule cannot contain more than one axis of this order. If a mirror plane is present, the moment will lie in this plane or along the line of intersection of several planes. The presence of an inversion center eliminates the presence of a dipole moment for the molecule.

17.20 MOLECULAR TRANSLATIONAL MOTION

The matrix expressions given in Table 17-3 are applicable to the translational motion of a rigid molecule and by using *(17.6)* it is possible to find the sum of the irreducible representations that make up V_{trans}. Each of the x-, y- and z-components of the translational motion can be assigned to a specific V_i in the sum by equating the results of the various symmetry operations on the component to the results of the transformations effected by the matrices making up V_i. Because these assignments are a property of the point group and are valid for all molecules in the group, they are usually given in the character table.

An entry of x, y in a table has a different meaning than an entry of (x, y): the presence of parentheses indicates that x and y together give a two-dimensional irreducible representation, whereas the former notation means that both x and y are represented by the same one-dimensional irreducible representation.

EXAMPLE 17.16. Determine which irreducible representation corresponds to translation along the y-axis for a molecule in the C_{2v} point group.

In Example 17.14 it was shown that $V_{\text{trans}} = V_1 \oplus V_3 \oplus V_4$. To find which of these V_i corresponds to the y-component of the translational motion, the four operations of the group are performed on y giving

$$\hat{E} \times y = (+1)y \qquad \hat{C}_2 \times y = (-1)y \qquad \hat{\sigma}_v \times y = (-1)y \qquad \hat{\sigma}'_v \times y = (+1)y$$

which are the same as the transformations contained in V_4.

17.21 MOLECULAR ROTATIONAL MOTION

Each of the components of rotational motion—R_x, R_y and R_z for a nonlinear molecule, and R_x and R_y for a linear molecule (R_z is used for optional orientations)—can be assigned to a specific V_i in the character table. The simplest technique for finding these assignments is based on the values of the characters in the V_i for the corresponding translational motion: $\chi(V_{R_i}, \hat{R})$ will be given by $\chi(V_i, \hat{R})$ for $\hat{R} = \hat{E}$ and $\hat{C}_n$, and by $-\chi(V_i, \hat{R})$ for $\hat{R} = \hat{S}_n$, $\hat{\sigma}$ and $\hat{i}$. Because these assignments are a property of the point group and are valid for all molecules in the group, they are usually given in the character table.

EXAMPLE 17.17. Determine which irreducible representation corresponds to R_x, the rotation component about the x-axis, in the C_{2v} point group.

Applying the above rules to the characters given for V_3, to which is assigned the x-component of translation, gives

$$\chi(V_{R_x}, \hat{E}) = \chi(V_3, \hat{E}) = 1 \qquad \chi(V_{R_x}, \hat{\sigma}_v) = -\chi(V_3, \hat{\sigma}_v) = -1$$

$$\chi(V_{R_x}, \hat{C}_2) = \chi(V_3, \hat{C}_2) = -1 \qquad \chi(V_{R_x}, \hat{\sigma}'_v) = -\chi(V_3, \hat{\sigma}'_v) = -(-1) = 1$$

which corresponds to V_4 in Table 17-4.

17.22 VIBRATIONAL MOTION FOR POLYATOMIC MOLECULES

The symmetry and degeneracy of the normal modes of intramolecular vibration can be determined for a polyatomic molecule from the irreducible representations of its symmetry group. Rather than working with the complete matrices, it is necessary only to consider the characters of these matrices, where

$$\chi(V_{3\Lambda}, \hat{E}) = 3\Lambda_{\hat{E}} \tag{17.7a}$$

$$\chi(V_{3\Lambda}, \hat{C}_n^m) = \Lambda_{\hat{C}_n^m}\left[1 + 2\cos\frac{2\pi m}{n}\right] \tag{17.7b}$$

$$\chi(V_{3\Lambda}, \hat{S}_n^m) = \Lambda_{\hat{S}_n^m}\left[-1 + 2\cos\frac{2\pi m}{n}\right] \quad (m \text{ odd}) \tag{17.7c}$$

$$\chi(V_{3\Lambda}, \hat{i}) = -3\Lambda_{\hat{i}} \tag{17.7d}$$

$$\chi(V_{3\Lambda}, \hat{\sigma}) = \Lambda_{\hat{\sigma}} \tag{17.7e}$$

where $\Lambda_{\hat{R}}$ represents the number of unmoved nuclei for the operation $\hat{R}$ (e.g. $\Lambda_{\hat{E}} = \Lambda =$ number of nuclei in the molecule, $\Lambda_{\hat{i}} = 0$ or 1, etc.). Once the $\chi(V_{3\Lambda}, \hat{R})$ have been determined using (*17.7*), (*17.6*) is used to determine a sum of irreducible representations from which the six (for nonlinear) or five (for linear) translational and rotational contributions are subtracted, leaving the sum of irreducible representations that describe the vibrational motion, V_{vib}. Because this final sum depends on the number of atoms present in the molecule, rather than being a property of the group, it must be determined for each molecule and will not appear in a character table.

EXAMPLE 17.18. Describe the vibrational motion in water.

For a molecule in C_{2v}, equations (*17.7*) give

$$\chi(V_{3\Lambda}, \hat{E}) = 3(3) = 9 \qquad \chi(V_{3\Lambda}, \hat{C}_2) = (1)\left[1 + \cos\frac{2\pi(1)}{2}\right] = -1$$

$$\chi(V_{3\Lambda}, \hat{\sigma}_v) = 1 \qquad \chi(V_{3\Lambda}, \hat{\sigma}_v') = 3$$

Using (*17.6*) gives

$$v_1 = \frac{1}{4}[(9)(1) + (-1)(1) + (1)(1) + (3)(1)] = 3$$

$$v_2 = \frac{1}{4}[(9)(1) + (-1)(1) + (1)(-1) + (3)(-1)] = 1$$

$$v_3 = \frac{1}{4}[(9)(1) + (-1)(-1) + (1)(1) + (3)(-1)] = 2$$

$$v_4 = \frac{1}{4}[(9)(1) + (-1)(-1) + (1)(-1) + (3)(1)] = 3$$

or $V_{3\Lambda} = 3V_1 \oplus V_2 \oplus 2V_3 \oplus 3V_4$. Subtracting V_1 for z, V_2 for R_z, $2V_3$ for x and R_y, and $2V_4$ for y and R_x gives

$$V_{\text{vib}} = 2V_1 \oplus V_4$$

which means that the three modes of vibration for water are singly degenerate, with two of them being completely symmetrical and one being symmetric with respect to $\hat{E}$ and $\hat{\sigma}_v'$ but antisymmetric with respect to $\hat{C}_2$ and $\hat{\sigma}_v$. The normal modes are illustrated in Fig. 17-16.

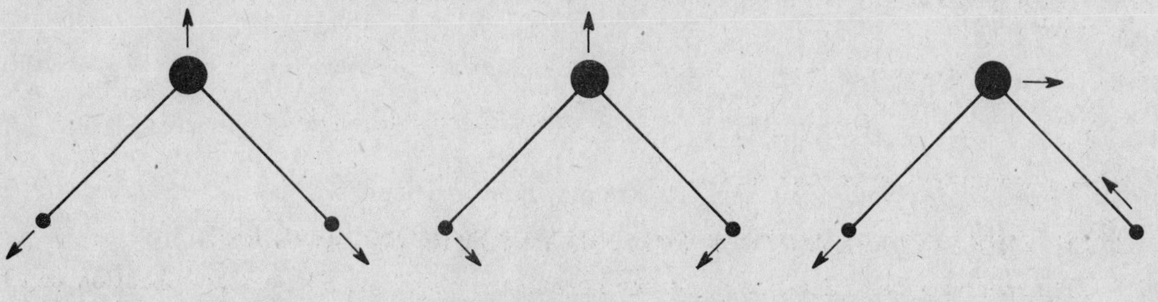

Fig. 17-16

EXAMPLE 17.19. The Mulliken convention for numbering the vibrational frequencies is to assign them according to the appearance of the corresponding irreducible representations in the character table. For modes of the same symmetry, the assignment is made according to decreasing frequency. An exception to this convention is made for linear triatomic molecules, where ν_2 has traditionally been assigned to the doubly-degenerate irreducible representation. Using this convention, assign the molecular vibrational frequencies for H_2O.

The results of Example 17.18 gave $V_{vib} = 2V_1 \oplus V_4$, so ν_1 would be assigned to the higher frequency corresponding to V_1 (symmetric stretch), ν_2 to the lower frequency corresponding to V_1 (bend) and ν_3 to V_4 (asymmetric stretch).

Solved Problems

Symmetry Elements and Operations

17.1. Diatomic and linear polyatomic molecules contain a C_∞ axis of rotation. Construct a perspective sketch for the points around this element.

The notation C_∞ is defined as an axis of proper rotation for which an infinite number of points are related to the original point by various angles ϕ, where $0 \leq \phi \leq 2\pi$. If the original (finite-sized) point is placed in a general position off the axis of rotation, a torus is generated which has no importance in discussing molecular and crystallographic symmetry. An alternate way of indicating a C_∞ axis is to place the point on the axis, see Fig. 17-17.

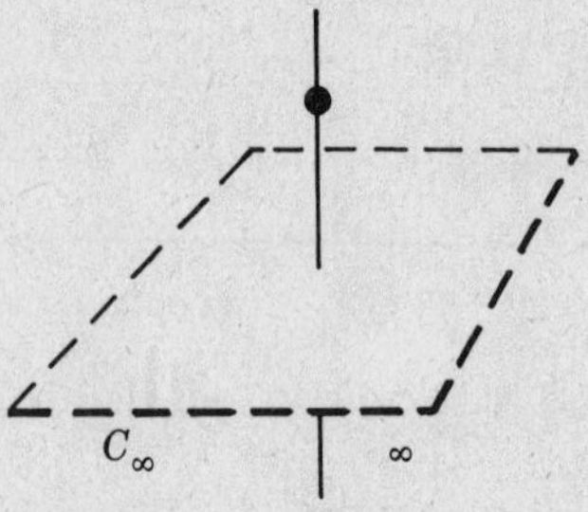

Fig. 17-17

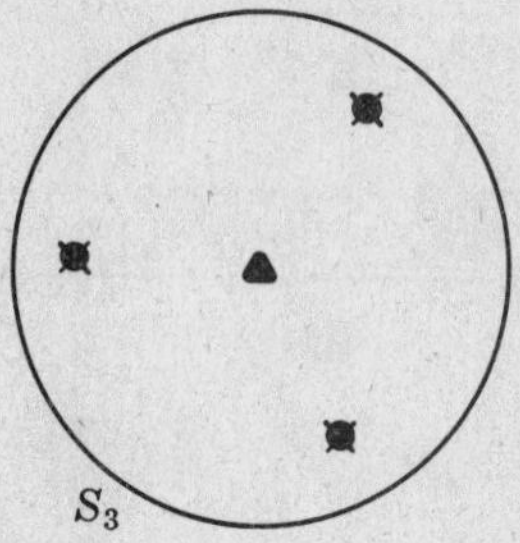

Fig. 17-18

17.2. Is $\hat{\sigma}^k$ distinct for all k?

As can be seen in Fig. 17-5, $\hat{\sigma}^1$ generates a point that cannot be generated in a less complicated manner and is therefore distinct; $\hat{\sigma}^2$ generates the original point—the result of $\hat{E}$— and is therefore not distinct; and $\hat{\sigma}^k$ for $k > 2$ generates one of the above points and is therefore not distinct.

17.3. Prepare an orthographic projection illustrating the points around the S_3 symmetry element.

The projection is shown in Fig. 17-18. The points are the images of the original point under the operations $\hat{S}_3^k$, $1 \leq k \leq 6$.

17.4. Prepare drawings for the points around the 4_3 element.

Based on the fundamental operation of rotation by 90° and translation by $3t/4$, the sketches shown in Fig. 17-9(*c*) result. After translating all points to similar positions within the distance t (see Example 17.6) and constructing the simplified diagram, it appears that 4_1 and 4_3 are *enantiomorphic* operations (i.e. they correspond to right- and left-hand screws of the same pitch).

17.5. Identify the symmetry elements present in (*a*) an ice-cream cone, (*b*) a donut, (*c*) a football, (*d*) a crescent and (*e*) the letter A.

From inspection of the figures mentioned: (*a*) C_∞, $\infty\sigma_v$, E; (*b*) C_∞, ∞C_2, $\infty\sigma_v$, σ_h, i, E; (*c*) C_∞, ∞C_2, $\infty\sigma_v$, σ_h, i, E; (*d*) C_2, σ_v, σ_v', E; (*e*) C_2, σ_v, σ_v', E.

Point Groups

17.6. Consider a molecule of ammonia (trigonal pyramid with the N at the apex). Determine the symmetry elements present.

The elements are E, C_3 and $3\sigma_v$.

17.7. Prepare a multiplication table of distinct operations in ammonia: $\hat{E}$, $\hat{C}_3$, $\hat{C}_3^2$, $\hat{\sigma}_{v1}$, $\hat{\sigma}_{v2}$ and $\hat{\sigma}_{v3}$.

See Table 17-6.

Table 17-6

C_{3v}	$\hat{E}$	$\hat{C}_3$	$\hat{C}_3^2$	$\hat{\sigma}_{v1}$	$\hat{\sigma}_{v2}$	$\hat{\sigma}_{v3} = \hat{B}$
$\hat{A} = \hat{E}$	$\hat{E}$	$\hat{C}_3$	$\hat{C}_3^2$	$\hat{\sigma}_{v1}$	$\hat{\sigma}_{v2}$	$\hat{\sigma}_{v3}$
$\hat{C}_3$	$\hat{C}_3$	$\hat{C}_3^2$	$\hat{E}$	$\hat{\sigma}_{v3}$	$\hat{\sigma}_{v1}$	$\hat{\sigma}_{v2}$
$\hat{C}_3^2$	$\hat{C}_3^2$	$\hat{E}$	$\hat{C}_3$	$\hat{\sigma}_{v2}$	$\hat{\sigma}_{v3}$	$\hat{\sigma}_{v1}$
$\hat{\sigma}_{v1}$	$\hat{\sigma}_{v1}$	$\hat{\sigma}_{v2}$	$\hat{\sigma}_{v3}$	$\hat{E}$	$\hat{C}_3$	$\hat{C}_3^2$
$\hat{\sigma}_{v2}$	$\hat{\sigma}_{v2}$	$\hat{\sigma}_{v3}$	$\hat{\sigma}_{v1}$	$\hat{C}_3^2$	$\hat{E}$	$\hat{C}_3$
$\hat{\sigma}_{v3}$	$\hat{\sigma}_{v3}$	$\hat{\sigma}_{v1}$	$\hat{\sigma}_{v2}$	$\hat{C}_3$	$\hat{C}_3^2$	$\hat{E}$

17.8. Determine the point group for (*a*) NH_3, (*b*) CH_4 and (*c*) C_6H_6.

The following analyses can be made using Fig. 17-14:

(*a*) NH_3: (1) are there ∞ C_∞ axes present? no; (2) is there a pentagonal dodecahedron or icosahedron present? no; (3) are there four C_3 axes at 54°44′? no; (4) is there at least one C_n where $n \geqq 2$? yes, C_3; (5) is there an S_{2n} present? no; (6) are there n C_2 axes perpendicular to C_n? no; (7) are there any σ_h planes present? no; (8) are there n σ_v planes present? yes, 3, therefore C_{3v}.

(*b*) CH_4: (1) are there ∞ C_∞ axes present? no; (2) is there a pentagonal dodecahedron or icosahedron present? no; (3) are there four C_3 axes at 54°44′? yes; (4) is there a C_4 axis present? no; (5) is there an S_4 axis present? yes, therefore $\mathcal{T}_d$.

(*c*) C_6H_6: (1) are there ∞ C_∞ axes present, no; (2) is there a pentagonal dodecahedron or icosahedron present? no; (3) are there four C_3 axes at 54°44′? no; (4) is there at least one C_n where $n \geqq 2$? yes, C_6; (5) is there an S_{2n} present? no; (6) are there n C_2 axes present perpendicular to C_n? yes, 6; (7) are there any σ_h planes perpendicular to C_n? yes, therefore $\mathcal{D}_{6h}$.

Representation of Groups

17.9. Considering the symmetry elements shown in Fig. 17-15 for the C_{2v} point group, show that $\hat{C}_2$ can be expressed as $\begin{pmatrix} -1 & 0 & 0 \\ 0 & -1 & 0 \\ 0 & 0 & 1 \end{pmatrix}$.

Assuming x_2, y_2 and z_2 to be the result of $\hat{C}_2$ operating on x_1, y_1 and z_1, then

$$x_2 = \hat{C}_2 \times x_1 = -x_1 \qquad y_2 = \hat{C}_2 \times y_1 = -y_1 \qquad z_2 = \hat{C}_2 \times z_1 = z_1$$

which can be restated as

$$x_2 = -1x_1 + 0y_1 + 0z_1$$
$$y_2 = 0x_1 - 1y_1 + 0z_1$$
$$z_2 = 0x_1 + 0y_1 + 1z_1$$

or in matrix form as

$$\begin{pmatrix} x_2 \\ y_2 \\ z_2 \end{pmatrix} = \begin{pmatrix} -1 & 0 & 0 \\ 0 & -1 & 0 \\ 0 & 0 & 1 \end{pmatrix} \begin{pmatrix} x_1 \\ y_1 \\ z_1 \end{pmatrix}$$

which is the desired result.

Another method would be to substitute $n = 2$ and $m = 1$ into the expression for $\hat{C}_2(z)^m$ in Table 17-3.

17.10. Confirm that $\hat{C}_2 \times \hat{\sigma}_v = \hat{\sigma}_v'$ for the C_{2v} point group using the respective matrix expressions.

Using $\hat{C}_2 \longrightarrow \begin{pmatrix} -1 & 0 & 0 \\ 0 & -1 & 0 \\ 0 & 0 & 1 \end{pmatrix}$, see Problem 17.9, and $\hat{\sigma}_v \longrightarrow \begin{pmatrix} 1 & 0 & 0 \\ 0 & -1 & 0 \\ 0 & 0 & 1 \end{pmatrix}$, see Example 17.11, the product is

$$\begin{pmatrix} -1 & 0 & 0 \\ 0 & -1 & 0 \\ 0 & 0 & 1 \end{pmatrix}\begin{pmatrix} 1 & 0 & 0 \\ 0 & -1 & 0 \\ 0 & 0 & 1 \end{pmatrix} = \begin{pmatrix} -1 & 0 & 0 \\ 0 & 1 & 0 \\ 0 & 0 & 1 \end{pmatrix}$$

which is the same as $\hat{\sigma}_v'$, see Problem 17.32.

17.11. Demonstrate that the elements of the irreducible representation V_2 for the C_{2v} point group multiply as the symmetry operations of the group.

A selection of the sixteen multiplications using

$$\hat{E} \longrightarrow (1) \qquad \hat{C}_2 \longrightarrow (1) \qquad \hat{\sigma}_v \longrightarrow (-1) \qquad \hat{\sigma}_v' \longrightarrow (-1)$$

are

$$\begin{array}{cccc} \hat{E} \times \hat{E} = \hat{E} & \hat{E} \times \hat{\sigma}_v' = \hat{\sigma}_v & \hat{\sigma}_v \times \hat{C}_2 = \hat{\sigma}_v' & \hat{\sigma}_v' \times \hat{\sigma}_v = \hat{C}_2 \\ \downarrow\ \ \downarrow\ \ \downarrow & \downarrow\ \ \downarrow\ \ \downarrow & \downarrow\ \ \downarrow\ \ \downarrow & \downarrow\ \ \downarrow\ \ \downarrow \\ (1)\times(1) = (1) & (1)\times(-1) = (-1) & (-1)\times(1) = (-1) & (-1)\times(-1) = (1) \end{array}$$

17.12. Find the characters of V_2 for the C_{2v} point group, given the incomplete character table

C_{2v}	$\hat{E}$	$\hat{C}_2$	$\hat{\sigma}_v$	$\hat{\sigma}_v'$
V_1	1	1	1	1
V_3	1	−1	1	−1
V_4	1	−1	−1	1

as determined from the irreducible representations found in Example 17.13.

The order of V_2 was determined as one-dimensional, which means $\chi(V_2, \hat{E}) = 1$. Applying *(17.3)* to V_1 and V_2 gives

$$0 = \chi(V_1, \hat{E})\chi(V_2, \hat{E}) + \chi(V_1, \hat{C}_2)\chi(V_2, \hat{C}_2) + \chi(V_1, \hat{\sigma}_v)\chi(V_2, \hat{\sigma}_v) + \chi(V_1, \hat{\sigma}_v')\chi(V_2, \hat{\sigma}_v')$$
$$= (1)(1) + (1)\chi(V_2, \hat{C}_2) + (1)\chi(V_2, \hat{\sigma}_v) + (1)\chi(V_2, \hat{\sigma}_v')$$

and to V_2 and V_3 and to V_2 and V_4 gives

$$0 = (1)(1) + (-1)\chi(V_2, \hat{C}_2) + (1)\chi(V_2, \hat{\sigma}_v) + (-1)\chi(V_2, \hat{\sigma}_v')$$

$$0 = (1)(1) + (-1)\chi(V_2, \hat{C}_2) + (-1)\chi(V_2, \hat{\sigma}_v) + (1)\chi(V_2, \hat{\sigma}_v')$$

Solving simultaneously gives $\chi(V_2, \hat{C}_2) = 1$, $\chi(V_2, \hat{\sigma}_v) = -1$ and $\chi(V_2, \hat{\sigma}_v') = -1$, which agrees with the entry in Table 17-4.

17.13. Demonstrate that the irreducible representations for C_{2v} obey (*17.3*) when $i = j$ and (*17.4*).

For $i = j = 1$, (*17.3*) gives for V_1

$$\chi(V_1, \hat{E})\chi(V_1, \hat{E}) + \chi(V_1, \hat{C}_2)\chi(V_1, \hat{C}_2) + \chi(V_1, \hat{\sigma}_v)\chi(V_1, \hat{\sigma}_v) + \chi(V_1, \hat{\sigma}_v')\chi(V_1, \hat{\sigma}_v')$$
$$= (1)(1) + (1)(1) + (1)(1) + (1)(1) = 4$$

and similarly for V_2, V_3 and V_4. Substituting the values of $\chi(V_i, \hat{E})$ from Table 17-4 into (*17.4*) gives

$$(1)^2 + (1)^2 + (1)^2 + (1)^2 = 4$$

17.14. Determine the Mulliken designations for the irreducible representations of C_{2v}.

Upon comparing the entries in Table 17-4 with the code given in Table 17-5, the letter A should be chosen for V_1 because $\chi(V_1, \hat{E}) = 1$ and $\chi(V_1, \hat{C}_2) = 1$, and the subscript 1 should be chosen because $\chi(V_1, \hat{\sigma}_v) = 1$; hence $V_1 = A_1$. Likewise, V_2 is designated as A_2 because $\chi(V_2, \hat{E}) = 1$, $\chi(V_2, \hat{C}_2) = 1$ and $\chi(V_2, \hat{\sigma}_v) = -1$; V_3 as B_1 because $\chi(V_3, \hat{E}) = 1$, $\chi(V_3, \hat{C}_2) = -1$ and $\chi(V_3, \hat{\sigma}_v) = 1$; and V_4 as B_2 because $\chi(V_4, \hat{E}) = 1$, $\chi(V_4, \hat{C}_2) = -1$ and $\chi(V_4, \hat{\sigma}_v) = -1$.

Applications of Group Theory to Molecular Properties

17.15. Which of the following two carbohydrates would be potentially optically active in the gas phase or in solution?

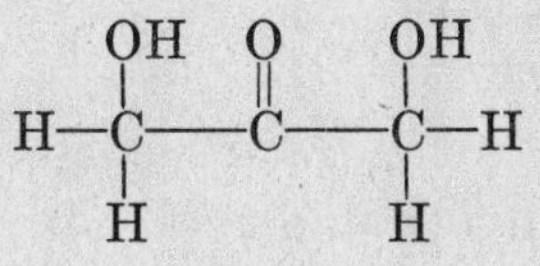

I

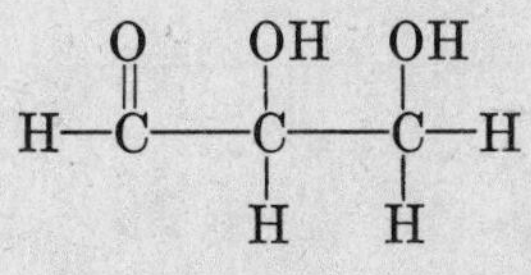

II

Even though there are conformations of *I* that would be optically active, the low energy necessary for rotation about the C—C single bonds would permit *I* to exist in essentially equal numbers in the various forms and the ensemble would be inactive. Because no $\hat{S}_n$ operation is allowed by *II*, it is potentially active in both phases.

17.16. Discuss the dipole moments of CH_4, CH_3Cl, CH_2Cl_2, $CHCl_3$ and CCl_4 using symmetry arguments.

Both CH_4 and CCl_4 belong to $\mathcal{T}_d$, which contains four C_3 axes, and thus they have no dipole moment. Both CH_3Cl and $CHCl_3$ belong to C_{3v}, which contains neither additional C_3 axes, a center of inversion, nor mirror planes other than σ_v, and thus they have a dipole moment which lies along the C_3 axis (and the intersection of the $3\sigma_v$). The molecule CH_2Cl_2 belongs to C_{2v}, which contains only E, C_2 and two types of σ_v, and thus it has a dipole moment which lies along the C_2 axis (and the intersection of the σ_v planes).

17.17. Determine which irreducible representations correspond to the x-, y- and z-components of translation for the $\mathcal{C}_{3v}$ point group.

Anticipating the results of Problem 17.36, the translational motion is the sum of V_1, a one-dimensional representation given by

$$\hat{E} \rightarrow (1) \qquad \hat{C}_3 \rightarrow (1) \qquad \hat{C}_3^2 \rightarrow (1) \qquad \hat{\sigma}_{v1} \rightarrow (1) \qquad \hat{\sigma}_{v2} \rightarrow (1) \qquad \hat{\sigma}_{v3} \rightarrow (1)$$

and V_3, a two-dimensional representation given by

$$\hat{E} \rightarrow \begin{pmatrix} 1 & 0 \\ 0 & 1 \end{pmatrix} \qquad \hat{C}_3 \rightarrow \begin{pmatrix} -0.500 & -0.866 \\ 0.866 & -0.500 \end{pmatrix} \qquad \hat{C}_3^2 \rightarrow \begin{pmatrix} -0.500 & 0.866 \\ -0.866 & -0.500 \end{pmatrix}$$

$$\hat{\sigma}_{v1} \rightarrow \begin{pmatrix} -1 & 0 \\ 0 & 1 \end{pmatrix} \qquad \hat{\sigma}_{v2} \rightarrow \begin{pmatrix} 0.500 & 0.866 \\ 0.866 & -0.500 \end{pmatrix} \qquad \hat{\sigma}_{v3} \rightarrow \begin{pmatrix} 0.500 & -0.866 \\ -0.866 & -0.500 \end{pmatrix}$$

Each of the symmetry operations leaves z invariant, which is the same as V_1. Thus z should be assigned to V_1 and (x, y) should be assigned to V_3.

17.18. Confirm the assignments of the R_i to the V_i shown in Table 17-7.

Applying the rules given in Section 17.21 to V_1, to which is assigned the z-component of translation, gives

$$\chi(V_{R_z}, \hat{E}) = \chi(V_1, \hat{E}) = 1 \quad \chi(V_{R_z}, 2\hat{C}_3(z)) = \chi(V_1, 2\hat{C}_3(z)) = 1 \quad \chi(V_{R_z}, 3\hat{\sigma}_v) = -\chi(V_1, 3\hat{\sigma}_v) = -1$$

which corresponds to V_2 in Table 17-7. Similarly, for V_3,

$$\chi(V_{R_{x,y}}, \hat{E}) = \chi(V_3, \hat{E}) = 2 \quad \chi(V_{R_{x,y}}, 2\hat{C}_3(z)) = \chi(V_3, 2\hat{C}_3(z)) = -1 \quad \chi(V_{R_{x,y}}, 3\hat{\sigma}_v) = -\chi(V_3, 3\hat{\sigma}_v) = 0$$

which corresponds to V_3 in Table 17-7.

Table 17-7

$\mathcal{C}_{3v}$ Representation	$\hat{E}$	$2\hat{C}_3(z)$	$3\hat{\sigma}_v$	Translation and Rotation
$V_1 = A_1$	1	1	1	z
$V_2 = A_2$	1	1	-1	R_z
$V_3 = E$	2	-1	0	(x, y), (R_x, R_y)

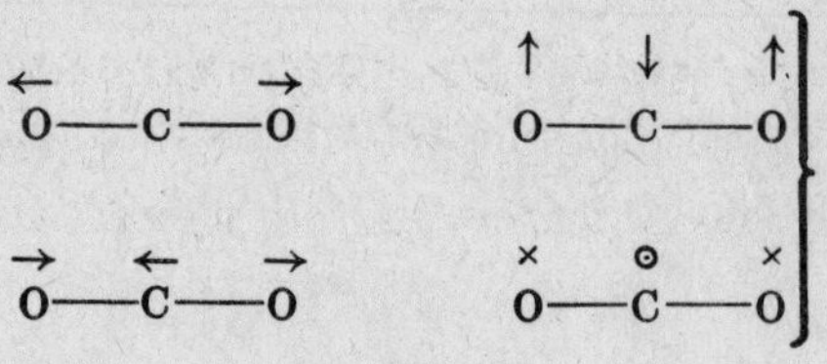

Fig. 17-19

17.19. CO_2 belongs to $\mathcal{D}_{\infty h}$, whose character table is Table 17-8. Discuss the normal modes of vibration for the molecule.

Using (*17.7*) gives

$$\chi(V_{3\Lambda}, \hat{E}) = 3(3) = 9 \qquad \chi(V_{3\Lambda}, \hat{C}_\infty^{\phi}) = 3[1 + 2\cos\phi] = 3 + 6\cos\phi$$

$$\chi(V_{3\Lambda}, \infty\hat{\sigma}_v) = 3 \qquad \chi(V_{3\Lambda}, \hat{i}) = -3(1) = -3 \qquad \chi(V_{3\Lambda}, \hat{\sigma}_h) = 1$$

$$\chi(V_{3\Lambda}, 2\hat{S}_\infty^{\phi}) = 1[-1 + 2\cos\phi] = -1 + 2\cos\phi \qquad \chi(V_{3\Lambda}, \infty\hat{C}_2) = 1\left[1 + 2\cos\frac{2\pi(1)}{2}\right] = -1$$

Because $h = \infty$ for this group, (*17.6*) is not applicable and $V_{3\Lambda}$ must be resolved by trial and error, giving $V_{3\Lambda} = V_1 \oplus 2V_2 \oplus V_5 \oplus 2V_6$. Subtracting $V_2 \oplus V_5 \oplus V_6$, which represents the contributions to $V_{3\Lambda}$ for x, y, z, R_x and R_y, gives

$$V_{\text{vib}} = V_1 \oplus V_2 \oplus V_6$$

The interpretation of this result is that there is one symmetrical stretch, one asymmetrical stretch and one doubly-degenerate bend, see Fig. 17-19.

Table 17-8

$\mathcal{D}_{\infty h}$ Representation	$\hat{E}$	$2\hat{C}_{\infty}^{\phi}$	$\hat{\sigma}_v$	$\hat{i}$	$\hat{\sigma}_h$	$2\hat{S}_{\infty}^{\phi}$	$\infty\hat{C}_2$	Translation and Rotation
$V_1 = A_{1g} = \Sigma g^+$	1	1	1	1	1	1	1	
$V_2 = A_{1u} = \Sigma u^+$	1	1	1	−1	−1	−1	−1	z
$V_3 = A_{2g} = \Sigma g^-$	1	1	−1	1	1	1	−1	R_z
$V_4 = A_{2u} = \Sigma u^-$	1	1	−1	−1	−1	−1	1	
$V_5 = E_{1g} = \Pi g$	2	$2\cos\phi$	0	2	−2	$-2\cos\phi$	0	(R_x, R_y)
$V_6 = E_{1u} = \Pi u$	2	$2\cos\phi$	0	−2	2	$2\cos\phi$	0	(x, y)
⋮	⋮	⋮	⋮	⋮	⋮	⋮	⋮	⋮

Supplementary Problems

Symmetry Elements and Operations

17.20. Construct perspective and orthographic drawings for C_1 (or 1). Is $\hat{C}_1$ distinct?

Ans. See Fig. 17-2; no, $\hat{C}_1 = \hat{E}$.

17.21. Construct perspective sketches and orthographic projections for the equivalent points around the C_3 and 6 symmetry elements.

Ans. Drawings are similar to Fig. 17-3(*e*) except three and six points appear, respectively.

17.22. List the distinct operations for $\hat{i}^k$. *Ans.* $\hat{i}$

17.23. Equate $\bar{3}$ and $\bar{6}$ to $\tilde{3}$ and $\tilde{6}$. *Ans.* $\bar{3} = \tilde{6}$, $\bar{6} = \tilde{3}$

17.24. Prepare a list of $\hat{S}_n^k$ that are distinct, where $n = 1, 2, 3, 4$ and 6.

Ans. $\hat{S}_3$, $\hat{S}_3^5$, $\hat{S}_4$, $\hat{S}_4^3$, $\hat{S}_6$, $\hat{S}_6^5$

17.25. What type of array is formed after $\hat{t}'$ has operated on the result of $\hat{t}$ operating on a motif, assuming many such operations and that the axes along which $\hat{t}$ and $\hat{t}'$ are performed are not collinear?

Ans. two-dimensional array (net)

17.26. Construct perspective sketches for the 3_1 and 3_2 elements. What is the relation between these elements?

Ans. See Fig. 17-20; 3_1 shows a clockwise rotation and 3_2 simplifies to a counterclockwise rotation.

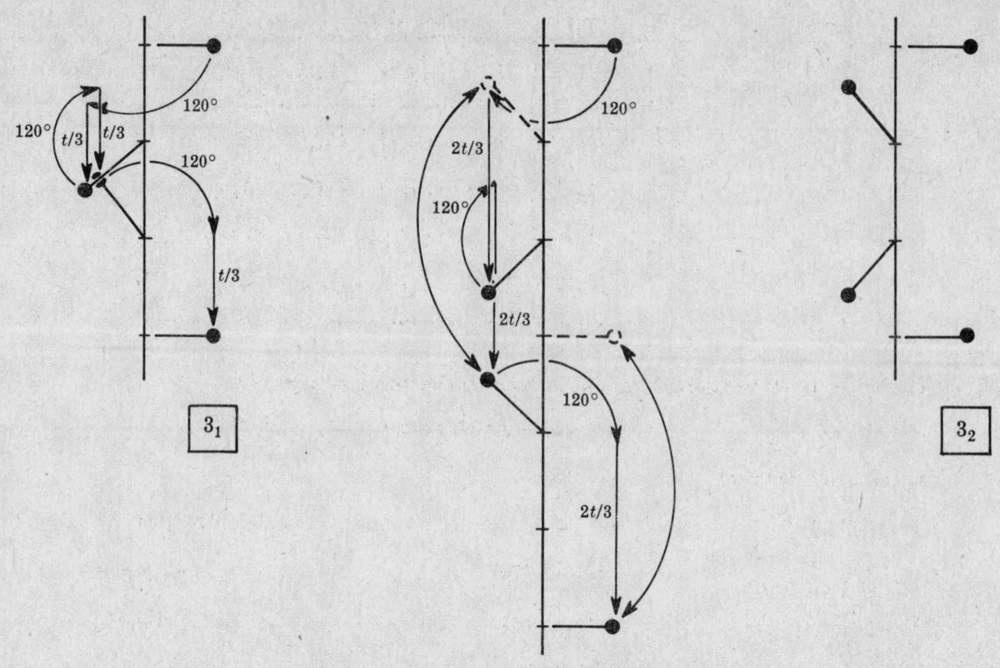

Fig. 17-20

17.27. Identify the symmetry elements present in (*a*) a die; (*b*) the letter B, assuming both lobes to be the same size; (*c*) the sign ×; and (*d*) a softball, including the stitching.

Ans. (*a*) E; (*b*) C_2, σ_v, σ_v', E; (*c*) C_4, $2C_2$, $2C_2'$, $2\sigma_v$, $2\sigma_v'$, σ_h, i, E; (*d*) S_4, σ_v, σ_v', C_2, i, E.

17.28. Give a geometrical proof that only 1-, 2-, 3-, 4-, and 6-fold axes are permitted in the solid state.

Ans. Interior angle of regular n-gon $= \dfrac{(n-2)\pi}{n} = \dfrac{2\pi}{k}$

Point Groups

17.29. Determine the symmetry elements present in a benzene molecule.

Ans. C_6; $3C_2$ which pass through the center of the molecule and through 2 C's and 2 H's; $3C_2'$ which pass through the center of the molecule and bisect the C—C bonds; σ_h; $3\sigma_v$ and $3\sigma_v'$ which bisect the angles formed by the C_2 and C_2' axes, respectively, and thus are $3\sigma_d$ and $3\sigma_d'$; i; E

17.30. Prepare multiplication tables for $\mathcal{C}_3$, $\mathcal{C}_{2h}$ and $\mathcal{D}_2$. *Ans.* See Tables 17-9, 17-10, 17-11.

Table 17-9

$\mathcal{C}_3$	$\hat{E}$	$\hat{C}_3$	$\hat{C}_3^2 = \hat{B}$
$\hat{A} = \hat{E}$	$\hat{E}$	$\hat{C}_3$	$\hat{C}_3^2$
$\hat{C}_3$	$\hat{C}_3$	$\hat{C}_3^2$	$\hat{E}$
$\hat{C}_3^2$	$\hat{C}_3^2$	$\hat{E}$	$\hat{C}_3$

Table 17-10

$\mathcal{C}_{2h}$	$\hat{E}$	$\hat{C}_2$	$\hat{\sigma}_h$	$\hat{i} = \hat{B}$
$\hat{A} = \hat{E}$	$\hat{E}$	$\hat{C}_2$	$\hat{\sigma}_h$	$\hat{i}$
$\hat{C}_2$	$\hat{C}_2$	$\hat{E}$	$\hat{i}$	$\hat{\sigma}_h$
$\hat{\sigma}_h$	$\hat{\sigma}_h$	$\hat{i}$	$\hat{E}$	$\hat{C}_2$
$\hat{i}$	$\hat{i}$	$\hat{\sigma}_h$	$\hat{C}_2$	$\hat{E}$

Table 17-11

$\mathcal{D}_2$	$\hat{E}$	$\hat{C}_2(x)$	$\hat{C}_2(y)$	$\hat{C}_2(z) = \hat{B}$
$\hat{A} = \hat{E}$	$\hat{E}$	$\hat{C}_2(x)$	$\hat{C}_2(y)$	$\hat{C}_2(z)$
$\hat{C}_2(x)$	$\hat{C}_2(x)$	$\hat{E}$	$\hat{C}_2(z)$	$\hat{C}_2(y)$
$\hat{C}_2(y)$	$\hat{C}_2(y)$	$\hat{C}_2(z)$	$\hat{E}$	$\hat{C}_2(x)$
$\hat{C}_2(z)$	$\hat{C}_2(z)$	$\hat{C}_2(y)$	$\hat{C}_2(x)$	$\hat{E}$

17.31. Classify the following molecules according to the point group:

(*a*) C_2H_4
(*b*) *p*-dichlorobenzene
(*c*) SiF_6^{2-}
(*d*) H_2S
(*e*) naphthalene
(*f*) PCl_5
(*g*) hexachlorobenzene
(*h*) HOCl
(*i*) I_3^-
(*j*) CH_2ClF
(*k*) coronene, $C_{24}H_{12}$
(*l*) CO_3^{2-}
(*m*) HCO_3^-
(*n*) S_8
(*o*) H_2O_2
(*p*) C_2H_6, staggered
(*q*) C_2H_6, eclipsed

Ans. (*a*) $\mathcal{D}_{2h}$ (*b*) $\mathcal{D}_{2h}$ (*c*) $\mathcal{O}_h$ (*d*) C_{2v} (*e*) $\mathcal{D}_{2h}$ (*f*) $\mathcal{D}_{3h}$ (*g*) $\mathcal{D}_{6h}$ (*h*) C_s (*i*) $\mathcal{D}_{\infty d}$ (*j*) C_s (*k*) $\mathcal{D}_{6h}$ (*l*) $\mathcal{D}_{3h}$ (*m*) C_s (*n*) $\mathcal{D}_{2h}$ (*o*) C_2 (*p*) $\mathcal{D}_{3d}$ (*q*) $\mathcal{D}_{3h}$

Representation of Groups

17.32. Show that $\hat{E}$ and $\hat{\sigma}_v'$ can be expressed as

$$\begin{pmatrix} 1 & 0 & 0 \\ 0 & 1 & 0 \\ 0 & 0 & 1 \end{pmatrix} \quad \text{and} \quad \begin{pmatrix} -1 & 0 & 0 \\ 0 & 1 & 0 \\ 0 & 0 & 1 \end{pmatrix}$$

respectively, for C_{2v} by performing the respective operations on a point having coordinates x_1, y_1 and z_1 and converting to matrix notation.

17.33. Confirm the expressions for $\hat{E}$ and $\hat{\sigma}_v'$ given in Problem 17.32 by using Table 17-3.

17.34. Using the matrix expressions given in Example 17.13 for the operations in C_{2v}, confirm the entries in Table 17-1 for $\hat{C}_2 \times \hat{\sigma}_v'$, $\hat{\sigma}_v \times \hat{C}_2$, $\hat{\sigma}_v \times \hat{\sigma}_v$, $\hat{\sigma}_v \times \hat{\sigma}_v'$, $\hat{\sigma}_v' \times \hat{C}_2$ and $\hat{\sigma}_v' \times \hat{\sigma}_v$.

17.35. Demonstrate that the elements of V_3 for the C_{2v} point group multiply as the symmetry operations of the group.

17.36. The six distinct operations in C_{3v} are $\hat{E}$, $\hat{C}_3$, $\hat{C}_3^2$, $\hat{\sigma}_{v1}$, $\hat{\sigma}_{v2}$ and $\hat{\sigma}_{v3}$, and they fall into the classes $\hat{E}$, $2\hat{C}_3$ and $3\sigma_v$. Show that the representation for this group provided by Table 17-3 is reducible. Determine the two obvious irreducible representations for the group and the dimension of the third.

Ans. $\hat{E} \rightarrow \left(\begin{array}{cc|c} 1 & 0 & 0 \\ 0 & 1 & 0 \\ \hline 0 & 0 & 1 \end{array}\right)$ $\qquad \hat{\sigma}_{v1} \rightarrow \left(\begin{array}{cc|c} -1 & 0 & 0 \\ 0 & 1 & 0 \\ \hline 0 & 0 & 1 \end{array}\right)$

$\hat{C}_3 \rightarrow \left(\begin{array}{cc|c} -0.500 & -0.866 & 0 \\ 0.866 & -0.500 & 0 \\ \hline 0 & 0 & 1 \end{array}\right)$ $\qquad \hat{\sigma}_{v2} \rightarrow \left(\begin{array}{cc|c} 0.500 & 0.866 & 0 \\ 0.866 & -0.500 & 0 \\ \hline 0 & 0 & 1 \end{array}\right)$

$\hat{C}_3^2 \rightarrow \left(\begin{array}{cc|c} -0.500 & 0.866 & 0 \\ -0.866 & -0.500 & 0 \\ \hline 0 & 0 & 1 \end{array}\right)$ $\qquad \hat{\sigma}_{v3} \rightarrow \left(\begin{array}{cc|c} 0.500 & -0.866 & 0 \\ -0.866 & -0.500 & 0 \\ \hline 0 & 0 & 1 \end{array}\right)$

$3^2 > 6$, therefore reducible; V_1 is the one-dimensional subset and V_3 is the two-dimensional subset of the matrices as blocked-out above; $\ell = (6 - 1^2 - 2^2)^{1/2} = 1$

17.37. Find the characters of the irreducible representations blocked-out in Problem 17.36. Recognizing that (*17.3*) is valid, find $\chi(V_2, \hat{R})$ for this group.

Ans. $\chi(V_2, \hat{E}) = 1,\ \chi(V_2, \hat{C}_3) = \chi(V_2, \hat{C}_3^2) = 1,\ \chi(V_2, \hat{\sigma}_{v1}) = \chi(V_2, \hat{\sigma}_{v2}) = \chi(V_2, \hat{\sigma}_{v3}) = -1$

17.38. Using V_3 as given in Problem 17.36, show that (*17.5*) is valid.

Ans. $\chi(V_3, \hat{C}_3) = \chi(V_3, \hat{C}_3^2) = -1,\ \chi(V_3, \hat{\sigma}_{v1}) = \chi(V_3, \hat{\sigma}_{v2}) = \chi(V_3, \hat{\sigma}_{v3}) = 0$

17.39. For C_{3v} find the characters of the irreducible representations corresponding to the Mulliken symbols E, A_1 and A_2. *Ans.* See Table 17-7.

Applications of Group Theory to Molecular Properties

17.40. The unit cell of cinnabar, HgS, belongs to the 32 point group. Is this mineral potentially optically active? *Ans.* yes

17.41. Using symmetry arguments, discuss the dipole moment in NH_3.

Ans. It lies along C_3 which is the intersection of the σ_v's.

17.42. Determine which irreducible representations correspond to the translations along the z- and x-axes for a water molecule. *Ans.* See Table 17-4.

17.43. Verify the assignments of translation components given in Table 17-12 for $\mathcal{D}_{2h}$, e.g. C_2H_4.

Table 17-12

$\mathcal{D}_{2h}$ Representation	$\hat{E}$	$\hat{\sigma}(xy)$	$\hat{\sigma}(xz)$	$\hat{\sigma}(yz)$	$\hat{i}$	$\hat{C}_2(z)$	$\hat{C}_2(y)$	$\hat{C}_2(x)$	Translation and Rotation
$V_1 = A_g$	1	1	1	1	1	1	1	1	
$V_2 = A_u$	1	−1	−1	−1	−1	1	1	1	
$V_3 = B_{1g}$	1	1	−1	−1	1	1	−1	−1	R_z
$V_4 = B_{1u}$	1	−1	1	1	−1	1	−1	−1	z
$V_5 = B_{2g}$	1	−1	1	−1	1	−1	1	−1	R_y
$V_6 = B_{2u}$	1	1	−1	1	−1	−1	1	−1	y
$V_7 = B_{3g}$	1	−1	−1	1	1	−1	−1	1	R_x
$V_8 = B_{3u}$	1	1	1	−1	−1	−1	−1	1	x

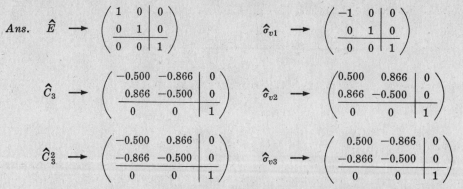

17.44. Confirm the assignments of R_y and R_z for C_{2v}.

17.45. Verify the assignments of rotation components given in Table 17-12 for $\mathcal{D}_{2h}$.

17.46. Discuss the symmetry of the vibrations of ONO, a nonlinear molecule.

Ans. C_{2v} (see Fig. 17-11)

17.47. Describe the vibrational motion in the linear molecules HCN and NNO.

Ans. Both belong to $C_{\infty v}$ (see Table 17-13) and can be shown to have a symmetrical stretch V_1, an asymmetrical stretch V_1, and a doubly-degenerate bend V_3, see Fig. 17-19.

17.48. Discuss the symmetry of the vibrations of (*a*) nonplanar AB_3, (*b*) C_2H_4 and (*c*) planar *WXYZ* chain.

Ans. (*a*) C_{3v} (see Table 17-7) having a symmetrical stretch V_1, symmetrical deformation V_1, degenerate stretch V_3 and degenerate deformation V_3

(*b*) $\mathcal{D}_{2h}$ (see Table 17-12) having $3V_1 \oplus V_2 \oplus 2V_3 \oplus V_4 \oplus V_5 \oplus 2V_6 \oplus 2V_8$

(*c*) C_s (see Table 17-14) having $5V_1 \oplus V_2$

Table 17-13

$C_{\infty v}$ Representation	$\hat{E}$	$2\hat{C}_{\infty}^{\phi}$	$\infty\hat{\sigma}_v$	Translation and Rotation
$V_1 = A_1 = \Sigma^+$	1	1	1	z
$V_2 = A_2 = \Sigma^-$	1	1	−1	R_z
$V_3 = E_1 = \Pi$	2	$2\cos\phi$	0	$(x, y), (R_x, R_y)$
$V_4 = E_2 = \Delta$	2	$2\cos 2\phi$	0	
$V_5 = E_3 = \Phi$	2	$2\cos 3\phi$	0	
⋮	⋮	⋮	⋮	

Table 17-14

C_s Representation	$\hat{E}$	$\hat{\sigma}(xy)$	Translation and Rotation
$V_1 = A'$	1	1	x, y, R_z
$V_2 = A''$	1	−1	z, R_x, R_y

Chapter 18

Intermolecular Bonding

Extended Covalent Bonding

18.1 COVALENT BONDING

Two types of substances have large networks of covalent bonds holding the atoms together in the condensed phases: (1) nonmetallic elements such as carbon for which the bonding arrangement satisfies electron deficiencies on the individual atoms and (2) compounds such as silicon dioxide which undergo energetically-favorable rearrangements of the electrons in the molecules that are stable in the gas phase. Because these bonds are no different than those described in Chapters 13 and 15, these substances will have intermediate to relatively high values for the melting and boiling points and for the heats of sublimation and vaporization, because these values depend on the thermal energy necessary to break the intermolecular bond.

If the covalent bonding is three-dimensional and if all bonds are equivalent, the substance will be isotropic, i.e. its properties will be the same in all directions. If the bonding varies within the substance or is not three-dimensional, the substance will be anisotropic, i.e. certain properties will depend on the direction of observation. Lower melting and boiling points can be expected for anisotropic materials.

18.2 HYDROGEN BONDING

The electronegativity differences between some elements and hydrogen are large enough that the hydrogen will form a weak coordinate covalent bond with an unshared pair of electrons on another molecule, giving a chain or three-dimensional network of molecules. For compounds containing F, O, N or Cl with H, these weak hydrogen bonds significantly increase the melting and boiling points of the compounds over the values predicted in the absence of these additional bonds.

Metallic Bonding

18.3 THE FREE-ELECTRON MODEL

In this theory of the bonding between the atoms in a metal, the kernels are placed in the physical arrangement found in the solid state, e.g. hexagonal or cubic closest-packed crystal structure, and the electrons act as freely moving particles in a three-dimensional box of uniform potential energy. The metallic bonds formed between the positively charged kernels and negatively charged electrons are rather strong, giving intermediate to high values for the melting and boiling points and for the heats of sublimation and vaporization.

At absolute zero, all the electrons will be in the lowest available quantum states with paired spins. The energy of the highest filled level predicted by (*11.45*) is

$$E_F = \frac{h^2}{8m_e}\left(\frac{3N}{\pi V}\right)^{2/3} \qquad (18.1)$$

where E_F is known as the *Fermi energy*, N is the number of conduction or valence electrons per mole of metal and V is the molar volume of the metal. At temperatures above absolute zero, the electronic kinetic energy per mole is given by

$$E = \frac{3}{5}NE_F\left[1 + \frac{5\pi^2}{12}\left(\frac{kT}{E_F}\right)^2 + \cdots\right] \qquad (18.2)$$

EXAMPLE 18.1. Find E_F for Na if $d = 0.97 \times 10^3$ kg m^{-3}. What is the electronic contribution to the thermal energy at 25 °C?

Substituting the molar volume,

$$V = \frac{M}{d} = \frac{(23.0 \text{ g mol}^{-1})(10^{-3} \text{ kg g}^{-1})}{0.97 \times 10^3 \text{ kg m}^{-3}} = 2.37 \times 10^{-5} \text{ m}^3 \text{ mol}^{-1}$$

into *(18.1)* gives

$$E_F = \frac{(6.626 \times 10^{-34} \text{ J s})^2}{8(9.11 \times 10^{-31} \text{ kg})}\left[\frac{3(6.022 \times 10^{23} \text{ mol}^{-1})}{\pi(2.37 \times 10^{-5} \text{ m}^3 \text{ mol}^{-1})}\right]^{2/3} = 5.04 \times 10^{-19} \text{ J}$$

The thermal energy (Section 2.1) becomes

$$E(\text{thermal}) = E - E_0 = \frac{\pi^2 N k^2 T^2}{4E_F} \qquad (18.3)$$

Substituting values for Na gives

$$E(\text{thermal}) = \frac{\pi^2(6.022 \times 10^{23} \text{ mol}^{-1})(1.3806 \times 10^{-23} \text{ J K}^{-1})^2(298 \text{ K})^2}{4(5.04 \times 10^{-19} \text{ J})} = 49.9 \text{ J mol}^{-1}$$

18.4 THE BAND THEORY

Instead of the uniform potential-energy function used in Section 18.3, the band theory assumes potential-energy wells centered at each kernel of the metal atom. For N atoms, bands of closely spaced energy levels are generated which are available for the valence electrons to occupy. Conduction occurs if a partially filled band passes over the walls of the barriers.

EXAMPLE 18.2. Prepare an energy diagram predicting the conductivity of Li.

Figure 18-1(*a*) shows the regularly spaced Li kernels and 1*s* electrons deep in the grand potential-energy well and the half-filled 2*s* band near the top of the well. The top of the band passes over the walls, hence Li should be a conductor.

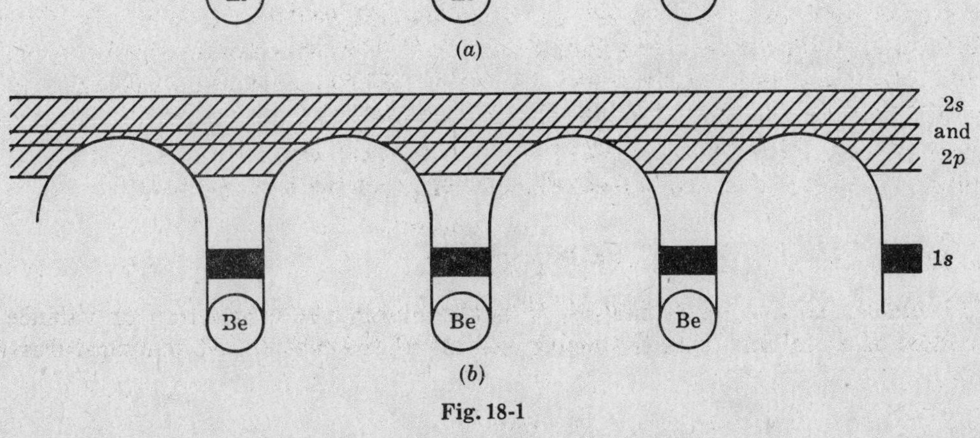

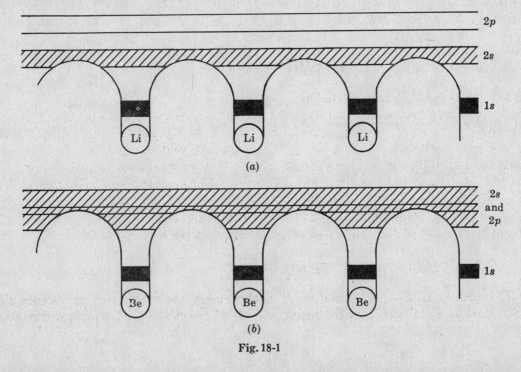

Fig. 18-1

EXAMPLE 18.3. Consider the n-type semiconductor diagramed in Fig. 18-2(a). What does the vertical arrow represent? Describe the mechanism for conduction if the impurity has 5 electrons.

The arrow represents the promotion of the "loose" fifth electron of the impurity by thermal energy. If the band into which this electron is promoted lies above the walls of the wells, conduction occurs.

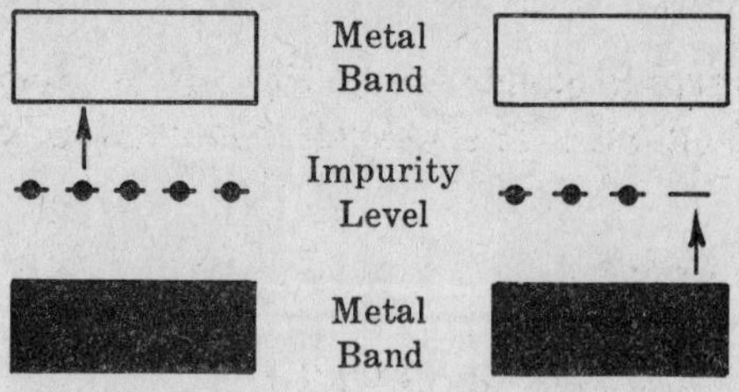

Fig. 18-2

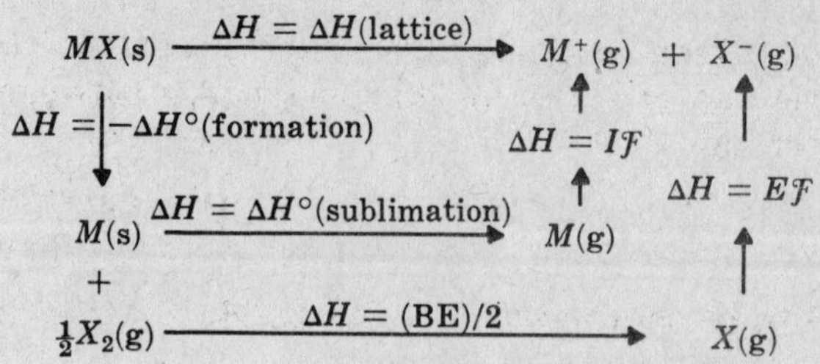

Fig. 18-3

Ionic Bonding

18.5 BORN-HABER CYCLE

The *lattice energy* of one mole of an ionic compound is the value of ΔH for the reaction

$$M_aX_b(\text{s}) = aM^{b+}(\text{g}) + bX^{a-}(\text{g})$$

The lattice energy between ions is strong enough that most ionic compounds have relatively high melting and boiling points, as well as high heats of sublimation and vaporization.

If MX is the halide of a Group I metal, the *Born-Haber cycle*, shown in Fig. 18-3, gives the lattice energy as

$$\Delta H(\text{lattice}, MX) = -\Delta H^\circ(\text{formation}, MX, \text{s}) + \Delta H^\circ(\text{sublimation}, M) + \frac{\text{BE}}{2} + I\mathcal{F} + E\mathcal{F} \tag{18.4}$$

where BE is the bond energy of the halogen in J mol^{-1}, I is the ionization potential of the metal in eV, E is the electron affinity of the halogen in eV, and $\mathcal{F} = 96{,}484.56$ C mol^{-1} is Faraday's constant. If the dissociation energy is used instead of the bond energy for the halogen, the term $\frac{1}{2}RT$ must be added to the right side of (*18.4*). The equation is also valid for an oxide of a Group II metal.

EXAMPLE 18.4. Calculate the lattice energy for NaCl at 25 °C if ΔH°(formation, NaCl, s) $= -98.260$ kcal mol^{-1}, ΔH°(sublimation, Na) $= 25.755$ kcal mol^{-1}, BE $= 57.844$ kcal mol^{-1} for Cl_2, $I = 5.138$ eV for Na and $E\mathcal{F} = -84.822$ kcal mol^{-1} for Cl.

Using (*18.4*) gives

$$\begin{aligned}\Delta H(\text{lattice}) &= -(-98.260)(4.184) + (25.755)(4.184) + \left(\frac{57.844}{2}\right)(4.184) \\ &\quad + (5.138 \text{ eV})(96.48456 \text{ kJ mol}^{-1}\text{ eV}^{-1}) + (-84.822)(4.184) \\ &= 780.74 \text{ kJ mol}^{-1}\end{aligned}$$

18.6 POTENTIAL-ENERGY FUNCTIONS

The attraction between each ion and its neighbors in a crystal gives rise to the molar potential

$$U_{\text{att}} = -\frac{L\mathcal{M}q^2}{4\pi\epsilon_0 r} \tag{18.5}$$

where the dimensionless number $\mathcal{M}$ is the *Madelung constant* for a given crystal configuration, q is the ionic charge, r is the shortest cation-anion distance in the crystal and $4\pi\epsilon_0$ is the permittivity constant ($4\pi\epsilon_0 = 1.11265 \times 10^{-10}\ \mathrm{C^2\ N^{-1}\ m^{-2}}$). Once the ion approaches another ion, a repulsive force described by the molar potential

$$U_{\mathrm{rep}} = Be^{-r/\rho} \quad \text{or} \quad U_{\mathrm{rep}} = B'r^{-n} \tag{18.6}$$

takes effect, resulting from the interaction of electronic clouds, etc. Here B, B' and ρ are constants and n is an integer usually between 6 and 12. The overall potential energy is given by

$$U = -\frac{L\mathcal{M}q^2}{4\pi\epsilon_0 r} + Be^{-r/\rho} \tag{18.7}$$

It can be shown, see Problem 18.24, that for the sodium chloride structure

$$B = \frac{4L\mathcal{M}q^2\rho e^{a/2\rho}}{4\pi\epsilon_0 a^2} \tag{18.8}$$

where a is the unit cell length. Combining (*18.8*) with (*18.7*) evaluated at $r = a/2$ gives for the sodium chloride structure

$$\Delta H(\text{lattice}) = \frac{2L\mathcal{M}q^2}{4\pi\epsilon_0 a}\left(1 - \frac{2\rho}{a}\right) + 2RT \tag{18.9}$$

where $2RT$ is added to convert the energy to an enthalpy.

EXAMPLE 18.5. Calculate ΔH(lattice) for NaCl at 25 °C using (*18.9*) if $a = 5.6402$ Å, $\rho = 0.34$ Å and $\mathcal{M} = 1.74756$. Compare this value to that determined in Example 18.4.

$$\Delta H(\text{lattice}) = \frac{2(6.022 \times 10^{23}\ \mathrm{mol^{-1}})(1.74756)(1.6022 \times 10^{-19}\ \mathrm{C})^2}{(1.11265 \times 10^{-10}\ \mathrm{C^2\ N^{-1}\ m^{-2}})(5.6402 \times 10^{-10}\ \mathrm{m})}\left[1 - \frac{2(0.34)}{5.6402}\right]$$
$$+ 2(8.314\ \mathrm{J\ mol^{-1}\ K^{-1}})(298\ \mathrm{K})$$
$$= (8.610 \times 10^5\ \mathrm{J\ mol^{-1}})(1 - 0.1206) + 4955\ \mathrm{J\ mol^{-1}} = 762.1\ \mathrm{kJ\ mol^{-1}}$$

which agrees well with the value calculated using the Born-Haber cycle.

Van der Waals Forces

18.7 DIPOLE MOMENTS

Coulomb's law describing the force between two electrical charges separated by a distance r within a dielectric is given by

$$f = \frac{q_1 q_2}{4\pi\epsilon r^2} = \frac{q_1 q_2}{(\epsilon/\epsilon_0)4\pi\epsilon_0 r^2} \tag{18.10}$$

where ϵ/ϵ_0 is the *dielectric constant*. The *molar polarization* of a substance is related to ϵ/ϵ_0 by

$$\mathcal{P} = \frac{(\epsilon/\epsilon_0) - 1}{(\epsilon/\epsilon_0) + 2}\frac{M}{d}(4\pi\epsilon_0) \tag{18.11}$$

The units of $\mathcal{P}$ are $\mathrm{C\ m^2\ V^{-1}\ mol^{-1}}$ in the SI system. Reported values of $\mathcal{P}$ in units of $\mathrm{cm^3\ mol^{-1}}$ or $\mathrm{m^3\ mol^{-1}}$ can be converted by multiplying by $4\pi\epsilon_0$. Considering the polarization of the molecule to result from permanent and induced dipole moments, it can be shown that

$$\mathcal{P} = \frac{4\pi L}{3}\left(\alpha + \frac{\mu^2}{3kT}\right) \tag{18.12}$$

where α is the *polarizability* of the molecule in units of C m^2 V^{-1} and μ is the permanent dipole moment of the molecule in units of C m (1 debye = 3.33564×10^{-30} C m). A plot of $\mathcal{P}$ against $1/T$ will have a slope proportional to μ and an intercept proportional to α.

Recalling the discussion given in Section 13.6 for diatomic molecules, a polyatomic molecule will have a dipole moment if it has the center of negative charge separated from the center of positive charge. Very frequently the determination of the molecular shape, see Sections 15.9 through 15.11, is a prerequisite to predicting whether a substance is polar or not.

If the dipole moment for a particular bond in a molecule is known, it is often possible to predict semiquantitatively the dipole moment for a molecule containing two such bonds by vectorial analysis (see Problem 18.10).

EXAMPLE 18.6. The dielectric constant for $CHCl_3$ at 20 °C is 4.806. If $-d\log(\epsilon/\epsilon_0)/dT = 0.160 \times 10^{-2}$, find α and μ. The density of $CHCl_3$ is 1.4832×10^3 kg m^{-3} at 20 °C.

At 20 °C the polarization is given by *(18.11)* as

$$\mathcal{P} = \frac{4.806-1}{4.806+2}\,\frac{(119.38\ \text{g mol}^{-1})(10^{-3}\ \text{kg g}^{-1})}{1.4832 \times 10^3\ \text{kg m}^{-3}}(1.11265 \times 10^{-10}\ \text{C}^2\ \text{N}^{-1}\ \text{m}^{-2})$$

$$= 5.008 \times 10^{-15}\ \text{C m}^2\ \text{V}^{-1}\ \text{mol}^{-1}$$

The dielectric constant at 25 °C = 298 K is found by integrating the temperature-dependence function, giving

$$\log(\epsilon/\epsilon_0)_{298} = \log(\epsilon/\epsilon_0)_{293} - (0.160 \times 10^{-2})(298-293)$$

$$= \log(4.806) - (0.160 \times 10^{-2})(5) = 0.6738$$

or

$$(\epsilon/\epsilon_0)_{298} = 4.718$$

Assuming an insignificant change in density, the polarization at 25 °C, calculated as above, is 4.956×10^{-15} C m^2 V^{-1} mol^{-1}.

Although a plot of $\mathcal{P}$ against $1/T$ could be prepared, it is simpler to substitute the two values of $\mathcal{P}$ and T into *(18.12)* and solve for α and μ directly. The results are

$$\mu = 3.89 \times 10^{-30}\ \text{C m} = 1.16\ \text{D} \qquad \alpha = 7.50 \times 10^{-40}\ \text{C m}^2\ \text{V}^{-1}$$

18.8 POTENTIAL-ENERGY FUNCTIONS

The weak, attractive *London forces* between the atoms, molecules or ions of any substance are described by the molar potential-energy function

$$U_L = \frac{(-1.8 \times 10^{-18}\ \text{J})\alpha^2 L}{(4\pi\epsilon_0)^2 r^6} \tag{18.13}$$

These forces alone cause the condensation of a gas to a liquid or solid for substances such as the noble gases, which do not have additional potential energies resulting from dipole-dipole interactions, ionic bonding, metallic bonding or covalent bonding. Such substances have relatively low melting and boiling points, as well as small heats of sublimation and vaporization.

The potential energy for a polar substance is the sum of a term for the dipole-dipole interaction and a term for the induced dipole effect, giving

$$U_d = -\frac{2\mu^2[(\mu^2/3kT)+\alpha]L}{(4\pi\epsilon_0)^2 r^6} \tag{18.14}$$

As in cases of ionic and covalent bonding, the potential-energy curve generated by the sum of *(18.6)* *(18.13)* and *(18.14)* passes through a minimum. Van der Waals radii have been assigned for several elements, which may be used to estimate the minimizing distance for different substances. Usually the sum of van der Waals radii is of the order of 3.5 to 5.5 Å.

EXAMPLE 18.7. Compare U_L and U_d for $CHCl_3$ at 25 °C using the data in Example 18.6.

Taking the ratio of *(18.14)* to *(18.13)* and substituting data gives

$$\frac{U_d}{U_L} = \frac{2\mu^2[(\mu^2/3kT) + \alpha]}{(1.8 \times 10^{-18})\alpha^2}$$

$$= \frac{2(3.89 \times 10^{-30})^2\{[(3.89 \times 10^{-30})^2/3(1.3807 \times 10^{-23})(298)] + 7.50 \times 10^{-40}\}}{(1.8 \times 10^{-18})(7.50 \times 10^{-40})^2}$$

$$= 0.059$$

Solved Problems

Extended Covalent Bonding

18.1. Several of the elements in Group IVA of the periodic table, e.g. C(dia), Si, Ge and gray tin, satisfy the four-electron deficiency on each atom by undergoing sp^3 hybridization and forming a three-dimensional network of covalent bonding in which each atom is bonded to four others. If the heats of formation of C(dia) and C(g) at 25 °C are 0.4533 and 171.291 kcal mol^{-1}, respectively, calculate the average C—C bond energy in diamond. Compare this value to 331 kJ mol^{-1}, which is the average value in organic compounds.

The energy necessary to sublime one mole of diamond is given by *(3.7)* as

$$\Delta H = [(1)(171.291) - (1)(0.4533)](4.184) = 714.785 \text{ kJ}$$

On the average, two C—C bonds must be broken to sublime a given carbon atom, giving an average energy of $714.785/2 = 357.392$ kJ mol^{-1}, about the same as in organic compounds.

18.2. The elements in Group VA of the periodic table, e.g. red P, black P, As, Sb and Bi, require three electrons to complete the "octet" of the outer-shell electrons. Describe the bonding in the condensed phases of these elements. Compare the melting points of the Group VA elements to those in Group IVA.

These elements form networks of puckered six-membered rings. Although the bonds between rings are very strong, the bonding between the networks is quite weak and these substances will melt and boil at lower temperatures than the Group IVA elements.

18.3. Assuming the absence of hydrogen bonding, predict the boiling points of HF and NH_3 by plotting boiling points against atomic number for the other compounds in each family having a similar formula and extrapolating to the proper atomic number. If the actual boiling points are 19.54 °C for HF and −33.35 °C for NH_3, which hydrogen bond is stronger? Is this in agreement with the electronegativities of the elements?

If a plot of −35.38 °C for HI, −67.0 °C for HBr and −84.9 °C for HCl against atomic number were prepared and extrapolated to HF, the predicted boiling point would be about −100 °C. Likewise the value for NH_3 is about −100 °C as determined by plotting 22 °C for H_3Bi, −17 °C for SbH_3, −55 °C for H_3As and −87.4 °C for PH_3. The increase for HF is about twice as much as that for NH_3, so the HF bond is stronger. The result agrees with the fact that F is more electronegative than N.

Metallic Bonding

18.4. The band theory diagram for a p-type semiconductor is shown in Fig. 18-2(b). Describe the mechanism for conduction if the impurity has three valence electrons.

The thermal energy promotes a metal electron to the impurity level, producing the required partially-filled band which can conduct if the energy level of the band is above the walls.

18.5. Find η in (*2.20*) for Ag.

Using the molecular weight and density for Ag, the molar volume is

$$V = \frac{(107.868\ \text{g mol}^{-1})(10^{-3}\ \text{kg g}^{-1})}{10.5 \times 10^{3}\ \text{kg m}^{-3}} = 1.03 \times 10^{-5}\ \text{m}^3\ \text{mol}^{-1}$$

which upon substitution into (*18.1*) gives

$$E_F = \frac{(6.626 \times 10^{-34}\ \text{J s})^2}{8(9.11 \times 10^{-31}\ \text{kg})}\left[\frac{3(6.022 \times 10^{23}\ \text{mol}^{-1})}{\pi(1.03 \times 10^{-5}\ \text{m}^3\ \text{mol}^{-1})}\right]^{2/3} = 8.80 \times 10^{-19}\ \text{J}$$

Anticipating the results of Problem 18.17 gives

$$\eta = \frac{\pi^2 Rk}{2E_F} = \frac{\pi^2(8.314\ \text{J mol}^{-1}\ \text{K}^{-1})(1.3807 \times 10^{-23}\ \text{J K}^{-1})}{2(8.80 \times 10^{-19}\ \text{J})}$$
$$= 6.44 \times 10^{-4}\ \text{J K}^{-2}\ \text{mol}^{-1}$$

Ionic Bonding

18.6. Assuming the melting point to be proportional to ΔH(lattice), qualitatively predict the melting points for NaCl and BaO if $a = 5.6402$ Å for NaCl and 5.50 Å for BaO. Both substances crystallize in the same crystal configuration, giving identical values of $\mathcal{M}$ in (*18.19*). Assume $\rho = 0.34$ Å for both substances.

The difference in the values of ΔH(lattice) for these substances will arise primarily from the difference in q. Because q^2 is four times as large for BaO than for NaCl, BaO is predicted to have the higher melting point. The actual values are 801 °C for NaCl and 1923 °C for BaO.

18.7. Find the expression for ΔH(lattice) using (*18.5*) and the second form for U_{rep} given in (*18.6*). Using $n = 6$ and 12, find ΔH(lattice) at 25 °C for NaCl and compare these values to those found in Examples 18.4 and 18.5.

The overall potential energy is given by

$$U = -\frac{L\mathcal{M}q^2}{4\pi\epsilon_0 r} + B'r^{-n}$$

For a minimum at $r = a/2$,

$$\left.\frac{\partial U}{\partial r}\right|_{r=a/2} = \frac{L\mathcal{M}q^2}{4\pi\epsilon_0(a/2)^2} - nB'(a/2)^{-n-1} = 0$$

whence

$$B' = \frac{L\mathcal{M}q^2(a/2)^{n-1}}{4\pi\epsilon_0 n}$$

The expression for U becomes

$$U = -\frac{L\mathcal{M}q^2}{4\pi\epsilon_0}\left[\frac{1}{r} - \frac{(a/2)^{n-1}}{nr^n}\right]$$

and

$$\Delta H(\text{lattice}) = \frac{L\mathcal{M}q^2}{4\pi\epsilon_0}\left[\frac{1}{r} - \frac{(a/2)^{n-1}}{nr^n}\right] + 2RT$$

Upon substitution of $r = a/2$ and the data from Example 18.5, for $n = 6$

$$\Delta H(\text{lattice}) = \frac{(6.022 \times 10^{23}\ \text{mol}^{-1})(1.74756)(1.6022 \times 10^{-19}\ \text{C})^2}{1.11265 \times 10^{-10}\ \text{C}^2\ \text{N}^{-1}\ \text{m}^{-2}} \left[\frac{5}{6}\left(\frac{1}{2.8201 \times 10^{-10}\ \text{m}}\right)\right]$$
$$+ 2(8.314\ \text{J K}^{-1}\ \text{mol}^{-1})(298\ \text{K})$$
$$= 722.5\ \text{kJ mol}^{-1}$$

and for $n = 12$, $\Delta H(\text{lattice}) = 794.2\ \text{kJ mol}^{-1}$. Both values are close to those determined in Examples 18.4 and 18.5, with the higher value of n giving better agreement.

Van der Waals Forces

18.8. Predict which molecules in Fig. 15-16 will have significant dipole moments.

Using the three-dimensional sketches given in Fig. 15-17, the following can be predicted:

(*a*) The polar covalent bonds in n-C_8H_{18} give rise to small dipole moments depending on the orientation of the carbon atoms, but the effect is not large.

(*b*) The planar molecule BF_3 has the bonds arranged such that the polar nature of the bonds cancels, giving a nonpolar molecule.

(*c*) The symmetrical molecule S_8 has no polar nature.

(*d*) The planar molecule C_2H_4 is symmetrical, giving a nonpolar molecule.

(*e*) The linear molecule C_2H_2 is symmetrical, giving a nonpolar molecule.

(*f*) There is a displacement of positive and negative centers of charge in HCNO, giving a dipole moment.

(*g*) The nonsymmetrical linear molecule N_2O has a dipole moment.

(*h*) The octahedral symmetry of $CrCl_6^{3-}$ makes the center of the molecule the center of both the positive and negative charge, so that the molecule is nonpolar. However, the presence of an ionic charge makes this determination purely an academic exercise.

(*i*) The square planar configuration of XeF_4 is a nonpolar configuration.

18.9. The dipole moment of HCl is 1.03 D, of HBr is 0.78 D and of HI is 0.38 D. If the dielectric constants of the gases at 1 atm are 1.0046 for HCl at 0 °C and 1.00313 for HBr at 20 °C , find the values of α for these substances. Assuming α to be proportional to the number of electrons present, qualitatively predict α for HI. Check this prediction by calculating α from the dielectric constant of 1.00234 at 100 °C for the gas.

Solving (*1.19*) for M/d and substituting into (*18.11*) gives for the gases

$$\mathcal{P} = \frac{(\epsilon/\epsilon_0) - 1}{(\epsilon/\epsilon_0) + 2} \frac{RT}{P} (4\pi\epsilon_0) \qquad (18.15)$$

Substituting the data for HBr gives

$$\mathcal{P} = \frac{1.00313 - 1}{1.00313 + 2} \frac{(8.21 \times 10^{-5}\ \text{m}^3\ \text{atm K}^{-1}\ \text{mol}^{-1})(293\ \text{K})}{1\ \text{atm}} (1.11265 \times 10^{-10}\ \text{C}^2\ \text{N}^{-1}\ \text{m}^2)$$
$$= 2.79 \times 10^{-15}\ \text{C m}^2\ \text{V}^{-1}\ \text{mol}^{-1}$$

Using (*18.12*) gives

$$2.79 \times 10^{-15} = (25.22 \times 10^{23}) \left[\alpha + \frac{(0.78)^2(3.33564 \times 10^{-30})^2}{3(1.3807 \times 10^{-23})(293)}\right]$$

which upon solving gives $\alpha = 5.5 \times 10^{-40}\ \text{C m}^2\ \text{V}^{-1}$. Similarly for HCl, $\mathcal{P} = 3.82 \times 10^{-15}$, giving $\alpha = 4.7 \times 10^{-40}$.

According to the number of electrons, the predicted value for HI should be greater than the values for HCl and HBr. Repeating the calculations confirms this prediction: $\mathcal{P} = 1.95 \times 10^{-15}$ and $\alpha = 7.73 \times 10^{-40}$.

18.10. The dipole moment of chlorobenzene is 1.69 D. Predict the dipole moments for *o*-, *m*- and *p*-dichlorobenzene.

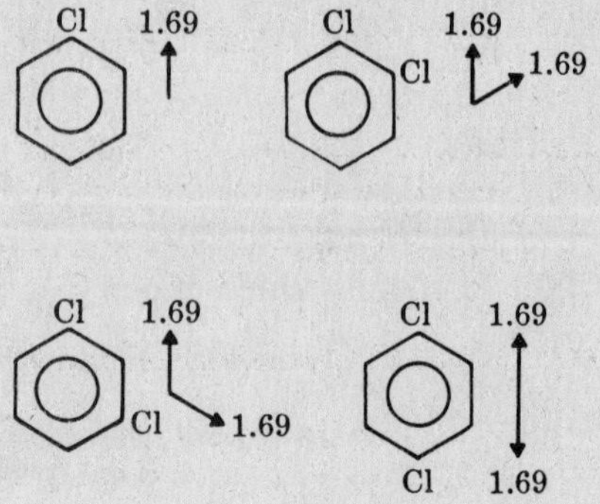

Fig. 18-4

Consider the sketches of the molecules shown in Fig. 18-4. For *o*-dichlorobenzene, the vectorial summing process gives

$$\mu_x = 1.69 \cos 30° + 1.69 \cos 90° = 1.46$$

$$\mu_y = 1.69 \sin 30° + 1.69 \sin 90° = 2.54$$

$$\mu = (\mu_x^2 + \mu_y^2)^{1/2} = [(1.46)^2 + (2.54)^2]^{1/2}$$

$$= 2.93 \text{ D}$$

which is a little higher than the actual 2.50 D. For *m*-dichlorobenzene,

$$\mu_x = 1.69 \cos(-30°) + 1.69 \cos 90° = 1.46$$

$$\mu_y = 1.69 \sin(-30°) + 1.69 \sin 90° = 0.85$$

$$\mu = [(1.46)^2 + (0.85)^2]^{1/2} = 1.69 \text{ D}$$

which is a little higher than the actual value of 1.58 D. For *p*-dichlorobenzene, $\mu = \mu_x = \mu_y = 0$, which agrees with the experimental value.

18.11. The dielectric constant for He is 1.0000684 at 1 atm and 140 °C, and for Ar is 1.000545 at 1 atm and 23°C. (*a*) Using (*18.12*) with $\mu = 0$, find α for these elements. (*b*) Assuming a van der Waals radius of 2 Å for each element, calculate U_L and qualitatively predict the boiling points of these substances.

(*a*) Using (*18.15*) gives

$$\mathcal{P}_{\text{He}} = \frac{1.0000684 - 1}{1.0000684 + 2} \frac{(8.21 \times 10^{-5})(413)}{1}(1.11265 \times 10^{-10}) = 8.60 \times 10^{-17} \text{ C m}^2 \text{ V}^{-1} \text{ mol}^{-1}$$

$$\mathcal{P}_{\text{Ar}} = 4.91 \times 10^{-16} \text{ C m}^2 \text{ V}^{-1} \text{ mol}^{-1}$$

Then, from (*18.12*),

$$\alpha_{\text{He}} = \frac{3\mathcal{P}}{4\pi L} = (3.964 \times 10^{-25})\mathcal{P} = (3.964 \times 10^{-25})(8.60 \times 10^{-17}) = 3.41 \times 10^{-41} \text{ C m}^2 \text{ V}^{-1}$$

a very low value, and $\alpha_{\text{Ar}} = 1.95 \times 10^{-40}$ C m² V⁻¹.

(*b*) With $r = 4$ Å, (*18.13*) gives

$$(U_L)_{\text{He}} = \frac{(-1.8 \times 10^{-18} \text{ J})(3.41 \times 10^{-41} \text{ C m}^2 \text{ V}^{-1})^2(6.022 \times 10^{23} \text{ mol}^{-1})}{(1.11265 \times 10^{-10} \text{ C}^2 \text{ N}^{-1} \text{ m}^{-2})^2(4 \times 10^{-10} \text{ m})^6} = -24.9 \text{ J mol}^{-1}$$

and $(U_L)_{\text{Ar}} = -813$ J mol^{-1}. The values of U_L indicate that much more energy is needed to boil Ar than He, neglecting repulsive forces, which agrees with the experimental values of $\Delta H°$(vaporization) = 1558 cal mol^{-1} for Ar at 87.29 K and 20 cal mol^{-1} for He at 4.22 K. Note that at 4.22 K,

$$(24.9 \text{ J mol}^{-1}) + 2RT = 95.1 \text{ J mol}^{-1}$$

for He, a value very close to the experimental value of 84 J mol^{-1}.

Supplementary Problems

Extended Covalent Bonding

18.12. The elements in Group VIA of the periodic table, e.g. S, Se and Te, require two electrons to complete the outer-shell "octet" of electrons. Describe the bonding in the condensed phases of these elements. Compare the melting points of the Group VIA elements to those in Groups IVA and VA.

Ans. networks of chains or single rings; lower, similar

18.13. Find the average Ge—Ge bond energy if the heat of sublimation for Ge is 106.4 kcal mol^{-1}. Why would the energy of a Ge—Ge bond be predicted as less than that of a C—C bond?

Ans. 222.6 kJ mol^{-1}; bonding electrons farther from the nucleus in Ge

18.14. Would ΔH for the phase transition

$$SiO_2(\alpha\text{-qtz}) = SiO_2(\alpha\text{-tridymite})$$

be large? In both structures each Si is bonded to four O's in a large three-dimensional network.

Ans. no

18.15. Discuss the bonding in diamond and graphite. Which substance will show the following properties: (*a*) very hard, (*b*) soft, (*c*) electrical insulator, (*d*) electrical conductor along two crystallographic axes, (*e*) absorption of gases and (*f*) oxidation?

Ans. Diamond has sp^3-hybridized atoms forming four equivalent bonds; graphite has sp^2 atoms forming covalent bonds in layers and weak forces between layers. (*a*) Bonds in diamond are hard to break. (*b*) Bonds between graphite layers are easy to break. (*c*) No available electrons in diamond. (*d*) Electrons between graphite layers move easily. (*e*) Layers of graphite are widely spaced and electrons provide mechanism for absorption. (*f*) Both oxidize under extreme conditions.

18.16. The boiling points for the hydrogen-containing compounds of Group VIA are −2 °C for H_2Te, −41.5 °C for H_2Se and −68.7 °C for H_2S. (*a*) Predict the boiling point for H_2O assuming the absence of hydrogen bonding. (*b*) Based on electronegativities, predict the relative strengths of hydrogen bonding in NH_3, H_2O and HF. (*c*) Why does water seemingly violate this order?

Ans. (*a*) About −80 °C. (*b*) HF > H_2O > NH_3. (*c*) H_2O can form three-dimensional networks of bonds, whereas HF and NH_3 can only form chains.

Metallic Bonding

18.17. Find the electronic contribution to the heat capacity by differentiating (*18.3*) with respect to *T*. Evaluate η in (*2.20*) for Na.

Ans. $C_{V,\text{electronic}} = \pi^2 RkT/2E_F$; using $E_F = 5.04 \times 10^{-19}$ J gives $\eta = 5.62 \times 10^{-4}$ J mol^{-1} K^{-2}

18.18. Find E_F and η for Al and compare the latter value to that found in Example 2.8. The density of Al is 2.702×10^3 kg m^{-3}.

Ans. $E_F = 8.98 \times 10^{-19}$ J, $\eta = 6.30 \times 10^{-4}$ J mol^{-1} K^{-2};
about 54% low, but correct order of magnitude

18.19. Prepare an energy diagram demonstrating the conductivity of Be, given that the $2p$ band overlaps the $2s$ band. *Ans.* See Fig. 18-1(*b*).

18.20. A photoconductor has an unfilled band near a filled band. Describe the mechanism for conduction.

Ans. Light quanta excite electrons, giving two partially filled bands; the upper band or both may conduct depending on the height of the barrier.

Ionic Bonding

18.21. Qualitatively predict the melting points for BaO and MgO if $a = 5.50$ Å and 4.213 Å, respectively, assuming equivalent crystal configurations.

Ans. MP $\propto \Delta H(\text{lattice}) \propto q^2/a$, giving MgO > BaO based on a; actual values are 1923 °C and 2800 °C

18.22. Using (*18.4*), calculate the lattice energy for periclase, MgO, at 25 °C if $\Delta H°$(formation, MgO, s) = -143.700 kcal mol^{-1}, $\Delta H°$(sublimation, Mg) = 35.281 kcal mol^{-1}, BE = 119.118 kcal mol^{-1} for O_2, $I = 22.675$ eV for Mg and $E\mathcal{F} = 156$ kcal mol^{-1} total for O. If $a = 4.213$ Å, $\rho = 0.34$ Å and $\mathcal{M} = 1.74756$, calculate ΔH(lattice) using (*18.9*). *Ans.* 3839 and 3866 kJ mol^{-1}

18.23. Combining (*18.7*) and (*18.8*) gives

$$U = -\frac{2L\mathcal{M}q^2}{4\pi\epsilon_0 a}\left\{\frac{a}{2r} - \frac{2\rho}{a}e^{[(a/2)-r]/\rho}\right\}$$

Prepare a plot of U against r for values of r between 1 and 10 Å for MgO, if $a = 4.213$ Å and $\rho = 0.34$ Å.

Ans. typical potential-energy well with minimum of -3866 kJ mol^{-1} at 4.213 Å

18.24. Show that (*18.8*) is the correct expression for B for the halite structure by differentiating (*18.7*) with respect to r, setting the result equal to zero at $r = a/2$ and solving for B.

Van der Waals Forces

18.25. Predict which molecules in Fig. 15-22 will have significant dipole moments.

Ans. H_2O_2, $SnCl_2$, $COCl_2$, $SeBr_4$

18.26. Calculate ϵ/ϵ_0 for water vapor at STP if $\alpha/4\pi\epsilon_0 = 1.44 \times 10^{-30}$ m^3 and $\mu = 1.82$ D.

Ans. $\mathcal{P} = 8.626 \times 10^{-15}$ C m^2 V^{-1} mol^{-1}; $\epsilon/\epsilon_0 = 1.0104$

18.27. If $\epsilon/\epsilon_0 = 2.238$ and $d = 1.5954 \times 10^3$ kg m^{-3} for CCl_4(liq) and 1.70 and 0.466×10^3 kg m^{-3} for CH_4(liq), find α for these substances. Arrange CCl_4, CH_4 and $CHCl_3$ (see Example 18.6) in order of increasing α. Predict where CH_3Cl and CH_2Cl_2 would fit into this sequence.

Ans. $\mathcal{P} = 3.134 \times 10^{-15}$ C m^2 V^{-1} mol^{-1} for CCl_4 and 7.337×10^{-16} for CH_4,
$\alpha = 12.4 \times 10^{-40}$ C m^2 V^{-1} for CCl_4 and 2.91×10^{-40} for CH_4;
$CH_4 < CH_3Cl < CH_2Cl_2 < CHCl_3 < CCl_4$

18.28. The dipole moment of chlorobenzene is 1.69 D and of nitrobenzene is 4.22 D. Predict the dipole moments for *o*-, *m*- and *p*-chloronitrobenzene using vectorial analysis.

Ans. 5.27, 3.67 and 2.53 (actual are 4.64, 3.73 and 2.83)

18.29. The boiling point of *n*-C_5H_{12} is 36.07 °C and of neopentane is 9.5 °C. If neither molecule has any appreciable intermolecular bonding except London forces, why is there such a large difference in the boiling points?

Ans. The "linear" *n*-C_5H_{12} molecules have large parallel overlap, allowing stronger London forces than the "spherical" neopentane molecules which have very little overlap.

18.30. The dielectric constant for N_2(g) is 1.000580 at 23 °C and 1.00 atm, and for CO(g) is 1.00070 under the same conditions. If the molecules are 3 Å apart, calculate α and the attractive potential energy for these substances. Which will have the higher boiling point and heat of vaporization? The dipole moment of CO is 0.112 D.

Ans. $\mathcal{P} = 5.23 \times 10^{-16}$ C m^2 V^{-1} mol^{-1} for N_2 and 6.31×10^{-16} for CO;
$\alpha = 2.07 \times 10^{-40}$ C m^2 V^{-1} for N^2 and 2.39×10^{-40} for CO;
$U_L = -5120$ J mol^{-1} for N_2 and -6860 J mol^{-1} for CO, $U_d = -4.64$ J mol^{-1} for CO;
$U = -5120$ J mol^{-1} for N_2 and -6860 J mol^{-1} for CO (the dipole moment contribution is insignificant); CO is predicted to have the higher boiling point and heat of vaporization (actual values are 1.444 kcal mol^{-1} at 81.66 K for CO and 1.333 kcal mol^{-1} at 77.34 K for N_2).

18.31. Predict the major contributions to the intermolecular bonding in:

(*a*) Mg	(*g*) Si	(*m*) *p*-xylene
(*b*) Br_2	(*h*) PCl_5	(*n*) Ne
(*c*) HF	(*i*) PCl_3	(*o*) $SnBr_4$
(*d*) HBr	(*j*) H_2Te	(*p*) *trans*-$PtCl_2Br_2$
(*e*) C_2H_6	(*k*) SO_2	(*q*) *cis*-$PtCl_2Br_2$
(*f*) AgCl	(*l*) NO_2	

Ans.

(*a*) metallic	(*g*) covalent	(*m*) London
(*b*) London	(*h*) London	(*n*) London
(*c*) hydrogen bonding	(*i*) London	(*o*) London
(*d*) dipole and London	(*j*) dipole and London	(*p*) London
(*e*) London	(*k*) London	(*q*) dipole and London
(*f*) ionic	(*l*) dipole (bent molecule) and London	

Chapter 19

Crystals

Unit Cell

19.1 INTRODUCTION

The constituents of a crystalline solid, whether atoms, molecules or ions, are arranged in an ordered, repetitive fashion in three dimensions. The array is called a (*space*) *lattice*. It is possible to choose a group of atoms to serve as a model of the crystal just as it is possible to select the repeated motif on wallpaper to serve as the representation of the entire roll. The representative atoms chosen for the model are collectively called the *unit cell* of the crystal. If the unit cell is properly chosen, it is possible to generate the entire lattice by repeating the structure of the unit cell.

Consider the three-dimensional arrangement of points in Fig. 19-1, which might correspond to the location of the constituents of a metallic crystal. An acceptable unit cell for this crystal is in bold outline. By translating this unit cell along the three axes shown in the diagram, the entire crystal pattern can be generated.

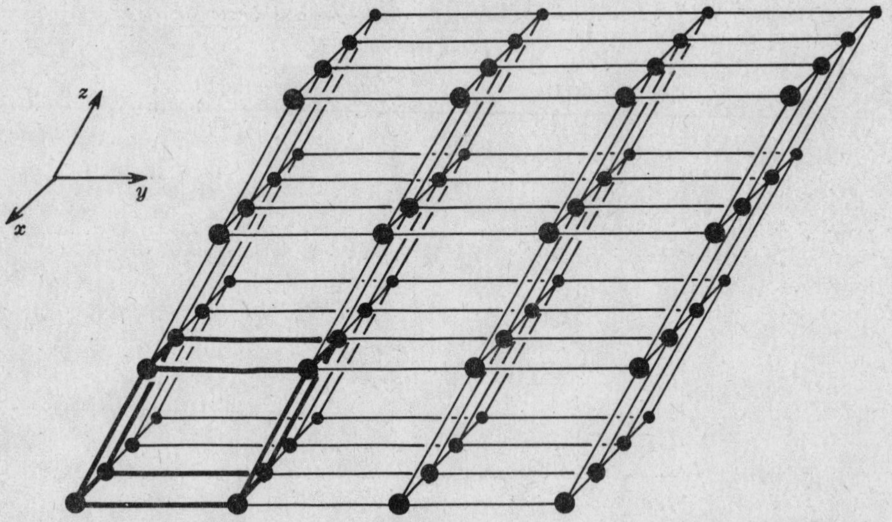

Fig. 19-1 (*after Metz, STRC–051,* Modular Laboratory Program, *Willard Grant Press, Inc.*)

Although any three noncoplanar rows will define a unit cell, by convention the preferred unit cell is one that represents the symmetry of the crystal, is as nearly orthogonalized as possible, and is minimal in content of atoms. The translational distances (Section 17.8) defining the lengths of the unit cell in the x-, y-, and z-directions are designated a, b and c, respectively, and the angles between these edges are α (between b and c), β (between a and c) and γ (between a and b). By convention, c usually lies parallel to the highest-order rotation axis in the unit cell, and a and b lie parallel or perpendicular to other symmetry elements, if present. Under these restrictions, usually $c \leqq a \leqq b$, and α and $\beta \geqq 90°$.

The seven *crystal systems* (the rhombohedral system is sometimes listed as a subsystem of the hexagonal system, giving six) are given in Table 19-1. (Optional conventions are shown in parentheses.) The fourteen *Bravais lattices* are also listed in Table 19-1. These are the only possible arrangements of identical points in space which retain the full symmetry of the system such that the entire crystal may be generated by translation. The symbol P means a primitive lattice in the shape defined by the geometric requirements of the system (R means a primitive rhombohedron and H is sometimes used to describe a primitive hexagonal unit cell); C, B or A means the centering of an atom only in the faces defined by the a- and b-axes, the a- and c-axes or the b- and c-axes, respectively; F means face-centering on all faces; and I means body-centering.

Table 19-1

Crystal System	Geometry of System	Bravais Lattices	Point Groups		Minimum Symmetry
triclinic	$a \neq b \neq c$†	P	$\bar{1}$	C_i	C_1
	$\alpha \neq \beta \neq \gamma$†		1	C_1	
monoclinic	$a \neq b \neq c$†	P; B or A	$2/m$	C_{2h}	C_2 or σ
	$\alpha = \beta = 90°$, $\gamma > 90°$	(C or A)	m	C_s (C_{1h}, C_{1v}, C_v)	
	($\alpha = \gamma = 90°$, $\beta > 90°$)		2	C_2	
orthorhombic	$a \neq b \neq c$	P; C, B or A;	$2/m\,2/m\,2/m$ (mmm)	$\mathcal{D}_{2h}$	$3 \perp C_2$
	$\alpha = \beta = \gamma = 90°$	F; I	$2mm$ ($mm2$)	C_{2v}	or C_2 and 2σ
			222	$\mathcal{D}_2$	
tetragonal	$a = b \neq c$ ($a_1 = a_2 \neq c$)	P; I	$4/m\,2/m\,2/m$ ($4/m\,mm$)	$\mathcal{D}_{4h}$	C_4 or $\bar{4}$
	$\alpha = \beta = \gamma = 90°$		422 (42)	$\mathcal{D}_4$	
			$4mm$	C_{4v}	
			$\bar{4}2m$ ($\bar{4}m2$)	$\mathcal{D}_{2d}$	
			$4/m$	C_{4h}	
			4	C_4	
			$\bar{4}$	$\mathcal{S}_4$	
hexagonal††	$a = b \neq c$ ($a_1 = a_2 = -a_3 \neq c$)	P (H)	$6/m\,2/m\,2/m$ ($6/m\,mm$)	$\mathcal{D}_{6h}$	C_6 or $\bar{6}$
	$\alpha = \beta = 90°$, $\gamma = 120°$		622 (62)	$\mathcal{D}_6$	
			$6mm$	C_{6v}	
			$\bar{6}m2$ ($\bar{6}2m$)	$\mathcal{D}_{3h}$	
			$6/m$	C_{6h}	
			6	C_6	
			6 ($3/m$)	C_{3h} ($\mathcal{S}_3$)	
rhombohedral (trigonal)	$a = b = c$ ($a_1 = a_2 = a_3$)	R (P)	$\bar{3}\,2/m$ ($\bar{3}m$)	$\mathcal{D}_{3d}$	C_3 or $\bar{3}$
	$120° > \alpha = \beta = \gamma \neq 90°$		32	$\mathcal{D}_3$	
	($a_1 = a_2 \neq c$, $\alpha = \beta = 90°$,		$3m$	C_{3v}	
	$\gamma = 120°$)		$\bar{3}$	C_{3i}	
			3	C_3	
cubic (isometric)	$a = b = c$ ($a_1 = a_2 = a_3$)	P; F; I	$4/m\,\bar{3}\,2/m$ ($m3m$)	O_h	$4C_3$ at 54°44′
	$\alpha = \beta = \gamma = 90°$		432 (43)	O	
			$\bar{4}3m$	$\mathcal{T}_d$	
			$2/m\,\bar{3}$ ($m3$)	$\mathcal{T}_h$	
			23	$\mathcal{T}$	

† Fortuitous equalities do not place the lattice in a system of higher symmetry.

†† The hexagonal system is often overdetermined by including a_3, which is a linear combination of a_1 and a_2 (see Fig. 19-6).

The point groups listed for each crystal system in Table 19-1 reflect the unique combinations of the various symmetry elements allowed in each system. Although each of these 32 point groups could be represented by a single symbol using the Schönflies system (see Chapter 17), crystallographers use the Hermann-Mauguin system which usually consists of (1) a symbol describing the symmetry element along the c-axis; (2) a symbol describing the symmetry element, if any, along one of the other axes or at an angle of $54°44'$ to the c-axis in the cubic system; and (3) a symbol describing the symmetry element, if any, along the third axis or at an angle of 30° or 45° to the second axis in the hexagonal and tetragonal systems, respectively. The equivalencies between the Schönflies and Hermann-Mauguin systems are given in Table 19-1, as well as the minimum symmetry requirements for a unit cell to belong to that system.

If the allowed symmetry elements include glide planes and screw axes, and if centering is permitted, 230 space groups are generated The symbol for a space group consists of the centering followed by an abbreviated Hermann-Mauguin symbol; e.g. $P2_12_12_1$ is a primitive unit cell in the orthorhombic system in which the two-fold axes are two-fold screw axes, and $Fm3m$ (complete symbol is $F4/m\,3\,2/m$) is a face-centered unit cell in the cubic system. Because very careful X-ray analysis and other tests are required to distinguish the various space groups, they will not be considered further.

19.2 UNIT CELL CONTENT

The *unit cell content, Z,* is the number of points contained within the unit cell. A primitive unit cell has points only at the corners of the parallelepiped, whereas a multiple unit cell contains additional points which are edge-centered, face-centered or body-centered. A point on a corner is being shared by several unit cells and thus contributes only a fraction of its volume and mass to the unit cell under consideration; the total contribution from all corners is $Z = 1$. A point that is centered on a face of a unit cell is being shared by exactly two unit cells and thus contributes $\frac{1}{2}$ of its volume and mass to the unit cell under consideration. A point that is centered within the unit cell is not being shared and thus contributes its entire volume and mass. A point that is centered along an edge of the unit cell is being shared by three or four unit cells; the total contribution of these points will be an integer.

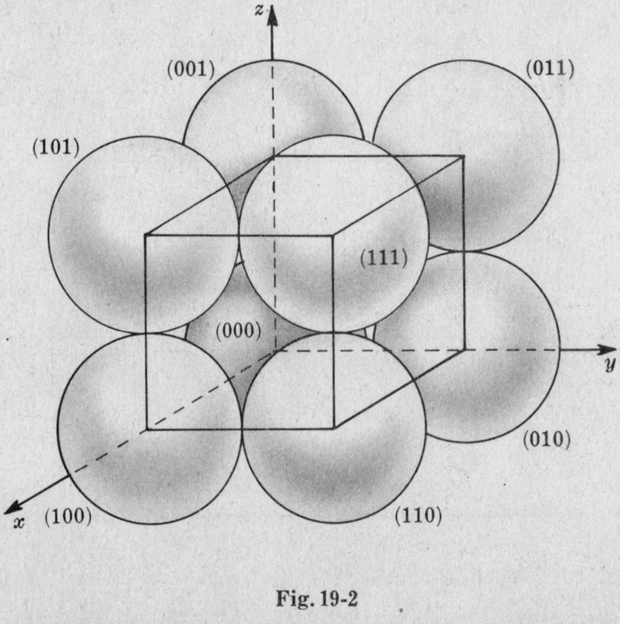

Fig. 19-2

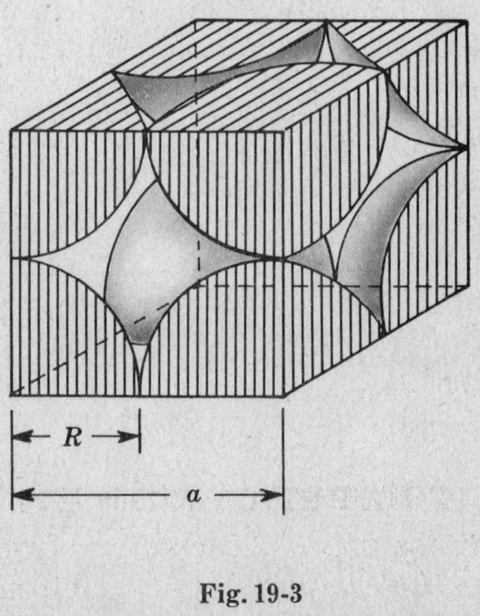

Fig. 19-3

EXAMPLE 19.1. Consider the primitive cubic unit cell shown in Fig. 19-2. Each corner is shared by eight unit cells and thus a given corner atom contributes only 1/8 of its volume and mass to the unit cell under consideration, see Fig. 19-3. The corners contribute a total of $8(1/8) = 1 = Z$ for this unit cell.

19.3 UNIT CELL COORDINATES

Each atom of the unit cell may be located by assigning x-, y- and z-coordinates to the atom. Consider the primitive cubic unit cell shown in Fig. 19-2. If the atom in the rear lower left-hand corner of the unit cell is taken as the origin of a three-dimensional Cartesian coordinate system, its coordinates (given as multiples of a, b and c) would be (000), those of the atom on the same body diagonal would be (111), etc. The coordinates of all eight atoms are given in Fig. 19-2. The letters u, v and w are often used to describe decimal fractions. A bar over a number or letter, e.g. $\bar{u}$, means the negative, which can be equally interpreted as $1-u$.

By convention, the set of coordinates (000) stands for the locations of all eight corners, i.e. (100), (111), (101), (110), (001), (011), (010) and (000); the set of coordinates $(00\frac{1}{2})$ stands for $(00\frac{1}{2})$, $(10\frac{1}{2})$, $(01\frac{1}{2})$ and $(11\frac{1}{2})$; the set given by $(\frac{1}{2}\frac{1}{2}0)$ stands for $(\frac{1}{2}\frac{1}{2}0)$ and $(\frac{1}{2}\frac{1}{2}1)$; etc. The minimum number of coordinate sets necessary to express the location of all atoms in the unit cell will be equal to Z.

19.4 CRYSTALLOGRAPHIC PROJECTIONS

A crystallographic projection, or view of the unit cell looking along one of the crystallographic axes, shows the shape of the unit cell in two dimensions, with the three-dimensional information being given by the coordinate of each constituent along that axis. If the projection is made along the z-axis, the combined symbol (1) represents an atom in the xy-plane (the plane of the paper) and an atom above the xy-plane by one unit length c. Only one projection is required for a cubic crystal. For crystals in the hexagonal, monoclinic and tetragonal systems, two projections are required as a minimum and for crystals in the other systems, three projections are necessary.

EXAMPLE 19.2. Prepare a crystallographic projection for the primitive cubic unit cell (Fig. 19-2).

The two-dimensional shape will be a square with atoms at each corner. The three-dimensional information for the cell is contained in the symbols (1). See Fig. 19-4. Clearly, only one projection is required.

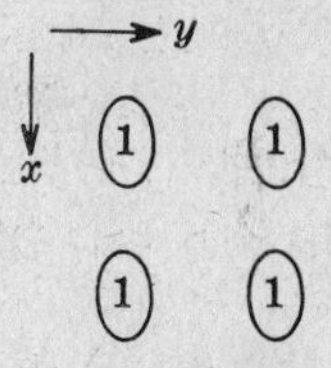

Fig. 19-4

19.5 COORDINATION NUMBER

The *coordination number*, CN, of an atom in a crystal is the number of nearest-neighbor atoms. All atoms in the Bravais lattice have the same CN.

EXAMPLE 19.3. Determine CN for an atom in the primitive cubic unit cell.

If the primitive cubic unit cell were translated to generate several unit cells as shown in Fig. 19-5, around any given atom there would be six equally-spaced nearest-neighbor atoms at a distance a. Thus $CN = 6$. Any other atoms in the crystal lattice will be at a distance greater than a from the atom under consideration.

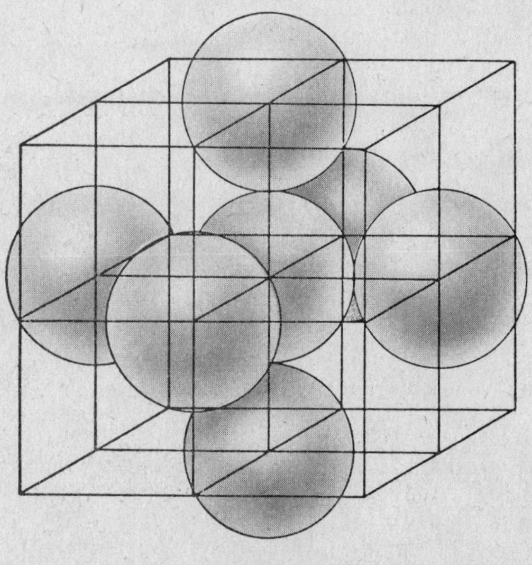
Fig. 19-5

19.6 THEORETICAL DENSITY

If the unit cell dimensions are known, the *theoretical density* for a substance can be calculated from

$$d = \frac{ZM}{LV} \tag{19.1}$$

where M is the molecular weight, L is Avogadro's number, and

$$V = abc(1 - \cos^2\alpha - \cos^2\beta - \cos^2\gamma + 2\cos\alpha\cos\beta\cos\gamma)^{1/2} \tag{19.2a}$$

For unit cells having 90° angles between edges, (*19.2a*) simplifies to

$$V = abc \tag{19.2b}$$

EXAMPLE 19.4. Polonium is the only element known to crystallize in a primitive cubic unit cell under room conditions. If $a = 3.36$ Å, find the theoretical density.

Using (*19.2b*) gives $V = (3.36\text{ Å})^3$ for the cubic unit cell, which upon substitution into (*19.1*) gives

$$d = \frac{(1)(209\text{ g mol}^{-1})(10^{-3}\text{ kg g}^{-1})}{(6.022\times 10^{23}\text{ mol}^{-1})(3.36\times 10^{-10}\text{ m})^3} = 9.15\times 10^3\text{ kg m}^{-3}$$

19.7 CRYSTAL RADII

If the spheres representing the atoms in a unit cell are assumed to touch along an edge, a face diagonal, a body diagonal, etc., the *crystal radius of the atom*, R, can be calculated from the unit cell dimensions.

EXAMPLE 19.5. Find the relationship between a and R for a primitive cubic unit cell and calculate R for Po if $a = 3.36$ Å.

Figure 19-3 shows that $a = 2R$, giving $R = 1.68$ Å.

19.8 SEPARATION OF ATOMS

The distance between two atoms in a unit cell, ℓ, can be calculated from their coordinates $(x_1y_1z_1)$ and $(x_2y_2z_2)$ as

$$\ell = [a^2(x_2-x_1)^2 + b^2(y_2-y_1)^2 + c^2(z_2-z_1)^2 - 2ab(x_2-x_1)(y_2-y_1)\cos\gamma - 2ac(x_2-x_1)(z_2-z_1)\cos\beta - 2bc(y_2-y_1)(z_2-z_1)\cos\alpha]^{1/2} \tag{19.3a}$$

which simplifies to

$$\ell = [a^2(x_2-x_1)^2 + b^2(y_2-y_1) + c^2(z_2-z_1)^2]^{1/2} \tag{19.3b}$$

for an orthogonal unit cell and to

$$\ell = a[(x_2-x_1)^2 + (y_2-y_1)^2 + (z_2-z_1)^2]^{1/2} \tag{19.3c}$$

for a cubic unit cell.

EXAMPLE 19.6. Find the distance between two Po atoms that lie along a body diagonal if $a = 3.36$ Å.

Substituting (000) and (111) into (*19.3c*) gives

$$\ell = a[(1-0)^2 + (1-0)^2 + (1-0)^2]^{1/2} = a(3)^{1/2} = (3.36\text{ Å})(3)^{1/2} = 5.82\text{ Å}$$

Crystal Forms

19.9 METALLIC CRYSTALS

Most metals crystallize in either the *hexagonal closest-packed* or *cubic closest-packed* unit cells, where CN = 12. These unit cells are a hexagonal body-centered cell (see Example 19.7) and the cubic face-centered cell, respectively, and have the highest packing density for simple lattices, as well as a great stability because of the high CN. Several of the alkali metals crystallize in the body-centered cubic unit cell, where CN = 8. Very few metals use the remaining twelve Bravais lattices because of the inefficient packing.

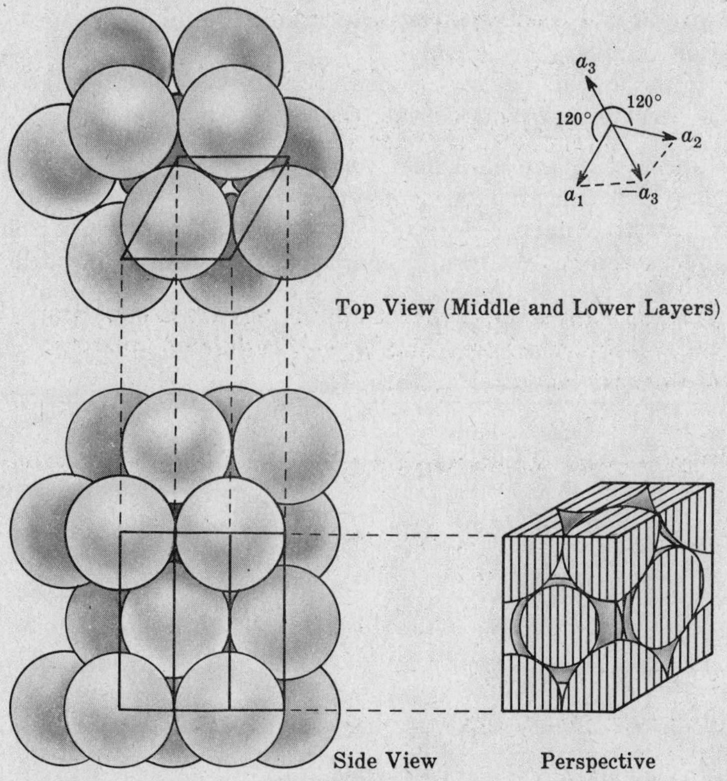

Fig. 19-6

EXAMPLE 19.7. Calculate the efficiency of packing in the hexagonal closest-packed unit cell, see Fig. 19-6.

The diagrams in Fig. 19-6 show that $Z = 2$ for the unit cell. If a radius of R is assumed for the metal atom, the total volume occupied by the metal atoms is

$$V_{\text{occ}} = 2\left(\frac{4}{3}\pi R^3\right) = 8.38\,R^3$$

By looking at the diagrams, $a_1 = a_2 = 2R$. By careful inspection of the geometry of the system, it can be shown that $c = 2(2/3)^{1/2}a = 1.633\,a$. Using (*19.2a*) for the volume of the unit cell gives

$$V_{\text{cell}} = a^2c(1-\cos^2\gamma)^{1/2} = a^2c\sin\gamma = (2R)^2(1.633)(2R)(\sin 120^\circ) = 11.31\,R^3$$

The packing efficiency is given by

$$\frac{V_{\text{occ}}}{V_{\text{cell}}} = \frac{8.38\,R^3}{11.31\,R^3} = 74.1\%$$

19.10 COVALENTLY BONDED CRYSTALS

As discussed in Section 18.1, the elements of Group IVA of the periodic table crystallize in networks of three-dimensional equivalent covalent bonds.

19.11 IONIC CRYSTALS

To this point, all unit cells have been assumed to have identical constituents. With some modifications, the previous treatment applies to ionic crystals, in which the constituents are charged ions. The content Z now refers to the number of ion groups, as specified by the empirical formula for the substance, present in the unit cell; the ratio of Z_+ to Z_- will be the ratio of subscripts in the empirical formula. Sets of coordinates must be assigned to each type of ion present; crystallographic projections should distinguish between types of ions; the coordination numbers CN_+ and CN_- (each defined as the number of oppositely-charged nearest neighbors) will be in the inverse ratio of the subscripts in the empirical formula; and the unit cell length will be related to two radii, R_+ and R_-.

For ionic substances with the empirical formula MX that crystallize in the cubic system, the unit cell can be predicted from the radius ratio R_+/R_-, see Table 19-2. Common noncubic unit cells for the empirical formula MX include the wurtzite and PbO structures in the hexagonal and tetragonal systems, respectively. Common unit cells for the empirical formula M_2X or MX_2 include the cuprite and fluorite structures in the cubic system and the rutile structure in the tetragonal system.

Table 19-2

Empirical Formula	Radius Ratio	CN	Structure If Cubic
	$0.225 < R_+/R_- < 0.414$	4	sphalerite (wurtzite, if hexagonal)
MX	$0.414 < R_+/R_- < 0.732$	6	halite
	$0.732 < R_+/R_- < 1.000$	8	CsCl
MX_2	$0.225 < R_+/R_- < 0.414$	4 and 2	SiO_2 and Cu_2O
or	$0.414 < R_+/R_- < 0.732$	6 and 3	TiO_2, CdI_2, NiS_2 and FeS_2
M_2X	$0.732 < R_+/R_- < 1.000$	8 and 4	CaF_2

EXAMPLE 19.8. AgCl crystallizes in the NaCl structure, see Fig. 19-7. Describe the unit cell in terms of interpenetrating Bravais lattices. What are the coordinates of the ions? If $R = 1.26$ Å for Ag^+ and 1.81 Å for Cl^-, show that this structure is predicted by the radius ratio rule. What are the values of CN for each ion? Determine Z_+, Z_- and Z for the unit cell and calculate the theoretical density if $a = 5.5491$ Å. Prepare a crystallographic projection for this unit cell.

AgCl can be described as two interpenetrating face-centered cubic structures, one of Ag^+ located at (000) and the second of Cl^- located at $(\frac{1}{2}00)$. The coordinates of the Ag^+ ions are identical to those of a face-centered cube: (000), $(\frac{1}{2}\frac{1}{2}0)$, $(\frac{1}{2}0\frac{1}{2})$ and $(0\frac{1}{2}\frac{1}{2})$. The coordinates of the Cl^- ions are $(\frac{1}{2}00)$, $(0\frac{1}{2}0)$, $(\frac{1}{2}\frac{1}{2}\frac{1}{2})$ and $(00\frac{1}{2})$.

The radius ratio is

$$\frac{R_+}{R_-} = \frac{1.26}{1.81} = 0.696$$

which falls into the NaCl structure range in Table 19-2. Around any given Ag^+, there are six Cl^- ions as nearest neighbors, giving $CN_+ = 6$. Likewise around a given Cl^- there are six Ag^+ ions as nearest neighbors, giving $CN_- = 6$. The ratio CN_+/CN_- is 1 : 1, which is inverse to the 1 : 1 ratio in the empirical formula.

Because both sets of ions are face-centered cubic, $Z_+ = Z_- = 4$ and $Z = 4$. The ratio Z_+/Z_- is 1 : 1 as in the empirical formula. The theoretical density is given by (*19.1*) and (*19.2b*) as

$$d = \frac{(4)(143.32)(10^{-3})}{(6.022 \times 10^{23})(5.5491 \times 10^{-10})^3} = 5.571 \times 10^3 \text{ kg m}^{-3}$$

Because there are two types of ions, the projection should distinguish between these. A common technique is to use the symbol * after the coordinate of one type of ion (Cl^- in Fig. 19-8).

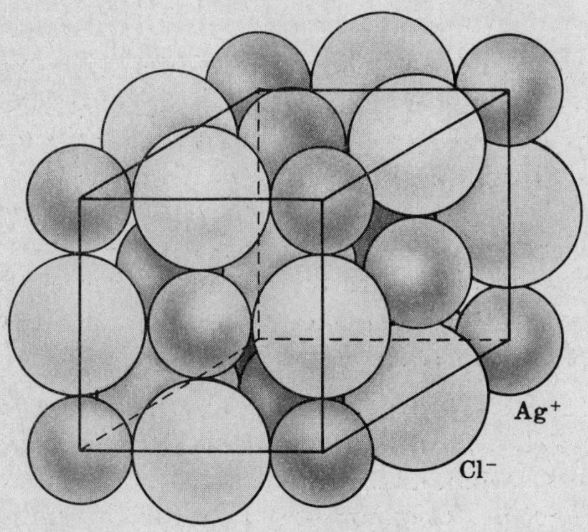

Fig. 19-7 (*after Metz, STRC–051*, Modular Laboratory Program, *Willard Grant Press, Inc.*)

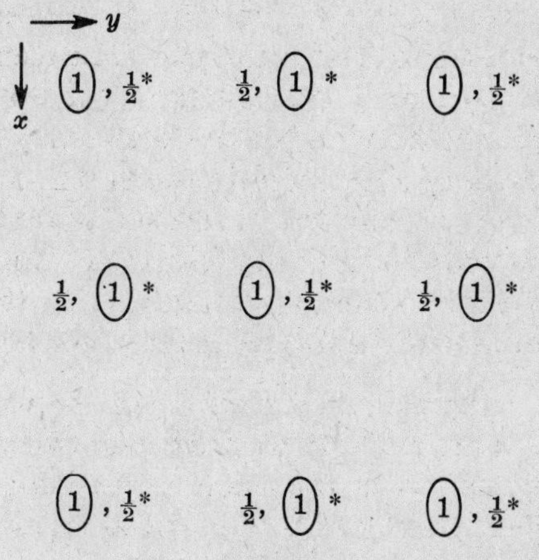

Fig. 19-8

19.12 MOLECULAR CRYSTALS

The molecules in these crystals are held together by van der Waals forces or hydrogen bonds, see Chapter 18.

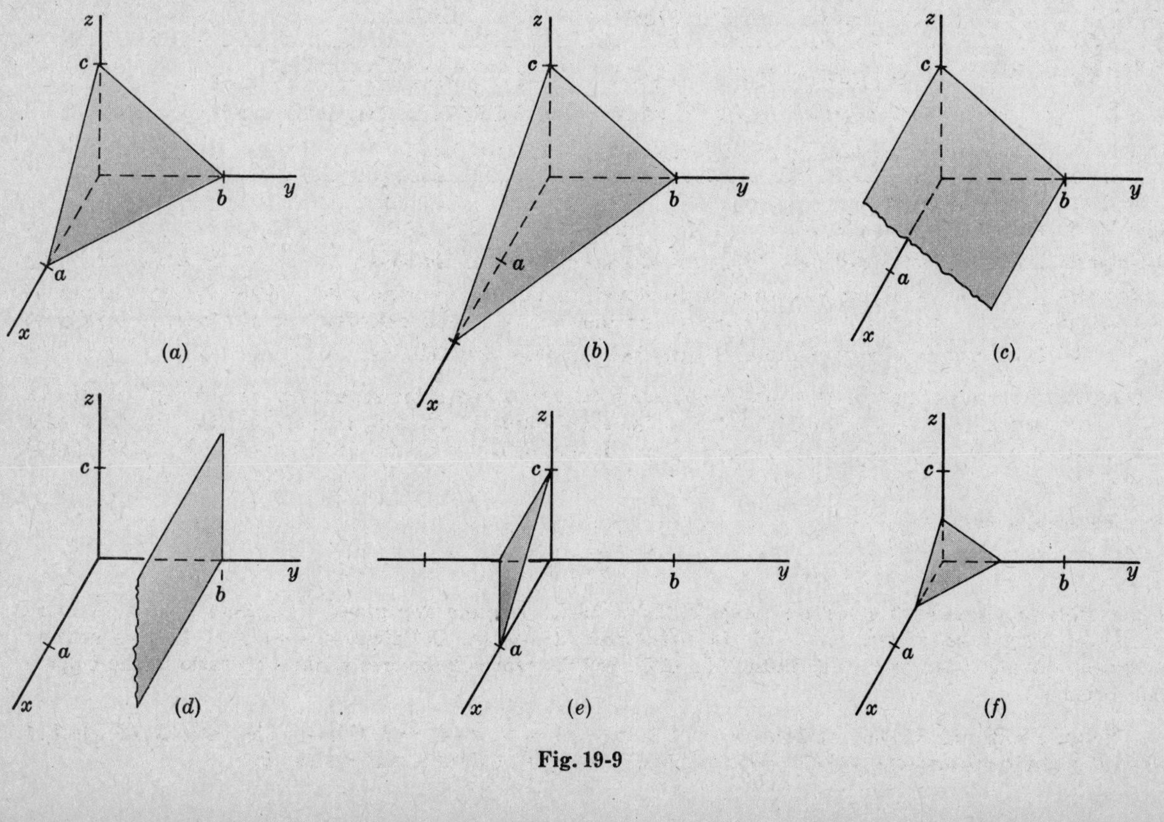

Fig. 19-9

Table 19-3   (*after Berry and Mason,* Mineralogy, *W. H. Freeman and Co.*)

TRICLINIC	hkl		MONOCLINIC	$hkl, h0l, 0kl$	001	010, 100, $hk0$
1	pinacoid(2)		2/m	prism(4)	pinacoid(2)	pinacoid(2)
$\bar{1}$	pedion(1)		2	sphenoid(2)	pedion(1)	pinacoid(2)
			m	dome(2)	pinacoid(2)	pedion(1)

ORTHORHOMBIC	hkl	$0kl, h01$	$hk0$
2/m 2/m 2/m	rhombic dipyramid(8)	rhombic prism(4)	rhombic prism(4)
222	rhombic disphenoid(4)	rhombic prism(4)	rhombic prism(4)
2mm	rhombic pyramid(4)	dome(2)	rhombic prism(4)

	001	010, 100
	pinacoid(2)	pinacoid(2)
	pinacoid(2)	pinacoid(2)
	pedion(1)	pinacoid(2)

TETRAGONAL	hkl	hhl	$h0l$
4/m 2/m 2/m	ditetragonal dipyramid(16)	tetragonal dipyramid(8)	tetragonal dipyramid(8)
422	tetragonal trapezohedron(8)	tetragonal dipyramid(8)	tetragonal dipyramid(8)
4mm	ditetragonal pyramid(8)	tetragonal pyramid(4)	tetragonal pyramid(4)
$\bar{4}$2m	tetragonal scalenohedron(8)	tetragonal disphenoid(4)	tetragonal dipyramid(8)

	$hk0$	100, 110	001
	ditetragonal prism(8)	tetragonal prism(4)	pinacoid(2)
	ditetragonal prism(8)	tetragonal prism(4)	pinacoid(2)
	ditetragonal prism(8)	tetragonal prism(4)	pedion(1)
	ditetragonal prism(8)	tetragonal prism(4)	pinacoid(2)

HEXAGONAL	$hk(\overline{h+k})l$	$h0\bar{h}l, 0h\bar{h}l$	$hh\overline{2h}l$
6/m 2/m 2/m	dihexagonal dipyramid(24)	hexagonal dipyramid(12)	hexagonal dipyramid(12)
622	hexagonal trapezohedron(12)	hexagonal dipyramid(12)	hexagonal dipyramid(12)
6mm	dihexagonal pyramid(12)	hexagonal pyramid(6)	hexagonal pyramid(6)
$\bar{6}$m2	ditrigonal dipyramid(12)	trigonal dipyramid(6)	hexagonal dipyramid(12)
6/m	hexagonal dipyramid(12)	hexagonal dipyramid(12)	hexagonal dipyramid(12)
6	hexagonal pyramid(6)	hexagonal pyramid(6)	hexagonal pyramid(6)
$\bar{6}$	trigonal dipyramid(6)	trigonal dipyramid(6)	trigonal dipyramid(6)

	$hk(\overline{h+k})0$	$10\bar{1}0, 01\bar{1}0$	$11\bar{2}0$	0001
	dihexagonal prism(12)	hexagonal prism(6)	hexagonal prism(6)	pinacoid(2)
	dihexagonal prism(12)	hexagonal prism(6)	hexagonal prism(6)	pinacoid(2)
	dihexagonal prism(12)	hexagonal prism(6)	hexagonal prism(6)	pedion(1)
	ditrigonal prism(6)	trigonal prism(3)	hexagonal prism(6)	pinacoid(2)
	hexagonal prism(6)	hexagonal prism(6)	hexagonal prism(6)	pinacoid(2)
	hexagonal prism(6)	hexagonal prism(6)	hexagonal prism(6)	pedion(1)
	hexagonal prism(6)	trigonal prism(3)	hexagonal prism(6)	pinacoid(2)

RHOMBOHEDRAL	$hk(\overline{h+k})l$	$hh\overline{2h}l$	$h0\bar{h}l, 0h\bar{h}l$
$\bar{3}$ 2/m	trigonal scalenohedron(12)	hexagonal dipyramid(12)	rhombohedron(6)
32	trigonal trapezohedron(6)	trigonal dipyramid(6)	rhombohedron(6)
3m	ditrigonal pyramid(6)	hexagonal pyramid(6)	trigonal pyramid(3)
$\bar{3}$	rhombohedron(6)	rhombohedron(6)	rhombohedron(6)
3	trigonal pyramid(3)	trigonal pyramid(3)	trigonal pyramid(3)

	$hk(\overline{h+k})0$	$10\bar{1}0, 01\bar{1}0$	$11\bar{2}0$	0001
	dihexagonal prism(12)	hexagonal prism(6)	hexagonal prism(6)	pinacoid(2)
	ditrigonal prism(6)	hexagonal prism(6)	trigonal prism(3)	pinacoid(2)
	ditrigonal prism(6)	trigonal prism(3)	hexagonal prism(6)	pedion(1)
	hexagonal prism(6)	hexagonal prism(6)	hexagonal prism(6)	pinacoid(2)
	trigonal prism(3)	trigonal prism(3)	trigonal prism(3)	pedion(1)

CUBIC	hkl	hkk	hhk
4/m $\bar{3}$ 2/m	hexoctahedron(48)	trapezohedron(24)	trisoctahedron(24)
432	gyroid(24)	trapezohedron(24)	trisoctahedron(24)
$\bar{4}$3m	hextetrahedron(24)	tristetrahedron(12)	deltohedron(12)
2/m $\bar{3}$	diploid(24)	trapezohedron(24)	trisoctahedron(24)
23	tetartoid(12)	tristetrahedron(12)	deltohedron(12)

	$hk0$	111	110	100
	tetrahexahedron(24)	octahedron(8)	dodecahedron(12)	cube(6)
	tetrahexahedron(24)	octahedron(8)	dodecahedron(12)	cube(6)
	tetrahexahedron(24)	tetrahedron(4)	dodecahedron(12)	cube(6)
	pyritohedron(12)	octahedron(8)	dodecahedron(12)	cube(6)
	pyritohedron(12)	tetrahedron(4)	dodecahedron(12)	cube(6)

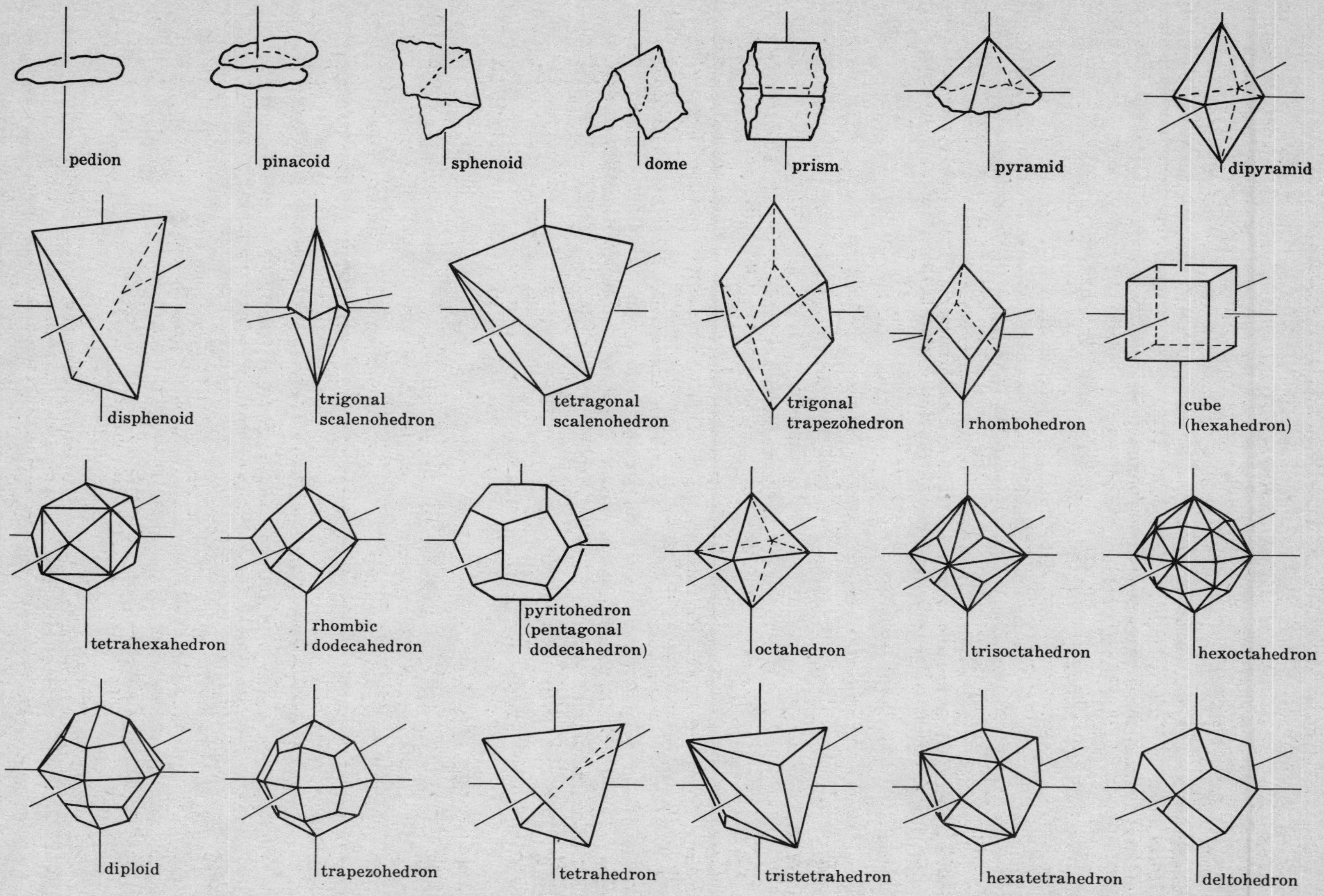

Fig. 19-10 (*after Berry and Mason,* Mineralogy, *W. H. Freeman and Co.*)

Crystallography

19.13 MILLER INDICES

The *Miller indices* are a set of integers hkl [or $hk(\overline{h+k})l$ for hexagonal crystals], which is used to describe a given plane in a crystal. The procedure for determining the Miller indices for a plane is: (1) prepare a three-column table with the unit cell axes at the tops of the columns, (2) enter in each column the intercept (expressed as a multiple of a, b or c) of the plane with that axis, (3) invert all numbers, and (4) clear fractions to obtain h, k and l.

From this it is easy to see that the Miller indices fix the direction of the plane. In particular, the normal to the plane has direction-cosines proportional to h/a, k/b and l/c.

EXAMPLE 19.9. Consider the plane shown in Fig. 19-9(a) which intersects the x-, y- and z-axes at a, b and c, the unit cell dimensions, respectively. What are the Miller indices for this plane?

Preparing the table as described above:

a	b	c	
1	1	1	intercepts
1	1	1	reciprocals
1	1	1	clear fractions

gives the indices as 111.

19.14 d-SPACINGS

When the intercepts of a plane are all doubled, tripled, etc., its Miller indices do not change. Therefore it is possible to construct a family of planes with identical values of hkl which are all parallel and separated by a constant distance d_{hkl}. This interplanar distance is related to the unit cell dimensions and angles by

$$\frac{1}{d_{hkl}^2} = \frac{h^2+k^2+l^2}{a^2} \tag{19.4a}$$

$$\frac{1}{d_{hkl}^2} = \frac{h^2+k^2}{a^2} + \frac{l^2}{c^2} \tag{19.4b}$$

$$\frac{1}{d_{hkl}^2} = \frac{h^2}{a^2} + \frac{k^2}{b^2} + \frac{l^2}{c^2} \tag{19.4c}$$

. . . .

$$\frac{1}{d_{hkl}^2} = \frac{(h^2/a^2)\sin^2\alpha + (k^2/b^2)\sin^2\beta + (l^2/c^2)\sin^2\gamma + (2hk/ab)(\cos\alpha\cos\beta - \cos\gamma) + (2kl/bc)(\cos\beta\cos\gamma - \cos\alpha) + (2lh/ca)(\cos\gamma\cos\alpha - \cos\beta)}{1 - \cos^2\alpha - \cos^2\beta - \cos^2\gamma + 2\cos\alpha\cos\beta\cos\gamma} \tag{19.4g}$$

for cubic, tetragonal, orthorhombic, . . ., and triclinic crystals, respectively. Formula (*19.4g*) includes the others as special cases.

19.15 POINT GROUP SYMMETRY

Crystal faces on a macroscopic crystal are related by symmetry operations which produce the forms given in Table 19-3. The numbers of related faces are shown in parentheses.

Note that the forms depend on both the symmetry elements present in the point group and the Miller indices for the face. Perspective sketches for many of these forms are given in Fig. 19-10.

Several forms do not define polyhedra that completely enclose space: (1) a pedion has no other face related to it by symmetry; (2) a pinacoid usually intersects only one axis and has a parallel face related to it; (3) a face on a sphenoid or dome has an intersecting face related to it producing a wedge or roof-like figure; (4) a prism face is parallel to an axis and has several faces related to it, the number depending on the cross-sectional shape of the prism (see Fig. 19-11); (5) a face on a pyramid intersects all axes and has several faces (depending on the cross section of the pyramid) related to it which all intersect at a vertex.

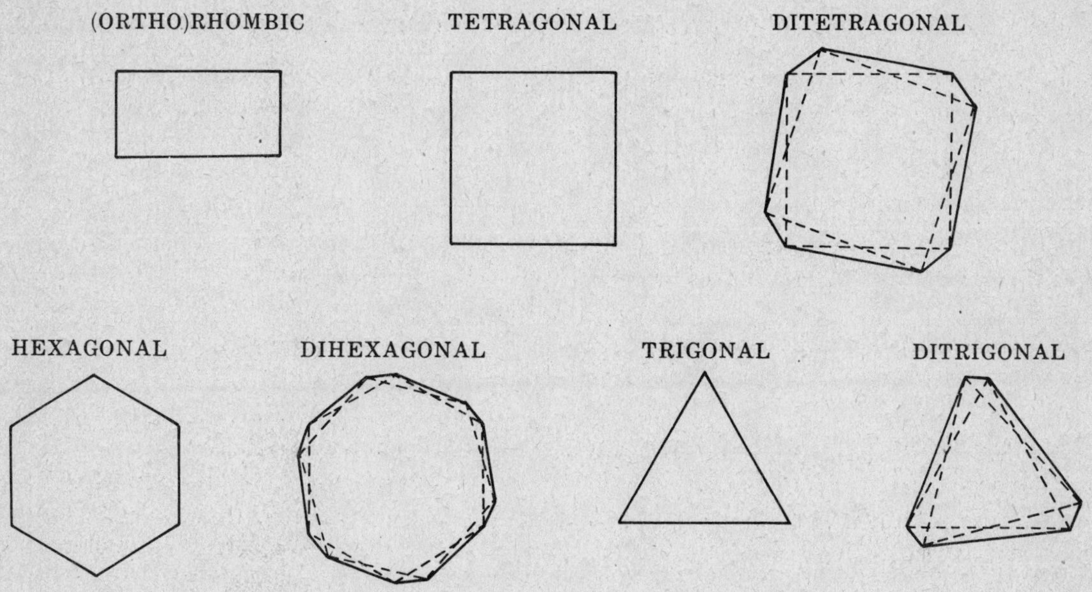

Fig. 19-11

The simple polyhedra that completely enclose space are generated by: (1) a triangle related by symmetry to three additional faces of which three intersect at a given vertex, giving a disphenoid; (2) a triangle related both to a set of faces all of which intersect at a given vertex, generating a pyramid, and to a second set of faces which generates an identical, common-based pyramid, giving a dipyramid; (3) a trapezium (quadrilateral having no parallel sides) related to additional faces, giving a trapezohedron; (4) a rhombus (parallelogram having four equal sides) related to five additional faces of which three intersect at a vertex, giving a rhombohedron; (5) an equilateral triangle, forming a special disphenoid known as the tetrahedron; (6) a square, forming a special rhombohedron known as the cube or hexahedron; and (7) an equilateral triangle, forming a special tetragonal dipyramid known as the octahedron.

The faces in the cubic system generate rather complicated polyhedra including: (1) a rhombic dodecahedron containing 12 rhombi of which 3 intersect at a vertex; (2) a pyritohedron (pentagonal dodecahedron) containing 12 pentagons of which 3 intersect at a vertex; (3) a tristetrahedron which appears to be formed by placing a trigonal pyramid on each face of a tetrahedron giving 12 trigonal faces; (4) a tetrahexahedron which is produced by placing tetragonal pyramids on each face of a cube, giving 24 trigonal faces; and (5) a trisoctahedron which is produced by placing a trigonal pyramid on each face of an octahedron, giving 24 trigonal faces.

A crystal may be assigned to a point group by use of the flow chart in Fig. 17-14. The point group for the unit cell of the crystal will be the same if the crystal has developed enough forms to allow it to be classified in only one point group. For example, a cube of pyrite could be classified in any one of the cubic point groups, but the presence of an octahedron reduces the possible point groups to 3 and the presence of a pyritohedron reduces the possible point groups to 2, with only one in common: $2/m\,\bar{3}$. If a crystal has extensive twinning (composite crystals related by additional symmetry elements), it may be mistakenly classified in a point group of higher symmetry. To avoid these problems of pseudosymmetry, various crystals should be inspected, etchings made, X-ray data taken, etc.

EXAMPLE 19.10. Determine the point groups for the etched cubes shown in Figs. 19-12(a) through 19-12(d). All cubes but (d) have opposite faces the same.

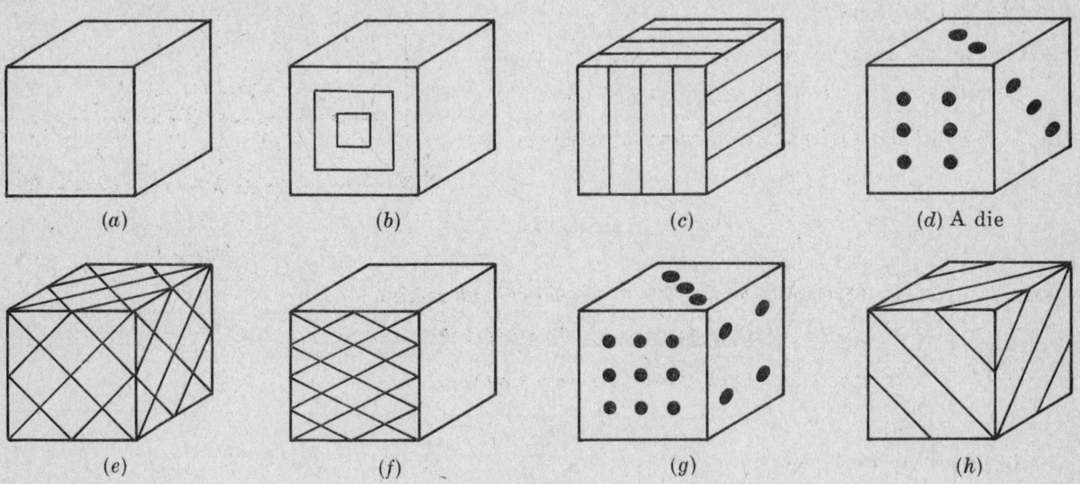

Fig. 19-12

For the cube shown in Fig. 19-12(a), the following analysis can be made using Fig. 17-14: (1) are there four C_3 axes at 54°44′? yes; (2) is there a C_4 axes? yes; (3) is there a σ_h perpendicular to C_4? yes, therefore O_h or $4/m\,\bar{3}\,2/m$.

For the cube shown in Fig. 19-12(b): (1) are there four C_3 axes at 54°44′? no; (2) is there at least one C_n where $n \geqq 2$? yes, C_4; (3) is there an S_{2n} present? no; (4) are there n C_2 axes perpendicular to C_n? yes; (5) is there a σ_h perpendicular to C_n? yes, therefore $\mathcal{D}_{4h}$ or $4/m\,2/m\,2/m$.

For the cube shown in Fig. 19-12(c): (1) are there four C_3 axes at 54°44′? yes; (2) is there a C_4 axis? no; (3) is there an S_4 present? no; (4) is there a σ_h perpendicular to C_2? yes, therefore $\mathcal{T}_h$ or $2/m\,\bar{3}$.

For the cube in Fig. 19-12(d): (1) are there four C_3 axes at 54°44′? no; (2) is there a C_n axis where $n \geqq 2$? no; (3) is there a σ present? no; (4) is i present? no, therefore $\mathcal{C}_1$ or 1.

X-Ray Spectra

19.16 BRAGG EQUATION

A crystal plane will "reflect" a beam of X-rays when

$$n\lambda = 2d_{hkl}\sin\theta \tag{19.5}$$

where n is an integer known as the *order of reflection* and λ is the wavelength of the radiation. The angle θ is the angle of reflection from the hkl plane (although in most experiments the angle 2θ is measured). Usually n is reduced to unity by incorporating the order of reflection into the value of hkl. [According to equations (*19.4*), this can be done by multiplying h, k and l by n.]

19.17 EXTINCTIONS

If a nonprimitive unit cell is used to describe a substance, certain reflections are not allowed. For example, if a body-centered unit cell is chosen, the values of hkl that are permitted are those which satisfy $h+k+l=$ even; if an end-centered cell designated as C is chosen, $h+k=$ even (with analogous criteria for A and B cells); and if a face-centered unit cell is chosen, all indices must be even or all must be odd. Additional extinctions are present for the various glide planes and screw axes.

EXAMPLE 19.11. Consider the C-centered orthorhombic unit cell, two of which are shown in Fig. 19-13. Prepare the matrix of transformation between the preferred orthorhombic unit cell and the primitive monoclinic unit cell indicated. Show that $h+k=$ even must be satisfied for a reflection to occur.

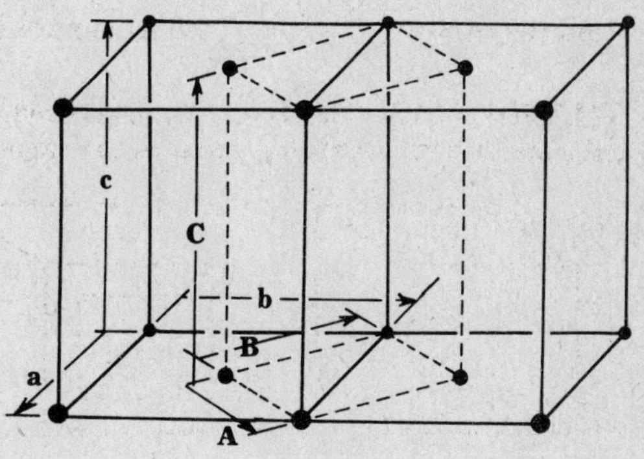

Fig. 19-13

Assuming the unit cell axes to be vectors,

$$\mathbf{a} = \mathbf{A}-\mathbf{B} \qquad \mathbf{b} = \mathbf{A}+\mathbf{B} \qquad \mathbf{c} = \mathbf{C}$$

which gives the following matrix of transformation:

$$\begin{pmatrix} 1 & -1 & 0 \\ 1 & 1 & 0 \\ 0 & 0 & 1 \end{pmatrix}$$

This matrix also describes the transformation of Miller indices giving

$$h = H-K \qquad k = H+K \qquad l = L$$

from which it can be seen that $h+k=2H$, an even number.

19.18 METHOD OF ITO

The *method of Ito* is a technique for indexing the X-ray powder pattern of a substance and inferring the dimensions of the unit cell. If

$$Q_{hkl} = \frac{1}{d_{hkl}^2} \tag{19.6}$$

the Bragg equation becomes

$$Q_{hkl} = \frac{4\sin^2\theta}{\lambda^2} \tag{19.7}$$

For orthogonal crystal systems, equations (*19.4*) give

$$Q_{hkl} = h^2a^{*2}+k^2b^{*2}+l^2c^{*2} \tag{19.8}$$

where $a^*=a^{-1}$, $b^*=b^{-1}$ and $c^*=c^{-1}$. Thus, by assigning values of hkl to the observed Q's (that is, to the observed θ's), a set of equations can be obtained for a^*, b^* and c^*. See Problem 19.18.

19.19 INTENSITIES

The *structure factor* for a plane hkl is defined as

$$F(hkl) = \sum_j f_j e^{2\pi i(hx_j+ky_j+lz_j)} \tag{19.9}$$

where the summation is performed over all the atoms in the unit cell; f_j is the *scattering factor,* which is related to the number of electrons and $(\sin\theta)/\lambda$; and the x_j, y_j and z_j are the unit cell coordinates of the atoms (Section 19.3). The intensity of the scattered X-ray beam is proportional to $F(hkl)^*F(hkl)$.

EXAMPLE 19.12. Determine the structure factor for the 200 plane in NaCl assuming Na^+ ions at (000), $(\frac{1}{2}\frac{1}{2}0)$, $(\frac{1}{2}0\frac{1}{2})$ and $(0\frac{1}{2}\frac{1}{2})$ and Cl^- ions at $(0\frac{1}{2}0)$, $(\frac{1}{2}00)$, $(00\frac{1}{2})$ and $(\frac{1}{2}\frac{1}{2}\frac{1}{2})$. For the experimental values of θ and λ, $f_+ = 8.8$ and $f_- = 13.7$.

Using (*19.9*) with $k = l = 0$ gives

$$\begin{aligned} F(200) &= 8.8\{e^{2\pi i[(2)(0)]} + e^{2\pi i[(2)(1/2)]} + e^{2\pi i[(2)(1/2)]} + e^{2\pi i[(2)(0)]}\} \\ &\quad + 13.7\{e^{2\pi i[(2)(1/2)]} + e^{2\pi i[(2)(0)]} + e^{2\pi i[(2)(1/2)]} + e^{2\pi i[(2)(0)]}\} \\ &= 8.8(2 + 2e^{\pi i}) + 13.7(2 + 2e^{2\pi i}) = 45.0(1 + e^{2\pi i}) = 45.0(1+1) = 90.0 \end{aligned}$$

where $e^{2\pi i}$ was evaluated from

$$e^{ix} = \cos x + i \sin x \qquad (19.10)$$

Solved Problems

Unit Cells

19.1. Determine Z for the body-centered cubic unit cell shown in Fig. 19-14.

The contribution of the eight corners is $8(1/8) = 1$, and that of the body-centered atom is 1, giving $Z = 1+1 = 2$.

19.2. Determine the coordinates of the atoms shown in Fig. 19-14.

The eight corners will be represented by (000). The coordinates of the atom in the center of the unit cell are $(\frac{1}{2}\frac{1}{2}\frac{1}{2})$. The required two sets of coordinates agrees with the unit cell content as determined in Problem 19.1.

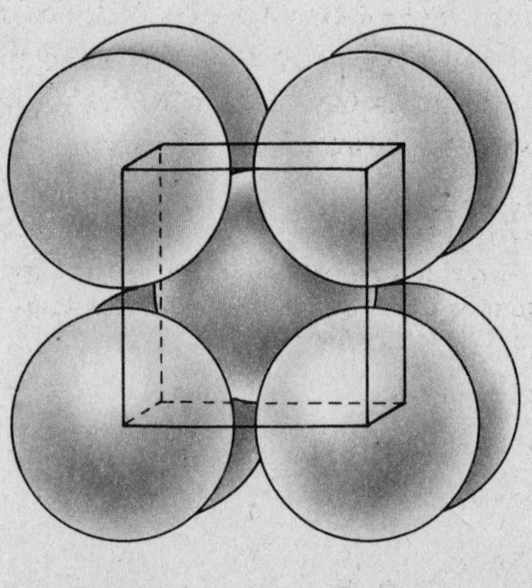

Fig. 19-14

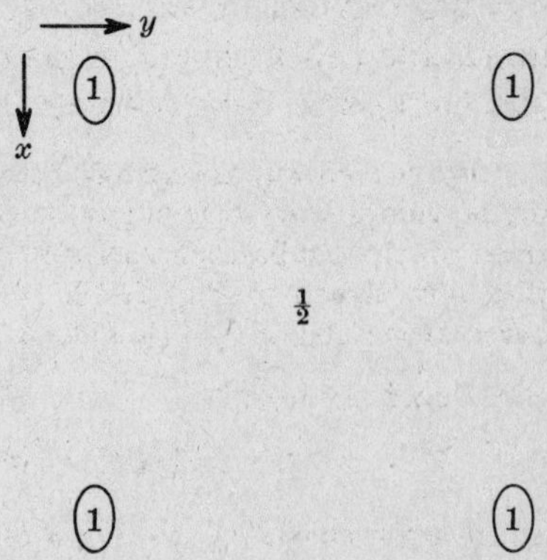

Fig. 19-15

19.3. Prepare a crystallographic projection for the body-centered cubic unit cell.

The eight corner atoms will be represented by four (1) symbols at the corners of a square and the body-centered atom will be represented by a $\frac{1}{2}$ in the center of the square, see Fig. 19-15.

19.4. Determine CN for an atom in the body-centered cubic unit cell.

Considering the atom in the center of the unit cell shown in Fig. 19-14, it is surrounded by 8 nearest-neighbor atoms, the corners of the cube. Thus $CN = 8$.

19.5. Sodium crystallizes in the body-centered cubic structure with $a = 4.24$ Å. Calculate the theoretical density of Na.

From Problem 19.1, $Z = 2$. Using (*19.2b*) gives $V = (4.24 \times 10^{-10}\text{ m})^3$, which upon substitution into (*19.1*) gives

$$d = \frac{(2)(23.0\text{ g mol}^{-1})(10^{-3}\text{ kg g}^{-1})}{(6.022 \times 10^{23}\text{ mol}^{-1})(4.24 \times 10^{-10}\text{ m})^3} = 1.00 \times 10^3\text{ kg m}^{-3}$$

19.6. Find the relationship between a and R for a body-centered cubic unit cell and calculate R for Na if $a = 4.24$ Å.

The spheres in this unit cell are touching along a body diagonal. The length of the body diagonal in terms of a is $a(3)^{1/2}$, and in terms of R is $4R$, giving

$$R = \frac{a(3)^{1/2}}{4}$$

Substituting the data for Na gives

$$R = \frac{(4.24\text{ Å})(3)^{1/2}}{4} = 1.84\text{ Å}$$

19.7. Find the distance between the body-centered atom and one corner atom in Na if $a = 4.24$ Å.

Substitution of the coordinates (000) and $(\frac{1}{2}\frac{1}{2}\frac{1}{2})$ into (*19.3c*) gives

$$\ell = (4.24\text{ Å})[(\tfrac{1}{2} - 0)^2 + (\tfrac{1}{2} - 0)^2 + (\tfrac{1}{2} - 0)^2]^{1/2} = (4.24)(3/4)^{1/2} = 3.67\text{ Å}$$

19.8. Metallic zinc crystallizes in a hexagonal closest-packed unit cell, see Fig. 19-6, with $a = 2.665$ Å and $c = 4.949$ Å. Give the coordinates of the atoms and prepare crystallographic projections for the unit cell. What is CN? Find the theoretical density of the metal and the distances between atoms contained in the basal parallelogram.

By convention, the coordinates (000) account for all eight corners. The coordinates of the atom in the center can be found to be $(\frac{1}{3}\frac{1}{3}\frac{1}{2})$ by recognizing that the center of this atom lies at the centroid of the equilateral triangle formed by three of the atoms in the parallelogram. The projections are shown in Fig. 19-16. A given atom is touching six others in the same plane as well as three above and three below the plane, hence $CN = 12$ for this unit cell.

Using (*19.2a*) gives

$$V = a^2c(1 - \cos^2\gamma)^{1/2} = a^2c\sin\gamma = (2.665\text{ Å})^2(4.949\text{ Å})(\sin 120°) = 30.44 \times 10^{-30}\text{ m}^3$$

which upon substitution into (*19.1*) gives

$$d = \frac{(2)(65.37 \times 10^{-3})}{(6.022 \times 10^{23})(30.44 \times 10^{-30})} = 7.132 \times 10^3\text{ kg m}^{-3}$$

There are two interatomic distances in the basal parallelogram. The shorter is that between any three adjacent atoms and has the value $\ell = a = 2.665$ Å. The longer is that between the far corners of the parallelogram and is given by (*19.3a*) (or the law of cosines) as

$$\begin{aligned}\ell &= [a^2(1-0)^2 + a^2(1-0)^2 + c^2(0-0)^2 - 2a^2(1-0)(1-0)(\cos 120°) - 0 - 0]^{1/2} \\ &= a(2 - 2\cos 120°)^{1/2} = a(3)^{1/2} = 4.616\text{ Å}\end{aligned}$$

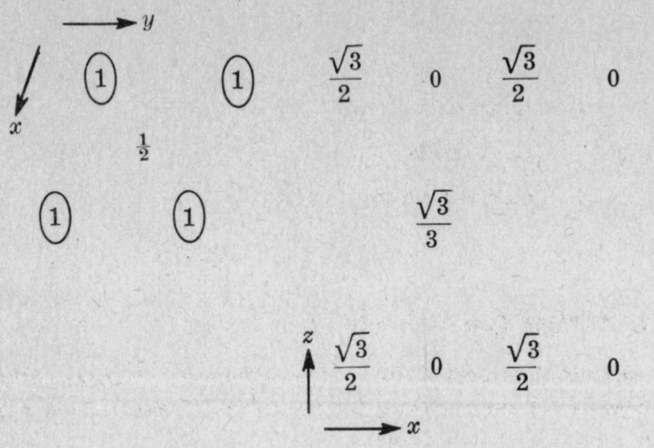

Fig. 19-16

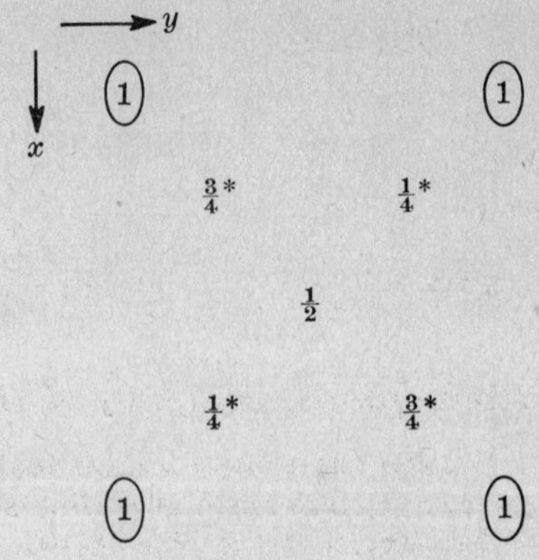

Fig. 19-17

Crystal Forms

19.9. Diamond has C atoms located at (000), $(\frac{1}{2}\frac{1}{2}0)$, $(\frac{1}{2}0\frac{1}{2})$, $(0\frac{1}{2}\frac{1}{2})$, $(\frac{1}{4}\frac{1}{4}\frac{1}{4})$, $(\frac{1}{4}\frac{3}{4}\frac{3}{4})$, $(\frac{3}{4}\frac{1}{4}\frac{3}{4})$ and $(\frac{3}{4}\frac{3}{4}\frac{1}{4})$. If $a = 3.5670$ Å, find the covalent radius of a carbon atom and the theoretical density of diamond.

The body diagonal of the unit cell is equal to $8R$, giving $a = 8R/(3)^{1/2}$ and hence

$$R = \frac{a(3)^{1/2}}{8} = \frac{(3.5670\ \text{Å})(3)^{1/2}}{8} = 0.772\ \text{Å}$$

Recognizing that $Z = 8$, *(19.1)* and *(19.2b)* give

$$d = \frac{(8)(12.011 \times 10^{-3})}{(6.022 \times 10^{23})(3.5670 \times 10^{-10})^3} = 3.516 \times 10^3\ \text{kg m}^{-3}$$

19.10. The cuprite unit cell can be described as a face-centered cubic unit cell of Cu^+ ions with its origin at $(\frac{1}{4}\frac{1}{4}\frac{1}{4})$ interpenetrating a body-centered cubic unit cell of O^{2-} ions with its origin at (000). Only a portion of the Cu^+ cubic unit cell is contained in the cuprite unit cell and thus appears as a tetrahedron of Cu^+ ions. Prepare a crystallographic projection of this unit cell. Find the coordinates of all the ions. If $a = 4.2696$ Å, determine the theoretical density of Cu_2O.

The face-centered cubic structure implies that $Z_+ = 4$ and the body-centered structure implies $Z_- = 2$, which is in agreement with the empirical formula. The coordinates of the Cu^+ are $(\frac{1}{4}\frac{1}{4}\frac{1}{4})$, $(\frac{1}{4}\frac{3}{4}\frac{3}{4})$, $(\frac{3}{4}\frac{3}{4}\frac{1}{4})$, $(\frac{3}{4}\frac{1}{4}\frac{3}{4})$ and of O^{2-} are (000) and $(\frac{1}{2}\frac{1}{2}\frac{1}{2})$. $CN_+ = 2$ and $CN_- = 4$, which is in agreement with the empirical formula. See Fig. 19-17 for the projection (* indicates Cu^+).

Using *(19.1)* and *(19.2b)* gives

$$d = \frac{(2)(143.08 \times 10^{-3})}{(6.022 \times 10^{23})(4.2696 \times 10^{-10})^3} = 6.105 \times 10^3\ \text{kg m}^{-3}$$

19.11. Consider the portion of the unit cell for ice shown in Fig. 4-6. Each water molecule is held in place by hydrogen bonding between four additional molecules. Determine CN for the H and the O atoms assuming all O—H distances to be the same.

Around a given H there are two O's and around a given O there are four H's, giving $CN_H = 2$ and $CN_O = 4$, which are in the inverse ratio of the formula subscripts.

Crystallography

19.12. Determine the indices for the plane shown in Fig. 19-9(*c*).

The table,

a	b	c	
∞	1	1	intercepts
0	1	1	reciprocals
0	1	1	clear fractions

gives 011.

19.13. Indicate the intercepts of the plane having the indices $1\bar{2}1$.

The value $h = 1$ means that the x-axis is intersected at a, the value $k = \bar{2}$ means that the y-axis is intersected at $-0.5\,b$, and the value $l = 1$ means that the z-axis is intersected at c, giving the plane shown in Fig. 19-9(e).

19.14. Find the spacing between the planes with indices 101 in NaCl if $a = 5.6402$ Å.

Using (*19.4a*) gives

$$\frac{1}{d_{101}^2} = \frac{1^2 + 0^2 + 1^2}{(5.6402\ \text{Å})^2} \qquad \text{or} \qquad d_{101} = \frac{5.6402}{(2)^{1/2}} = 3.9882\ \text{Å}$$

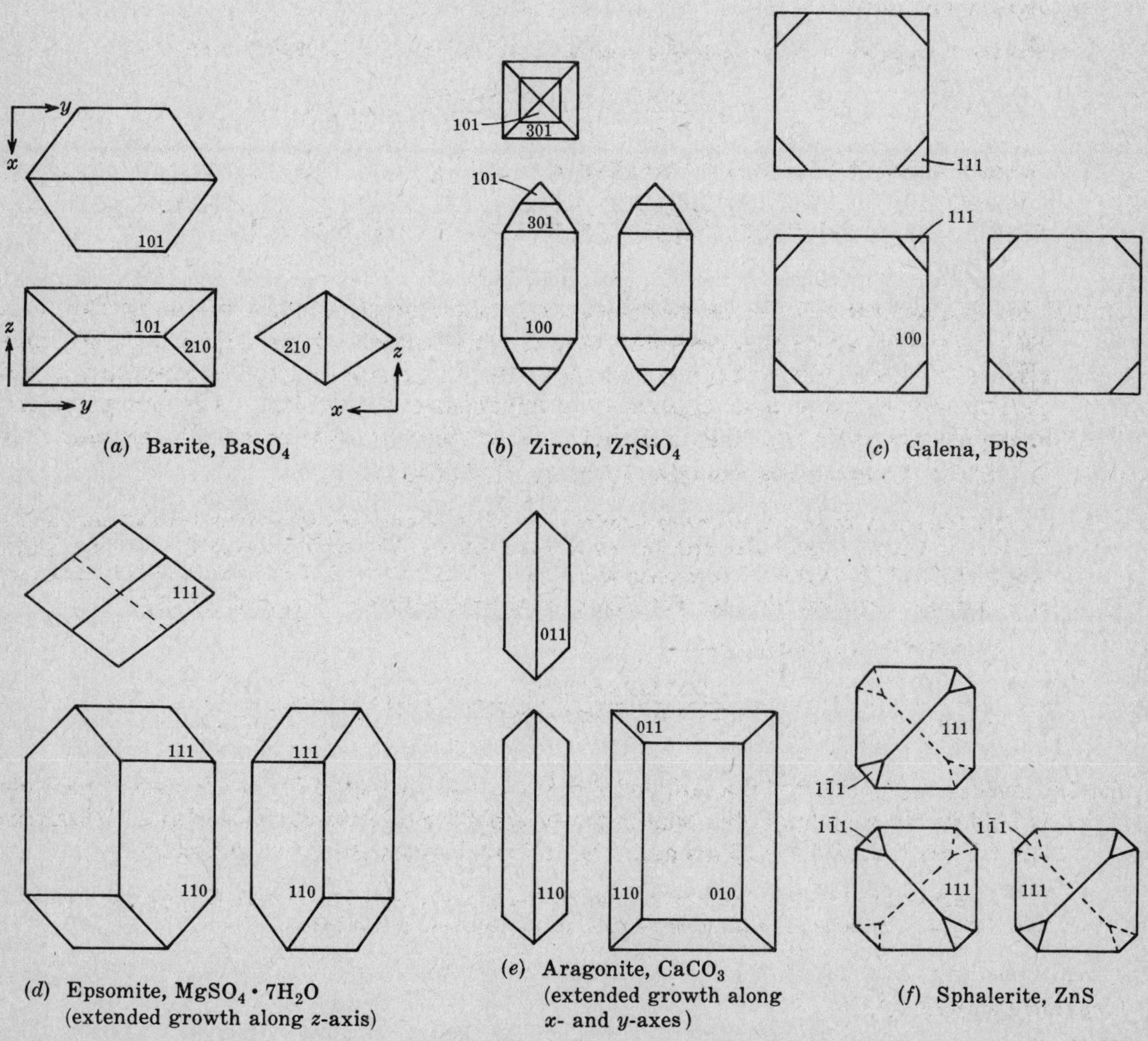

Fig. 19-18 (*after Berry and Mason,* Mineralogy, *W. H. Freeman and Co.*)

19.15. Using Fig. 17-14, determine the point groups for the crystals shown in Figs. 19-18(*a*) through 19-18(*c*). Describe the prominent crystal forms.

(*a*) Barite: (1) are there four C_3 axes at 54°44′? no; (2) is there at least one C_n with $n \geqq 2$? yes, C_2; (3) is there an S_{2n} present? yes, but other elements too; (4) are there n C_2 axes perpendicular to C_n? yes; (5) is there a σ_h perpendicular to C_n? yes, therefore $\mathcal{D}_{2h}$ or $2/m\,2/m\,2/m$ with 101 and 210 rhombic prisms present.

(*b*) Zircon: (1) are there four C_3 axes at 54°44′? no; (2) is there at least one C_n with $n \geqq 2$? yes, C_4; (3) is there an S_{2n} present? yes, but other elements too; (4) are there n C_2 axes perpendicular to C_n? yes; (5) is there a σ_h perpendicular to C_n? yes, therefore $\mathcal{D}_{4h}$ or $4/m\,2/m\,2/m$ with a 100 tetragonal prism and two tetragonal dipyramids (101 and 301).

(*c*) Galena: (1) are there four C_3 axes at 54°44′? yes; (2) is there a C_4 axis? yes; (3) is there a σ_h perpendicular to C_4? yes, therefore O_h or $4/m\,\bar{3}\,2/m$ with a 100 cube and 111 octahedron.

X-Ray Spectra

19.16. If $\lambda = 1.5418$ Å for filtered Cu radiation, at what angle would the maximum reflection by the 200 plane of AgCl occur, assuming that $a = 5.5491$ Å?

Using (*19.4a*) gives

$$\frac{1}{d_{200}^2} = \frac{2^2 + 0^2 + 0^2}{(5.5491\ \text{Å})^2} \quad \text{or} \quad d_{200} = 2.7746\ \text{Å}$$

Then (*19.5*) gives

$$\sin\theta = \frac{1.5418\ \text{Å}}{(2)(2.7746\ \text{Å})} = 0.278 \quad \text{or} \quad \theta = 16.1°$$

19.17. Which of the following indices are allowed in the pattern of AgCl: 100, 010, 001, 200, 020, 002, 110, 101, 011, 120, 102, 012, 210, 201, 021, 220, 202, 022, 111, 222, 221, 212, 122, 211, 121, 112?

Recalling that AgCl has a face-centered cubic unit cell, the only allowed reflections are those in which all indices are even or all are odd, giving: 200, 020, 002, 220, 202, 022, 111 and 222. Because $a = b = c$, $200 = 020 = 002$ and $220 = 202 = 022$, so that really only four peaks will be observed: 200, 220, 111 and 222.

19.18. The powder pattern of halite using filtered Cu radiation, $\lambda = 1.5418$ Å, shows six peaks. The values of 2θ and the relative intensities for these spectral lines are 27.1°(10%), 31.5°(100%), 45.2°(45%), 53.6°(5%), 56.3°(10%) and 65.9°(5%). If halite is known to crystallize in the cubic system, determine a for the mineral and index the lines.

Converting the various values of 2θ to Q using (*19.7*) gives

$$Q_1 = \frac{4\sin^2(27.1°/2)}{(1.5418)^2} = 0.0924$$

$Q_2 = 0.1240$, $Q_3 = 0.249$, $Q_4 = 0.342$, $Q_5 = 0.375$ and $Q_6 = 0.498$. Recalling the results of Section 19.17, none of these Q's correspond to a $100 = 010 = 001$ d-spacing. Assuming Q_2, the most intense peak, to be for the $200 = 020 = 002$ plane, (*19.8*) gives

$$Q_{100} = \frac{Q_{200}}{4} = \frac{0.1240}{4} = 0.0310$$

Using $Q_{100} = 0.0310$, Q_{111} is given by

$$Q_{111} = (1^2 + 1^2 + 1^2)Q_{100} = (3)(0.0310) = 0.0930 = Q_1$$

Continuing by trial and error gives $Q_{300} = 0.279$, $Q_{400} = 0.496 = Q_6$, $Q_{120} = 0.1550$, $Q_{121} = 0.1860$, $Q_{220} = 0.248 = Q_3$, $Q_{222} = 0.372 = Q_5$ and $Q_{113} = 0.341 = Q_4$. Summarizing, the peaks correspond to the 111, 200, 220, 113, 222 and 400 planes. Using (*19.8*) gives $a^{*2} = 0.0310$, which converts to $a = 5.69$ Å. Based on the extinctions, the unit cell must be face-centered cubic.

19.19. Calculate the intensity of the 220 peak relative to that of the 200 peak for NaCl using the results of Example 19.12 and Problem 19.51.

Using $F(200) = 90.0$ and $F(220) = 69.6$, the relative intensity will be

$$\frac{I(220)}{I(200)} = \frac{F(220)^* F(220)}{F(200)^* F(200)} = \frac{(69.6)^2}{(90.0)^2} \times 100\% = 59.8\%$$

The actual value is about 45%.

Supplementary Problems

Unit Cells

19.20. Determine Z for the face-centered cubic unit cell shown in Fig. 19-19.

Ans. $8(1/8) + 6(1/2) = 4$

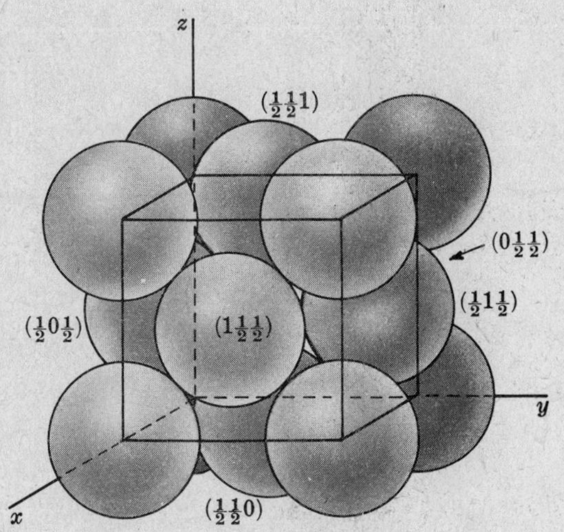

Fig. 19-19

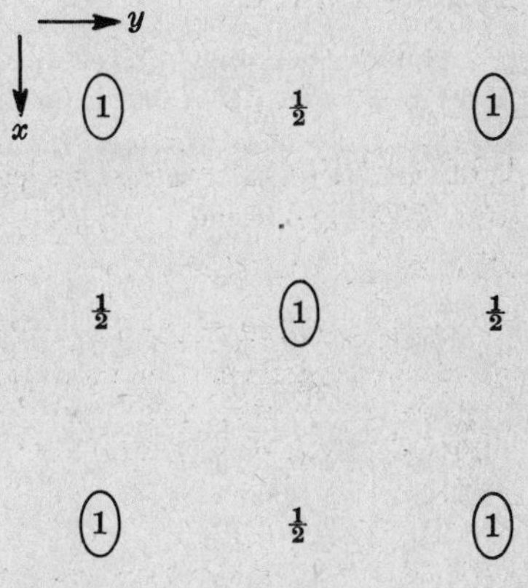

Fig. 19-20

19.21. Determine the coordinates of the atoms shown in Fig. 19-19.

Ans. (000), $(\frac{1}{2}0\frac{1}{2})$, $(\frac{1}{2}\frac{1}{2}0)$, $(0\frac{1}{2}\frac{1}{2})$

19.22. Prepare a crystallographic projection for the face-centered cubic unit cell.

Ans. See Fig. 19-20.

19.23. Determine CN for the face-centered cubic unit cell. *Ans.* 12

19.24. Platinum crystallizes in the face-centered cubic structure with $a = 3.923$ Å. Calculate the theoretical density of Pt. *Ans.* 21.5×10^3 kg m^{-3}

19.25. Find the relation between a and R for a face-centered cubic unit cell. Calculate R for Pt assuming $a = 3.923$ Å. *Ans.* $a(2)^{1/2}/4$; 1.39 Å

19.26. Find the distance between two of the face-centered atoms on adjacent sides of Pt if $a = 3.923$ Å.

Ans. $a/(2)^{1/2}$, 2.774 Å

19.27. Using the data in Problem 19.8, show that the lengths of the two types of body diagonals (000 to 111 and 100 to 011) in zinc are 6.767 Å and 5.621 Å. Show that in the ideal case $c = 2a(2/3)^{1/2}$.

Crystal Forms

19.28. Calculate the packing efficiency in the cubic closest-packed unit cell (face-centered cubic) and compare it to the answer for Example 19.7.

Ans. $V_{\text{cell}} = 64R^3/2^{3/2}$, $V_{\text{occ}} = 16\pi R^3/3$; 74.1% (same)

19.29. Calculate the packing efficiencies in the primitive and body-centered cubic unit cells. Compare these answers to those found in Problem 19.28 for the other Bravais lattices.

Ans. $\dfrac{\pi}{6} = 52.4\%$, $\dfrac{\pi(3)^{1/2}}{8} = 68.0\%$; FCC and HCP most efficient

19.30. Repeat Problem 19.9 for Si ($a = 5.4305$ Å). *Ans.* 1.177 Å, 2.330×10^3 kg m^{-3}

19.31. The fluorite structure can be described as a face-centered cubic unit cell of Ca^{2+} ions interpenetrated by a complete primitive cube of F^-. What are the coordinates of the ions? Find CN_+ and CN_-. Prepare a crystallographic projection for this unit cell.

Ans. (000), $(0\frac{1}{2}\frac{1}{2})$, $(\frac{1}{2}0\frac{1}{2})$ and $(\frac{1}{2}\frac{1}{2}0)$ for Ca^{2+} and $(\frac{1}{4}\frac{1}{4}\frac{1}{4})$, $(\frac{1}{4}\frac{3}{4}\frac{3}{4})$, $(\frac{3}{4}\frac{1}{4}\frac{3}{4})$, $(\frac{3}{4}\frac{3}{4}\frac{1}{4})$, $(\frac{3}{4}\frac{3}{4}\frac{3}{4})$, $(\frac{1}{4}\frac{1}{4}\frac{3}{4})$, $(\frac{1}{4}\frac{3}{4}\frac{1}{4})$ and $(\frac{3}{4}\frac{1}{4}\frac{1}{4})$ for F^-; $CN_+ = 8$, $CN_- = 4$; see Fig. 19-21(*a*).

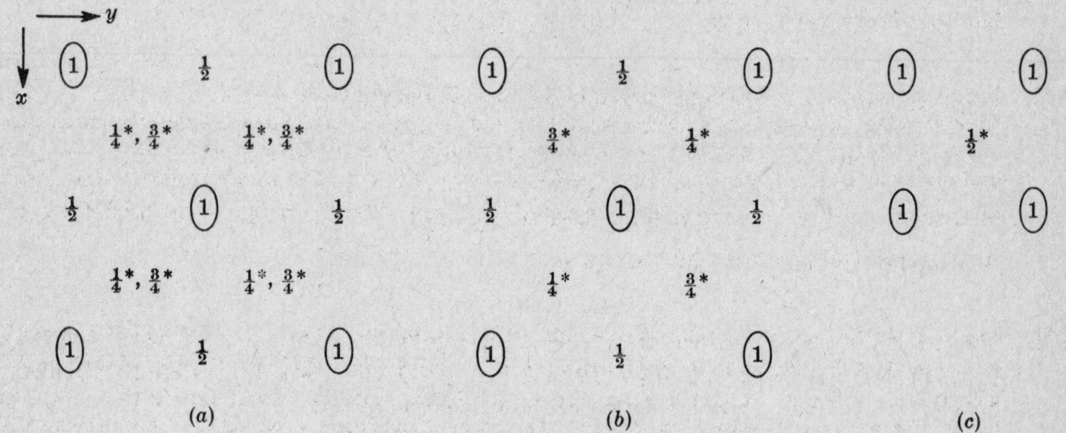

Fig. 19-21

19.32. The coordinates of the ions in the sphalerite unit cell are (000), $(\frac{1}{2}\frac{1}{2}0)$, $(0\frac{1}{2}\frac{1}{2})$, $(\frac{1}{2}0\frac{1}{2})$ for Zn^{2+} and $(\frac{1}{4}\frac{1}{4}\frac{1}{4})$, $(\frac{1}{4}\frac{3}{4}\frac{3}{4})$, $(\frac{3}{4}\frac{1}{4}\frac{3}{4})$, $(\frac{3}{4}\frac{3}{4}\frac{1}{4})$, for S^{2-}. Describe the unit cell in terms of interpenetrating Bravais lattices. What are Z and CN for the ions and the unit cell? Prepare a crystallographic projection for the unit cell.

Ans. Recalling that the tetrahedron of S^{2-} is an alternative way of describing a face-centered cube, see Problem 19.10, there are two face-centered cubes, one at (000) and the second at $(\frac{1}{4}\frac{1}{4}\frac{1}{4})$; $Z_+ = Z_- = Z = 4$; $CN_+ = CN_- = 4$; see Fig. 19-21(*b*).

19.33. The coordinates of the ions in the CsCl unit cell are (000) for Cs^+ and $(\frac{1}{2}\frac{1}{2}\frac{1}{2})$ for Cl^-. Describe the unit cell in terms of interpenetrating Bravais lattices and prepare a crystallographic projection.

Ans. Two primitive cubes, one of Cs^+ at (000) and the second of Cl^- at $(\frac{1}{2}\frac{1}{2}\frac{1}{2})$; see Fig. 19-21(*c*).

19.34. Using the values of R_+ and R_- given below, predict the crystal structures for the alkali metal halides and the alkaline-earth chalkogenides, assuming the radius ratio rule to be valid and that the crystals are cubic.

Li^+	0.68 Å			O^{2-}	1.32 Å	F^-	1.33 Å
Na^+	0.97	Mg^{2+}	0.66 Å	S^{2-}	1.84	Cl^-	1.81
K^+	1.33	Ca^{2+}	0.99	Se^{2-}	1.91	Br^-	1.96
		Sr^{2+}	1.12			I^-	2.20
Cs^+	1.67	Ba^{2+}	1.34				

Ans. Sphalerite structure: LiCl, LiBr, LiI, MgS and MgSe. Halite structure: LiF, Na*X*, (KCl), KBr, KI, MgO, CaS, CaSe, SrS, SrSe, BaS and BaSe. CsCl structure: KF, KCl, Cs*X*, CaO, SrO and BaO.

19.35. The red oxide of lead, litharge, crystallizes in the tetragonal crystal system with Pb^{2+} at $(0\frac{1}{2}u)$ and $(\frac{1}{2}0\bar{u})$, where $u = 0.24$, and O^{2-} at (000) and $(\frac{1}{2}\frac{1}{2}0)$. Describe the unit cell.

Ans. O^{2-} in *C*-centered tetragonal with Pb^{2+} in tetragonal disphenoid (distorted tetrahedron) with the corners on the faces of the unit cell, see Fig. 19-22.

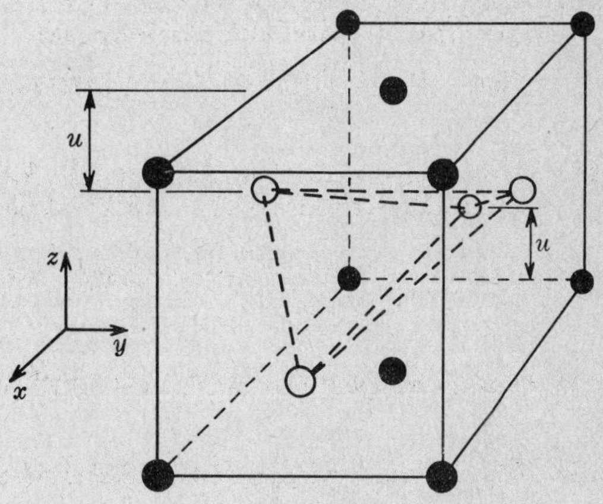

Fig. 19-22

19.36. Ti_2O(rutile) crystallizes in the tetragonal system with Ti^{4+} at (000) and $(\frac{1}{2}\frac{1}{2}\frac{1}{2})$ and O^{2-} at $(\bar{u}u0)$, $(uu0)$, $(\frac{1}{2}+u\ \frac{1}{2}-u\ \frac{1}{2})$ and $(\frac{1}{2}-u\ \frac{1}{2}+u\ \frac{1}{2})$, where $u = 0.305$. If $a = 4.5937$ Å and $c = 2.9618$ Å, calculate the theoretical density. *Ans.* $Z = 2$; 4.246×10^3 kg m^{-3}

19.37. ZnS is known to be polymorphic, crystallizing in both the sphalerite and wurtzite (zincite) structures. The wurtzite structure can be described as two interpenetrating hexagonal closest-packed unit cells, one of Zn^{2+} and the other of S^{2-}. The penetration is such that the coordinates of Zn^{2+} are (000) and $(\frac{1}{3}\frac{2}{3}\frac{1}{2})$ and of S^{2-} are $(00u)$ and $(\frac{1}{3}\frac{2}{3}\ \frac{1}{2}+u)$ where $u = 3/8$. Calculate the theoretical densities of these minerals if $a = 5.4093$ Å for sphalerite and if $a = 3.8230$ Å and $c = 6.2565$ Å for wurtzite.

Ans. 4.09×10^3 kg m^{-3}, 4.09×10^3 kg m^{-3}

19.38. The coordinates of Ca^{2+} in the calcite unit cell are (000) and $(\frac{1}{2}\frac{1}{2}\frac{1}{2})$, of C are $(\frac{1}{4}\frac{1}{4}\frac{1}{4})$ and $(\frac{3}{4}\frac{3}{4}\frac{3}{4})$, and of O are $(\frac{1}{4}+u\ \frac{1}{4}\ \frac{1}{4}-u)$, $(\frac{1}{4}+u\ \frac{1}{4}-u\ \frac{1}{4})$, $(\frac{1}{4}\ \frac{1}{4}+u\ \frac{1}{4}-u)$, $(\frac{3}{4}-u\ \frac{3}{4}\ \frac{3}{4}+u)$, $(\frac{3}{4}\ \frac{3}{4}-u\ \frac{3}{4}+u)$ and $(\frac{3}{4}-u\ \frac{3}{4}+u\ \frac{3}{4})$ where $u = 0.243$. Find Z_+ and Z_- from these coordinates. If the calcite structure is considered in terms of a hexagonal unit cell instead of the above rhombohedral cell, $Z = 6$ for the new cell with $a = 4.9899$ Å and $c = 17.064$ Å. Calculate the density of calcite.

Ans. $Z_+ = 2$, $Z_- = 2$ for $CO_3{}^{2-}$; 2.710×10^3 kg m^{-3}

19.39. Calculate the theoretical density of (ortho)rhombic S if $a = 10.4646$ Å, $b = 12.8660$ Å and $c = 24.4860$ Å. $Z = 128$ for this unit cell. *Ans.* 2.067×10^3 kg m^{-3}

Crystallography

19.40. Determine the Miller indices for the planes shown in Fig. 19-9(*b*) and 19-9(*d*).

Ans. 122, 010

19.41. Sketch the plane having the indices 222. *Ans.* See Fig. 19-9(*f*).

19.42. Find the spacing between the family of planes having the indices 202 in NaCl if $a = 5.6402$ Å. Compare with the result of Problem 19.14. *Ans.* 1.9941 Å (half the 101 spacing)

19.43. Determine the point groups for the etched cubes shown in Figs. 19-12(*e*) through 19-12(*h*).
Ans. (*e*) O_h or $4/m\,\bar{3}\,2/m$; (*f*) $\mathcal{D}_{2h}$ or $2/m\,2/m\,2/m$; (*g*) $\mathcal{C}_{2h}$ or $2/m$; (*h*) $\mathcal{C}_{3v}$ or $3m$

19.44. Determine the point groups for the crystals shown in Figs. 19-18(*d*) through 19-18(*f*). Describe the prominent crystal forms.
Ans. (*d*) $\mathcal{D}_2$ or 222, 110 rhombic prism and 111 rhombic disphenoid
(*e*) $\mathcal{D}_{2h}$ or $2/m\,2/m\,2/m$, 110 and 011 rhombic prisms and 010 pinacoid
(*f*) $\mathcal{T}_d$ or $\bar{4}3m$, 111 and $1\bar{1}1$ tetrahedrons

19.45. Identify the point groups to which the crystals shown in Fig. 19-23 belong. Describe the prominent forms on the crystals. Note that other samples of the quartz shown in Fig. 19-23(*d*) do not show the σ_h and σ_d planes that this crystal does.
Ans. (*a*) $\mathcal{T}_h$ or $2/m\,\bar{3}$, 210 pyritohedron
(*b*) $\mathcal{C}_{6v}$ or $6mm$, $10\bar{1}0$ hexagonal prism, $10\bar{1}1$ hexagonal pyramid, $000\bar{1}$ pedion
(*c*) $\mathcal{D}_{2h}$ or $2/m\,2/m\,2/m$, 001 pinacoid, 210, 011 and 101 rhombic prisms
(*d*) pseudosymmetry of $\mathcal{D}_{3h}$, correctly as $\mathcal{D}_3$ or 32, $10\bar{1}0$ hexagonal prism, two rhombohedrons, $01\bar{1}1$ and $10\bar{1}1$ and $2\bar{1}\bar{1}1$ trigonal dipyramid

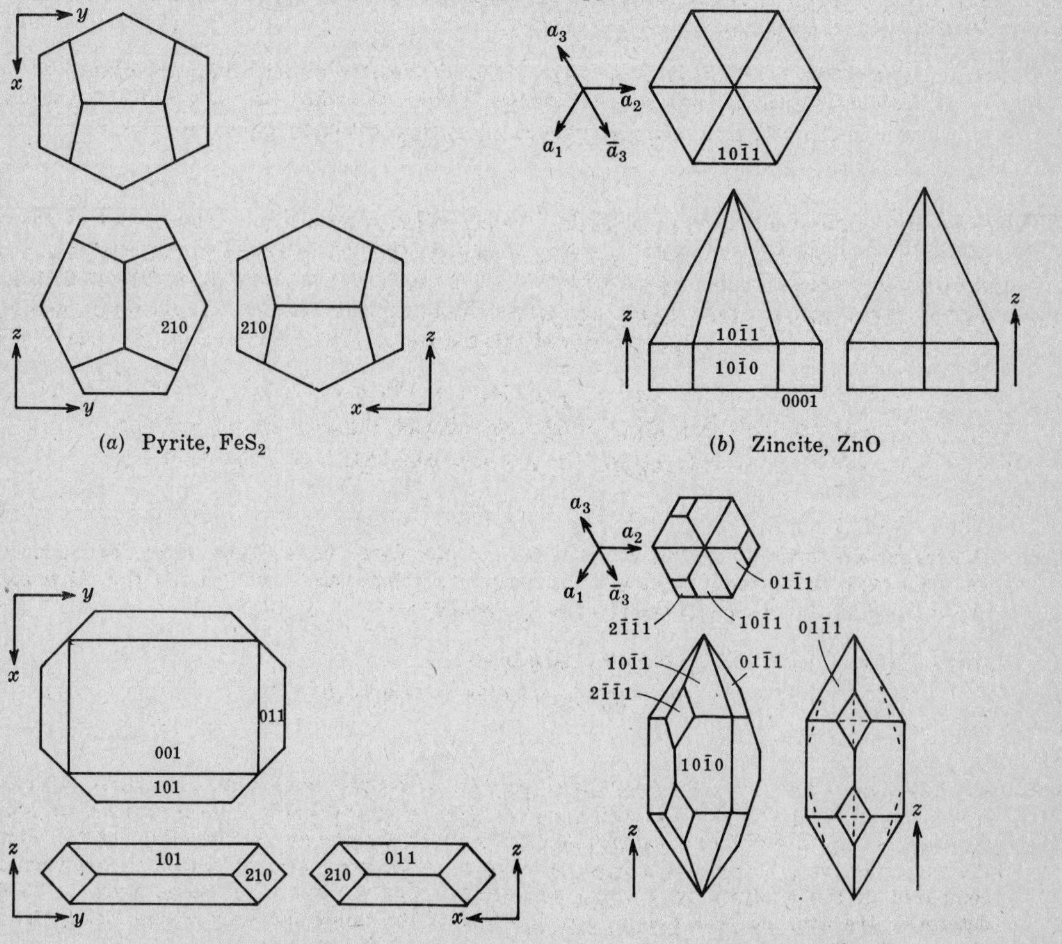

(*a*) Pyrite, FeS_2

(*b*) Zincite, ZnO

(*c*) Barite, $BaSO_4$

(*d*) α-Quartz, SiO_2

Fig. 19-23 (*after Berry and Mason,* Mineralogy, *W. H. Freeman and Co.*)

19.46. Four crystals were prepared as geometrical cubes, polished and etched to develop the true symmetry. The results were as follows: (*a*) no etch pattern showing; (*b*) vertical striations on all four side faces and no pattern on the top and bottom; (*c*) vertical striations on the side faces, horizontal striations on the front and back, and no pattern on the top and bottom; and (*d*) square designs on a pair of parallel and opposite faces. Classify these crystals.

Ans. (*a*) O_h or $4/m\,\bar{3}\,2/m$ (*c*) $\mathcal{D}_{2h}$ or $2/m\,2/m2/m$

(*b*) $\mathcal{D}_{4h}$ or $4/m\,2/m\,2/m$ (*d*) $\mathcal{D}_{4h}$ or $4/m\,2/m\,2/m$

X-Ray Spectra

19.47. Repeat Problem 19.16 for the 111 plane. *Ans.* $d_{111} = 3.2038$ Å; $\theta = 13.9°$

19.48. Which of the possible indices listed in Problem 19.17 are allowed for CsCl?

Ans. body-centered cubic;
200 = 020 = 002, 110 = 101 = 011, 220 = 202 = 022, 222, and 211 = 121 = 112

19.49. The powder pattern for sylvite using filtered Cu radiation, $\lambda = 1.5418$ Å, shows six peaks. The values of 2θ and the relative intensities for these lines are 28.3°(100%), 40.5°(55%), 50.2°(20%), 58.6°(5%), 66.3°(15%) and 73.6°(10%). If sylvite is known to crystallize in the cubic system, determine a for the mineral and index the lines.

Ans. The values 100, 110, 111, 200, 210 and 211, which will work for the spectrum, must be discarded because these correspond to a primitive cubic cell, which is not possible for a compound. Hence 200, 220, 222, 400, 420 and 422 with $Q_{100} = 0.0251$, giving $a = 6.31$ Å.

19.50. Sparteine sulfate pentahydrate, $C_{15}H_{26}N_2 \cdot H_2SO_4 \cdot 5H_2O$, crystallizes in the monoclinic crystal system with $a = 8.03$ Å, $b = 15.2$ Å, $c = 8.84$ Å and $\beta = 91°30'$. Index the following intense lines of the powder pattern as reported by Metz: d = 8.9446, 8.0932, 7.6748, 7.1320, 5.7936, 5.6755, 5.4733, 4.7714, 4.6718, 4.4313, 4.3204, 4.0458, 3.9139, 3.8371, 3.7078, 3.6201, 3.5090, 3.4528, 3.3532 and 3.2639 Å. If $Z = 2$, calculate the theoretical density of this compound. The observed density is $1.28 \times 10^3\ \mathrm{kg\,m^{-3}}$.

Ans. 001; 100; 011 and 020; 110; 021 and 101; $11\bar{1}$; 120 and 111; $12\bar{1}$; 121; 002 and 031;
012 and 130; 200; 210, $13\bar{1}$ and $10\bar{2}$; 102, $11\bar{2}$, 040, 131 and 022; $20\bar{1}$ and 112;
201 and $21\bar{1}$; 041, 211 and 220; 140 and 122; 032; 221; $d = 1.30 \times 10^3\ \mathrm{kg\ m^{-3}}$

19.51. Determine the structure factors for the 111 and 220 planes in NaCl, see Example 19.12. Assume $f_+ = 7.4$ and $f_- = 10.0$ for the 220 plane and $f_+ = 9.2$ and $f_- = 14.4$ for the 111 plane. Find the ratio of the intensities of the 111 and 220 peaks.

Ans. $F(220) = 17.4(1 + 2e^{2\pi i} + e^{4\pi i}) = 69.6,$
$F(111) = 9.2(1 + 3e^{2\pi i}) + 14.4(3e^{\pi i} + e^{3\pi i}) = -20.8;$ 8.9%

19.52. Quantitative X-ray analysis of mixtures can be performed if a calibration curve is determined. Using the $2\theta = 28.3°$ peak for sylvite and the 31.5° peak for halite, known samples were analyzed for peak heights five different times to obtain a statistical average. A plot of ($\text{height}_{28.3}/\text{height}_{31.5}$) or ($\text{height}_{31.5}/\text{height}_{28.3}$) against composition gives a calibration curve to which an unknown may be compared in the analysis by working backwards. For the known mixtures given in Table 19-4, determine the average peak height, calculate one of the ratios and make a calibration plot. Using the data for the unknown, determine the composition of the mixture.

Ans. 49 wt% NaCl

Table 19-4

wt% Halite	wt% Sylvite	Trial 1		Trial 2		Trial 3		Trial 4		Trial 5	
		28.3	31.5	28.3	31.5	28.3	31.5	28.3	31.5	28.3	31.5
80.0	20.0	20	59	21	56	20	55	20	55	22	58
60.0	40.0	79	89	68	86	85	93	77	87	76	95
50.0	50.0	74	64	79	69	83	57	76	66	75	58
40.0	60.0	61	27	63	27	62	29	62	26	62	25
20.0	80.0	71	10	61	12	60	10	73	11	63	11
Unknown		59	41	52	37	52	39	52	40	57	40

Chapter 20

Liquids

Critical Point

A substance cannot exist as a liquid at any pressure unless its temperature is below the critical temperature, see Section 1.11. One way to determine the critical temperature and density of a material that does not associate in the liquid phase is to use the Rectilinear Diameter Law of Cailletet and Mathias, which can be stated as

$$\frac{1}{2}(d_{\text{liq}} + d_{\text{gas}}) = A + BT' + C(T')^2 + \cdots \tag{20.1}$$

where A, B and C are constants and T' is the temperature in °C. This law implies that plots of the orthobaric densities of the gas and of the liquid will intersect at the critical point, giving

$$d_c = A + BT'_c + C(T'_c)^2 + \cdots \tag{20.2}$$

EXAMPLE 20.1. Estimate the critical temperature for a substance having gaseous densities of 1.03×10^3, 1.07×10^3, 1.14×10^3 and 1.25×10^3 kg m^{-3} and liquid densities of 1.46×10^3, 1.43×10^3, 1.39×10^3 and 1.33×10^3 kg m^{-3} at 100°, 290°, 450° and 540 °C, respectively.

The plot of these densities, see Fig. 20-1, shows that the curves converge at about 560 °C = T'_c. The point of intersection can be identified more easily by extrapolation of the $(d_{\text{liq}} + d_{\text{gas}})/2$ plot.

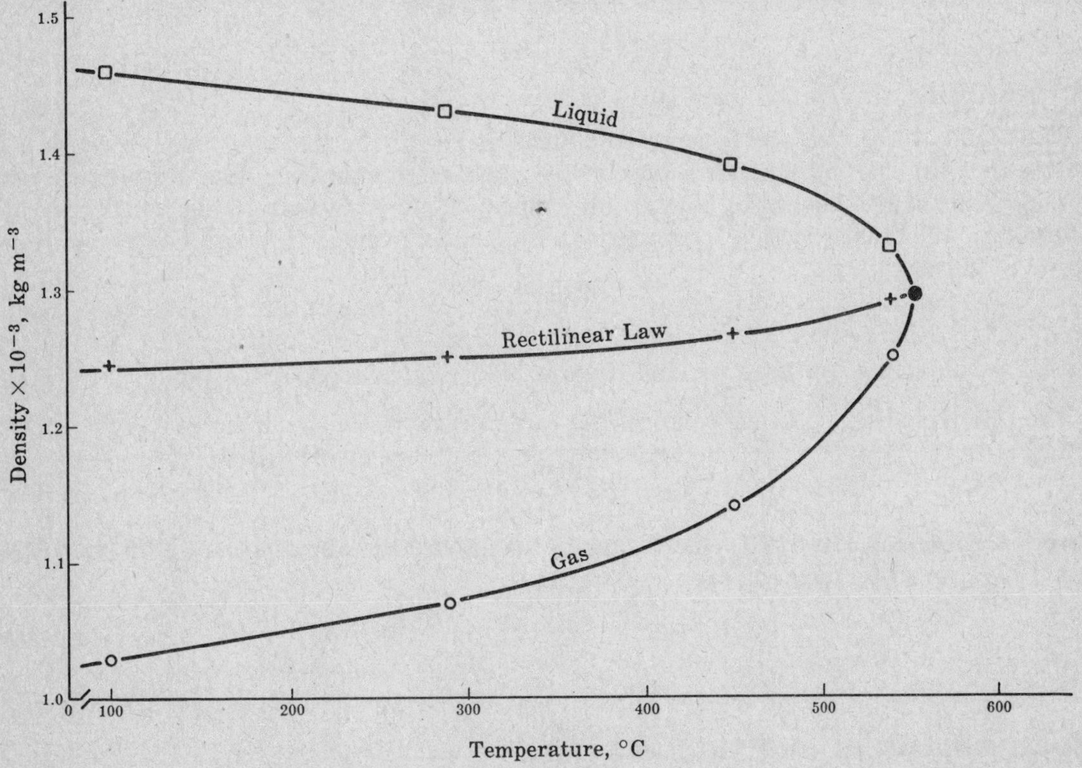

Fig. 20-1

Viscosity

20.1 FLOW

The flow of a fluid through a pipe of radius R has associated with it a *Reynolds number*, RN, given by

$$\mathrm{RN} = \frac{2R\bar{v}d}{\eta} \tag{20.3}$$

where $\bar{v}$ is the average or bulk velocity of the fluid, d is the density and η is the coefficient of viscosity. If RN is greater than 4000, the flow is turbulent and if less than 2100, the flow is laminar. In laminar flow a velocity profile given by

$$v = \frac{\Delta P}{4\eta\ell}(R^2 - r^2) \tag{20.4}$$

is observed in the pipe, where ΔP is the pressure drop over a length ℓ and r is the distance from the axis of the pipe.

The volume of liquid flowing through a fixed cross section in time t is given by

$$V = \frac{\pi R^4(\Delta P)t}{8\eta\ell} \tag{20.5}$$

EXAMPLE 20.2. The cgs unit of viscosity is the *poise* ($1\ \mathrm{g\ cm^{-1}\ s^{-1}}$). Show that $1\ \mathrm{poise} = 0.1\ \mathrm{N\ s\ m^{-2}}$.

Converting the cgs units to SI units gives

$$(1\ \mathrm{poise})(1\ \mathrm{g\ cm^{-1}\ s^{-1}/poise})(10^{-3}\ \mathrm{kg\ g^{-1}})(10^2\ \mathrm{cm\ m^{-1}})(1\ \mathrm{N/1\ kg\ m\ s^{-2}}) = 0.1\ \mathrm{N\ s\ m^{-2}}$$

The unit *poiseuille* (Pl) has been assigned to represent $1\ \mathrm{N\ s\ m^{-2}}$.

20.2 MEASUREMENT OF VISCOSITY

The coefficient of viscosity is commonly measured with the *Ostwald viscometer* (or some revision) or with the *falling-sphere viscometer*. In the Ostwald technique, the time required for a given amount of liquid to flow at low values of RN is measured and (*20.5*) is used to calculate η. In actual practice, a comparison method is often used to bypass the determination of R and ℓ, giving

$$\frac{\eta_1}{\eta_0} = \frac{d_1 t_1}{d_0 t_0} \tag{20.6}$$

where the subscripts are used to identify the unknown and reference liquids.

The falling-sphere technique balances the force of gravitation against viscous drag, giving

$$\eta = \frac{2r_b^2(d_b - d)g}{9v} \tag{20.7}$$

where the subscript b refers to the dropping sphere or bead and g is the gravitational constant. If comparison methods are used,

$$\frac{\eta_1}{\eta_0} = \frac{(d_b - d_1)t_1}{(d_b - d_0)t_0} \tag{20.8}$$

20.3 TEMPERATURE DEPENDENCE

A plot of $\log \eta$ against $1/T$, where T is the absolute temperature, is linear over moderate temperature intervals:

$$\log \eta = \frac{A}{T} + B \tag{20.9}$$

Here A and B are constants for a given material. Taking antilogarithms gives

$$\eta = B' e^{\Delta E(\text{viscosity})/RT} \tag{20.10}$$

where $A = \Delta E(\text{viscosity})/2.303\,R$. For many substances, $\Delta E(\text{viscosity}) \approx 0.3\,\Delta E(\text{vaporization})$.

EXAMPLE 20.3. Glycerin has the following viscosities:

T, °C	−42	−25	−10.8	0	20	30
η, N s m^{-2}	6710	262	35.5	12.11	1.49	0.629

Find $\Delta E(\text{viscosity})$ and calculate η at 25 °C.

Preparing a plot of $\log \eta$ against $1/T$ gives a straight line with slope $A = 3.53 \times 10^3$ K, see Fig. 20-2. Then

$$\Delta E(\text{viscosity}) = 2.303\,RA = (2.303)(8.314 \text{ J mol}^{-1} \text{ K}^{-1})(3.53 \times 10^3 \text{ K}) = 67.6 \text{ kJ mol}^{-1}$$

The value of B can best be calculated using one of the data pairs, e.g. that for 20 °C, giving

$$B = \log \eta - \frac{A}{T}$$

$$= \log 1.49 - \frac{3.53 \times 10^3 \text{ K}}{293 \text{ K}} = -11.87$$

At 25 °C, (*20.9*) gives

$$\log \eta = \frac{3.53 \times 10^3 \text{ K}}{298 \text{ K}} - 11.87$$

$$= -0.024$$

and taking antilogarithms gives $\eta = 0.945$ N s m^{-2}.

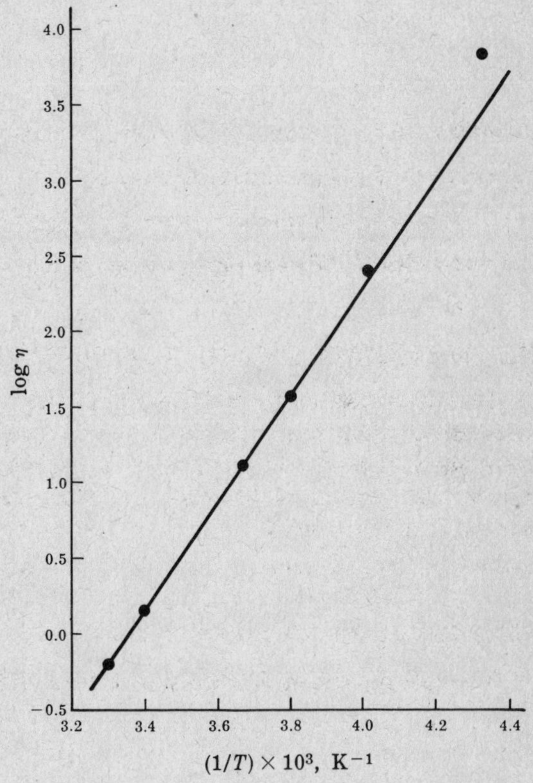

Fig. 20-2

Surface Tension

20.4 MEASUREMENT OF SURFACE TENSION

The surface tension of a liquid, γ, was defined in (*2.7b*). In the *capillary-tube method* of measuring γ, the liquid in the tube of radius r will rise or be depressed a distance ℓ given by

$$\ell = \frac{2\gamma}{drg} \tag{20.11}$$

where g is the gravitational constant. If a comparison method is used,

$$\frac{\gamma_1}{\gamma_0} = \frac{d_1\ell_1}{d_0\ell_0} \tag{20.12}$$

In the *drop-weight method*, γ is determined from the mass of the drop which forms on the end of a capillary tube before falling off. In the *bubble-pressure method*, γ is determined by measuring the pressure required to produce a bubble of a gas in the liquid at the end of a capillary tube. In the *ring method*, γ is related to the force necessary to lift a ring from the surface of the liquid.

EXAMPLE 20.4. The surface tension of water at 20 °C is 72.75×10^{-3} N m^{-1}. A 33.24-vol% solution of ethanol has $\gamma = 33.24 \times 10^{-3}$ N m^{-1} at this same temperature. If $d = 0.9614 \times 10^3$ kg m^{-3} for the solution and 0.9982×10^3 kg m^{-3} for water, how much less in the same capillary tube will the alcohol solution rise?

Using (*20.12*) gives

$$\frac{\ell_1}{\ell_0} = \frac{\gamma_1}{\gamma_0}\frac{d_0}{d_1} = \frac{33.24 \times 10^{-3}}{72.75 \times 10^{-3}}\frac{0.9982 \times 10^3}{0.9614 \times 10^3} = 0.474$$

Thus the solution will rise only 47.4% as far as pure water.

20.5 WETTING

Consider a drop of liquid on a solid (or on another liquid with which it is mutually insoluble). Defining the *contact angle* θ as the angle that the surface of the drop makes with the solid,

$$\gamma_s = \gamma_{\text{s-liq}} + \gamma_{\text{liq}} \cos\theta \qquad (20.13)$$

The subscript s-liq refers to the surface tension (*interfacial tension*) between the liquid and solid.

EXAMPLE 20.5. "Wetting" is arbitrarily defined as $\theta < 90°$. Determine the relationship between γ_s and $\gamma_{\text{s-liq}}$ for wetting to occur.

For $\theta < 90°$, $\cos\theta$ is positive and so $\gamma_s > \gamma_{\text{s-liq}}$, as in the case of water on glass.

20.6 PARACHOR

The *parachor*, $\{P\}$, is defined as

$$\{P\} = \frac{10^3 M(\gamma \times 10^3)^{1/4}}{d_{\text{liq}} - d_{\text{gas}}} \qquad (20.14)$$

where M is the molecular weight (g mol^{-1}), γ is the surface tension (N m^{-1}) and d is the density (kg m^{-3}). The parachor is an additive property depending on the elements present in the compound and the configuration of the atoms. By working from known values and from predicted values for $\{P\}$, it is often possible to determine certain structural properties of compounds.

EXAMPLE. 20.6. Predict the parachor and γ for $CH_3C_6H_4CN$ if the parachor equivalent for C is 4.8; H, 17.1; N, 12.5; double bond, 23.2; triple bond, 46.6; and six-membered ring, 6.1. The average density of the three isomers is 0.985×10^3 kg m^{-3} for the liquids and d_{gas} can be assumed to be negligible.

The predicted parachor is the sum of the equivalents, giving

$$\{P\} = 8(4.8) + 7(17.1) + 1(12.5) + 46.6 + 6.1 + 3(23.2) = 292.9$$

Using (*20.14*) gives

$$(\gamma \times 10^3)^{1/4} = \frac{\{P\}d}{M10^3} = \frac{(292.9)(0.985 \times 10^3)}{(117.14)(10^3)} = 2.46$$

whence $\gamma = 36.6 \times 10^{-3}$ N m^{-1}.

20.7 VAPOR PRESSURE OF DROPLETS

For a very small droplet of radius r, the vapor pressure P_s is given by

$$\ln\frac{P_s}{P} = \frac{2\gamma M}{rdRT} \qquad (20.15)$$

where P is the vapor pressure of large (bulk) samples of the substance. The heat of vaporization is related to P via (*3.14*).

EXAMPLE 20.7. Determine P_s/P for a drop of water at 25 °C that has $r = 0.1$ cm. At this temperature $\gamma = 71.97 \times 10^{-3}$ N m^{-1} and $d = 0.997044 \times 10^3$ kg m^{-3}.

Using (*20.15*) gives

$$\ln\frac{P_s}{P} = \frac{2(71.97\times10^{-3}\text{ N m}^{-1})(18.01\text{ g mol}^{-1})(10^{-3}\text{ kg g}^{-1})}{(1\times10^{-3}\text{ m})(0.997044\times10^{3}\text{ kg m}^{-3})(8.314\text{ J mol}^{-1}\text{ K}^{-1})(298\text{ K})} = 1.05\times10^{-6}$$

Taking antilogarithms, see Problem 1.20, gives $P_s/P = 1.00000105$, an insignificant change.

Solved Problems

Critical Point

20.1. The densities of liquid and gaseous CCl_4 are 0.7634×10^3 and 0.3597×10^3 kg m^{-3} at 280 °C and 0.8666×10^3 and 0.2710×10^3 kg m^{-3} at 270 °C. Find A and B in (*20.1*). If $T_c' = 283.2$ °C, find d_c and the molar volume at the critical point.

Using the density table data in (*20.1*) gives

$$\frac{1}{2}(0.7634\times10^3 + 0.3597\times10^3) = A + B(280)$$

$$\frac{1}{2}(0.8666\times10^3 + 0.2710\times10^3) = A + B(270)$$

which upon solving simultaneously gives $A = 0.7632 \times 10^3$ kg m^{-3} and $B = -0.72$ kg m^{-3} (°C)$^{-1}$. Using $T_c' = 283.2$ °C, (*20.2*) gives

$$d_c = (0.7632\times10^3\text{ kg m}^{-3}) + [-0.72\text{ kg m}^{-3}\,(°\text{C})^{-1}](283.2\text{ °C}) = 0.5593\times10^3\text{ kg m}^{-3}$$

The critical molar volume is given by

$$V_c = \frac{M}{d_c} = \frac{(153.82\text{ g mol}^{-1})(10^{-3}\text{ kg g}^{-1})}{0.5593\times10^3\text{ kg m}^{-3}} = 2.75\times10^{-4}\text{ m}^3\text{ mol}^{-1} = 275\text{ cm}^3\text{ mol}^{-1}$$

Viscosity

20.2. Consider the flow of water through a horizontal pipe with $R = 1$ in. and $\bar{v} = 3$ cm s^{-1}. If $\eta = 1.202$ centipoise at 13 °C and $d = 0.999377 \times 10^3$ kg m^{-3}, find RN. What is v at $r = 0$, at $r = 0.5\,R$ and at $r = R$? If the water is being pumped through a length of pipe equivalent to 300 ft, what pressure must the pump be able to produce for the desired flow rate?

Using (*20.3*) gives

$$\text{RN} = \frac{2(1\text{ in.})(2.54\times10^{-2}\text{ m in}^{-1})(3\times10^{-2}\text{ m s}^{-1})(0.999377\times10^3\text{ kg m}^{-3})}{(1.202\times10^{-2}\text{ poise})(0.1\text{ N s m}^{-2}\text{ poise}^{-1})} = 1267$$

which means the flow is laminar. The volume of liquid flowing in time t is given by

$$V/t = \pi R^2\bar{v} = \pi(2.54\times10^{-2}\text{ m})^2(3\times10^{-2}\text{ m s}^{-1}) = 6.08\times10^{-5}\text{ m}^3\text{ s}^{-1}$$

which combined with (*20.5*) gives the pumping pressure as

$$\Delta P = \frac{(V/t)8\eta\ell}{\pi R^4}$$

$$= \frac{(6.08\times10^{-5}\text{ m}^3\text{ s}^{-1})(8)(1.202\times10^{-2}\text{ poise})(0.1\text{ N s m}^{-2}\text{ poise}^{-1})(300\text{ ft})(12\text{ in. ft}^{-1})(2.54\times10^{-2}\text{ m in}^{-1})}{\pi(2.54\times10^{-2}\text{ m})^4}$$

$$= 40.9\text{ N m}^{-2} = 4.04\times10^{-4}\text{ atm}$$

Combining (*20.4*), (*20.5*) and the expression for V/t gives

$$v = 2\bar{v}\left[1 - \left(\frac{r}{R}\right)^2\right] = (6\text{ cm s}^{-1})\left[1 - \left(\frac{r}{R}\right)^2\right]$$

Hence the velocities at $r = 0, \frac{1}{2}R$ and R are 6, 4.5 and 0 cm s^{-1}, respectively.

20.3. An Ostwald viscometer was calibrated using water at 25 °C ($\eta = 0.89$ centipoise and $d = 1.00 \times 10^3$ kg m^{-3}). The same viscometer was used at −193 °C (volume changes, etc., neglected) to determine the viscosity of liquid air ($d = 0.92 \times 10^3$ kg m^{-3}). If $t_1/t_0 = 0.193$, find η_1.

Using (*20.6*) gives

$$\eta_1 = \eta_0 \frac{d_1}{d_0}\frac{t_1}{t_0} = (0.89\text{ centipoise})\left(\frac{0.92 \times 10^3}{1.00 \times 10^3}\right)(0.193) = 0.16\text{ centipoise} = 1.6 \times 10^{-4}\text{ N s m}^{-2}$$

20.4. The times that a steel "bb" ($d_b = 7.80 \times 10^3$ kg m^{-3}) required to drop through water and a commercial shampoo were 1 s and 7 s, respectively. If the densities are 1.00×10^3 and 1.03×10^3 kg m^{-3}, respectively, find η_1/η_0.

Using (*20.8*) gives

$$\frac{\eta_1}{\eta_0} = \frac{(7.80 \times 10^3 - 1.03 \times 10^3)(7)}{(7.80 \times 10^3 - 1.00 \times 10^3)(1)} = 7$$

20.5. The viscosity of molten sodium is 0.450 centipoise at 200 °C and 0.212 centipoise at 600 °C. Find ΔE(viscosity) and predict η at 400 °C.

For two temperatures, (*20.9*) gives

$$\log \eta_2 - \log \eta_1 = \frac{\Delta E(\text{viscosity})}{2.303\,R}\left(\frac{1}{T_2} - \frac{1}{T_1}\right)$$

which upon substitution of the data gives

$$\Delta E(\text{viscosity}) = \frac{(2.303)(8.314\text{ J mol}^{-1}\text{ K}^{-1})[\log(0.212) - \log(0.450)]}{\dfrac{1}{873\text{ K}} - \dfrac{1}{473\text{ K}}}$$

$$= \frac{(2.303)(8.314)(-0.327)}{-0.969 \times 10^{-3}} = 6.46\text{ kJ mol}^{-1}$$

Using the above equation for η_2 gives

$$\log \eta_2 = \log(0.450) + \frac{6460}{(2.303)(8.314)}\left(\frac{1}{673} - \frac{1}{473}\right)$$

$$= -0.347 + \frac{(6460)(-0.628 \times 10^{-3})}{(2.303)(8.314)} = -0.559$$

which upon taking antilogarithms gives $\eta_2 = 0.276$ centipoise $= 2.76$ N s m^{-2}. The actual value is 0.278 centipoise.

Surface Tension

20.6. A capillary tube was calibrated at 20 °C using water and the water rose 8.37 cm before it came to equilibrium. A sample of mercury was depressed 3.67 cm using the same capillary. If $d = 0.9982 \times 10^3$ kg m^{-3} for water and 13.5939×10^3 kg m^{-3} for Hg, find γ for mercury if $\gamma = 72.75$ dyne cm^{-1} $= 72.75 \times 10^{-3}$ N m^{-1} for water. What is the nominal size of the capillary tubing used?

Using (*20.12*) gives

$$\gamma_1 = (72.75 \times 10^{-3}\ \text{N m}^{-1}) \frac{(13.5939 \times 10^3\ \text{kg m}^{-3})(3.67\ \text{cm})}{(0.9982 \times 10^3\ \text{kg m}^{-3})(8.37\ \text{cm})} = 0.434\ \text{N m}^{-1}$$

Rearranging (*20.11*) gives

$$r = \frac{2\gamma}{dgl} = \frac{2(72.75 \times 10^{-3}\ \text{N m}^{-1})}{(0.9982 \times 10^3\ \text{kg m}^{-3})(9.8\ \text{m s}^{-2})(8.37 \times 10^{-2}\ \text{m})} = 1.78 \times 10^{-4}\ \text{m}$$

or a nominal size of 0.2 mm.

20.7. The interfacial tension between H_2O and *n*-octyl alcohol at 20 °C is 8.5 dyne cm^{-1}. If $\gamma = 27.53$ dyne cm^{-1} for the alcohol and 75.75 dyne cm^{-1} for H_2O at this temperature, predict whether wetting occurs for a drop of water in contact with a pool of *n*-octyl alcohol.

Substituting the data into (*20.13*) gives (the units are irrelevant):

$$\cos\theta = \frac{27.53 - 8.5}{75.75} = 0.251$$

which corresponds to the angle $\theta = 75.5°$, a wetting situation.

20.8. The density of paraldehyde is 0.9943×10^3 kg m^{-3}, $M = 132.16$ g mol^{-1} and the surface tension is 25.9 dyne cm^{-1} = 25.9×10^{-3} N m^{-1}. Calculate $\{P\}$. Calculate the parachor for acetaldehyde using parachor equivalents of 4.8 for C, 17.1 for H, 20.0 for O and 23.2 for a double bond. If paraldehyde is a trimer of acetaldehyde containing a six-membered ring (additional parachor equivalent of 6.1) of carbon and oxygen, describe the bonding ring.

Neglecting d_{gas}, the value of $\{P\}$ for paraldehyde is given by (*20.14*) as

$$\{P\} = \frac{10^3(132.16)(25.9)^{1/4}}{0.9943 \times 10^3} = 300$$

Summing the contributions for acetaldehyde gives

$$\{P\} = 2(4.8) + 4(17.1) + 1(20.0) + 1(23.2) = 121.2$$

Assuming a trimer ring of acetaldehyde, $\{P\}$ would be $3(121.2) + 6.1 = 369.7$, which is too high. Assuming a trimer ring without double bonding, $\{P\}$ would be $3(121.2) + 6.1 - 3(23.2) = 300.1$, which agrees with the value determined using (*20.14*).

Vapor Pressure

20.9. What is the minimum size of water droplets such that the vapor pressure does not differ by more than 1% from the bulk value?

Substituting $P_s = 1.01\,P$ and the necessary data for water into (*20.15*) gives

$$r = \frac{2(71.97 \times 10^{-3}\ \text{N m}^{-1})(18.01\ \text{g mol}^{-1})(10^{-3}\ \text{kg g}^{-1})}{(0.997044 \times 10^3\ \text{kg m}^{-3})(8.314\ \text{J mol}^{-1}\ \text{K}^{-1})(298\ \text{K})(\ln 1.01)} = 1.05 \times 10^{-7}\ \text{m}$$

Supplementary Problems

Critical Point

20.10. If

$$d_{gas} = 20.0 + 0.1750\,T' + 1.500 \times 10^{-4}(T')^2$$

$$d_{liq} = 1000.0 - 0.5000\,T' - 2.000 \times 10^{-4}(T')^2$$

both in units of kg m^{-3}, find T'_c, d_c, A, B and C.

Ans. 967 °C, 329.5 kg m^{-3}, 510.0 kg m^{-3}, -0.1625 kg m^{-3} (°C)$^{-1}$, -2.50×10^{-5} kg m^{-3} (°C)$^{-2}$

Viscosity

20.11. Repeat the calculations of Problem 20.2 at 25 °C where

$$\eta = 0.8904 \text{ centipoise} \quad \text{and} \quad d = 0.997044 \times 10^3 \text{ kg m}^{-3}$$

If the same pump is used, compare the values of v.

Ans. RN = 1707; ΔP = 30.3 N m^{-2}; $\bar{v}$ and v same as before.
For ΔP = 40.9 N m^{-2}, $\bar{v}$ = 3(1.202/0.8904) cm s^{-1} and velocities are increased by 34.9%.

20.12. If light machinery oil has η = 50 centipoise and $d = 0.97 \times 10^3$ kg m^{-3} at 25 °C, how long will it take for a sample to pass through a viscometer if water under the same conditions takes 1 min?

Ans. 57.9 min assuming $d = 1.00 \times 10^3$ kg m^{-3} and η = 0.89 centipoise

20.13. The viscosity of a 20-wt% aqueous solution of ethanol is 2.183 centipoise and the density is 0.97139×10^3 kg m^{-3}. If an olive is dropped into a tall glass of this solution, what will be the velocity once equilibrium between the gravitational and viscous forces has been established? Assume r_b = 0.9 cm, $d_b = 1.10 \times 10^3$ kg m^{-3} and g = 9.8 m s^{-2}. *Ans.* 10.4 m s^{-1}

20.14. If η = 1.307 centipoise at 10.0 °C and 0.5468 centipoise at 50.0 °C, find ΔE(viscosity) for water. At 25 °C, ΔH(vaporization) = 10.514 kcal mol^{-1} for water. Is the relationship ΔE(viscosity) = 0.3 ΔE(vaporization) valid for water?

Ans. A = 865 K, ΔE(viscosity) = 16.56 kJ mol^{-1};

ΔE(vaporization) = 43.99 − RT = 41.51 kJ mol^{-1} by (*3.2*);

ΔE(viscosity)/ΔE(vaporization) = 0.4 (reasonably valid)

20.15. For glycerin it was shown in Example 20.3 that ΔE(viscosity) = 67.6 kJ mol^{-1}. If ΔH(vaporization) = 31.7 kcal mol^{-1}, does the approximate relationship ΔE(viscosity) = 0.3 ΔE(vaporization) hold true for this substance? *Ans.* 0.52 would be a better factor.

20.16. The viscosity of a 60-wt% aqueous solution of sucrose is 238 centipoise at 0 °C and 43.86 centipoise at 25 °C. If the density of the solution changes insignificantly over this temperature range, test the adage "As slow as molasses in January." *Ans.* t_0/t_{25} = 5.43

Surface Tension

20.17. Molten LiCl wets BN. If γ = 12.5 dyne cm^{-1} at 800 °C and $d = 1.417 \times 10^3$ kg m^{-3}, describe what will happen if a BN tube having a radius of 1 mm and height of 1 cm is placed in a sample of LiCl(liq). *Ans.* ℓ = 1.80 cm (fountain effect)

20.18. The value of $\gamma_{\text{s-liq}}$ for Hg on glass is large enough that $\gamma_s - \gamma_{\text{s-liq}}$ is negative. Will wetting occur?

Ans. No: $\theta > 90°$.

20.19. The interfacial tension between CCl_4 and H_2O is 45 dyne cm^{-1}. If γ = 26.95 dyne cm^{-1} for CCl_4 and 72.75 dyne cm^{-1} for water, find the contact angle between water and CCl_4 for a drop of water on a pool of CCl_4. Does wetting occur? *Ans.* $\theta = 104°$; no

20.20. The parachor equivalent for C is 4.8; for H, 17.1; and for O, 20.0. (*a*) Predict the parachors for methanol and ethanol. (*b*) Calculate the parachors if $\gamma = 22 \times 10^{-3}$ N m^{-1} for each alcohol and if $d = 0.7914 \times 10^3$ kg m^{-3} for methanol and 0.7893×10^3 kg m^{-3} for ethanol. (*c*) The parachor defect in these substances is related to the amount of hydrogen bonding between molecules. In which substance is this effect more significant?

Ans. (*a*) 93.2 for methanol and 132.2 for ethanol

(*b*) 87.6 for methanol and 126.2 for ethanol

(*c*) defect is 5.6 for methanol and 6.0 for ethanol, suggesting more hydrogen bonding in ethanol

Vapor Pressure

20.21. The vapor pressure of glycerin is 10 torr at 167.2 °C and 100 torr at 220.1 °C. Find ΔH(vaporization).

Ans. 78.63 kJ mol^{-1}

20.22. Determine P_s/P for a drop of water at 25 °C that has $r = 10^{-6}$ cm.

Ans. 1.111 (a significant change)

Chapter 21

Nuclear Chemistry

Nuclei

21.1 NUCLEAR CONSTITUENTS

Many particles have been found in the nucleus, but only the few given in Table 21-1 will be considered in this chapter.

Table 21-1

Particle	Symbol	Mass (u)	Charge (e)
neutron	n or ${}^{1}_{0}n$	1.0086654	0
proton	p or ${}^{1}_{1}\mathrm{H}$	1.0072766	+1
electron	β^- or ${}^{\ 0}_{-1}\beta$	0.0005486	−1
positron	β^+ or ${}^{\ 0}_{+1}\beta$	0.0005486	+1

EXAMPLE 21.1. The (unified) atomic mass unit, u, is defined such that the mass of the particular carbon atom having six neutrons and six protons is exactly 12.00000 u. Calculate the conversion factor between u and g.

This species of carbon has molecular weight 12.00000 g mol^{-1}. Hence, using Avogadro's number,

$$1 = \frac{(12.00000\ \mathrm{u})(6.022045 \times 10^{23}\ \mathrm{mol}^{-1})}{12.00000\ \mathrm{g\ mol}^{-1}} = 6.022045 \times 10^{23}\ \mathrm{u\ g}^{-1}$$

or 1.660565×10^{-24} g u^{-1}.

21.2 TERMINOLOGY

The *atomic number, Z,* of a nuclide is equal to the number of protons present in the nucleus; the *neutron number, N,* is equal to the number of neutrons in the nucleus; and the *mass number, A,* is given by $N + Z$ and represents the number of nucleons in the nucleus. A given nuclide is represented by the symbol ${}^{A}_{Z}X$ (or ${}_{Z}X^{A}$) where X is the elemental chemical symbol corresponding to the value of Z.

EXAMPLE 21.2. List (*a*) isotopes, (*b*) isobars and (*c*) isotones among the following nuclides:

$${}^{15}_{8}\mathrm{O},\ {}^{14}_{7}\mathrm{N},\ {}^{13}_{6}\mathrm{C},\ {}^{12}_{5}\mathrm{B},\ {}^{14}_{8}\mathrm{O},\ {}^{13}_{7}\mathrm{N},\ {}^{15}_{7}\mathrm{N},\ {}^{16}_{8}\mathrm{O},\ {}^{18}_{9}\mathrm{F},\ {}^{17}_{9}\mathrm{F}$$

(*a*) *Isotopes* are nuclides having the same value of Z. Hence: ${}^{13}_{7}\mathrm{N}$, ${}^{14}_{7}\mathrm{N}$ and ${}^{15}_{7}\mathrm{N}$; ${}^{14}_{8}\mathrm{O}$, ${}^{15}_{8}\mathrm{O}$ and ${}^{16}_{8}\mathrm{O}$; and ${}^{17}_{9}\mathrm{F}$ and ${}^{18}_{9}\mathrm{F}$.

(*b*) *Isobars* are nuclides having the same value of A. Hence: ${}^{13}_{6}\mathrm{C}$ and ${}^{13}_{7}\mathrm{N}$, ${}^{14}_{7}\mathrm{N}$ and ${}^{14}_{8}\mathrm{O}$, and ${}^{15}_{7}\mathrm{N}$ and ${}^{15}_{8}\mathrm{O}$.

(*c*) *Isotones* are nuclides having the same value of N. Hence: ${}^{13}_{7}\mathrm{N}$ and ${}^{14}_{8}\mathrm{O}$; ${}^{12}_{5}\mathrm{B}$, ${}^{13}_{6}\mathrm{C}$, ${}^{14}_{7}\mathrm{N}$ and ${}^{15}_{8}\mathrm{O}$; and ${}^{15}_{7}\mathrm{N}$, ${}^{16}_{8}\mathrm{O}$ and ${}^{17}_{9}\mathrm{F}$.

21.3 NUCLEAR SIZE

An empirical formula which may be used to predict the radius of a nucleus is

$$r = (1.5 \times 10^{-15}\ \mathrm{m})A^{1/3} \tag{21.1}$$

where A is the mass number.

21.4 BINDING ENERGY

The *total binding energy* of a nucleus is defined as the energy for the reaction

$${}^{A}_{Z}X = Z\,{}^{1}_{1}\mathrm{H} + (A-Z)\,{}^{1}_{0}n$$

as calculated from the difference in the rest masses of products and reactants ($\Delta E = c^2\,\Delta m$). Two useful conversion factors are $1\ \mathrm{u} = 931.5017\ \mathrm{MeV} = 1.492442 \times 10^{-10}\ \mathrm{J}$ and $1\ \mathrm{MeV} = 1.6021892 \times 10^{-13}\ \mathrm{J}$. The *average binding energy* for a nucleus is the total binding energy divided by the value of A.

The *mass excess,* $M - A$, is the mass of the nuclide in u less the mass number. The *packing fraction* is given by

$$\mathrm{pf} = \frac{(M-A)10^4}{A} \tag{21.2}$$

Radioactive Decay

21.5 TYPES OF DECAY

The common modes of decay are summarized in Table 21-2 (EC = electron capture, IT = internal transition). These modes can be represented by plotting energy against the atomic number, see Fig. 21-1.

Table 21-2

Type of Decay	Z	N	A	General Equation
α	−2	−2	−4	${}^{A}_{Z}X = {}^{A-4}_{Z-2}Y + {}^{4}_{2}\alpha$
β^-	+1	−1	0	${}^{A}_{Z}X = {}_{Z+1}^{A}Y + {}_{-1}^{0}\beta$
β^+	−1	+1	0	${}^{A}_{Z}X = {}_{Z-1}^{A}Y + {}^{0}_{1}\beta$
EC	−1	+1	0	${}^{A}_{Z}X + {}_{-1}^{0}e = {}_{Z-1}^{A}Y$
IT or γ	0	0	0	${}^{A}_{Z}X^* = {}^{A}_{Z}X + \gamma$

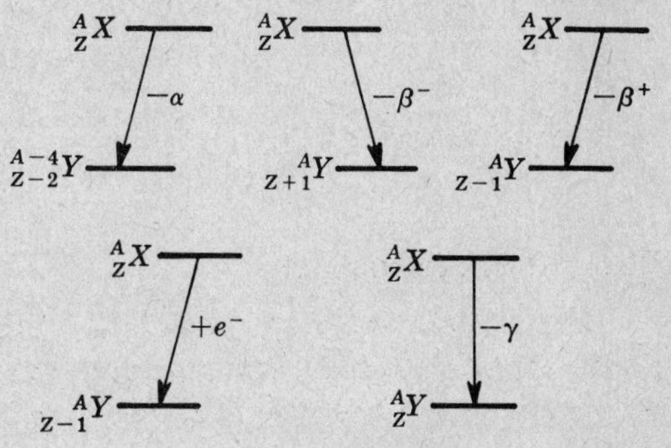

Fig. 21-1

EXAMPLE 21.3. ${}^{203}_{83}\mathrm{Bi}$ undergoes positron emission, electron capture and alpha emission. Write equations showing the products of each type of decay.

In writing equations, it is necessary that the sums of the Z's and of the A's on both sides of the reaction be equal. Using the symbols for the particles given in Table 21-2, the reactions are

$${}^{203}_{83}\mathrm{Bi} = {}_{+1}^{0}\beta + {}^{203}_{82}\mathrm{Pb}, \quad {}^{203}_{83}\mathrm{Bi} + {}_{-1}^{0}\beta = {}^{203}_{82}\mathrm{Pb}, \quad {}^{203}_{83}\mathrm{Bi} = {}^{4}_{2}\alpha + {}^{199}_{81}\mathrm{Tl}$$

21.6 DECAY SCHEMES

Usually there are several types and energies of radiation observed during the decay of a parent nucleus into a daughter nuclide. An analysis of these data can be diagramed using a decay scheme similar to those shown in Fig. 21-1 for the modes of decay.

EXAMPLE 21.4. ${}^{23}_{10}Ne$ undergoes β^- decomposition to ${}^{23}_{11}Na$. An analysis of the β^- radiation showed that 1% of the particles had an energy of 2.4 MeV, 32% had 3.95 MeV and 67% had 4.39 MeV. The analysis of the gamma radiation showed that a 0.436-MeV gamma was coincident with the 3.95-MeV β^- and that a 1.65-MeV gamma was coincident with both the 2.4-MeV β^- and 0.436-MeV gamma radiation. Construct a decay scheme from these data.

The diagram given in Fig. 21-2 agrees with the data. From the reaction

$${}^{23}_{10}Ne = {}^{0}_{-1}\beta + {}^{23}_{11}Na$$

the top and bottom lines were drawn, the latter to the right of the diagram because of the increase in Z. Three arrows were drawn from the top line to the bottom line and lines above the bottom line, in agreement with the three β's observed. Vertical arrows are drawn between the isomers of ${}^{23}_{11}Na$, corresponding to the two γ's observed. The total energy along any path is nearly the same: 4.39, $3.95 + 0.436 = 4.39$ and $2.4 + 1.65 + 0.436 = 4.49$ MeV. The numbers to the right of the diagram represent the nuclear energy levels above the ground state of the daughter.

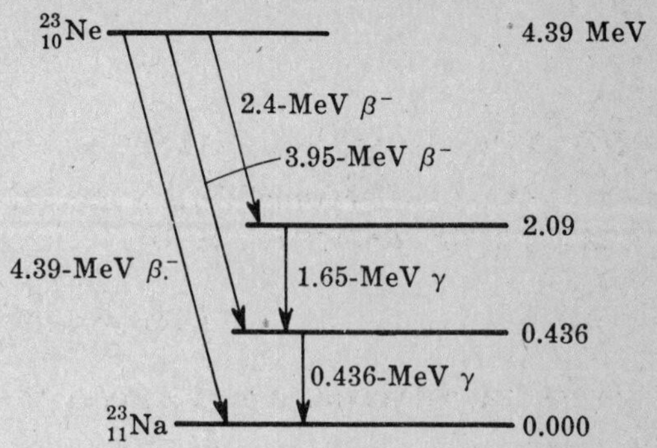

Fig. 21-2

21.7 DECAY SERIES

If the daughter of one decay happens to be radioactive and undergoes further decay, a decay series is created.

EXAMPLE 21.5. ${}^{238}_{92}U$ belongs to the series known as the $4n + 2$ *decay series* because all the values of A for the successive daughters are equal to four times an integer plus two. Using a suitable reference such as the Table of Isotopes found in a recent edition of the *Handbook of Chemistry and Physics*, list the first eight members of the series.

The Table of Isotopes lists ${}^{238}_{92}U$ as an α emitter, giving ${}^{238}_{92}U = {}^{4}_{2}He + {}^{234}_{90}Th$. The daughter is a β^- emitter, so ${}^{234}_{90}Th = {}^{0}_{-1}\beta + {}^{234}_{91}Pa$. ${}^{234}_{91}Pa$ is also a β^- emitter, so ${}^{234}_{91}Pa = {}^{0}_{-1}\beta + {}^{234}_{92}U$. This daughter is an α emitter, so ${}^{234}_{92}U = {}^{4}_{2}He + {}^{230}_{90}Th$. This is an α emitter, so ${}^{230}_{90}Th = {}^{4}_{2}He + {}^{226}_{88}Ra$. ${}^{226}_{88}Ra$ is an α emitter, so ${}^{226}_{88}Ra = {}^{4}_{2}He + {}^{222}_{86}Rn$. Again after emitting an α, ${}^{222}_{86}Rn = {}^{4}_{2}He + {}^{218}_{84}Po$.

21.8 DECAY CONSTANT AND HALF-LIFE

Radioactive decay follows first-order kinetics, see Section 10.3, in which the number of nuclei undergoing decay is directly proportional to the number present. Expressing this mathematically gives

$$-\frac{dN}{dt} = \lambda N \tag{21.3}$$

where N is the number of radioactive nuclei at time t and λ is the *decay constant*. The integrated form of (*21.3*) is

$$\ln \frac{N}{N_0} = -\lambda t \tag{21.4}$$

The *activity*, A, is defined as

$$A = c\lambda N \tag{21.5}$$

where c, the *detection coefficient*, depends on the detection instrument, geometrical arrangement of experiment, etc., and in the ideal case is unity. Substituting (*21.5*) into (*21.4*) gives

$$\ln \frac{A}{A_0} = -\lambda t \tag{21.6}$$

EXAMPLE 21.6. Find the relationship between λ and the *half-life* of a radioactive nuclide.

The half-life, $t_{1/2}$, is defined as the time at which $A = A_0/2$. Substituting into (*21.6*) gives

$$\ln\left(\frac{A_0/2}{A_0}\right) = -0.69315 = -\lambda t_{1/2}$$

or

$$\lambda t_{1/2} = 0.69315 \qquad (21.7)$$

21.9 SUCCESSIVE DECAYS

If the daughter nuclide is a member of a decay series, then the number present at time t is given by, see Section 10.10,

$$N_2 = \lambda_1 N_{0,1} \frac{e^{-\lambda_1 t} - e^{-\lambda_2 t}}{\lambda_2 - \lambda_1} + N_{0,2} e^{-\lambda_2 t} \qquad (21.8)$$

where the subscripts 1 and 2 refer to the parent and daughter nuclides, respectively.

Three special cases of (*21.8*) are often considered: (1) *transient equilibrium*, in which the parent has a longer half-life than the daughter ($\lambda_1 < \lambda_2$) and

$$\frac{N_1}{N_2} \approx \frac{\lambda_2 - \lambda_1}{\lambda_1} \qquad (21.9)$$

(2) *secular equilibrium*, in which the activity of the parent does not decrease much during several half-lives of the daughter ($\lambda_1 \ll \lambda_2$) and

$$\frac{N_1}{N_2} \approx \frac{\lambda_2}{\lambda_1} \qquad (21.10)$$

and (3) disequilibrium, in which case the daughter outlives the parent ($\lambda_1 > \lambda_2$) and (*21.8*) must be used.

21.10 UNITS OF RADIOACTIVITY

The *curie*, c, is the unit of radioactivity defined as the quantity of nuclide necessary to generate 3.700×10^{10} disintegrations per second.

EXAMPLE 21.7. Another commonly used radioactive unit is the *Rutherford*, rd, which is defined as the amount of material necessary to generate 1.000×10^6 disintegrations per second. Clearly,

$$1 \text{ c} = 3.700 \times 10^4 \text{ rd}$$

Interaction of Radiation with Matter

21.11 CHARGED PARTICLES

Charged particles such as α particles and protons form ion pairs within the absorber as they pass through the material. The mechanism of beta absorption is similar except that the number of ions formed in a given length of absorber is less and hence electrons have a greater penetrating power.

EXAMPLE 21.8. The range of an ion with a charge q (in units of e), mass M (in units of u), and energy E is equal to M/q^2 times the range of a proton with energy E/M. What is the ratio of the range of an alpha to that of a proton having the same velocity?

Putting the relationship described into mathematical form gives

$$R_{\alpha,E} = \frac{M}{q^2} R_{p,E/M} \tag{21.11}$$

Substituting 2 and 4 for q and M, respectively, gives

$$\frac{R_{\alpha,E}}{R_{p,E/4}} = \frac{4}{2^2} = 1$$

(Note that M is replaced by A in many equations.) The ratio of the kinetic energies is

$$\frac{E_\alpha}{E_p} = \frac{\frac{1}{2}A_\alpha v^2}{\frac{1}{2}A_p v^2} = 4$$

Thus the ranges are equal.

21.12 GAMMA RADIATION

There are three mechanisms by which γ's can lose their energy: (1) production of an ion or excited atom by low-energy γ's, (2) Compton scattering for moderate energy radiation, and (3) electron-positron pair formation for energies greater than 1.022 MeV. These processes give rise to an exponential decay within the absorber, described by

$$A = A_0 e^{-\mu x} \tag{21.12}$$

where A is the γ flux at a depth x within the material, A_0 is the incident γ flux, and μ is the *absorption coefficient*. The ratio of μ to the density is known as the *mass absorption coefficient*. The *half-thickness* of a material is defined as the depth at which $A = A_0/2$ and is given by

$$x_{1/2} = \frac{0.693}{\mu} \tag{21.13}$$

21.13 NEUTRONS

Neutrons usually interact with the nuclei of the absorber, producing nuclear transformations (Sections 21.15–21.17).

21.14 UNITS OF ABSORPTION

A *roentgen*, r, is the amount of radiation that will produce about 1.61×10^{15} ion pairs per kilogram of air; more exactly, $1\ \text{r} = 2.57976 \times 10^{-4}\ \text{C kg}^{-1}$. It is used primarily for measuring incident γ flux. As the definition is based on incident radiation in air, and does not reflect the amount of energy absorbed by the target, a more meaningful unit is the *rad*, which is equal to 1.00×10^{-2} J of energy actually absorbed by 1 kg of target material. The rad is used for all types of radiation. Because energy release is not the only factor to consider as causing damage to tissue, each type of radiation has its *relative biological effectiveness*, rbe: $\beta^- =$ X-ray $= 1$, thermal neutron $= 3$, $p =$ fast neutron $= 10$, and $\alpha = 20$. The *roentgen-equivalent-man*, rem, is equal to the product of the dose in rads times the rbe.

EXAMPLE 21.9. If 1.5 rem is considered a maximum weekly dose for the hands and forearms, how long would it take for a man to receive this dose from a 10-mc source emitting a 2.5-MeV gamma? Assume that negligible radiation is absorbed by the air and that the hands are about 10 cm from the sample.

From the definition of the curie, the number of γ's being emitted is

$$N = (10 \times 10^{-3}\ \text{c})(3.7 \times 10^{10}\ \text{s}^{-1}\ \text{c}^{-1}) = 3.7 \times 10^{8}\ \text{s}^{-1}$$

The flux or amount reaching the hands is

$$\frac{N}{4\pi r^2} = \frac{3.7 \times 10^8}{4\pi(0.1)^2} = 2.9 \times 10^9 \ s^{-1}\ m^{-2}$$

The corresponding energy flux is

$$(2.9 \times 10^9\ \text{s}^{-1}\ \text{m}^{-2})(2.5\ \text{MeV}) = 7.3 \times 10^9\ \text{MeV s}^{-1}\ \text{m}^{-2} = 1.2 \times 10^{-3}\ \text{J s}^{-1}\ \text{m}^{-2}$$

Assuming an area of 800 cm^2 gives the dosage rate as

$$(1.2 \times 10^{-3}\ \text{J s}^{-1}\ \text{m}^{-2})(0.08\ \text{m}^2) = 9.6 \times 10^{-5}\ \text{J s}^{-1}$$

From the definition of the rem and the fact that the rbe is 1,

$$(1.5\ \text{rem})/1 = 1.5\ \text{rad} = 1.5 \times 10^{-2}\ \text{J kg}^{-1}$$

Assuming the hands and forearms to be about 4 kg gives

$$(1.5 \times 10^{-2}\ \text{J kg}^{-1})(4\ \text{kg}) = 6 \times 10^{-2}\ \text{J}$$

for the permitted dose. Dividing this by the dosage rate gives the time as

$$\frac{6 \times 10^{-2}\ \text{J}}{9.6 \times 10^{-5}\ \text{J s}^{-1}} = 6.3 \times 10^2\ \text{s} = 10.5\ \text{min}$$

Nuclear Reactions

21.15 EQUATIONS AND NOTATION

The shorthand notation that is commonly used for a transformation reaction reads:

TARGET NUCLIDE(PROJECTILE,EJECTED PARTICLES)PRODUCT NUCLIDE

21.16 ENERGY CONSIDERATIONS

The energy for a nuclear transformation reaction is calculated by subtracting the sum of the rest masses of the reactants from the sum of the rest masses of the products. The energy can similarly be calculated using the respective mass excesses. The Q, or yield, of the reaction is defined as the negative of the energy.

If the conservation of kinetic energy is considered, the projectile for a reaction with a positive value of Δ(mass) must supply the threshold energy given by

$$E_{\text{thr}} = \frac{(M_{\text{proj}} + M_{\text{targ}})\Delta(\text{mass})}{M_{\text{targ}}} \tag{21.14}$$

Mass numbers are often substituted for the actual masses in (*21.14*).

In order for a positively charged particle to approach the nucleus, it must overcome a potential barrier resulting from the coulombic repulsion between the target and projectile. For an alpha particle this potential barrier can be expressed as

$$U_{\text{proj}} = U_\alpha = \frac{(1.92\ \text{MeV})Z_{\text{targ}}}{A_{\text{targ}}^{1/3} + 1.59} \tag{21.15a}$$

and for a proton projectile

$$U_{\text{proj}} = U_p = \frac{(0.96\ \text{MeV})Z_{\text{targ}}}{A_{\text{targ}}^{1/3} + 1} \tag{21.15b}$$

where the nuclear sizes are assumed to be given by (*21.1*)

The total energy required by a projectile because of the conservation of kinetic energy is given by

$$E_{\text{proj}} = \frac{(M_{\text{proj}} + M_{\text{targ}})U_{\text{proj}}}{M_{\text{targ}}} \qquad (21.16)$$

where E_{proj} is assumed to be larger than the value of E_{thr}; if not, E_{thr} must be used.

EXAMPLE 21.10. Calculate Q, E_{thr} and E_{proj} for the reaction $^{58}_{26}\text{Fe}(^{3}_{2}\text{He},^{2}_{1}\text{H})^{59}_{27}\text{Co}$ if the masses are 57.9333, 3.01603, 2.0140 and 58.9332 u, respectively.

The change in mass is

$$\Delta(\text{mass}) = (58.9332 + 2.0140) - (57.9333 + 3.01603) = -0.0021 \text{ u}$$

which gives

$$Q = -\Delta(\text{mass}) = 0.0021 \text{ u} = 1.96 \text{ MeV}$$

Because Δ(mass) is negative, E_{thr} has no meaning.

The potential barrier for $^{3}_{2}\text{He}$ is given by

$$U_{\text{proj}} = \frac{(1.92 \text{ MeV})Z_{\text{targ}}}{A_{\text{targ}}^{1/3} + 1.44} = \frac{(1.92)(26)}{58^{1/3} + 1.44} = 9.40 \text{ MeV}$$

and using (21.16),

$$E_{\text{proj}} = \frac{(3 + 58)(9.40)}{58} = 9.89 \text{ MeV}$$

21.17 CROSS SECTIONS

The probability of a reaction taking place depends on the *cross section*, σ, of the target particle for the particular type of radiation being used as projectiles. The integrated form of the equation describing the number of reactions per second, $I_0 - I$, is

$$I_0 - I = I_0(1 - e^{-N\sigma x}) \qquad (21.17)$$

where I and I_0 represent the intensity of the beam after traveling a distance x and the initial intensity, respectively, and N is the number of atoms per m^3 of the target. The values for σ are often given in the unit of *barns*, where 1 barn = 10^{-28} m^2.

Miscellaneous Considerations

21.18 NUCLEAR FISSION

If $^{235}_{92}\text{U}$ is exposed to a beam of thermal neutrons, the nuclide $^{236}_{92}\text{U}$ is formed which undergoes fission into two unequal fragments having values of Z and A of the order of 50 and 100, respectively. The reaction can be written in two steps:

$$^{1}_{0}n + ^{235}_{92}\text{U} = ^{236}_{92}\text{U} \qquad ^{236}_{92}\text{U} = ^{A_1}_{Z_1}X + ^{A_2}_{Z_2}Y + 2.43\,^{1}_{0}n$$

The fragments X and Y usually have too many neutrons for stability and undergo β^- emission.

21.19 NUCLEAR FUSION

This process is essentially the opposite of fission because smaller nuclei are used to produce larger ones.

EXAMPLE 21.11. Calculate the thermonuclear energy released in a hydrogen bomb consisting of 1 mol of deuterium, if the reaction is

$$2\,{}^{2}_{1}\mathrm{H} = {}^{3}_{1}\mathrm{H} + {}^{1}_{1}\mathrm{H}$$

The energy change for two atoms reacting is

$$\Delta(\text{mass}) = (3.01605 + 1.007825) - 2(2.0140) = -0.0041\ \mathrm{u} = -3.82\ \mathrm{MeV}$$

or a Q of 0.0021 u per atom. Scaling up to 1 mol gives

$$(0.0021\ \mathrm{u})(6.022 \times 10^{23}\ \mathrm{mol^{-1}})(1.4924 \times 10^{-10}\ \mathrm{J\ u^{-1}}) = 1.9 \times 10^{11}\ \mathrm{J\ mol^{-1}}$$

21.20 RADIOACTIVE DATING

For determining the age of once-living, carbon-containing materials up to 60,000 years old, ${}^{14}_{6}\mathrm{C}$ dating is used. The initial activity per unit mass is assumed to be 12.6 $\mathrm{min^{-1}\ g^{-1}}$ and the half-life is 5730 y.

Geological dating of potassium-bearing rocks can be done by measuring the ratio of atoms of ${}^{40}_{18}\mathrm{Ar}$ to atoms of ${}^{40}_{19}\mathrm{K}$ in the sample. Because ${}^{40}_{19}\mathrm{K}$ undergoes two types of decay, (*21.6*) becomes

$$t = \frac{1}{\lambda_{\mathrm{EC}} + \lambda_{\beta^-}} \ln\left[1 + \frac{(\lambda_{\mathrm{EC}} + \lambda_{\beta^-})N_{40,\mathrm{Ar}}}{\lambda_{\mathrm{EC}} N_{40,\mathrm{K}}}\right] \qquad (21.18)$$

where $\lambda_{\mathrm{EC}} = 5.85 \times 10^{-11}\ \mathrm{y^{-1}}$ and $\lambda_{\beta^-} = 4.72 \times 10^{-10}\ \mathrm{y^{-1}}$.

If a rock contains uranium, its age can be determined by the *lead-lead technique*, which (assuming no loss of lead or intermediates in the decay series) gives

$$\frac{N_{207,\mathrm{Pb}}}{N_{206,\mathrm{Pb}}} = (7.25 \times 10^{-3}) \frac{e^{\lambda_{235}t} - 1}{e^{\lambda_{238}t} - 1} \qquad (21.19)$$

where $t_{1/2,235} = 7.1 \times 10^{8}$ y and $t_{1/2,238} = 4.51 \times 10^{9}$ y. This procedure is not good for ages less than 10^9 y.

EXAMPLE 21.12. One sample of rock #12013 from the Apollo 12 exploration contained an extremely large amount of $^{40}\mathrm{Ar}$. If the moon rock contains 1.66% by weight of K and if there is $81.9 \times 10^{-7}\ \mathrm{m^3}$ of $^{40}\mathrm{Ar}$ at STP per kilogram of rock, calculate the age of the rock.

The number of moles of $^{40}\mathrm{Ar}$ in 1 kg of rock is calculated using the ideal gas law, (*1.6*):

$$n = \frac{(1\ \mathrm{atm})(81.9 \times 10^{-7}\ \mathrm{m^3\ kg^{-1}})}{(8.21 \times 10^{-5}\ \mathrm{m^3\ atm\ K^{-1}\ mol^{-1}})(273\ \mathrm{K})} = 3.65 \times 10^{-4}\ \mathrm{mol\ kg^{-1}}$$

and the number of atoms is

$$N_{40,\mathrm{Ar}} = (3.65 \times 10^{-4})L$$

Not all of the $^{40}\mathrm{Ar}$ present in the sample originated from the $^{40}\mathrm{K}$ decay. Experimentally for this sample, the $^{40}\mathrm{Ar}/^{36}\mathrm{Ar}$ ratio was determined as 52,700 whereas in normal Ar the ratio is 296. Applying a correction factor of

$$(52{,}700 - 296)/52{,}700 = 0.994$$

to $(3.65 \times 10^{-4})L$ gives the amount of $^{40}\mathrm{Ar}$ formed from the $^{40}\mathrm{K}$ as

$$(0.994)(3.65 \times 10^{-4})L = 3.63 \times 10^{-4}\ L$$

The number of moles of potassium in the 1-kg sample is given by

$$\frac{(1.66 \times 10^{-2})(1000\ \mathrm{g})}{39.1\ \mathrm{g\ (mol\ K)^{-1}}} = 0.425\ \mathrm{mol\ K}$$

Of this, a fraction 1.18×10^{-4} is $^{40}\mathrm{K}$. Hence, the number of $^{40}\mathrm{K}$ atoms per kg of rock is

$$N_{40,\mathrm{K}} = (0.425)(L)(1.18 \times 10^{-4}) = (5.01 \times 10^{-5})L$$

Equation (*21.18*) now gives

$$t = \frac{1}{5.31 \times 10^{-10}} \ln \left[1 + \frac{(5.31 \times 10^{-10})(3.63 \times 10^{-4} L)}{(5.85 \times 10^{-11})(5.01 \times 10^{-5} L)} \right]$$

$$= \frac{1}{5.31 \times 10^{-10}} \ln (1 + 65.8) = 7.9 \times 10^{9} \text{ y}$$

Comparison of this answer to that for Problems 21.20 and 21.53 indicates that possibly a sampling error was present.

21.21 ISOTOPE DILUTION

Suppose that a mixture has a component X that cannot be completely separated by quantitative methods. If a known mass of radioactive X (i.e. a radioactive isotope of X or radioactive-tagged X) is added to the mixture and then a partial extraction of the component is made, the extract will have the same proportions of radioactive and nonradioactive X atoms as the whole enriched mixture. Thus the mass of X originally present can be inferred from the *dilution factor*

$$\text{df} = \frac{A_{\text{orig}}}{A_{\text{dil}}} \qquad (21.20)$$

where A_{orig} and A_{dil} are respectively the activities per unit mass of the added material and of the extract. See Problem 21.21.

Solved Problems

Nuclei

21.1. On an older atomic mass scale, the mass of $^{16}_{8}O$ was taken as exactly 16.00000 amu; on this scale $^{12}_{6}C$ had a mass of 12.00382 amu. On the current physical scale, these masses are 15.99491 u and 12.000000 u, respectively. Calculate an average scale factor to convert between amu and u.

Since

$$(16.00000 - 12.00382) \text{ amu} = (15.99491 - 12.00000) \text{ u}$$

the desired conversion factor is

$$1 = \frac{(16.00000 - 12.00382) \text{ amu}}{(15.99491 - 12.00000) \text{ u}} = \frac{3.99618 \text{ amu}}{3.99491 \text{ u}} = 1.000318 \text{ amu u}^{-1}$$

21.2. The natural abundance of neon is 90.92% $^{20}_{10}Ne$ (19.99244 u), 0.257% $^{21}_{10}Ne$ (20.99395 u) and 8.82% $^{22}_{10}Ne$ (21.99138 u). Calculate the average atomic weight for natural neon gas.

Dividing the sum of the products of the percentages times the atomic weights by the sum of the percentages gives

$$\frac{(0.9092)(19.99244) + (0.00257)(20.99395) + (0.0882)(21.99138)}{(0.9092) + (0.00257) + (0.0882)} = 20.171 \text{ u}$$

21.3. The mass of an atom of hydrogen having one proton and one electron is 1.0072766 + 0.0005486 = 1.0072852 u. What fraction of the total mass of a hydrogen atom is contained within the nucleus? Contrast this answer to that for the fraction of the atomic volume ($r = 0.529$ Å) occupied by the nucleus if (*21.1*) is valid.

The fraction of atomic mass is

$$\frac{1.0072766}{1.0078252}(100\%) = 99.94557\%$$

and the fraction of volume is

$$\frac{[(1.5 \times 10^{-15})(1)]^3}{(0.529 \times 10^{-10})^3}(100\%) = 2.3 \times 10^{-12}\%$$

The answers imply that the nucleus is a very dense object.

21.4. Calculate the total and average binding energies and the packing fraction for ${}^{12}_{6}C$.

For the reaction

$${}^{12}_{6}C = 6\,{}^{1}_{1}H + 6\,{}^{1}_{0}n$$

the change in mass is

$$\Delta(\text{mass}) = 6(1.007825) + 6(1.008665) - 12.000000 = 0.098940\text{ u} = 92.163\text{ MeV}$$

and the average binding energy is

$$\frac{92.163\text{ MeV}}{12} = 7.680\text{ MeV}$$

Since $M = A$ for this nuclide, pf $= 0$.

Radioactive Decay

21.5. ${}^{27}_{12}Mg$ undergoes β^- emission to form ${}^{27}_{13}Al$. An analysis of the β^- radiation showed that 58% of the particles had an energy of 1.75 MeV and 42% had 1.59 MeV. The analysis of the gamma radiation showed that a 0.834-MeV gamma was coincident with the 1.75-MeV β^- and that a 1.015-MeV gamma was coincident with the 1.59-MeV β^-. Construct a decay scheme from these data.

Figure 21-3 agrees with the data. From the reaction

$${}^{27}_{12}Mg = {}^{0}_{-1}\beta + {}^{27}_{13}Al$$

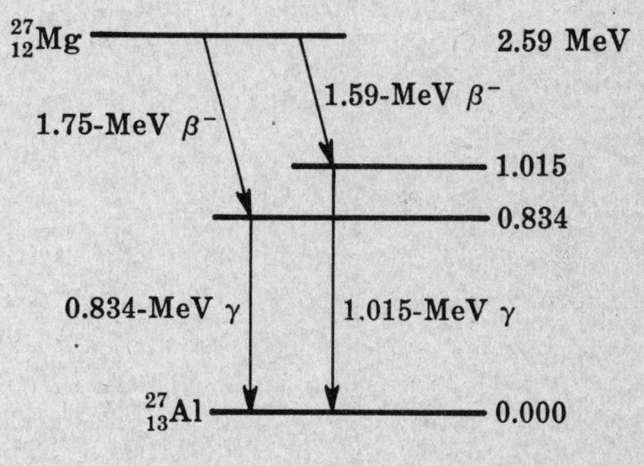

Fig. 21-3

the top and bottom lines were drawn, with the latter to the right of the diagram. The arrows representing the β and γ decays show that there are three isomers of ${}^{27}_{13}Al$ and a direct transition between the ground states of ${}^{27}_{12}Mg$ and ${}^{27}_{13}Al$ does not occur.

21.6. For a short period of time, each isotope of the various elements had an individual name. Three such names are still commonly used: *protium, deuterium* and *tritium* —the three isotopes of hydrogen. Identify the element "Ionium" if it is a member of the ${}^{238}_{92}U$ decay series and is produced after two different α's and two different β^-'s have been released.

The daughter generated after the release of an α, two β^-'s and an α is ${}^{230}_{90}Th$ according to the reactions given in Example 21.5.

21.7. Calculate the ratio of N/N_0 after an hour has passed, for a material having a half-life of 47.2 s.

Using (*21.7*) gives

$$\lambda = \frac{0.693}{47.2\ \text{s}} = 1.47 \times 10^{-2}\ \text{s}^{-1}$$

and (*21.4*) gives

$$\ln \frac{N}{N_0} = -(1.47 \times 10^{-2}\ \text{s}^{-1})(1\ \text{hr})(3600\ \text{s hr}^{-1}) = -52.9$$

$$\log \frac{N}{N_0} = \frac{-52.9}{2.303} = -23.0$$

$$\frac{N}{N_0} = 1 \times 10^{-23}$$

21.8. If $N = 0.798\, N_0$ for a sample at the end of 4.2 days, calculate $t_{1/2}$.

Substituting the data into (*21.4*) gives

$$\lambda = -\frac{\ln (0.798)}{4.2\ \text{d}} = 0.054\ \text{d}^{-1}$$

which upon substitution into (*21.7*) gives

$$t_{1/2} = \frac{0.693}{0.054} = 12.8\ \text{d}$$

21.9. The half-life of ${}^{212}_{82}\text{Pb}$, which decays to ${}^{212}_{83}\text{Bi}$, is 10.6 hr. The half-life of ${}^{212}_{83}\text{Bi}$ is 60.5 min. Describe the activity in a sample of ${}^{212}_{82}\text{Pb}$ after equilibrium has been established.

The total activity of the sample will decay with a half-life equal to 10.6 hr, and the ratio of parent to daughter will be given by (*21.9*) as

$$\frac{N_1}{N_2} = \frac{(0.693/t_{1/2,2}) - (0.693/t_{1/2,1})}{(0.693/t_{1/2,1})}$$

$$= \frac{(60/60.5) - (1/10.6)}{1/10.6} = 9.51$$

21.10. What mass of ${}^{220}_{86}\text{Rn}$ having $t_{1/2} = 54.5$ s is equivalent to 1 mc?

Using (*21.7*) to determine λ gives

$$\lambda = \frac{0.693}{54.5\ \text{s}} = 1.27 \times 10^{-2}\ \text{s}^{-1}$$

The definition of a curie gives for the millicurie

$$-\frac{dN}{dt} = 3.7 \times 10^{7}\ \text{s}^{-1}$$

Solving (*21.3*) for N and substituting values gives

$$N = \frac{3.700 \times 10^{7}\ \text{s}^{-1}}{1.27 \times 10^{-2}\ \text{s}^{-1}} = 2.91 \times 10^{9}$$

which can be converted to moles and mass by

$$\frac{2.91 \times 10^{9}}{6.022 \times 10^{23}\ \text{mol}^{-1}}(220\ \text{g mol}^{-1}) = 1.06 \times 10^{-15}\ \text{kg}$$

Interaction of Radiation with Matter

21.11. Calculate the penetration of a 1.0-MeV β^- particle if it produces 6.1 ion pairs per mm in air. Assume that 2.86×10^{4} ion pairs must be produced to stop the radiation.

Dividing the required number of ion pairs by the rate that they are being formed gives

$$\frac{2.86 \times 10^4}{6.1} = 4690 \text{ mm air} = 4.69 \text{ m}$$

21.12. The mass absorption coefficient of Pb for 3.0-MeV γ's corresponds to a "half-thickness" of 16 g cm^{-2}. Calculate the percent decrease in activity at a depth of 1 cm. The density of Pb is $11.3 \times 10^3 \text{ kg m}^{-3}$.

The mass absorption coefficient has the value

$$\frac{0.693}{16 \text{ g cm}^{-2}} = 4.33 \times 10^{-2} \text{ cm}^2 \text{ g}^{-1} = 4.33 \times 10^{-3} \text{ m}^2 \text{ kg}^{-1}$$

Multiplying by the density gives

$$\mu = (4.33 \times 10^{-3} \text{ m}^2 \text{ kg}^{-1})(11.3 \times 10^3 \text{ kg m}^{-3}) = 48.9 \text{ m}^{-1}$$

Using (*12.12*) gives

$$A = A_0 e^{-(48.9 \text{ m}^{-1})(1 \times 10^{-2} \text{ m})} = 0.613 A_0$$

The decrease in A is 38.7%.

Nuclear Reactions

21.13. Complete the shorthand notations for the following reactions by writing equations for the processes shown: (*a*) ^{9}B(n,p)____, (*b*)____(d,t)^{18}O and (*c*) ^{30}P(____,p)^{33}S.

The sums of A and Z must be the same on both sides of the reaction.

(*a*)
$$^{9}_{5}\text{B} + {}^{1}_{0}n = {}^{9}_{4}\text{Be} + {}^{1}_{1}p$$

so $^{9}_{4}$Be is the product nuclide.

(*b*)
$$^{19}_{8}\text{O} + {}^{2}_{1}d = {}^{18}_{8}\text{O} + {}^{3}_{1}t$$

so $^{19}_{8}$O is the target nuclide.

(*c*)
$$^{30}_{15}\text{P} + {}^{4}_{2}\alpha = {}^{33}_{16}\text{S} + {}^{1}_{1}p$$

so an α particle is the projectile.

21.14. Calculate the threshold energy for ^{34}S(p,n)^{34}Cl if $Q = -6.203$ MeV.

The change in mass is

$$\Delta(\text{mass}) = -Q = 6.203 \text{ MeV}$$

which upon substitution into (*21.14*) gives

$$E_{\text{thr}} = \frac{(1 + 34)(6.203 \text{ MeV})}{34} = 6.4 \text{ MeV}$$

21.15. Calculate the barrier potential and the total energy that an α particle must have to penetrate a ^{14}N nucleus and compare it to the 1.54 MeV threshold energy.

Using (*21.15a*) gives the value of the barrier potential as

$$U_\alpha = \frac{(1.92)(7)}{14^{1/3} + 1.59} = 3.36 \text{ MeV}$$

and using (*21.16*) gives the total energy as

$$E_{\text{proj}} = \frac{(4 + 14)(3.36)}{14} = 4.32 \text{ MeV}$$

Because of their charge, α projectiles must have about three times as much kinetic energy for nuclear penetration as would uncharged projectiles with the same mass.

21.16. Consider a flux of thermal neutrons equal to $10^8\ s^{-1}\ cm^{-2}$ falling on a lead foil 1 cm^2 in area and 1 mm thick. If $\sigma = 0.18$ barn and $d = 11.3 \times 10^3\ kg\ m^{-3}$ for lead, calculate the number of radioactive nuclei formed per second.

The number of nuclei per m^3 is

$$N = \frac{(11.3 \times 10^3\ kg\ m^{-3})(6.022 \times 10^{23}\ mol^{-1})}{(207\ g\ mol^{-1})(10^{-3}\ kg\ g^{-1})} = 3.29 \times 10^{28}\ m^{-3}$$

The intensity of the incident beam is

$$I_0 = (\text{flux})(\text{area}) = (10^8\ s^{-1}\ cm^{-2})(1\ cm^2) = 10^8\ s^{-1}$$

which upon substitution into (*21.17*) gives

$$I_0 - I = (10^8)[1 - e^{-(3.29\times 10^{28}\ m^{-3})(0.18\times 10^{-28}\ m^2)(1\times 10^{-3}\ m)}]$$

$$= (10^8)(1 - e^{-5.9\times 10^{-4}}) = 5.9 \times 10^4\ s^{-1}$$

Miscellaneous Considerations

21.17. Estimate the energy released if the fragments of the fission process described in Section 21.18 are $^{94}_{38}Sr$ and $^{140}_{54}Xe$.

The separate decays are

$$^{236}_{92}U = {}^{94}_{38}Sr + {}^{140}_{54}Xe + 2\,{}^{1}_{0}n$$

$$^{94}_{38}Sr = {}^{94}_{40}Zr + 2\,{}^{0}_{-1}\beta$$

$$^{140}_{54}Xe = {}^{140}_{58}Ce + 4\,{}^{0}_{-1}\beta$$

giving the overall reaction

$$^{236}_{92}U = {}^{94}_{40}Zr + {}^{140}_{58}Ce + 6\,{}^{0}_{-1}\beta + 2\,{}^{1}_{0}n$$

Hence

$$\Delta(\text{mass}) = [93.9061 + 139.9053 + 6(0.00055) + 2(1.00867)] - 236.0457$$

$$= -0.2137\ u = -199\ MeV$$

or $Q = 199$ MeV. Only 95% of this energy is available for useful purposes.

21.18. Which is the better nuclear fuel on a weight basis, ^{235}U or ^{2}H?

For about 235 u of U, about 199 MeV of energy is released, see Problem 21.17; and for about 4 u of H, about 3.82 MeV of energy is released, see Example 21.11. Taking a ratio gives

$$\frac{Q_U}{Q_H} = \frac{199/235}{3.82/4} = 0.89$$

(About the same.)

21.19. A sample of wood from an Egyptian tomb gave a ^{14}C activity per unit mass of 7.3 $min^{-1}\ g^{-1}$. What is the age of the wood?

Using (*21.7*) gives

$$\lambda = \frac{0.693}{5730} = 1.21 \times 10^{-4}\ y^{-1}$$

and using (*21.6*) gives

$$\ln\frac{7.3}{12.6} = -0.546 = -1.21 \times 10^{-4} t$$

which upon solving gives $t = 4510$ y.

21.20. A current nuclear theory suggests that $^{235}U/^{238}U$ was nearly unity at the time of the formation of the elements. If the current ratio is 7.25×10^{-3}, calculate the age of the elements.

Using (*21.7*) for the isotopes gives

$$\lambda_{235} = \frac{0.693}{7.1 \times 10^8} = 9.76 \times 10^{-10}\ y^{-1}$$

and $\lambda_{238} = 1.54 \times 10^{-10}\ y^{-1}$. The exponential form of (*21.4*) gives for the current ratio

$$7.25 \times 10^{-3} = (1)e^{-(\lambda_{235}-\lambda_{238})t} = e^{-8.22 \times 10^{-10}\,t}$$

Solving for t gives

$$t = -\ln \frac{7.25 \times 10^{-3}}{8.22 \times 10^{-10}} = 6.0 \times 10^9\ y$$

21.21. Suppose that the activity per unit mass of the added material in an isotope dilution procedure was $12.5\ s^{-1}\ g^{-1}$ and the activity per unit mass of the dilute sample was $2.5\ s^{-1}\ g^{-1}$. Calculate the dilution factor and the amount of original material, assuming $m_* = 100$ mg of radioactive material was added.

Using (*21.20*) gives

$$df = \frac{12.5}{2.5} = 5.0$$

If the activity per unit mass has decreased by a factor of 5, then the mass must have increased by a factor of 5. Thus the original amount, m_0, is given by

$$m_0 + m_* = 5.0\, m_*$$

or

$$m_0 = (5.0 - 1)m_* = (5.0 - 1)(100\ \text{mg}) = 400\ \text{mg}$$

Supplementary Problems

Nuclei

21.22. Mercury consists of 0.146% ^{196}Hg (195.9658 u), 10.02% ^{198}Hg (197.9668 u), 16.84% ^{199}Hg (198.9683 u), 23.13% ^{200}Hg (199.9683 u), 13.22% ^{201}Hg (200.9703 u), 29.80% ^{202}Hg (201.9706 u) and 6.85% ^{204}Hg (203.9735 u). Calculate the average atomic weight. *Ans.* 200.60 u

21.23. Chlorine has an atomic weight of 35.45 u. If the ^{35}Cl mass is 34.97 u and the ^{37}Cl mass is 36.98 u, calculate the percent ^{35}Cl in naturally occurring chlorine. *Ans.* 76.1%

21.24. Estimate the ratio of the radii of the nuclei of ^4_2He and ^1_1H. *Ans.* $r_{He}/r_H = 1.6$

21.25. Using (*21.1*) and the data in Table 21-1, calculate the density of a neutron.

Ans. $1.2 \times 10^{17}\ kg\ m^{-3}$

21.26. Calculate the total and average binding energies and the packing fraction for ^7_4Be. Assume the actual nuclide weight to be 7.0169 u. *Ans.* 37.6 MeV, 5.37 MeV, 24.14

21.27. Plot average binding energy against A and packing fraction against A for the following nuclides. STABLE NUCLIDES: ^{23}Na (22.99714 u), ^{40}Ar (39.97510 u), ^{60}Ni (59.94948 u), ^{110}Cd (109.9391 u), ^{110}Pd (109.9410 u), ^{194}Pt (194.0240 u) and ^{209}Bi (209.0455 u). UNSTABLE NUCLIDES: ^{23}Mg (23.0011 u), ^{23}Ne (23.00168 u), ^{40}K (39.97658 u), ^{60}Co (59.95250 u), ^{60}Cu (59.9561 u), ^{110}Ag (109.9422 u), ^{194}Ir (194.0264 u), ^{209}Po (209.0475 u) and ^{209}Pb (209.0462 u). Comment on the plots.

Ans. On the plot of a.b.e. against A, there are two sets of points, the stable isotopes having more binding energy than the unstable; on the plot of pf against A the radioactive nuclei lie above the stable nuclei.

Radioactive Decay

21.28. $^{68}_{31}$Ga undergoes positron decay as well as electron capture. Compare the products of these alternate paths. *Ans.* Daughter nuclides are the same, $^{68}_{30}$Zn.

21.29. Construct a decay scheme for ^{24}Ne from the following data: 8% of the nuclei decay by emitting a 1.10-MeV β^- and 92% with a 1.98-MeV β^-. There is a 0.472-MeV gamma coincident with the 1.98-MeV β^- and also a 0.878-MeV gamma. *Ans.* See Fig. 21-4.

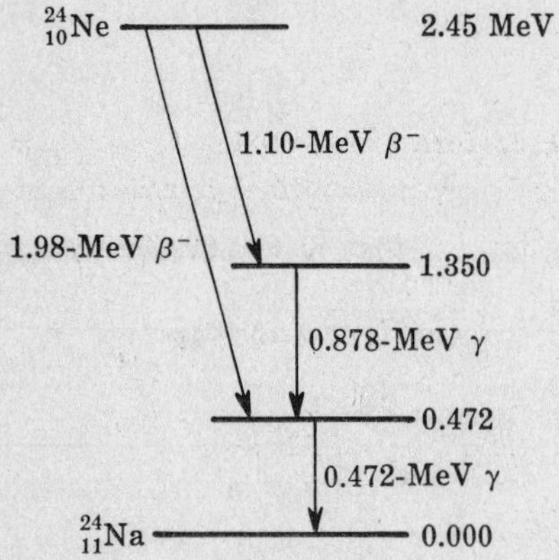

Fig. 21-4

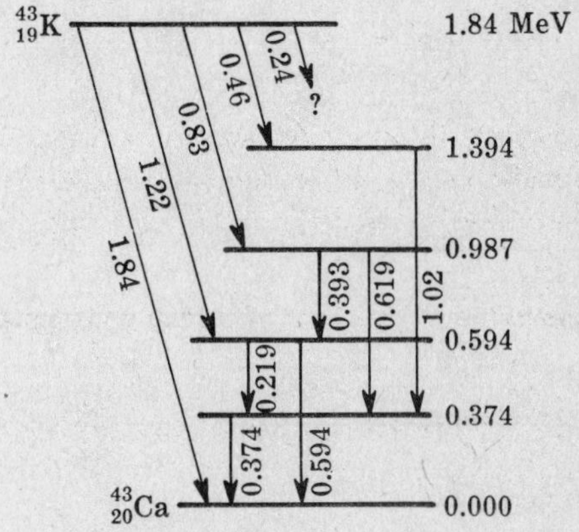

Fig. 21-5

21.30. Construct a decay scheme for ^{43}K from the following data: 5% of the nuclei decay by emitting a 0.24-MeV β^-, 5% by 0.46-MeV β^-, 83% by 0.83-MeV β^-, 5% by 1.22-MeV β^- and 2% by 1.84-MeV β^-. There is a 1.02-MeV γ coincident with a 0.374-MeV γ, a 0.619-MeV γ coincident with a 0.374-MeV γ, and a 0.393-MeV γ coincident either with a 0.219-MeV γ and a 0.374-MeV γ or with a 0.594 MeV γ.

Ans. See Fig. 21-5.

21.31. Prepare a decay scheme for ^{230}U from the following data: 67.2% of the nuclei decay with a 5.884-MeV α, 32.1% with a 5.813-MeV α and 0.7% with a 5.658-MeV α. There is gamma radiation at 0.07213, 0.1543, 0.158 and 0.232 MeV. *Ans.* See Fig. 21-6.

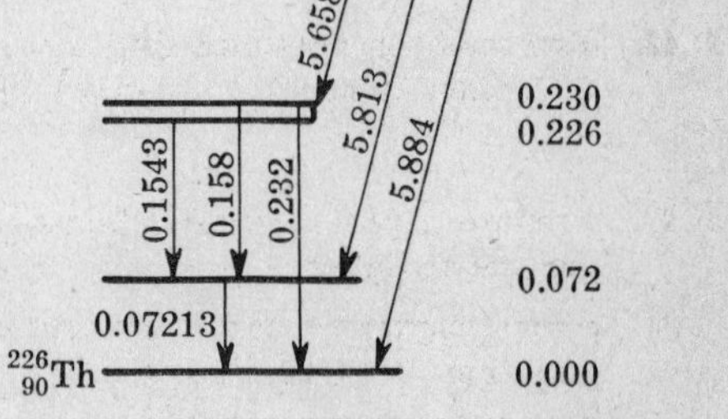

Fig. 21-6

21.32. Prepare a flow chart representing the $4n$ decay series beginning with $^{232}_{90}$Th and ending with a stable isotope. Use a suitable reference such as the Table of Isotopes in the *Handbook of Chemistry and Physics* to identify the modes of decay for the daughters.

Ans. $^{232}_{90}\text{Th} \xrightarrow{-\alpha} {}^{228}_{88}\text{Ra} \xrightarrow{-\beta} {}^{228}_{89}\text{Ac} \xrightarrow{-\beta} {}^{228}_{90}\text{Th} \xrightarrow{-\alpha} {}^{224}_{88}\text{Ra} \xrightarrow{-\alpha} {}^{220}_{86}\text{Rn} \xrightarrow{-\alpha} {}^{216}_{84}\text{Po} \xrightarrow{-\alpha} {}^{212}_{82}\text{Pb} \xrightarrow{-\beta} {}^{212}_{83}\text{Bi} \xrightarrow{-\beta} {}^{212}_{84}\text{Po} \xrightarrow{-\alpha} {}^{208}_{82}\text{Pb}$,

with a side branch $^{212}_{83}\text{Bi} \xrightarrow{-\alpha} {}^{208}_{81}\text{Tl} \xrightarrow{-\beta} {}^{208}_{82}\text{Pb}$

21.33. The elements RaC and RaC′ are radioactive daughters of $^{218}_{84}Po$ in the $4n+2$ series. If these are produced by the emission of α and β^- and α, $\beta^-$and β^-, respectively, identify these elements.

Ans. $^{214}_{83}Bi$, $^{214}_{84}Po$

21.34. Find the amount of time, expressed in units of $t_{1/2}$, at which $A/A_0 = 0.125$. *Ans.* 3

21.35. Compare the fractions of various radioactive Na nuclei left after 1 hr, if $t_{1/2} = 0.39$ s, 23 s, 2.602 yr, 15.0 hr, 60 s and 1 s for ^{20}Na, ^{21}Na, ^{22}Na, ^{24}Na, ^{25}Na and ^{26}Na, respectively.

Ans. 10^{-2777}, 8×10^{-48}, 0.9999696, 0.9549, 9×10^{-19}, 10^{-1083}

21.36. From the following data, prepare a plot of $\log A$ against t and determine the half-life for the isotope.

A, s^{-1}	86	63	45	33	24	17	13
t, min	0	2	4	6	8	10	12

Ans. slope is $(-\lambda/2.303)$; $t_{1/2} = 4.39$ min

21.37. $^{224}_{88}Ra$ having $t_{1/2} = 3.64$ day emits an alpha particle to form $^{220}_{86}Rn$ which has $t_{1/2} = 54.5$ s. If the molar volume of radon under these conditions is 35.2 dm^3, what volume of radon is in secular equilibrium with 1 g of radium? *Ans.* 2.72×10^{-8} m^3

21.38. What mass of ^{14}C with $t_{1/2} = 5730$ y is equal to 1 c? *Ans.* 1.92×10^{-4} kg

21.39. Find the ratio of 1 μc of $^{226}_{88}Ra$ ($t_{1/2} = 1622$ y) to 1 μc of $^{222}_{86}Rn$ ($t_{1/2} = 3.825$ d).

Ans. 1.58×10^5

Interaction of Radiation with Matter

21.40. Assuming that 35 eV of energy is dissipated by an alpha particle for each ion pair formed in air, calculate the number of ion pairs produced by a 1.00-MeV alpha. *Ans.* 2.86×10^4

21.41. Using the data from Problem 21.11 for β^- particles and an estimate that an α particle produces 3000 ion pairs per mm air, find the ratio of penetration for β^- to that for α.

Ans. 500/1

21.42. How many more times thick does a shield have to be to reduce the radiation passing through it by 99% than by 50%? *Ans.* 6.64

21.43. Prepare a plot of $\log A$ against x for the data below and calculate the half-thickness of the foil for the radiation.

x, mm	0.00	0.1	0.2	0.3	0.4	0.5	0.6	0.7	0.8	0.9	1.0	1.5	2.0	4.0
A, min^{-1}	1102	726	490	335	244	176	139	112	95	81	70	51	40	16

Ans. Curve consists of two lines. Slope for α or β is -2.05 mm^{-1} giving $\mu = 4.72$ mm^{-1} and for γ is -0.200 mm^{-1} giving $\mu_\gamma = 0.461$ mm^{-1}; $x_{1/2} = 0.150$ mm for α or β and 1.50 mm for γ.

21.44. If the maximum permissible dose of 0.1 rem per week is not to be exceeded for the overall body, what size sample of $^{23}_{10}Ne$ (assuming 4.38-MeV radiation) can be used safely? See Example 21.4 for radiation data. Assume that the worker (150 lb, 70 in. tall, 20 in. wide) will work an eight-hour day shift for five days a week and will never approach the radiation source any closer than 5 ft.

Ans. 1×10^{-3} J kg^{-1}, 6.81×10^{-2} J; 4.73×10^{-7} J s^{-1}, 5.24×10^{-7} J s^{-1} m^{-2}; 7.47×10^{5} s^{-1} m^{-2}, 2.18×10^{7} s^{-1}; 5.9×10^{-4} c

Nuclear Reactions

21.45. Complete the shorthand notation for the reactions: (*a*) $^{37}Ar(d,\_\_\_)^{38}Ar$, (*b*) $^{46}Ca(^{3}He,\alpha)\_\_\_$ and (*c*) $^{51}V(n,\_\_\_)^{52}V$. *Ans.* (*a*) *p*, (*b*) ^{45}Ca, (*c*) γ

21.46. Calculate Q for $^{58}Fe(p,\alpha)^{55}Mn$ given that the mass excesses of ^{58}Fe and ^{55}Mn are -0.0667 and -0.0619, respectively, and that the masses of a proton and an α particle are 1.0078 and 4.0026 u, respectively. *Ans.* 0.37 MeV

21.47. Calculate the threshold energy for $^{47}Ti(\alpha,t)^{48}V$ if $Q = -12.992$ MeV. *Ans.* 14.10 MeV

21.48. Calculate the ratio of total energy required for the penetration of a ^{14}N nucleus by an α particle to that required by a proton. *Ans.* 2.05/1

21.49. Write the equation corresponding to the reaction $^{31}P(n,d)^{30}Si$. Calculate the energy of the reaction and the threshold energy. The atomic masses are 30.97376, 1.00866, 2.0140 and 29.97376 u, respectively.

Ans. $^{31}_{15}P + ^{1}_{0}n = ^{2}_{1}H + ^{30}_{14}Si$; 4.97 MeV; 5.13 MeV

21.50. Repeat the calculations of Problem 21.16 using potassium as the absorber, which has a value of $\sigma = 1.97$ barn and a density of 0.86×10^{3} kg m^{-3}. Compare the results.

Ans. $I_0 - I = 2.6 \times 10^{5}$ s^{-1}. K gives about four times the decrease; increase of σ more important than decrease in N.

Miscellaneous Considerations

21.51. If 190 MeV is considered the possible useful energy from a fission reaction, how many kilowatt-hours would be generated by 1 gram of ^{235}U? *Ans.* 2.2×10^{4} kW-hr

21.52. A chip of paint from "Leif Ericson's ship" had a ^{14}C activity per unit mass of 12.0 min^{-1} g^{-1}. Comment. *Ans.* $t = 406$ y; fake (Ericson flourished 1000 A.D.)

21.53. Another sample of rock #12013 from Apollo 12 (see Example 21.12) had an argon content of 7.17×10^{-7} (m^3 STP) kg^{-1}. What is the age of this section?

Ans. $n = 3.20 \times 10^{-5}$, $N_{40,\,Ar} = 2.97 \times 10^{-5}L$; $t = 3.49 \times 10^{9}$ y

21.54. A 15-g sample of the enzyme ribonuclease ($M = 13{,}683$) was hydrolyzed and analyzed for analine ($M = 89$) using the isotope dilution technique: a sample of tagged analine was added to the hydrolysate and separation was effected using paper chromatography. If the dilution factor was 117 for adding 10 mg of tagged analine, what is the number of analine units in a molecule of ribonuclease?

Ans. 0.11×10^{-2} mol enzyme, 1.16 g $= 1.30 \times 10^{-2}$ mol original analine; 11.8 = 12 analine units

INDEX